# EATING DISORDERS AND OBESITY

# EATING DISORDERS AND OBESITY

## A Comprehensive Handbook

### SECOND EDITION

*Edited by*
CHRISTOPHER G. FAIRBURN
KELLY D. BROWNELL

THE GUILFORD PRESS
New York   London

© 2002 The Guilford Press
A Division of Guilford Publications, Inc.
72 Spring Street, New York, NY 10012
www.guilford.com

Printed in the United States of America

This book is printed on acid-free paper.

Last digit is print number:   9   8   7   6   5   4   3   2   1

**Library of Congress Cataloging-in-Publication Data**

Eating disorders and obesity : a comprehensive handbook / edited by
Christopher G. Fairburn, Kelly D. Brownell — 2nd ed.
    p.   cm.
  Includes bibliographical references and index.
  ISBN 1-57230-688-2 (hardcover)
  1. Eatings disorders—Handbooks, manuals, etc. 2. Obesity—
Handbooks, manuals, etc.   I. Fairburn, Christopher G.   II. Brownell,
Kelly D.

RC552.E18 E2825 2002
616.85′26—dc21

                           2001033077

# Contents

## PART I. FOUNDATION

### Basic Regulation of Eating and Body Weight

# PART II. EATING DISORDERS

## Clinical Characteristics of Eating Disorders

## Epidemiology and Etiology of Eating Disorders

## Medical and Physical Aspects of Eating Disorders

## Treatment and Prevention of Eating Disorders

## PART III. OBESITY

### Clinical Characteristics of Obesity

### Epidemiology, Etiology, and Course of Obesity

## Medical Aspects of Obesity and Weight Loss

## Treatment and Prevention of Obesity

# Preface

The first edition of this book had two main goals: to strengthen connections between the eating disorders and obesity fields, and to provide a comprehensive and authoritative account of knowledge in the two areas. To what extent were these goals realized? It is our view that we accomplished the second goal but were only partly successful in achieving the first—the separation between the fields remains too large. It is still the case that there is too little exchange between the two areas and it is still true that there are few people who are knowledgeable about both fields.

Yet many issues are common to the two areas. The first is the basic physiology and psychology of hunger and satiety, and the processes that underlie weight regulation. Much is known about these matters and knowledge is increasing. For example, one notable advance has been the discovery of leptin and the elucidation of its contribution to the regulation of energy balance (see Chapter 6), yet its clinical importance remains unclear. What is the contribution of leptin to the development and maintenance of obesity, and what is its relevance to eating disorders (see Chapter 48)? These fundamental questions remain to be answered.

Another area of common interest is binge eating. Here there has been more progress stimulated to a large extent by the provisional new eating disorder diagnosis "binge eating disorder" (see Chapter 31). It is now established that a subgroup of people with obesity have a frank eating disorder (although many people with binge eating disorder are not overweight) and these people appear to be especially prone to gain further weight. So in binge eating disorder we have a disorder that lies right on the interface between obesity and eating disorders.

Body image is a third common area. The overevaluation of body shape and weight is a central feature of most eating disorders (see Chapter 29) but body image concerns are also present among some people with obesity albeit generally to a lesser extent (see Chapter 72). In the eating disorder field, body image was the subject of much research in the 1980s, but this declined during the 1990s in part because of difficulties of conceptualization and measurement. There are now signs that research on body image is on the increase and we hope this will benefit both fields.

Cognitive-behavioral therapy is another potential link between the two fields. Cognitive-behavioral theory is well established as being relevant to the understanding of bulimia nervosa (see Chapter 54) and anorexia nervosa (see Chapter 55), and cognitive-behavioral therapy is the leading evidence-based treatment for bulimia nervosa (see Chapter 54). Cognitive-behavioral principles are also widely used in the treatment of other eating disorders. As yet, however, the relevance of cognitive-behavioral theory to the understanding of obesity is only just beginning to be explored and the value of cognitive-behavioral therapy has barely been tested (although there has been a tendency for behavioral treatments to be relabeled as "cognitive-behavioral"). This is a promising area for future research since cognitive processes underpin these patients' unrealistic weight goals and their body image concerns, and it is possible that they contribute to their marked tendency to relapse.

In the Preface to the first edition, we noted that dieting was the one issue that threatened to divide the two areas. In the eating disorder field, dieting was regarded as a public enemy, a threat to health, whereas in the obesity field it was viewed as the solution rather than as the problem. This seems less true today. Polemics against dieting are no longer *de rigueur* in the eating disorder field, possibly because their multifactorial etiology has become even better established over the past decade. Both risk factor research (see Chapter 44) and the findings of genetic epidemiological studies (see Chapter 42) challenge the simplistic notion that dieting is the major culprit in the development of eating disorders. Simultaneously, the obesity community has questioned dieting as the means for losing weight (see Chapter 109). At best, it works for only some people and usually only for a short time. Nevertheless, dieting remains a potential battle zone, for those who specialize in the prevention of eating disorders typically remain resolutely opposed to dieting (see Chapter 67), while to the general public dieting and weight loss remain conflated. The way forward must be better understanding of the mechanisms involved in the etiology of eating disorders and the persistence of obesity, and greater sophistication in analyzing the costs and benefits of dieting (see Chapter 17).

## THIS NEW EDITION

What about this second edition? Unlike new editions of many books, which are simple updates, this second edition of *Eating Disorders and Obesity* is entirely new. We took a fresh view of the two fields and started anew in constructing the book. However, in doing so, we made the major decision to retain the format of having multiple short but authoritative chapters since there was consensus that this worked well. Of course, many of the topics and contributors in this second edition are unchanged, but this is hardly surprising since we were covering the same two general fields and since (thankfully) the turnover in world experts is not very great!

We have taken three steps to further our goal of encouraging communication between the two fields. First, this time more than last, we have collections of chapters that straddle topics common to both areas. Obvious examples are the chapters on diets and dieting (Chapters 14, 15, 16, 17, 96, 97, 98, and 109), the chapters on binge eating (Chapters 18, 31, 63, 64, 73, and 94), and the chapters that address body image (Chapters 19, 21, 29, 72, and 108). Second, we have expanded the series of chapters in Part I on the basic processes that underpin the control of eating and weight. Third, we have taken pains to include extensive cross-referencing in the different sections of the book.

Some of the new chapters address topics that were not covered in the first edition, reflecting developments in the two fields. The three best examples are the chapters on molecular genetics (Chapters 5 and 43), leptin (Chapter 6), and binge eating disorder (Chapters 31, 63, and 64), but change in knowledge, understanding, and practice is evident throughout the book. In the eating disorder area, it is illustrated by the upsurge in knowledge about the etiology of eating disorders (see especially Chapters 42, 43, and 44) and in the large body of research on the treatment of bulimia nervosa (see Chapters 54, 57, and 58). In the obesity area, more is known about the social and psychological consequences of obesity (see Chapters 20, 70, and 71), genetic and environmental causes (see Chapters 3, 4, 5, and 78), pharmacological treatment (see Chapters 99 and 100), and the ever-vexing issue of maintaining the weight loss (see Chapters 106 and 107).

Like last time, we have learned a great deal in editing the book. Rarely, if ever, does one have the privilege of reading truly expert and up-to-date accounts of such a broad range of topics of relevance to one's interests. It is for this reason that the editing of this book has been such a pleasure and education. It is our great hope that our readers benefit similarly.

## ACKNOWLEDGMENTS

Few books are solo efforts, and this is certainly not one of them. We have over 100 contributors to thank for taking part in this enterprise. To them we express our very considerable gratitude for their contributions of knowledge and time. Several people have written more than one chapter and to them we are especially grateful; namely, G. Terence Wilson, David B. Allison, Cynthia M. Bulik, Gary D. Foster, Stanley Heshka, Steven B. Heymsfield, James O. Hill, Albert J. Stunkard, Thomas A. Wadden, B. Timothy Walsh, Denise E. Wilfley, David F. Williamson, Rena R. Wing, Rodolfo Valdez, and Walter Vandereycken.

For their help with the editing process, we want to thank Mara Catling, Rachel Hewitt, Marianne O'Connor, and Lorna Nelson, and for help with the indexing we thank Clare Farrell. CGF also wants to thank The Wellcome Trust for their personal support. And last, but certainly not least, we both want to thank Seymour Weingarten and his colleagues at The Guilford Press for their encouragement and help at every stage in the evolution of this second edition.

Christopher G. Fairburn
*University of Oxford*

Kelly D. Brownell
*Yale University*

# A Note for Readers

For readers who are new to *Eating Disorders and Obesity*, we thought that it might be helpful if we briefly explained something about the nature and use of this book.

In common with the first edition, our goal has been to create a book that provides comprehensive coverage of the main issues of relevance to the eating disorders and obesity fields. As a result, it encompasses a very broad range of topics and has 112 chapters. Its breadth of coverage and organizational structure are best seen in the Contents, which lists all the chapters across the three main sections (Part I, Foundation; Part II, Eating Disorders; and Part III, Obesity).

Another goal has been to ensure that the book is authoritative. Accordingly, we approached the leading international experts on each topic and, with very few exceptions, each agreed to contribute. Their names can be found in the list of contributors.

The task of the contributors was to write a succinct yet comprehensive account of the topic in question, highlighting what is known and what is not. As a result, the chapters are concise syntheses of current knowledge in a very specific area (with cross-references to other relevant chapters). In common with the first edition, the chapters do not include references; rather, each chapter concludes with a section titled "Further Reading," in which up to 10 key articles are listed, together with a brief commentary explaining why they have been chosen. Thus, this section is designed to help readers identify avenues of inquiry to pursue.

The omission of in-text references is a controversial and distinctive feature of the book. We believe that by asking the contributors not to incorporate references, we have helped them step back and write true overviews of their subject rather than the all-too-common litanies of important studies. And we think that an added benefit is that the text is more readable as a result, since it is not broken up by lists of authors and dates. The potential cost is loss of guidance as to the important studies in the area. We believe that this has been avoided by the inclusion of key studies in each chapter's Further Reading section. Since we envision a third edition, we would welcome readers' views on these and any other matters.

CGF
KDB

# About the Editors

**Christopher G. Fairburn, DM, FRCPsych, FMedSci,** is Wellcome Principal Research Fellow and Professor of Psychiatry at the University of Oxford. He specializes in research on the nature and treatment of eating disorders and obesity. His studies have addressed many aspects of eating disorders, including their diagnostic status, epidemiology, etiology, assessment, course, and treatment. Professor Fairburn has a particular interest in the development and evaluation of psychological treatments for eating disorders and obesity. He has held research grants in Great Britain and the United States, and he has published extensively in the area. Professor Fairburn has twice been a Fellow at the Center for Advanced Study in the Behavioral Sciences at Stanford University. He is also a Fellow of the Academy of Medical Sciences.

**Kelly D. Brownell, PhD,** is Professor of Psychology at Yale University, where he also serves as Professor of Epidemiology and Public Health and as Director of the Yale Center for Eating and Weight Disorders. He served from 1995 until 1999 as Director of Clinical Training, and is currently Director of Graduate Studies in the Department of Psychology. In 1994, he became Master of Silliman College at Yale, where he served until 2000. Dr. Brownell has served as president of the Society of Behavioral Medicine, the Association for Advancement of Behavior Therapy, and the Division of Health Psychology of the American Psychological Association, and has received the James McKeen Cattell Award from the New York Academy of Sciences, the award for Outstanding Contribution to Health Psychology from the American Psychological Association, and the Distinguished Alumni Award from Purdue University.

# Contributors

**David B. Allison, PhD,** Section on Statistical Genetics, Department of Biostatistics, and Clinical Nutrition Research Center, University of Alabama at Birmingham, USA

**Arnold E. Andersen, MD,** College of Medicine, University of Iowa, USA

**Reubin Andres, MD,** National Institute on Aging, Gerontology Research Center, Baltimore, USA

**Louis J. Aronne, MD,** Department of Medicine, Cornell University Medical Center, USA

**Robert I. Berkowitz, MD,** Department of Psychiatry, University of Pennsylvania, USA

**Joseph E. Beshay, MD,** Department of Surgery, Eastern Carolina University School of Medicine, USA

**Pierre J. V. Beumont, MD, MSc, MPhil, FRCP(E), FRACP, FRANZCP, FRCPsych,** Department of Psychological Medicine, University of Sydney, Australia

**Leann L. Birch, PhD,** Department of Human Development and Family Studies, Pennsylvania State University, USA

**Per Björntorp, MD, PhD,** Department of Heart and Lung Diseases, Sahlgren's Hospital, University of Göteborg, Sweden

**George L. Blackburn, MD, PhD,** Department of Surgery, Beth Israel Deaconess Medical Center, Boston, USA

**Steven N. Blair, PhD,** Division of Epidemiology and Clinical Applications, Cooper Institute for Aerobics Research, Dallas, USA

**John E. Blundell, PhD,** Department of Psychology, University of Leeds, United Kingdom

**Claude Bouchard, PhD,** Pennington Biomedical Research Institute, Louisiana State University, USA

**George A. Bray, MD,** Pennington Biomedical Research Institute, Louisiana State University, USA

**Kelly D. Brownell, PhD,** Departments of Psychology and Epidemiology and Public Health, Yale University, USA

**Rachel Bryant-Waugh, PhD,** Department of Psychological Medicine, Great Ormond Street Hospital, London, United Kingdom

**Cynthia M. Bulik, PhD,** Virginia Institute for Psychiatric and Behavioral Genetics, Virginia Commonwealth University, USA

**Susan M. Byrne, PhD,** Department of Psychiatry, University of Oxford, United Kingdom

**L. Arthur Campfield, PhD,** Department of Food Science and Human Nutrition, Colorado State University, USA

**Jacqueline C. Carter, DPhil, PhD,** Department of Psychiatry, University of Toronto, Canada

**Thomas F. Cash, PhD,** Department of Psychology, Old Dominion University, Virginia, USA

**David A. Collier, PhD,** Institute of Psychiatry, University of London, United Kingdom

**Christopher Dare, MD, FRCPsych,** Institute of Psychiatry, University of London, United Kingdom

**Jean-Pierre Després, PhD,** Quebec Heart Institute, Laval Hospital, Canada

**Michael J. Devlin, MD,** Department of Psychiatry, Columbia University, USA

**William H. Dietz, MD, PhD,** Division of Nutrition and Physical Activity, Centers for Disease Control and Prevention, Atlanta, USA

**Adam Drewnowski, PhD,** Nutritional Sciences Program, University of Washington, USA

**Johanna Dwyer, DSc, RD,** Frances Stern Nutrition Center, Tufts University School of Medicine, USA

**Ivan Eisler, PhD,** Institute of Psychiatry, University of London, United Kingdom

**Leonard H. Epstein, PhD,** Department of Pediatrics, State University of New York at Buffalo, USA

**Christopher G. Fairburn, DM, FRCPsych, FMedSci,** Department of Psychiatry, University of Oxford, United Kingdom

**Kevin R. Fontaine, PhD,** Department of Medicine, Johns Hopkins University School of Medicine, USA

**John P. Foreyt, PhD,** Nutrition Research Clinic, Baylor College of Medicine, USA

**Gary D. Foster, PhD,** Department of Psychiatry, University of Pennsylvania, USA

**Michael A. Friedman, PhD,** Department of Psychology, Rutgers University, USA

**Paul E. Garfinkel, MD, FRCP(C),** Centre for Addiction and Mental Health, University of Toronto, Canada

**David M. Garner, PhD,** River Centre Clinic, Sylvania, Ohio, USA

**James Gibbs, MD,** Bourne Laboratory, Cornell University Medical Center and New York Hospital, USA

**Gary S. Goldfield, PhD,** Department of Mental Health, Children's Hospital of Eastern Ontario Research Institute, Canada.

**Edward W. Gregg, PhD,** Division of Diabetes Translation, Centers for Disease Control, Atlanta, USA

**Carlos M. Grilo, PhD,** Yale Psychiatric Institute, Yale University School of Medicine, USA

**Katherine A. Halmi, MD,** New York Presbyterian Hospital–Westchester Division and Weill Medical College of Cornell University, USA

**David Heber, MD, PhD,** Center for Human Nutrition, University of California at Los Angeles, USA

**Stanley Heshka, MD,** Obesity Research Center, St. Luke's–Roosevelt Hospital Center and Columbia University, USA

**Steven B. Heymsfield, MD,** Obesity Research Center, St. Luke's–Roosevelt Hospital Center, USA

**Andrew J. Hill, PhD,** School of Medicine and Behavioural Sciences, University of Leeds, United Kingdom

**James O. Hill, PhD,** Center for Human Nutrition, University of Colorado Health Sciences Center, USA

**Hans Wijbrand Hoek, MD,** Parnassia The Hague Psychiatric Institute, The Netherlands

**Scott Holder, MA,** Division of Epidemiology and Clinical Applications, Cooper Institute for Aerobics Research, Dallas, USA

**W. Philip T. James, MD,** International Association for the Study of Obesity and International Obesity Task Force, London, United Kingdom

**Susan A. Jebb, PhD, FRD,** Dunn Clinical Nutrition Centre, Cambridge, United Kingdom

**Robert W. Jeffery, PhD,** Division of Epidemiology, University of Minnesota, USA

**Allan S. Kaplan, MD, MSc, FRCP(C),** Department of Psychiatry, University of Toronto, Canada

**Melanie A. Katzman, PhD,** Department of Psychiatry, Weill Cornell Medical Center, USA

**Walter H. Kaye, MD,** Western Psychiatric Institute and Clinic, University of Pittsburgh School of Medicine, USA

**MaryLou Klem, PhD,** Department of Psychiatry, University of Pittsburgh, USA

**Shiriki K. Kumanyika, PhD,** Center for Clinical Epidemiology and Biostatistics, University of Pennsylvania School of Medicine, USA

**Robert F. Kushner, MD,** Department of General Internal Medicine, Northwestern University Medical Center, USA

**Bryan Lask, DM, FRCPsych, MPhil,** Department of Psychiatry, St. George's Hospital Medical School, London, United Kingdom

**Sing Lee, FRCPsych,** Department of Psychiatry, The Chinese University of Hong Kong, Shatin, Hong Kong

**Rudolph L. Leibel, MD,** Department of Pediatrics, Columbia University, USA

**Sarah F. Leibowitz, PhD,** The Rockefeller University, New York, USA

**Timothy G. Lohman, PhD,** Department of Physiology, University of Arizona, USA

**Michael R. Lowe, PhD,** Department of Clinical and Health Psychology, MCP Hahnemann University, USA

**JoAnn E. Manson, MD,** Division of Preventive Medicine, Brigham and Women's Hospital, Harvard Medical School, USA

**Kathleen Melanson, PhD, RD,** Frances Stern Nutrition Center, Tufts University School of Medicine, USA

**James E. Mitchell, MD,** Department of Neuroscience, School of Medicine, University of North Dakota, USA

**Marion P. Olmsted, PhD,** Department of Psychiatry, University of Toronto, Canada

**Robert L. Palmer, DM, FRCPsych,** Academic Department of Psychiatry, Leicester General Hospital, United Kingdom

**Michael G. Perri, PhD,** Department of Clinical and Health Psychology, University of Florida, USA

**Katharine A. Phillips, MD,** Department of Psychiatry and Human Behavior, Brown University, USA

**Niva Piran, PhD,** Department of Applied Psychology, The Ontario Institute for Studies in Education, Canada

**F. Xavier Pi-Sunyer, MD,** Department of Medicine, St Luke's–Roosevelt Hospital Center and Columbia University, USA

**Janet Polivy, PhD,** Department of Psychology, University of Toronto, Canada

**Claire Pomeroy, PhD,** Department of Infectious Diseases, University of Kentucky Chandler Medical Center, USA

**Walter J. Pories, MD,** Department of Surgery, Eastern Carolina University School of Medicine, USA

**Andrew M. Prentice, PhD,** MRC International Nutrition Group, Public Health Nutrition Unit, London School of Hygiene and Tropical Medicine, United Kingdom

**Rebecca Puhl, MS,** Department of Psychology, Yale University, USA

**Eric Ravussin, PhD,** Pennington Biomedical Research Institute, Louisiana State University, USA

**Gary M. Rodin, MD,** Department of Psychiatry, Toronto General Hospital, Canada

**James C. Rosen, PhD,** Department of Psychology, University of Vermont, USA

**Stephan Rössner, MD,** Department of Medicine, Huddinge University Hospital, Sweden

**Brian E. Saelens, PhD,** Division of Psychology, Children's Hospital Medical Center, University of Cincinnati, USA

**James F. Sallis, PhD,** Department of Psychology, San Diego State University, USA

**Wim H. M. Saris, MD,** Department of Human Biology, University of Maastricht, The Netherlands

**Ulrike Schmidt, MD,** Institute of Psychiatry, University of London, United Kingdom

**Jacob C. Seidell, PhD,** Department of Chronic Disease Epidemiology, National Institute of Public Health and the Environment, Bilthoven, The Netherlands

**Roz Shafran, PhD,** Department of Psychiatry, University of Oxford, United Kingdom

**Lars Sjöström, MD, PhD,** Medical Department, Sahlgrenska University Hospital, Göteborg, Sweden

**Patrick J. Skerrett, MS,** Division of Preventive Medicine, Brigham and Women's Hospital, Harvard Medical School, USA

**Gerard P. Smith, MD,** Bourne Laboratory, Cornell University Medical Center, New York Hospital, USA

**Linda Smolak, PhD,** Department of Psychology, Kenyon College, USA

**Alan Stein, MD, MRCPsych,** Department of Psychiatry, University of Oxford, United Kingdom

**Eric Stice, PhD,** Department of Psychology, University of Texas at Austin, USA

**Sachiko T. St. Jeor, PhD, RD,** Nutrition Education and Research Program, University of Nevada School of Medicine, USA

**Ruth H. Striegel-Moore, PhD,** Department of Psychology, Wesleyan University, USA

**Michael Strober, PhD,** Department of Psychiatry/Behavioral Sciences, UCLA Neuropsychiatric Institute, USA

**Albert J. Stunkard, MD,** Department of Psychiatry, University of Pennsylvania, USA

**Patrick F. Sullivan, MD,** Department of Psychiatry, Virginia Institute for Psychiatric and Behavioral Genetics, Virginia Commonwealth University, USA

**Marja A. R. Tijhuis, PhD,** Department for Chronic Disease Epidemiology, National Institute of Public Health and the Environment, Bilthoven, The Netherlands

**Jarl S:son Torgerson, MD, PhD,** Medical Department, Sahlgrenska University Hospital, Göteborg, Sweden

**Janet Treasure, DM, FRCPsych,** Department of Psychiatry, Guys Hospital, London, United Kingdom

**Rodolfo Valdez, PhD,** Division of Diabetes Translation, Centers for Disease Control, Atlanta, USA

**Walter Vandereycken, MD, PhD,** Department of Psychiatry, Catholic University of Leuven, Belgium

**Kelly Bemis Vitousek, PhD,** Department of Psychology, University of Hawaii, USA

**Thomas A. Wadden, PhD,** Department of Psychiatry, University of Pennsylvania, USA

**Glenn Waller, PhD,** Department of Psychiatry, St. George's Hospital Medical School, London, United Kingdom

**B. Timothy Walsh, MD,** Department of Psychiatry, Columbia University, USA

**Roland L. Weinsier, MD, DrPH,** Department of Nutrition Sciences, University of Alabama at Birmingham, USA

**Denise E. Wilfley, PhD,** Department of Psychology, San Diego State University, USA

**Walter C. Willett, MD, DrPH,** Departments of Nutrition and Epidemiology, Harvard School of Public Health, USA

**David F. Williamson, PhD, MS,** Division of Diabetes Translation, Centers for Disease Control, Atlanta, USA

**G. Terence Wilson, PhD,** Graduate School of Applied and Professional Psychology, Rutgers University, USA

**Rena R. Wing, PhD,** Weight Control and Diabetes Research Center, Miriam Hospital, and Department of Psychiatry and Human Behavior, Brown Medical School, USA

**Anne M. Wolf, MS, RD,** Charlottesville, Virginia, USA

**Leslie G. Womble, PhD,** Department of Psychiatry, University of Pennsylvania, USA

**Stephen A. Wonderlich, PhD,** Department of Neuroscience, School of Medicine, University of North Dakota, USA

**D. Blake Woodside, MD,** Department of Psychiatry, University of Toronto, Canada

**Joel Yager, MD,** Department of Psychiatry, University of New Mexico School of Medicine, USA

**Susan Z. Yanovski, MD,** Obesity and Eating Disorders Program, National Institute of Diabetes and Digestive and Kidney Diseases/National Institutes of Health, Bethesda, USA

**Marion Zabinski, BA,** Joint Doctoral Program in Clinical Psychology, San Diego State University, USA

# PART I

# FOUNDATION

# Basic Regulation of Eating and Body Weight

# 1

# Central Physiological Determinants of Eating Behavior and Body Weight

## SARAH F. LEIBOWITZ

Nutritional and appetite disorders occur in epidemic proportions. Obesity and diabetes affect over 30% of our population, while eating disorders occur in up to 3% of adolescents and young adults. Disturbed eating patterns are a primary symptom of numerous psychiatric disorders, and loss of appetite and cachexia, during illness or in the elderly, preclude proper medical treatment for restoring good health or preserving life. Increased understanding of the systems of the body and brain related to energy and nutrient balance may help us treat and prevent these common problems.

## INTEGRATION OF DIVERSE SIGNALS

Researchers in neurobiology have used an integrative, interdisciplinary approach to study the multiple determinants of eating behavior, energy balance, and body weight. These include such diverse signals as (1) simple nutrients in the blood, including glucose, fatty acids, triglycerides, or amino acids; (2) classical neurotransmitter molecules for rapid, short-term communication; (3) larger neuropeptides for slower, more long-term action; and (4) circulating hormones for both neuromodulatory and metabolic processes. These signals derive from different peripheral organs, in particular, the adrenals, liver, pancreas, and gastrointestinal tract, and also from different areas of the central nervous system, from the hindbrain to the forebrain. Moreover, they are dynamic in nature, shifting across the daily cycle, developmental stages, the female estrous cycle, and seasonal periods.

### Systems in the Body

In the periphery, in both animals and humans, a variety of substances are believed to be involved, in the complex process of integrating physiological and behavioral systems geared toward energy and nutrient homeostasis (see Chapter 2). From the gastrointestinal tract, cholecystokinin and other peptides are released after a meal to coordinate several aspects of digestion, absorption, and metabolism, and to transmit information to the brain, via the vagus nerve, that signals meal termination and satiety. The pancreatic peptide hormone, insulin, has also been linked to satiety, in addition to the metabolism and utilization of food, while the adipocyte hormone, leptin, is released from and reflects the amount of body fat. The adrenal steroids, aldosterone and corticosterone, have different actions mediated by two different types of receptors. These are the mineralocorticoid receptors, which increase the ingestion and metabolism of fat, and glucocorticoid receptors, which predominantly influence carbohydrate intake and its metabolism. This glucoregulatory action occurs when the body's carbohydrate stores are low (e.g., at the start of the natural feeding cycle); thus, blood steroid levels are particularly high to mobilize and convert calories to glucose. The gonadal steroids (e.g., estrogen and progesterone) also introduce a major behavioral and metabolic signal at critical times of the estrous cycle and around puberty, when the body's fat stores must be enhanced for reproduction. Testosterone, the male steroid, is known to enhance protein ingestion while stimulating growth and muscle development.

## Systems in the Brain

In addition to these hormones, the process of integrating metabolic information from the periphery with neurochemical signals in the central nervous system requires specialized functions of multiple brain areas. These include the lower brainstem, in particular the dorsal vagal complex, which relays and integrates neural information between peripheral autonomic–endocrine organs and forebrain structures; the pons–midbrain and thalamus, which interpret this information in relation to the sensory properties of foods; the hypothalamus which, through its extensive vascularity and connections with the pituitary and hindbrain, remains closely linked to circulating metabolites and hormones as well as neural signals; and forebrain structures, such as the nucleus accumbens, amygdala and frontal cortex, which perform higher-order functions to integrate incoming information with various cognitive factors pertaining to the rewarding and aversive aspects of food.

The role of the hypothalamus in this process, relating hormones and metabolism to behavior, has received considerable attention and is the focus of this review. A number of neurochemical and neuroendocrine systems have been identified in this structure and are believed to be involved in controlling appetite for the macronutrients, carbohydrate, fat, and protein. They also modulate metabolism and contribute to the body's nutrient stores and, ultimately, weight gain and adiposity. These systems, which are closely linked to and controlled by circulating hormones and metabolites, are described with respect to their possible contribution to normal physiological functions. They are then evaluated in terms of their role in the development or maintenance of clinical eating and body weight disorders.

## MAINTENANCE OF CARBOHYDRATE BALANCE

Maintenance of the body's carbohydrate stores involves the coordinated effort of several brain neurochemicals and hormones. These substances translate metabolic signals, reflecting decreased carbohydrate stores and intracellular glucose utilization, into neural signals for promoting carbohydrate intake and metabolism. They include the amino acid, gamma-aminobutyric acid, the amine norepinephrine, the peptide neuropeptide Y, and the glucocorticoid actions of corticosterone. Their primary site of action is in the medial region of the hypothalamus, including the paraventricular nucleus, where the neurotransmitters and glucocorticoid receptors are known to be synthesized. Their local administration stimulates eating behavior, preferentially carbohydrate ingestion, causes an increase in the utilization of carbohydrate to promote fat storage, and reduces sympathetic activity to conserve energy.

The activity of these neurochemicals and their receptors sharply peaks at specific times (e.g., during the initial hours of the natural eating cycle), when the body's glycogen stores and blood glucose levels are particularly low. At this time, carbohydrate is strongly preferred by animals and humans, perhaps since it is most efficient in rapidly replenishing glucose stores in a hungry animal. Simultaneously, there occurs a natural rise in circulating levels of corticosterone, whose main function is to enhance the body's carbohydrate stores. This initiates a positive feedback loop, which involves a stimulatory effect of this steroid, via glucocorticoid receptors, on the synthesis and release of the neurochemicals in the hypothalamus and, in turn, a stimulatory action of these neurochemicals themselves on adrenal release of corticosterone. Brain substances involved in turning off this positive feedback loop include serotonin, its amino acid precursor, tryptophan, and the gut peptide, cholecystokinin, each of which are released by a carbohydrate-rich meal. In addition to suppressing carbohydrate ingestion, these neurochemicals stimulate metabolic rate and sympathetic activity, and reduce body weight and adiposity.

Much evidence suggests that disturbances in the endogenous activity of these neurochemicals and steroids contribute to the development or maintenance of abnormal patterns of eating and body weight gain. For example, when pharmacologically or surgically deprived of their natural neurotransmitter or steroid, animals fail to exhibit normal carbohydrate feeding, both in the initial hours of the active feeding cycle and in response to the physiological challenge of food deprivation. Conversely, with excessive hypothalamic infusions of norepinephrine, neuropeptide Y, or corticosterone, animals respond by overeating carbohydrate, which leads to an increase in fat deposition and body weight gain. In fact, animals that are genetically obese or that spontaneously overeat palatable, energy-rich diets have excessive levels of circulating corticosterone, and hypothalamic norepinephrine, and neuropeptide Y. These disturbances may be consequent to deficiencies in insulin sensitivity and, thus, glucose homeostasis.

## MAINTENANCE OF FAT BALANCE

A different set of substances in the hypothalamus controls the ingestion and deposition of fat. They include the peptide galanin, the opioid peptides, and the mineralocorticoid actions of corticosterone or aldosterone. These substances act within the medial hypothalamus to potentiate fat intake and are more abundant in animals with a strong natural preference for fat and, consequently, greater body weight and adiposity. In contrast to those controlling carbohydrate balance, these systems involved in fat balance exhibit greater activity during the middle-to-late hours of the natural feeding cycle. During this time, appetite for fat naturally rises, peptide synthesis is increased, and circulating corticosterone, remaining at low basal levels, binds specifically to mineralocorticoid receptors, which enhance the deposition as well as ingestion of fat. The catecholamine, dopamine, appears to be one neurochemical involved in turning off these anabolic signals. Its hypothalamic action is reflected in the inhibitory effect on fat intake and body weight produced by the drug, amphetamine, which releases dopamine, and also by phenylpropanolamine, a structurally similar product. The opposite effect, in contrast, is commonly seen with neuroleptic drugs (e.g., chlorpromazine) that antagonize dopamine receptors and are known to promote obesity.

## MAINTENANCE OF PROTEIN BALANCE

In rats and humans, appetite for protein, similar to that of fat, increases gradually over the course of the active feeding cycle, perhaps to enhance nutrient stores in preparation for an inactive period of little eating. The finding that the opioid peptides potentiate protein intake, in addition to fat ingestion, suggests that these neurochemicals may assist in balancing the intake and perhaps storage of these two nutrients. Another peptide, growth hormone releasing factor, may also function in the medial hypothalamus to coordinate behavioral and physiological functions related to protein balance. In addition to stimulating the release of growth hormone, which promotes protein synthesis and growth, this peptide, acting in part through opioid systems, potentiates the ingestion of food and, specifically, protein.

## DEVELOPMENTAL PATTERNS AND GENDER DIFFERENCES

In animals and humans, appetite before puberty is characterized by a stronger preference for carbohydrate in females and a stronger appetite for protein in males. This preference in females may be attributed to a natural, prepubertal surge in hypothalamic levels of neuropeptide Y in association with increased adrenal activity. The appetite for protein in males, in contrast, occurs in response to a rise in growth hormone releasing factor. After puberty, this pattern dramatically shifts, with a sharp increase in appetite for fat. This growing preference for fat-rich diets, associated with a rise in fat deposition and body weight gain, develops simultaneous to a sharp increase in hypothalamic levels of galanin and the opioids induced by a rise in gonadal steroids. This pattern, due to the actions of estrogen and progesterone, is observed earlier and more dramatically in females, who require fat stores for reproduction.

## RECENTLY DISCOVERED HYPOTHALAMIC PEPTIDES

Techniques of molecular biology have permitted the discovery of new peptides in the past few years. These peptides include the orexins, agouti-related peptide, and melanin-concentrating hormone. These peptides are heavily expressed in the hypothalamus. Furthermore, their injection into this region stimulates food intake in animals. The precise role of these peptides in the regulation of nutrient homeostasis has yet to be characterized. Recent findings, however, suggest that the orexins function similarly to galanin in relation to fat balance. Other work has led to the discovery of the hormone, leptin, which is produced in adipose tissue and found to control the production of these hypothalamic peptides that stimulate feeding behavior. Thus, leptin generates a signal from the periphery that, like insulin, provides a negative feedback message for reducing food intake.

## CLINICAL STUDIES OF EATING AND BODY WEIGHT DISORDERS

The ultimate goal of studies in animals is to determine whether these neurochemical and hormone systems also function in humans, and whether disturbances in these systems contribute to the development or maintenance of nutritional and body weight disorders. Remarkable similarities between humans and lower mammals are found in their responses to various pharmacological agents that affect eating and body weight, and in their diurnal rhythms and gender differences in nutrient selection. Moreover, drugs most commonly used today in the management of obesity, anorexia nervosa, and bulimia have their primary effect in modulating the balance between the monoamines, norepinephrine, serotonin and dopamine (see Chapters 99, 100).

There is some evidence to suggest that disturbances in brain neurochemical systems, together with neuroendocrine processes, may contribute to the development of abnormal patterns of eating and body weight gain in humans. For example, clinical studies have revealed altered levels of the amines and neuropeptides in the cerebrospinal fluid of patients with anorexia nervosa or bulimia and those with common eating problems, such as food cravings, seasonal appetite disturbances, and stress-related eating. The contribution of neuroendocrine disturbances is demonstrated by the reciprocal changes in fat balance observed in patients with Cushing's and Addison's disease, consequent to abnormal cortisol levels, and by the hyperphagia and increased weight gain in diabetics, due possibly to insufficient insulin-mediated control of hypothalamic peptide synthesis. A deficiency of the hormone, leptin, is also known to result in overeating and obesity. Understanding the dramatic rise in fat intake and fat deposition that occurs in women at puberty, and its relationship to estrogen-stimulated production of hypothalamic peptides, may help in identifying therapies for eating disorders that frequently develop around this time. These findings, in animals and humans, are now generating considerable excitement and hope that compounds affecting these brain neurochemical and neuroendocrine systems, in conjunction with nutritional and behavioral strategies, will have real therapeutic value in a range of eating and body weight disorders, and also for psychiatric disorders that have a strong nutritional component.

## ACKNOWLEDGMENTS

Research in the author's laboratory described in this article was support by Grant No. MH-43422 from the National Institute of Mental Health.

## FURTHER READING

Bray, G. A. (2000). Medicinal strategies in the treatment of obesity. *Nature, 404,* 672–677.— Review of drugs used in the long-term treatment of obesity.
Flier, J. S., & Maratos-Flier, E. (1998). Obesity and the hypothalamus: Novel peptides for new

pathways. *Cell, 92,* 437–440.—Minireview of hypothalamic peptide systems controlled by the hormone, leptin.

Hoebel, B. G., Leibowitz, S. F., & Hernandez, L. (1992). Neurochemistry of anorexia and bulimia. In G. H. Anderson & S. H. Kennedy (Eds.), *The biology of feast and famine* (pp. 22–45). New York: Academic Press.—Review of brain neurochemical processes related to eating disorders.

Inui, A. (1999, February). Neuropeptide Y: A key molecule in anorexia and cachexia in wasting disorders? *Molecular Medicine Today,* pp. 79–84.—A summary of evidence for and against a central role for neuropeptide Y and leptin in anorexia and cachexia.

Kaye, W. H. (1992). Neurotransmitter abnormalities in anorexia nervosa and bulimia nervosa. In G. H. Anderson & S. H. Kennedy (Eds.), *The biology of feast and famine* (pp. 22–45). New York: Academic Press.—Review of neurochemical disturbances in eating disorders.

Leibowitz, S. F. (1999). Hypothalamic galanin, dietary fat, and body fat. In G. Bray & D. Ryan (Eds.), *Nutrition, genetics and obesity* (Pennington Center Nutrition Series, Vol. 9, pp. 338–381). Baton Rouge: Louisiana State University Press.—Review focused on galanin in relation to dietary fat.

Leibowitz, S. F., & Hoebel, B. G. (1998). Behavioral neuroscience of obesity. In G. A. Bray, C. Bouchard, & W. P. T. James (Eds.), *Handbook of obesity* (pp. 313–358). New York: Marcel Dekker.—Comprehensive review of hypothalamic systems controlling food intake and body weight.

Walsh, B. T., & Devlin, M. J. (1999). Eating disorders: Progress and problems. *Science, 280,* 1387–1390.—Review article summarizing current thinking on the etiology and treatment of eating disorders.

Woods, S. C., Seeley, R. J., Porte, D., Jr., & Schwartz, M. W. (1999). Signals that regulate food intake and energy homeostasis. *Science, 280,* 1378–1383.—Review on hypothalamic signals that modulate food intake while integrating the body's immediate and long-term energy needs.

York, D. A. (1999). Regulation of feeding behavior: Advances in understanding from molecular and physiological approaches. In B. Guy-Grand & G. Ailhaud (Eds.), *Progress in obesity research* (Vol. 8, pp. 267–277). London: John Libbey.—Description of molecular approaches to the study of feeding behavior.

# 2

## Peripheral Physiological Determinants of Eating and Body Weight

GERARD P. SMITH
JAMES GIBBS

The relative importance of the peripheral controls of eating and body weight has increased significantly in the past 5 years. This has been due to the realization that peripheral controls function at every meal, that so-called long-term controls of food intake act by modulating the potency of the peripheral controls, and the discovery of a new genetic obesity in rats that is due to spontaneous mutation of a mechanism of a peripheral control. All of this is the result of using meals as the functional unit of nalysis for investigating the control of eating.

The experimental focus on the controls of eating has not only led to a better understanding of peripheral controls but also to a paradigm shift from seeing eating as a problem of how intake serves metabolism to seeing eating as a problem in behavioral neuroscience. Using this larger view, recent research has revealed a coherent neural network composed of peripheral feedbacks and central mechanisms for distributed processing that use amines, peptides, and steroids (see Chapter 1). This network is sensitive to genetic change, sexual differences, and prior experience. The new view also provides a more relevant basic science of eating for clinical eating disorders in which abnormally large meals can occur in patients with high, normal, or low body weight.

All of the recent progress has occurred in analyzing the controls of the size of meals (i.e., what maintains eating once it has begun and what terminates it). Much less has been discovered about the peripheral controls of meal number (i.e., what initiates eating).

### MEAL SIZE

Meal size is determined by the integration of the positive and negative feedbacks produced by ingested food stimuli (Figure 2.1). Positive feedback stimulates the central net-

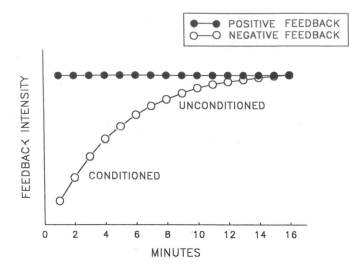

**FIGURE 2.1.** Temporal interaction of positive and negative feedback effects produced by ingested carbohydrate solutions during a scheduled meal. Eating stops and the meal ends when the potencies of the positive and negative feedbacks are judged to be equal by a comparator function(s) of the central networks for the control of eating. Note that the negative feedback effect during the early part of the meal is a conditioned orosensory effect, and the unconditioned effect in the later part of the meal is an unconditioned postingestive effect. From Smith, G. P., Davis, J. D., & Greenberg, D. (1996). The direct control of meal size in the Zucker rat. In G. A. Bray & D. H. Ryan (Eds.), *Molecular and genetic aspects of obesity* (Pennington Biochemical Medical Center Nutrition Series, Vol. 5, pp. 161–174). Baton Rouge: Louisiana State University Press. Copyright 1996 by Louisiana State University Press. Reprinted by permission.

work that controls eating and negative feedback inhibits it. Eating continues as long as the potency of the positive feedback to the central network exceeds the potency of the negative feedback. Eating stops when the potency of negative feedback equals or exceeds the potency of the positive feedback.

Both feedbacks are initiated by the *direct* contact of the mechanical and chemical stimuli of ingested food on preabsorptive receptors in the mouth, stomach, and small intestine. The relative potency of these feedbacks is determined not only by the potency of the peripheral feedbacks on neurons in the hindbrain but also by a number of other categories of central stimuli that affect the central processing of the afferent feedbacks. These categories are diverse and important. They include stimuli related to metabolic state, diurnal and ovarian rhythms, prior experience, social factors, and, in humans, cultural factors. Because none of these diverse stimuli contact the preabsorptive receptors directly, they are classified as indirect controls of meal size. Note that all indirect controls affect meal size by modulating the central potency of the direct controls.

That chronic decerebrate rats respond to direct controls, but not to indirect controls, provides a functional neurology for the controls of meal size: Indirect controls require intact neural connections between the forebrain and hindbrain in order to modulate the potency of the direct controls provided by the peripheral feedbacks. In contrast, the caudal brainstem has sufficient neural complexity to integrate the direct controls of meal size.

## Sites and Mechanisms of Positive Feedback

The mouth and nose (by retropharyngeal stimulation) are the principal sites of positive feedback. The intimate contact of mechanical and chemical stimuli with receptors in the mucosa of these regions means that the orosensory effects of food stimuli are mediated to the brain by afferent fibers of olfactory, gustatory, and somatosensory neurons of cranial nerves 1, 5, 7, 9, and 10. The mechanisms of transduction at specific peripheral receptors and the synaptic mechanisms in the central terminations of these afferent fibers are largely unknown. Central processing of this orosensory positive feedback involves dopaminergic and opioid mechanisms in the limbic system, because specific antagonists of these neuromodulators have been shown to decrease the potency of the positive feedback of carbohydrates and fats.

## Sites and Mechanisms of Negative Feedback

Food stimuli in the mouth, stomach, and small intestine produce negative feedback on eating. Because there is spatial and temporal synergism from these sites, the potency of negative feedback is strongest when these sites are stimulated sequentially, as occurs during a meal.

The afferent fibers of the vagus nerve mediate the inhibitory effects of gastric distension on food intake under certain circumstances. It is possible that peptides released by gastric stimuli, such as gastrin-releasing peptide, are also involved in mediating negative feedback from the stomach.

In contrast to the stomach, chemical stimuli of ingested food in the small intestine are more important for producing negative feedback than are mechanical stimuli. Chemical stimuli activate vagal afferent fibers directly. They also work indirectly through the release of cholecystokinin (CCK) from mucosal cells in the upper small intestine and through glucagon from the pancreas; these peptides then stimulate vagal afferent fibers.

The satiating effect of cholecystokinin released from the small intestine has been demonstrated to be a physiological function of the peptide in numerous animals and in humans. The variety of evidence required to prove the satiating effect of endogenous CCK provides a case study of how to evaluate the physiological function of a candidate peptide in the peripheral control of food intake. Pancreatic glucagon fulfills the physiological criteria in the rat; the evidence for amylin, apolipoprotein AIV, and enterostatin is growing.

## ANALYSIS OF A CHANGE IN MEAL SIZE

Because meal size is determined by the central modulation of afferent feedback information, any change in meal size produced by genetic, neural, physiological, pharmacological, or psychological factors must be due to a change in the potency of positive or negative feedbacks (see Chapter 8). Such changes in feedback potency can now be measured in animals and humans.

That all changes in meal size are due to a change in the potency of peripheral feedbacks led to the question of how insulin and leptin, signals of the indirect control by the mass of white adipose tissue, decrease meal size. The answer is by increasing the potency of the peripheral negative feedback from the small intestine mediated by CCK. Estrogen, the mediator of the indirect control exerted by the ovarian rhythm, also decreases meal size by increasing the potency of CCK.

The recent demonstration that the phenotype of rats with a spontaneous null mutation of the $CCK_A$ receptor that eliminates the negative feedback effect of CCK is increased meal size and obesity is complementary evidence for the importance of peripheral feedback control of eating in rodents.

Reports that bulimic patients release less CCK than control subjects in response to ingested food suggest that this abnormality contributes to the large meals characteristic of these patients.

As the molecular mechanisms of indirect and direct controls are identified, the meaning of the numerous peptides and amines in the brain that change meal size will become clear. Ultimately, all relevant molecules will be defined by the function they have in the central network for the control of eating.

## MEAL NUMBER

Three endogenous changes occur just before the initiation of meals in rodents: a small decrease of plasma glucose, a decrease of metabolism, and an increase in liver temperature. Although these changes have been correlated with meal initiation, they have not been proven to be causal. They are certainly not necessary for meal initiation, because the presentation of food or stimuli (temporal, sensory, or social) previously associated with food initiate a meal at times when the endogenous changes are not present. It is important to note that the initiation of a meal does not predict the size of a meal. This means that the controls of meal number are different from the controls of meal size.

## SUMMARY

Recent research has demonstrated the importance of peripheral positive and negative feedbacks for the control of meal size in rodents and humans. The mechanisms of these feedbacks provide the direct controls of meal size, and all other controls act by modulating the central potency of the direct controls. Because the sensory control of the feedbacks is possible in humans and rodents, the feedbacks can be exploited for the experimental investigation of any molecular, neural, physiological, or psychological control of eating.

## ACKNOWLEDGMENTS

We thank Laurel Torres for processing the manuscript. We are supported by Grant Nos. MH-40010 and DK-33248 from the National Institutes of Health.

## FURTHER READING

Devlin, M. J., Walsh, B. J., Guss, J. L., Kissileff, H. R., Liddle, R. A., & Petkova, E. (1997). Postprandial cholecystokinin release and gastric emptying in patients with bulimia nervosa. *American Journal of Clinical Nutrition, 65*, 114–120.—The most recent and careful study demonstrating decreased release of cholecystokinin from the small intestine by ingested food in bulimic patients. This decrease in negative feedback probably contributes to the abnormally large meals that are characteristic of this disorder.

French, S. J. (1999). The effects of specific nutrients on the regulation of feeding behaviour in human subjects. *Proceedings of the Nutrition Society, 58*, 533–539.—Good review of how the direct controls of meal size are being studied in humans.

Geary, N. (2000). Estradiol and appetite. *Appetite, 35*, 273–274.—A succinct overview of recent progress in the author's laboratory in understanding the inhibitory effects of estrogen on eating and body weight.

Moran, T. H., Katz, L. F., Plata-Salaman, C. R., & Schwartz,G. J. (1998). Disordered food intake and obesity in rats lacking cholecystokinin A receptors. *American Journal of Physiology, 274*, R618–R625.—First demonstration of hyperphagia and obesity resulting from a genetic mutation of a mechanism of a direct negative feedback control of meal size.

Ritter, R. C., Covasa, M., & Matson, C. A. (1999). Cholecystokinin: Proofs and prospects for involvement in control of food intake and body weight. *Neuropeptides, 33*, 387–399.—Intelligent review of the satiating effect of CCK, emphasizing new results that show that high-fat diets decrease its satiating potency, and that CCK can increase the inhibitory effect of leptin on body weight.

Smith, G. P. (Ed.). (1998). *Satiation: From gut to brain.* New York: Oxford University Press.—Authoritative monograph that contains nine critical chapters on the mechanisms of satiation.

Smith, G. P. (1999). Introduction to the reviews on peptides and the control of food intake and body weight. *Neuropeptides, 33*, 323–328.—Critical overview of the role of peripheral and central peptides in the control of intake and body weight that are discussed in detail in eleven reviews in the October 1999 issue of the journal.

Smith, G. P. (2000). The controls of eating: Brain meanings of food stimuli. In E. A. Mayer & C. B. Saper (Eds.), *The biological basis for mind body interactions* (pp. 173–186). New York: Elsevier.—Extensive review of the evidence for the theory of direct and indirect controls of meal size in animals and humans.

Smith, G. P. (2000). The controls of eating: a shift from nutritional homeostasis to behavioral neuroscience. *Nutrition, 16*, 814–820.—Discusses the evidence that produced the paradigm shift and the advantages of the theory of direct and indirect controls over previous theories of the control of eating.

# 3

# Genetic Influences on Body Weight

## CLAUDE BOUCHARD

How many overweight or obese individuals have developed their condition as a result of a major deficiency in one gene? How many are overweight or obese as a consequence of a strong genetic predisposition determined by DNA sequence variation at several genes? How many have only a slight genetic predisposition but have gained large amounts of body weight because they have poor nutritional habits and a sedentary lifestyle? How many do not have any genetic susceptibility but have nonetheless become overweight or obese? We cannot yet answer these questions, but in recent years, genetic epidemiology and molecular genetic studies have begun to generate data that allow us to formulate these questions in more relevant terms and to sketch some answers. This chapter examines the genetic epidemiology of the obesity epidemic. The molecular genetic issues are addressed in Chapter 5.

## HERITABILITY LEVEL

C. B. Davenport, from the Carnegie Institute, described in 1923 the first comprehensive attempt to understand the role of inheritance in human body mass for stature. Among his findings were that normal-weight parents sometimes have obese adult offspring, and that obese parents frequently have normal-weight adult descendants. In the aggregate, however, his study demonstrated that body mass index (BMI) values were more similar among family members than among unrelated persons.

Except for some rare Mendelian disorders, the vast majority of obese patients do not exhibit a clear pattern of Mendelian inheritance. Despite many studies on the familial aggregation and heritability of the obesity phenotypes, there is no unanimity among researchers regarding the importance of genetic factors.

Heritability is the fraction of the population variation in a trait (e.g., BMI) that can be explained by genetic transmission. It has been considered in a large number of twin, adoption, and family studies. The results depend on sampling strategy, sample size, and kinds of relatives upon which they are based. For instance, studies conducted with identical twins and fraternal twins, or identical twins reared apart, have yielded the highest heritability levels, with values clustering around 70% of the variation in BMI. In contrast, adoption studies have generated the lowest heritability estimates, 30% and less. The family studies have generally found levels of heritability intermediate between the twin and the adoption studies.

There are divergent views on the interpretation of these statistical genetic studies. Some see them as evidence for a strong genetic role in obesity, saying that heritability is of the order of 70–90% of the total population variance. Among the implications of such high heritability levels is that one expects to find a good number of predisposing genes or a few predisposing alleles at key genes present at high frequencies in human populations. Other scientists conclude that the heritability level reaches about one-third of the population variance. One implication is that the changes in lifestyle experienced in this century have played a dominant role in the current overweight and obesity epidemic. At present, it is not possible to establish whether one school of thought is closer to the truth than the other.

## FAMILIAL RISK OF OBESITY

The risk of becoming obese when a first-degree biological relative is overweight or obese can be quantified using a statistic called the lambda coefficient. This is the ratio of the risk of being obese when a biological relative is obese compared to the risk in the population at large (i.e., the prevalence of obesity in the same population). Estimates of lambda values based on BMI data were recently reported. Age and gender risk ratios were obtained from 2,349 first-degree relatives of 840 obese probands and 5,851 participants of the National Health and Nutrition Examination Survey III. The prevalence of obesity is twice as high in families of obese individuals than in the population at large. The risk increases with the severity of obesity in the proband. Thus, the risk of extreme obesity (BMI of 45 and above) is about seven to eight times higher in families of extremely obese subjects. Other large studies report similar trends.

These lambda values are accepted as evidence for a strong genetic effect for obesity, particularly severe obesity. However, the picture is more complex than originally suggested. For instance, Katzmarzyk and collaborators, using data from 15,245 participants, ages 7–69 years, from the 1981 Canada Fitness Survey, showed that the familial risk of obesity was five times higher for relatives in the upper 1% of the distribution of BMI values than in the general Canadian population. But the study suggested that the familial risk was not due entirely to genetic factors, as the risk was also markedly elevated in the spouse of the proband. Future studies need to consider not only a genetic hypothesis (i.e., assessing the familial risk in a first-degree relative of the proband) but also a mixed model in which the familial risk is assessed in a nonbiological but cohabitating relative of the same proband.

## GENOTYPE–ENVIRONMENT INTERACTIONS

A genotype–environment interaction (G × E) effect arises when the response of a phenotype to environmental changes depends on the genotype of the individual. It is known that there are interindividual differences in the responses to various dietary interventions or to exercise programs. However, few attempts have been made to verify whether these differences are genotype-dependent, particularly for obesity-related phenotypes.

Studies with identical twins strongly suggest that undetermined genetic characteristics may play an important role in the responsiveness to standardized alterations in energy balance. Experiments performed with monozygotic (MZ) twins revealed that the response to positive or negative energy balance is very heterogeneous among twin individuals but quite homogeneous within members of the same twin pair.

In one study, 12 pairs of male MZ twins ate a 4.2 MJ (1,000 kcal) per day caloric surplus, 6 days a week, during a period of 100 days, for a total caloric surplus of 353 MJ (84,000 kcal) over the energy cost of weight maintenance. Significant increases in body weight and fat mass were observed. There were considerable interindividual differences in the adaptation to excess calories, but the variation observed was not randomly distributed, as indicated by the significant within-pair resemblance in response. There was at least three times more variance in response between pairs than in response within pairs for the gains in body weight (Figure 3.1, left panel) and body fat. Some individuals are more at risk than others to gain fat when energy intake surplus is clamped at the same level for everyone, and when subjects are confined to a sedentary lifestyle. The amount of weight gained is likely influenced by the genotype.

In another experiment, seven pairs of young adult male identical twins completed a negative energy balance protocol during which they exercised on cycle ergometers twice a day, 9 out of 10 days, over a period of 93 days, while being kept on a constant daily energy and nutrient intake. The mean total energy deficit caused by exercise above the estimated energy cost of body weight maintenance reached 244 MJ (58,000 kcal). Mean body weight loss was 5.0 kg. Intrapair resemblance was observed for changes in body weight (Figure 3.1, right panel) and body fat content. Even though there were large individual differences, subjects with the same genotype were more alike than subjects with different genotypes.

The results of both experiments are remarkably similar. They demonstrate heterogeneous response to positive or negative energy balance. A two- to threefold range in response to the protocols was typically observed for body mass, body composition, and other obesity-related phenotypes. The experiments also reveal that being genetically identical translates into a similar pattern of adaptation. These studies provide highly suggestive evidence for G × E effects that are of critical importance for understanding predisposition to obesity and response to treatment. Replication is necessary with larger sample sizes to solidify these conclusions and to define the true magnitude of the G × E effects. Ultimately, we would like to know the genes and DNA sequence variants that are at the origin of this individuality in adaptation.

## OTHER CONSIDERATIONS

Several investigators have examined a maternal effect in risk for obesity. In the aggregate, the evidence is negative. Both parents seem to contribute more or less equally to the genetic risk. Moreover, there is no clear evidence for a role of non-Mendelian maternal inheritance, as would be the case if mitochondrial DNA were a major contributor to risk. Studies have not found that obese parents differ in the frequency of having obese boys or

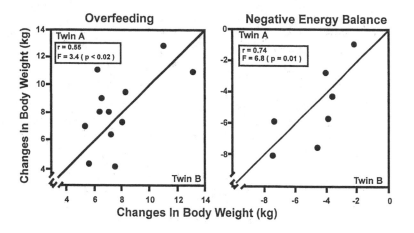

**FIGURE 3.1.** Intrapair resemblance in the response of identical twins to long-term changes in energy balance. *Left*: Twelve pairs of identical twins were submitted to an 84,000-kcal energy intake surplus over 100 days. *Right*: Seven pairs were subjected to a negative energy balance protocol caused by exercise. The energy deficit was 58,000 kcal over 93 days. From Bouchard, C., Tremblay, A., Després, J. P., Nadeau, A., Lupien, P. J. Thériault, G., Dussault, J., Moorjani, S., Pineault, S., & Fournier, G. (1990). The response to long-term overfeeding in identical twins. *New England Journal of Medicine*, *322*, 1477–1482; and Bouchard, C. (1994). The response to exercise with constant energy intake in identical twins. *Obesity Research*, *2*, 400–410. Copyright 1990 by *New England Journal of Medicine* and 1994 by North American Association for the Study of Obesity. Reprinted by permission.

girls. The transmission of risk from parents to offspring does not appear to be sex-specific.

In the Swedish Obese Subjects (SOS) study, the severely or morbidly obese proband is typically 10–15 BMI units heavier than his or her siblings. The same observation has been made in other studies of severely obese men and women. There is no good explanation for such a difference. However, the ratio of severely obese to other offspring in such families is around one out of three or four siblings. This is compatible with the ratio expected if a single recessive gene with a large effect were contributing to the risk. Under this scenario, the homozygotes for the recessive allele would be severely affected. Such a gene (and there may be several of them) has not been identified yet, but candidates have emerged recently.

Dozens of studies have reported a spousal correlation for BMI or adiposity phenotypes. In general, the correlation is low, at about 0.2 or less, although there are exceptions. Assortative mating may, however, be stronger at the upper end of the BMI distribution. This is exactly what has been found in some recent studies. This has led to speculation that adiposity genes are present at a higher frequency among heavy or obese parents, and that such genes are passed along to their offspring, increasing the genetic risk for obesity in this segment of the population. Two studies have provided confirming data. Childhood overweight and obesity were in both cases more frequent in families in which both parents were themselves obese. However, since obese parents may have reduced fertility, the true contribution of this phenomenon to the evolution of genetic risk in large populations remains unknown. Note that opposite forces may be acting at the other end of the distribution, although it is not yet clear from the existing studies. If this were the case, the effect would be to increase the frequency of the leanness genes in another segment of the population.

Finally, if current societal trends are maintained for generations, almost every individual living in a knowledge-based economy and well-developed society will eventually be living in an obesogenic environment (see Chapter 78). One consequence of such a trend will be that the genetic component of the resistance to, or the protection against, positive energy balance will increase. Another implication will be that those with some genetic predisposition to the disease will naturally evolve toward obesity.

## CONCLUSION

Excessive adiposity is a complex multifactorial trait evolving under the interactive influences of dozens of affectors from the social, behavioral, physiological, metabolic, cellular, and molecular domains. Segregation of the genes is not easily detected in familial or pedigree studies, and whatever the influence of the genotype on etiology, it is generally attenuated or exacerbated by nongenetic factors, particularly in the present obesogenic environment of the Western world.

The distinction between the genes causing obesity and those predisposing to obesity is particularly relevant. We have begun to make progress in the first category, perhaps because the effect of a major disruption in a gene is so evident that it attracts attention. Progress in the identification of the predisposing genes is much slower. However, populations of informative patients have been assembled. Geneticists and gene hunters are expected to move forward faster in the coming years and should be able to isolate many of these genes. It will nonetheless be a daunting task to define how genetic individuality interacts with factors in our environment to make some people resistant to obesity and others very much at risk of becoming obese. The task can be seen as even more complex when the phenomenon of gene–gene interactions is considered. We will need all the power of human genetics, experimental genetics, and molecular biology to unravel the genetic basis of the predisposition to obesity.

## FURTHER READING

Allison, D. B., Neale, M. C., Kezis, M. I., Alfonso, V. C., Heshka, S., & Heymsfield, S. B. (1996). Assortative mating for relative weight: Genetic implications. *Behavior Genetics*, 26, 103–111.—A discussion on assortative mating based on old and new evidence. The implications for population estimates of heritability are also highlighted.

Bouchard C. (1996). Genetic and energy balance interactions in humans. In C. D. Berdanier (Ed.), *Nutrients and gene expression: Clinical aspects* (pp. 83–100). Boca Raton, FL: CRC Press.—A review of several experimental twin studies designed to address the issue of gene–environment interactions under positive and negative energy balance conditions.

Bouchard, C., Pérusse, L., Rice, T., & Rao, D. C. (1998). The genetics of human obesity. In G. A. Bray, C. Bouchard, & W. P. T. James (Eds.), *Handbook of obesity* (pp. 157–190). New York: Marcel Dekker.—An overview of the human genetic studies of obesity, with an emphasis on genetic epidemiology issues.

Hebebrand, J., Wulftange, H., Goerg, T., Ziegler, A., Hinney, A., Barth, N., Mayer, H., & Remschmidt, H. (2000). Epidemic obesity: Are genetic factors involved via increased rates of assortative mating? *International Journal of Obesity and Related Metabolic Disorders, 24,* 345–353.—The first paper to suggest that assortative mating contributes to the increase in the prevalence of obesity.

Katzmarzyk, P. T., Perusse, L., Rao, D. C., & Bouchard, C. (1999). Familial risk of obesity and central adipose tissue distribution in the general Canadian population. *American Journal of Epidemiology, 149,* 933–942.—The first paper to provide evidence that the familial risk for obesity is likely to be caused by both genetic and nongenetic factors.

Lee, J. H., Reed, D. R., & Price, R. A. (1997). Familial risk ratios for extreme obesity: Implications for mapping human obesity genes. *International Journal of Obesity and Related Metabolic Disorders, 21,* 935–940.—Familial risks for increasing levels of obesity are presented and their implications discussed.

Maes, H. H., Neale, M. C., & Eaves, L. J. (1997). Genetic and environmental factors in relative body weight and human adiposity. *Behavior Genetics, 27,* 325–351.—A detailed review of twin, family, and adoption studies of the genetic component of obesity.

Perusse, L., Chagnon, J. C., & Bouchard, C. (1998). Etiology of massive obesity: Role of genetic factors. *World Journal of Surgery, 22,* 907–912.—A review of the familial aggregation and genetic determinants of massive obesity.

Price, J. H., Reed, D. R., & Price, R. A. (1998). Obesity-related phenotypes in families selected for extreme obesity and leanness. *International Journal of Obesity and Related Metabolic Disorders, 22,* 406–413.—A discussion of the advantage of sampling families with extremely obese siblings with a lean parent to address genetic questions.

Stunkard, A. J., Harris, J. R., Pedersen, N. L., & McClearn, G. E. (1990). The body-mass index of twins who have been reared apart. *New England Journal of Medicine, 322,* 1483–1487.—A study of fraternal and identical twin pairs reared apart, with the goal of estimating the heritability of BMI.

# 4

# Constitutional Thinness and Resistance to Obesity

CYNTHIA M. BULIK
DAVID B. ALLISON

In the wake of unprecedented economic growth; decreased infectious disease; nearly unlimited food supply; wide availability of high-fat, highly palatable, and preprepared foods; large portion sizes; and technological advances leading to a more sedentary lifestyle, modern westernized environments promote obesity (see Chapter 78). Despite the increasing prevalence of obesity, some individuals remain thin. In this chapter, we explore evidence supporting the study of constitutional thinness as a complementary and informative strategy for understanding the development and maintenance of obesity.

## THINNESS AND NATURAL SELECTION

Throughout human evolution, selection pressures may have favored efficient energy storage and moderate adiposity (see Chapter 83). Such traits would increase the chances of survival during periods of famine or exposure to the elements. Conversely, traits producing inefficient energy storage or high metabolism, which would resist weight gain and fat storage, may have been selected against, and via natural selection, may be relatively rare. A comprehensive understanding of individuals who remain thin in the presence of strong environmental factors may assist with preventing individuals who are genetically predisposed from becoming obese and, ultimately, with the development of effective treatments for obesity.

## WHAT IS THINNESS?

It is unclear whether thinness represents a distinct phenotype or merely the lower tail of the body mass index (BMI) distribution. Several factors must be considered. In order to perform preliminary analyses on extant data, we define thinness as having an age-, sex-, and ethnicity-adjusted BMI below the 10th percentile. This is a suboptimal definition because the 10th percentile will differ across populations and over time. The optimal definition of thinness should consider factors such as (1) *stability* over time, such that an individual has always been in the lower percentiles for age, sex, and ethnicity; (2) *age*, as some forms of obesity are only expressed in mid-life; (3) *parity* in women, given that pregnancy has been recognized as a life event related to the onset of obesity in some women (see Chapter 80); (4) regular dieting or weight loss efforts in order to maintain a low BMI (because, constitutionally, thin individuals should be protected against the need to diet); (5) behaviors and conditions that could give rise to thinness phenocopies such as medical conditions (e.g., cancer or AIDS), metabolic disorders, or disorders of the digestive system) that could lead to or mimic thinness, and psychiatric disorders or their subclinical forms associated with loss of appetite or weight (e.g., major depression, anorexia nervosa, or bulimia nervosa); and (6) the use of substances that can lead to weight loss (e.g. crack cocaine, heroin), or be used to prevent weight gain (e.g., nicotine).

## EVIDENCE SUPPORTING THINNESS AS A UNIQUE TRAIT

### Animal Studies

Animal studies support the existence of a unique thinness or leanness phenotype that is under genetic control, since animals can be selectively bred for these traits. For example, the pure-line "I" strain of inbred mice are unusually resistant to the development of dietary obesity. Recessive genes for extreme thinness or leanness, including the halothane gene in pigs and the double-muscling gene in cattle, have been identified. Similarly, a substrain of Sprague–Dawley rats has been bred for their *resistance* to the development of obesity even when maintained on a high-fat diet. In addition, knockout mice created for the RII beta subunit of protein kinase were healthy but had greatly diminished white adipose tissue despite normal food intake. These animals were protected against developing diet-induced obesity, thus becoming potential models for the humans in our society who stay thin *despite* an obesity-promoting environment.

### Studies of Humans

#### The Stability of Thinness

From adolescence through adulthood, obesity tracks over time, which might be due to the constant influence of an unchanging genotype. To what extent is thinness a persistent trait?

Figure 4.1 presents simple statistics that address the stability of thinness. The first statistic, $\gamma_t$, is the conditional probability of being thin (adjusted BMI < 10th percentile) at one point in time, given that one was thin at some previous point in time. Similarly, the second statistic, $\gamma_o$, is the conditional probability of being obese (adjusted BMI > 90th percentile) at one point in time, given that one was obese at some previous point in time.

The graph includes data from the National Longitudinal Study of Youth, the Framingham Heart Study, the China Health and Nutrition Survey, and the Russia Longitudinal Study. Across these various populations and time intervals, the stability is simi-

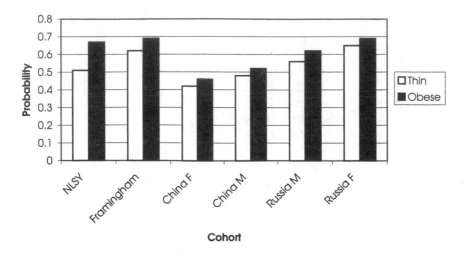

**FIGURE 4.1.** Conditional probability of being obese or thin at time 2 given the same BMI category at time 1.

larly high for obesity and thinness, suggesting that thinness observed at one point in time is a reasonable indicator of "true thinness propensity," just as obesity at one point in time is an indicator of "true obesity propensity."

### Familiality and Heritability of Thinness

We explored the extent to which thinness is familial using both family and twin data. Risch's lambda ($\lambda$) is defined as the risk to a relative of an affected individual divided by the population risk. Comparing lambda values for low BMI with lambda values for high BMI is therefore one way to assess the relative risks of obesity and thinness. The samples include African American, European American, Native American, and East Indian pairs. Across these varied populations, one can see in Figure 4.2 that the lambda values are similarly high for both thinness and obesity.

Twin studies can also address the heritability of thinness. Together with K. S. Kendler, we explored the question using a population-based sample of 591 monozygotic (MZ) female twin pairs and 432 dizygotic (DZ) female twin pairs from Virginia. Thinness was defined as a current BMI < 20 kg/m² (lowest 10th percentile for age) and no history of either anorexia or bulimia nervosa. Twin studies allow one to partition causal variance into three sources—additive genetic effects, shared environmental effects (to which both members of a twin pair are exposed, and which increase similarity between twins), and unique environmental effects (that act to increase differences between twins and to which only one member of a twin pair is exposed). Model fitting suggested a substantial contribution of additive genetic effects to thinness with 67% (95% confidence interval: 3–79%), a negligible contribution of shared environment (4%: 95% confidence interval: 0–36%), and the remaining variance attributable to individual-specific environmental factors (29%: 95% confidence interval: 21–39%). Together, these family and twin studies suggest that thinness is indeed familial and that the observed aggregation in families is primarily due to the additive effects of genes.

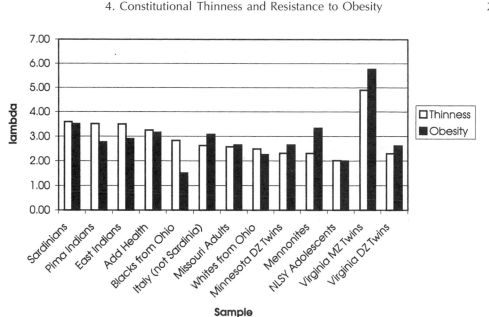

**FIGURE 4.2.** Sibling lambda values: thinness and obesity.

## CONCLUSIONS

In summary, evidence from animal studies strongly suggests that leanness and thinness are genetically influenced traits that can be bred. Sophisticated animal studies have revealed that certain genes confer resistance to the development of obesity even in the presence of an experimentally manipulated obesogenic diet. Studies of humans have shown that thinness appears to be stable over time, is familial, and may be substantially influenced by additive genetic effects. Intensive efforts directed toward understanding individuals who remain thin in an obesogenic environment may lead to important clues to the causes of and treatments for obesity.

## ACKNOWLEDGMENTS

Supported in part by National Institutes of Health Grant Nos. R01-DK51716, P30-DK26687, R01-DK51716, and K01-MH01553.

## FURTHER READING

Bulik, C. M., & Allison, D. B. (in press). Genetic epidemiology of thinness. *Obesity Reviews.*—A comprehensive review of the genetics and genetic epidemiology of thinness.
Treasure, J., Collier, D., & Campbell, I. (1997). Ill-fitting genes: The biology of weight and shape control in relation to body composition and eating disorders. *Psychological Medicine*, 27, 505–508.—An excellent review of the biology and genetics of body weight and shape.

# 5

# The Molecular Genetics of Body Weight Regulation

## RUDOLPH L. LEIBEL

That genes exist for body weight and composition in animals is apparent from the autosomal recessive and dominant obesity mutations in rodents, transgenic experiments in mice, single gene mutations affecting muscle mass in cattle and sheep, and strain-related differences in body composition in domesticated cattle, pigs, sheep, and other animals. The concordance of somatic phenotype among mono- and dizygous twins, and adopted children and their respective parents, as well as segregation analyses of relative adiposity in families, indicate a substantial genetic contribution to body fatness (see Chapters 3 and 4). Single gene/locus mutations that produce obesity in humans are also well documented (see below).

## GENES AND BODY COMPOSITION

The genes determining fatness must affect *energy intake*, *energy expenditure*, or *partitioning* (the molecular form; e.g., fat, glycogen, and proteins in which calories are stored in the body). Such genes can affect all three of these major phenotypes or may affect only one or two of them. Body mass and composition reflect the lifetime effects of these three phenotypes, so small imbalances persisting over time can have large effects. Therefore, despite potent genetic influences on body fat, it is difficult to implicate specific genes in any but the rare instances of obesity that are inherited in Mendelian fashion.

Most observed Mendelian variation in phenotype is due to DNA sequence variation in a single gene. For non-Mendelian, complex or polygenic traits, phenotype variation reflects allelic variation in several or many genes and their interactions with each other and the environment. The recent applications of linkage analysis and positional cloning to Mendelian phenotypes have succeeded where the correlations between single-locus genotype and phenotype are strong, and where the effect of genotype is large.

The genes responsible for control of body composition are likely to be substantial in number, possibly differing qualitatively and quantitatively among different populations and ethnic groups, with each having relatively small effects conditioned by nonadditive interactions with other genes (epistasis), and environmental and developmental effects. In inbred animal strains, genetic effects are seen on body composition when animals ingest a fixed number of calories, and in response an *ad libitum* high-calorie diet. Genetic mapping shows that the genes determining the latter effects may not account for the former. In many instances, neither are related to the Mendelian loci that influence body composition.

## MOLECULAR GENETICS OF THE LEPTIN AXIS

Leptin (LEP), synthesized in adipocytes in proportion to adipocyte mass and short-term energy fluxes, signals the hypothalamus regarding the status of somatic energy stores and metabolic flux (see Chapter 6). Molecular genetic analyses indicate how the leptin molecule interacts with the central nervous system (CNS).

The *db* mutation (*Lepr$^{db}$*) is a splice mutation that results in the inability to synthesize only the Rb (signal transducer and activator of transcription [STAT] domain containing) isoform of the leptin receptor (LEPR) in all tissues. The metabolic–behavioral phenotypes of animals homozygous for this mutation are not distinguishable from those of animals in which all isoforms of the receptor are eliminated, or from *ob* mice (*Lep$^{ob}$*) that are totally deficient in the ligand for the LEPR. Thus, we can infer that absence of the leptin signal transduction via STAT is the main mechanism for the changes in behavior and metabolism that characterize these animals. Furthermore, since LEPR-Rb is expressed primarily in the CNS (specifically, the hypothalamus), most of leptin's physiological effects are likely conveyed via the CNS. Very small amounts of leptin protein delivered to the third ventricle of *Lep$^{ob}$* (leptin-deficient) mice restores their phenotypes to normal. Recent experiments in which the Rb isoform of *Lepr* is transgenically restored only to the brain of mice otherwise totally deficient in the synthesis of the *Lepr* gene show substantial restoration of leptin-deficient phenotypes to normal.

*Lep$^{ob}$* mice display elevated expression of orexigenic peptides (NPY, AGRP, MCH, HCRT/Orexin) and decreased expression of anorexiant peptides (CRF, MCH, and POMC/MSH) in the hypothalamus. The administration of LEP systemically, or into the third ventricle, reverses these changes in neuropeptide gene expression and the obese phenotype. The hierarchy of signaling can be examined by assessing the phenotypes of animals with natural and experimental mutations of these molecular components of the neural pathways regulating energy homeostasis. The *Npy* knockout mouse, for example, is—contrary to expectation—of normal body composition and not hypophagic. However, homozygosity for the *Npy* knockout mutation mitigates some of the obesity of the *ob/ob* animal, indicating a role for NPY in the hyperphagia of the *ob/ob* animal. Conversely, animals with knockout of the melanocortin-4 receptor (*Mc4r*), which binds the anorexiant molecule α-MSH, are obese, and those with knockout of the oxrexiant melanocyte-concentrating hormone (*Mch*), are lean. This hierarchy of effects could reflect the relative importance of the respective molecules and/or redundancy of critical functions sufficient to cause compensation for developmental absence. For definitive analysis, facultative, organ-specific knockouts using Cre-loxP technologies are being used. The fact that all of these knockout animals respond to some extent to exogenous leptin, and that *Mc4r* knockout animals respond to anorexiant (e.g., corticotropin-releasing factor) and orexiant (e.g., NPY) molecules, indicates that the response processes are not simple daisy chains of neurons or molecules. The extreme biological importance of these pathways—integrating somatic energy stores with food seeking, neuroendocrine (reproduction, growth), and immune physiology—accounts for the redundancy of the components.

Animals lacking functional *Lep* or *Lepr* genes still respond to food deprivation with compensatory hyperphagia and declines in energy expenditure, indicating that the leptin axis is not the sole mediator of body weight regulation. Many physiological studies implicate neural, humoral, and substrate-specific pathways from the liver and gastrointestinal (GI) tract in energy homeostasis, and these are presumably largely intact in animals with interruptions of the leptin axis. For example, inhibition of fatty acid synthase in the brain reduces food intake in both wild type and *ob/ob* (leptin-deficient) mice.

Animals heterozygous for inactivating mutations of *Lep*, *Lepr,* and *Mc4r* have more body fat than animals with two functioning copies of these genes. The phenotypic effect of such haploinsufficiency suggests that moderate differences in rates of gene expression can have significant effects on quantitative phenotypes such as body fatness. These sorts of differences, due in many instances to allelic variations in promoter and regulatory regions of genes, will probably account for differences in quantitative traits such as fatness in humans and animals.

## QUANTITATIVE GENETICS IN RODENTS

Inbred rodent strains differ widely in adiposity. The responsible genes can be mapped by intercrossing inbred strains maximally divergent for body fat and looking for statistical associations between genetic intervals and specific phenotypes. The appearance of the same genetic interval in several such crosses strengthens confidence in the resulting inferences regarding molecular physiology. Such studies have generated over 70 regions linked to obesity in nearly 20 interstrain crosses. As in human studies, some mouse intervals contain strong candidate genes. Because mice are inherently easier to work with for molecular cloning, one strategy is to clone the responsible mouse genes and then test them by association and direct sequencing in humans.

Despite their evolutionary divergence about 60–100 million years ago, the mouse and human genomes retain close similarities in both general organization and the sequences of individual genes. The similarities in relative gene position ("synteny") extend over long (10 million bases) stretches of DNA and can be used to infer the positions of genes between the species. These transspecies maps are becoming increasingly refined as the respective genomes are physically mapped and sequenced. Instances in which an obesity-related phenotype maps to syntenic regions of two or more species may reinforce inferences regarding the biological role of genes in such intervals.

## MOLECULAR GENETICS OF HUMAN OBESITY

Intensive screenings of human populations for mutations in orthologs of the spontaneous rodent obesity mutations have shown that such mutations are extremely rare. They have been identified in *LEP* and *LEPR* in highly inbred families; mutations in *CPE* (fat), *TUB* (tubby), and agouti-signaling protein (*ASP*) (homologous to mouse *Yellow*) have not yet been implicated in human obesity. Other genes known by virtue of physiology or the phenotypes of knockout animals to participate in energy homeostasis have been implicated in human obesity: pro-opiomelanocortin (*POMC*), melanocortin-4 receptor (*MC4R*), and prohormone convertase 1 (*PCSK1*). Of these, *Mc4r* mutations are prevalent and found in 3–5% of patients with body mass index (BMI) > 40. However, not all individuals with *Mc4r* mutations are obese, suggesting that obesity may depend on genetic variation in other genes in these individuals.

The realization that the human and rodent genomes contain large amounts of apparently noncoding DNA sequence, and that random variation in such sequences can be used to track the segregation of specific intervals of DNA, revolutionized genetic mapping by replacing limited phenotypic variants (e.g., blood groups, major histocompatibility complex haplotypes) with a nearly limitless number of genetic polymorphisms that could be used to mark specific sites in the 3 billion base-pair haploid genomes of humans (or mice, rats, pigs, etc.). Use of these reagents in DNA of families segregating for highly penetrant single-gene mutations, such as cystic fibrosis and Huntington's disease, led to the spectacular successes of positional genetics in identifying the genetic bases for many Mendelian genetic disturbances in humans and animals (see http://www.ncbi.nlm.nih.gov). For rare types of "syndromic" human obesity (e.g., Prader–Labhardt–Willi, Bardet–Biedl, Alstrom, Cohen), specific regions of the genome have been implicated. However, when the segregation of "simple" human obesity either as a dichotomous (obese, nonobese) or continuous (BMI, percentage body fat, etc.) variable is examined by statistical techniques in extended or nuclear human families–sib pairs, single genes or regions of the genome cannot account for the majority of phenotypic variance. Some regions implicated contain intriguing candidate genes (e.g., *POMC* on chromosome 2p or cocaine-amphetamine-related transcript [*CART*] on chromosome 5p), and weaker signals have been obtained in the regions of *LEPR* (1p) and *LEP* (7q). However, close scrutiny of the coding sequences, and some of the regulatory regions of these genes, have as yet failed to identify the sequence variant(s) responsible for these statistical signals. A possible explanation is that the responsible sequence variant is in yet unidentified regulatory (e.g., promoter) DNA or in another gene that is closely linked to the positional candidate gene, or possibly both. The linkage for *POMC* (precursor molecule for α-MSH) has been detected in studies of Caucasians, Mexican Americans, and African Americans, supporting the likely role of a gene in this region in determining BMI and/or plasma leptin concentration. However, few of the other regions implicated in the four genome scans reported in humans have been replicated. This does not mean that the linkages are statistical artifacts, but more likely that the linkage is present in only selected ethnic groups or populations. Such results are not surprising if one considers the large number of genes that are already implicated in the regulation of body weight.

## PROVING THE PHENOTYPIC ROLES OF MODIFIER GENES

Efforts to "solve" the complex genetics of human obesity confront several imposing problems. The effects of any single gene are likely to be small, of different salience in different populations and environments, and dependent on developmental processes and epistatic interactions with other genes. The linkage signals, using conventional nonparametric techniques such as sib pairs and transmission distortion testing (TDT), are likely to be below the usual statistical thresholds set for such analyses (e.g., $p \leq 10^{-3}$). The sequence differences are, by definition, likely to be subtle variants in coding and regulatory sequence, not the highly penetrant mutations seen in Mendelian traits such as *ob*, *db*, *Yellow*, and so forth. Thus, even when plausible candidate genes are implicated by either genetic position or molecular physiology, it may be difficult to prove their functional relevance. Such proof may require combinations of *in vitro* expression studies, phenotyping of congenic lines in which the implicated sequence variants are segregating, and the development of new statistical strategies that will permit the investigation of the interactive roles of multiple sequence variants in multiple genes on phenotypes of interest. These analyses, in turn, will require the pooling of large data sets to permit the required grouping stratifications (by race, age, sex, etc.).

Within the next several years, there will be human SNP (single-nucleotide polymorphism) genetic maps (linked to radiation hybrid and physical maps) with over 2 million entries. Thus, molecular markers will be spaced at 1,500 bp intervals across the genome. These SNPs can be selected to favor coding sequences and known regulatory regions, so that a linkage or disequilibrium study can simultaneously examine locus–gene position and identify candidate sequence variants. The scoring of such dense SNP maps will constitute a first pass, selected resequencing experiment on each subject, generating huge amounts of sequence data that must be related to phenotype information. As in all linkage-type strategies, the quality of phenotypic data remains paramount. Access to complete sequence information of genes related to a phenotype enables, in theory, the digital "representation" of a continuous biological phenotype. For the proper multivariate correlations to be made, the phenotype(s) must be explicitly and accurately defined. The digital representation cannot exceed the fidelity of the phenotypes being analyzed.

The genetic control of body composition is paradigmatic of problems confronting efforts to work out the molecular genetics of physiological and medical phenotypes (e.g., blood pressure, osteoporosis, type 2 diabetes, psychiatric disorders) in which convergent phenotypes are caused by complex interactions of genes, development, and the environment. Successes in one or more of these areas will almost certainly provide "lessons" useful in the analysis of the others.

## FURTHER READING

Barsh, G. S., Farooqi, I. S., & O'Rahilly, S. (2000.) Genetics of body-weight regulation. *Nature*, *404*, 644–651.—This article, and others in this *Insight: Obesity* issue of *Nature*, review the genetics, neurophysiology, molecular genetics, and pharmacology of obesity.

Chung, W. K., Belfi, K., Chua, M., Wiley, J., Mackintosh, R., Nicolson, M., Boozer, C. N., & Leibel, R. L. (1998). Heterozygosity for *Lep^ob* or *Lepr^db* affects body composition and leptin homeostasis in adult mice. *American Journal of Physiology, 274*, R985–R990.—Demonstration of the subtle phenotypic effects of haploinsufficiency for the *Lep* and *Lepr* genes relevant to possible similar mechanisms in humans.

Comuzzie, A. G., & Allison, D. B. (1998). The search for human obesity genes. *Science, 280*, 1374–1377.—Descriptions of human genome scans for obesity-related genes.

Johnson, P. R., Stern, J. S., Greenwood, M. R., Zucker, L. M., & Hirsch, J. (1973). Effect of early nutrition on adipose cellularity and pancreatic insulin release in the Zucker rat. *Journal of*

*Nutrition, 103,* 738–743.—Powerful effects of environment and development on a highly penetrant obesity mutation in the leptin receptor, *Lepr^fa*.

Kowalski, T. J., Liu, S.-M., Leibel, R. L., & Chua, S. C. (2001). Transgenic complement of leptin receptor deficiency: Rescue of the obesity/diabetes phenotype of *Lepr*-null mice expressing a *Lepr-B* transgene. *Diabetes, 50,* 425–435.—Example of use of transgenic mice to analyze molecular physiology of weight regulation.

Leibel, R. L., Chua, S. C., & Rosenbaum, M. (2001). Obesity: The molecular physiology of weight regulation. In C. R. Scriver, A. L. Beaudet, W. S. Sly, & D. Valle (Eds.), *The metabolic and molecular bases of inherited disease* (8th ed., pp. 3965–4028). New York: McGraw Hill.—A detailed description of the physiology and genetics of the control of body composition.

Leibel, R. L., Chung, W. K., & Chua, S. C. (1997). The molecular genetics of rodent single gene obesities. *Journal of Biological Chemistry, 272,* 31937–31940.—Details the behavioral and metabolic phenotypes of the mouse single-gene mutations causing obesity.

Risch, N., & Merikangas, K. (1996). The future of genetic studies of complex human disease. *Science, 273,* 1516–1517.—Statistical strategies for analyzing complex genetic traits in humans.

Risch, N. J. (2000). Searching for genetic determinants in the new millennium. *Nature, 405,* 847–856.—Statistical strategies for analyzing complex genetic traits in humans.

West, D. B., Waguespack, J., & McCollister, S. (1995). Dietary obesity in the mouse: Interaction of strain with diet composition. *American Journal of Physiology, 268,* R658–R665.—Molecular mapping of mouse-quantitative trait loci related to body composition responses to diet composition.

# 6

# Leptin and Body Weight Regulation

## L. ARTHUR CAMPFIELD

Leptin (also known as OB protein) is a protein hormone, encoded by the *ob* gene, produced primarily by adipocytes and secreted into the circulation, where it binds to a family of binding proteins.*Leptin enters the brain through a specific receptor-mediated transport system in brain microvessels and acts on specific brain areas involved in the control of food intake and the regulation of energy balance. It acts through a specific membrane receptor, OB-$R_L$, to alter ongoing brain processes, descending autonomic nervous system activity, and gene expression of neuropeptides involved in the regulation of energy balance. The primary role of leptin is to coordinate the responses of brain neuropeptide and neurotransmitter pathways to provide a situationally appropriate regulation of food intake, metabolic rate, energy balance, and fat storage (see Chapters 1 and 2).

### BIOLOGY OF LEPTIN IN HUMANS

Clinical studies of circulating leptin concentration have revealed the basic facts: Obese subjects have *higher* serum leptin concentrations than lean individuals, and concentrations *increase* with increasing percentage of body fat. Women have higher leptin concentrations than men, even when corrected for percentage of body fat. When obese subjects lose weight by caloric restriction, leptin concentrations decrease. Serum leptin concentrations in patients with eating disorders are appropriate for their percent body fat; that is, patients with anorexia nervosa have very low leptin levels, while overweight patients with bulimia nervosa have elevated leptin levels. Thus, the decreased food intake or failure to eat characteristic of anorexia nervosa is *not* a result of suppression of food intake by high leptin levels.

Fasting (18–24 hours) is followed by a decrease in leptin concentration by as much as 90% in humans. Thus, prolonged fasting leads to the coordinated inhibition of leptin production from groups of individual fat cells in many regions of the body. Refeeding after a fast is followed by a return of circulating leptin concentrations to baseline concentrations. The regulation of leptin production in the fasting state and the mechanisms responsible remain to be determined.

## SOURCES OF LEPTIN

Leptin is produced and secreted from the following tissues: white fat; brown fat; bone marrow; placenta; and probably from fat within muscles and other peripheral organs, including the stomach. With the exception of the placenta and the stomach, the general rule appears to be that as fat content increases in fat cells within a tissue, the production and secretion of leptin also increases. When fat cells are devoid of lipid, the expression of the *ob* gene is severely reduced. When lipid is accumulated within fat cells, the OB and OB-R messenger RNA (mRNA) levels and the presence of leptin and OB-$R_L$ increase.

## LEPTIN-SENSITIVE NEURAL CIRCUIT THAT CONTROLS ENERGY BALANCE

Studies of neuronal activity indicate that multiple brain regions contain neurons that are responsive to leptin and involved in detection of its presence and in generation of its effects. Hyperpolarization of glucose-receptive, adenosine triphosphate (ATP)-sensitive potassium channels and stimulation and inhibition of firing rates have been reported in ventromedial and lateral neurons. Brain administration of leptin leads to neuronal activation in many brain areas known to be involved in the regulation of food intake and body energy balance, including the hypothalamus, periform cortex, and brown fat in the periphery. In addition, direct recording of efferent sympathetic fibers innervating organs in anesthetized rats demonstrate that intravenous administration of leptin increases sympathetic nerve activity to multiple target organs. These converging lines of evidence strongly suggest that, in addition to several nuclei of the hypothalamus (ventromedial, dorsomedial, paraventricular, and arcuate), other brain areas are involved in a distributed neural network within the brain including the periform cortex, the brainstem, the cerebellum, the basal ganglia, and the cortex.

## PERIPHERAL ACTIONS OF LEPTIN

Initial reports of direct peripheral effects of leptin were greeted with some skepticism due to the experimental difficulty of demonstrating the presence of OB-$R_L$, the long form of OB-R. However, strong support has accumulated for the following peripheral effects of leptin: (1) increased insulin sensitivity and glucose uptake; (2) decreased cholesterol and triglyceride concentrations, and improved lipid profile; (3) decreased plasma glucose concentration; (4) inhibition of insulin secretion; (5) inhibition of adrenal cortex glucocorticoid secretion; and (6) inhibition of steroidogenesis in ovaries. OB-$R_L$ has been identified in the peripheral nervous system and in several peripheral tissues, including the pancreas, the adrenal gland, the kidney, white and brown fat, the liver, the ovary, perivertebral ganglion cells, cells within the enteric nervous system, and pancreatic ganglion cells.

## EVIDENCE SUPPORTING THE IMPORTANCE OF THE LEPTIN PATHWAY IN HUMANS

The operation of the leptin pathway in humans has now been established. First, rare mutations in the leptin and OB-R genes that have been documented in a few obese humans are similar to those in leptin-deficient and -unresponsive mice. These humans are severely obese and have incomplete sexual maturation. Second, experimental treatment of obese humans with recombinant human leptin has been reported. Daily injections of leptin for 24 weeks in obese subjects resulted in weight loss that was significantly greater than placebo treatment. Third, the chronic treatment with daily leptin injections of the first human identified with a mutation in her leptin gene was reported. After a life dominated by continuous weight gain and ravenous hunger, sustained weight loss and reduction of hunger were observed during the treatment. Fourth, many studies in lean and obese humans have demonstrated that weight gain is associated with an increase in serum concentrations of leptin, while weight loss is associated with a decrease in circulating leptin concentrations.

## TIMESCALE OF EFFECTS OF LEPTIN CONCENTRATIONS AND ACTIONS

The time course of a specific experiment may limit our ability to conclude that leptin does or does not have a particular effect. Human studies have shown that leptin concentrations are not changed before or after meals of normal size or individual bouts of intense exercise. However, increases in energy intake or energy expenditure maintained for 3–4 days have been shown to increase or decrease circulating leptin concentrations, respectively. Similarly, actions of leptin can be considered to occur over different time periods, ranging from the rapid reduction of food intake (< 1 hour) to the slow changes in body fat and composition (days to weeks).

## DECREASED BRAIN RESPONSIVENESS TO LEPTIN IN OBESITY

The observation that almost all obese individuals have elevated circulating levels of leptin has prompted speculation that human obesity can arise from reduced brain responsiveness to leptin. This hypothesis is supported by studies of diet-induced obese (DIO) mice and rats. In comparison to lean animals, DIO animals require higher peripheral and central doses of leptin to alter food intake, metabolism, and body fat. Recent studies indicate that brain responsiveness to leptin is reduced in these obese animals and can be reversed by weight loss.

The level of leptin in the cerebrospinal fluid (CSF) of obese humans is much lower than expected and is not proportional to the elevated serum leptin concentration. This observation has led to the suggestion that the brain uptake of leptin and/or its appearance in the CSF compartment is defective in obese humans and may be a component of the decreased sensitivity to leptin.

## SUMMARY

Leptin acts as *chef d'orchestre* to coordinate a variety of neuropeptide and neurotransmitter responses to generate an appropriate whole-body response with respect to body energy balance given the current physiological and environmental conditions in nonobese individuals. In this way, coordinated whole-body response to undernutrition, overnutrition, increased energy demand, and decreased energy demand is generated. Additional advances in our knowledge of the leptin pathway, and its marked alterations in obesity, will surely lead to new pharmacological treatments for obesity, to be used as adjuncts to healthy eating and physical activity (see Chapter 100).

## FURTHER READING

Campfield, L. A. (1999). Multiple facets of OB protein (leptin) physiology: Integration of central and peripheral mechanisms in the regulation of energy balance. In B. Guy-Grand & G. Ailhaud (Eds.), *Progress in obesity research* (Vol. 8, pp. 327–335). London: Libbey.—Review of the central and peripheral effects of leptin in the regulation of energy balance. Both brain and peripheral mechanisms of leptin action are discussed. Unresolved questions and future directions in leptin research are identified.

Campfield, L. A., & Smith, F. J. (1998). Overview: neurobiology of OB protein (leptin). *Proceedings of the Nutrition Society, 57*, 429–440.—Reviews of the underlying brain mechanisms of the biological effects of leptin and the alterations seen in obese animals. Recent presentation of the *chef d'orchestre* or "orchestra conductor" role for leptin, first suggested by the authors in 1995, has been supported by several observations in different species. One of a series of excellent papers from a comprehensive symposium, "Leptin: Energy Regulation and Beyond" is published in this issue, pages 409–485.

Campfield, L. A., Smith, F. J., & Burn, P. (1998). Strategies and potential molecular targets for obesity treatment. *Science, 280*, 1383–1387.—A review of the current approaches to the treatment of obesity, classes of antiobesity drugs, and potential molecular targets of new medicine for obesity. The strong rationale for drugs that could activate the leptin pathway in obese patients is reviewed and discussed. Part of a very informative special issue, "Regulation of Body Weight," published on May 29, 1998, this article is an excellent introduction to advanced topics relating to obesity.

Considine, R. V., Sinha, M. K., Heiman, M. L., Kriauciunas, A., Stephens, T. W., Nyce, M. R., Ohannesian, J. P., Marco, C. C., McKee, L. J., Baur, T. L., & Caro, J. F. (1996). Serum immunoreactive-leptin concentrations in normal-weight and obese humans. *New England Journal of Medicine, 334*, 292–295.—Classic paper describing the first results of the measurement of serum leptin concentrations in humans, including the observation that obese humans have higher leptin concentrations than lean individuals.

Corp, E. S., Conze, D. B., Smith, F., & Campfield, L. A. (1998). Regional localization of specific [125I] leptin binding sites in rat forebrain. *Brain Research, 789*, 40–47.—Original and comprehensive analysis of the binding of leptin to sites in the rat brain.

Farooqi, I. S., Jebb, S. A., Langmack, G., Lawrence, E., Cheetham, C. H., Prentice, A. M., Hughes,

I. A., McCamish, M. A., & O'Rahilly, S. (1999). Effects of recombinant leptin therapy in a child with congenital leptin deficiency. *New England Journal of Medicine, 341*, 879–884.— Seminal study that presents the effects of treatment with recombinant leptin of the first human identified with a mutated leptin gene, demonstrating the importance of a functional leptin pathway in humans.

Friedman, J. M. (2000). Obesity in the new millennium. *Nature, 404*, 632–634.—Review by the leader of the team that cloned the OB gene and discovered leptin offers his perspective on leptin and its role in regulation of body weight.

Schwartz, M. W., Seeley, R. J., Campfield, L. A., Burn, P., & Baskin, D. G. (1996). Identification of targets of leptin action in rat hypothalamus. *Journal of Clinical Investigation, 98*, 1101–1106.—Classic, early identification of sites in the rat hypothalamus that respond to administered leptin.

Van Heek, M., Compton, D. S., France, C. F., Tedesco, R. P., Fawzi, A. B., Graziano, M. P., Sybertz, E. J., Strader, C. D., & Davis, H. R., Jr. (1997). Diet-induced obese mice develop peripheral, but not central, resistance to leptin. *Journal of Clinical Investigation, 99*, 385–390.—This classic study of decreased leptin responsiveness in diet-induced obesity of prolonged duration is a clear demonstration that leptin responsiveness is very reduced in obese animals with functional leptin and OB-R genes.

Woods, S. C., Seeley, R. J., Porte, D., Jr., & Schwartz, M. W. (1998). Signals that regulate food intake and energy homeostasis. *Science, 280*, 1378–1383.—An original and thoughtful integration of the multiple factors, including leptin, that control food intake and the regulation of energy balance.

# 7

## Energy Intake and Body Weight

### SUSAN A. JEBB

Energy intake is an especially critical element in the regulation of body weight because the flexibility in energy intake is very much greater than that in energy expenditure. Figure 7.1 illustrates that it is relatively easy to double energy intake on a single day but extremely difficult to make a similar increase in energy expenditure. It is possible for an individual to starve or consume little energy on some days, yet the energy expenditure of a sedentary individual cannot be reduced by more than about 30%. Day-to-day variability in energy expenditure is estimated to be about 8%, compared to 25% for energy intake. Changes in energy intake thus have considerable potential to influence body weight.

### CONTROL OF ENERGY INTAKE

The relative maintenance of body weight over prolonged periods of time has been cited as evidence that energy intake is regulated to match energy needs (see Chapter 8). Advances in basic science have revealed some components of this metabolic control system. The picture is complex, involving a network of gastrointestinal, metabolic, and hormonal signals that are integrated in the brain and trigger a coordinated cascade of neuropeptides that either stimulate or inhibit consumption (see Chapters 1, 2, and 6). These signals work across various time frames to bring an eating episode to a conclusion, to trigger the next meal, or to influence overall energy intake in the longer term over days, weeks, or even months.

Although most research on the control of energy intake has been conducted in small animals, there is good evidence that many of the pathways act in a similar manner in humans. However, the complexity of the system in humans is enhanced by a variety of additional cognitive factors that can in many circumstances override the innate physiological control of food intake. The nature of these cognitive factors is a product of various environmental factors, social and emotional influences, and learned experiences. Humans have the capacity to eat when they are not actually hungry or in need of food, perhaps

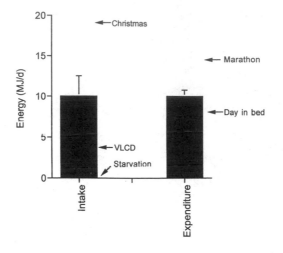

**FIGURE 7.1.** Flexibility of daily energy intake and expenditure. Error bars indicate within-subject coefficient of variation.

prompted by a social occasion, or to reject some foods even at a time of hunger, if they consider them to be unpalatable or are attempting to restrain their intake.

## CROSS-SECTIONAL STUDIES OF ENERGY INTAKE

Studies in the latter half of the 20th century frequently showed that heavier people tended to consume the same, or even less energy, than their lighter counterparts. This precipitated detailed studies of the energy needs of these apparently thrifty individuals. However, measurements of energy expenditure in both controlled experimental (using whole-body calorimeters) and free-living conditions (using doubly labeled water) showed conclusively that energy needs are proportionally greater in obese people, reflecting their greater body size and tissue mass. Figure 7.2 shows the measured energy expenditure and self-reported energy intake over a 2-week period in two groups of lean and obese subjects. This and similar studies have provided clear evidence of the trend toward underreporting of food intake, which is most marked in obese and weight-conscious people, such as formerly obese people who have successfully lost weight. Snacks are more likely to be omitted from food records than main meals, and protein intake may be more accurately recorded that other macronutrients, leading to relative overreporting. Although much less researched, it is also apparent that individuals with anorexia nervosa may misreport their intake. Here, there is more individual variability, with reports of both over- and underestimation of food intake.

The accuracy of food intake records appears to be a characteristic of the individual under consideration rather than the method of data collection (see Chapter 23). The most accurate methods to record energy intake, such as the 7-day weighed food record, are invasive and may change habitual intake during the recording period. Simpler methods, such as the 24-hour recall, may aid compliance but provide no guarantee that subjects

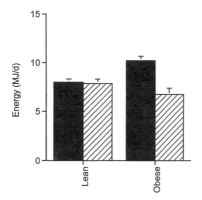

**FIGURE 7.2.** Measured energy expenditure (solid bars) and self-reported energy intake (hatched bars) in lean and obese women. Mean ± *SE*.

provide a representative record of their food intake. Studies have shown that the ranking of individuals by energy intake is broadly similar across different measurement techniques, although the absolute values may differ.

These difficulties in obtaining reliable records of food intake and the nonrandom nature of measurement error can lead to substantial errors in quantitative calculation of energy and nutrient intake. This is an important consideration in any studies of the relationship between energy intake and body weight.

## SECULAR TRENDS IN ENERGY INTAKE

Mean body weight is rising in populations throughout the world, leading to increased prevalence of obesity. However, most studies of energy intake do not show a clear relationship between energy intake and weight gain. Indeed, studies in the United Kingdom, where there is a good longitudinal record of changes in body weight and household food intake, show that, over the last 30 years, energy intake has been in decline. Although the absolute magnitude of the decrease may be exaggerated by an increase in underreporting and the failure to account adequately for the increasing proportion of food eaten outside the home, there is no evidence that the rise in obesity can be simply attributed to an increase in energy intake. A consideration of the secular trends in energy expenditure suggests that, at a population level, the decline in physical activity may have reduced energy needs at an even greater pace than the decline in energy intake. The rise in body weight can therefore be explained by a failure to down-regulate energy intake sufficiently to match the low energy needs (see Chapter 83).

## MACRONUTRIENT INTAKE

Over the last 50 years, many countries have seen a steady rise in the proportion of fat in the diet at the expense of carbohydrate. Recent dietary surveys show that this trend may now be in reverse, but food disappearance records suggest that fat intake may be continuing to increase and the apparent decline may be due to specific underreporting of fat intake as a consequence of intensive health promotion campaigns to eat less fat.

There is now good evidence that the macronutrient composition of the diet has important implications for body weight regulation. Ecological studies show a positive association between the proportion of fat in the diet and the prevalence of obesity; this is confirmed by many cross-sectional analyses within populations. There are a number of potential mechanisms to explain this effect. In metabolic terms, fat is more readily absorbed and assimilated into body fat stores and less rapidly oxidized than other macronutrients. However, quantitatively, more important effects are observed in relation to appetite and the control of subsequent food intake.

Subjects fed a high-fat meal under experimental conditions exhibit lower levels of satiety and consume more energy at a subsequent meal than following an isoenergetic low-fat–high-carbohydrate meal. When allowed to eat *ad libitum* over the course of one or more days, subjects almost invariably consume more energy as the proportion of fat in the diet increases. Fat, containing 9 kcal/g, relative to only 4 kcal/g for protein and carbohydrate, is the most energy-dense nutrient, and high-fat diets therefore usually have a high energy density. Thus, subjects may eat a similar portion of high- or low-fat food but consume more total energy as a consequence of the higher energy density of the high-fat food. This phenomenon has been described as "passive overconsumption." Figure 7.3 shows the change in body fat stores relative to a nominal zero at the start of the study in a group of male volunteers studied on three occasions in which the fat content of their food was manipulated to provide 20%, 40%, or 60% energy as fat, with reciprocal changes in carbohydrate. Subjects were allowed to eat *ad libitum* throughout. On the 20% fat diet, they experienced a modest decrease in body fat, whereas on the 60% fat diet, they gained around 0.5 kg body fat in 1 week. Modest weight loss on a low-fat diet is also observed

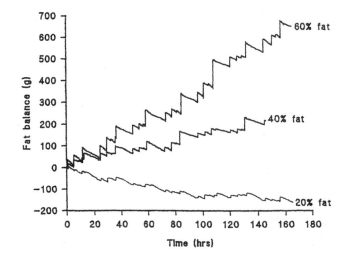

**FIGURE 7.3.** Changes in fat balance during *ad libitum* consumption of diets with 20%, 40%, or 60% energy as fat.

in a number of dietary intervention studies. However, this is rarely sustained in the medium- to long-term without additional dietary control strategies. Whether the attenuation of weight loss is due to compensatory increases in appetite or reduced compliance to the low fat diet is unclear.

The precise mechanism underpinning the effect of macronutrients on energy intake is unclear, but it is believed to include both pre- and postabsorptive effects (see Chapters 1 and 2). Further research is under way to establish whether passive overconsumption is specific to fat per se or simply a consequence of its energy density. This has clear public health implications given the introduction of low-fat foods onto the market that have a similar energy density to their high-fat counterparts.

## EATING FREQUENCY

Recent changes in eating habits have led to a decline in traditional meal eating and an increase in snacking, with multiple eating episodes spread throughout each day. Epidemiological analyses of the relationship between eating frequency and body weight often show that snacking is associated with leanness. However, the accurate interpretation of these data sets is confounded by the extent of underreporting of total energy intake and the difficulties in establishing a causal relationship. Obese people may appear to have fewer eating episodes either because of a failure to accurately report all eating occasions or because snacking has been eliminated as a weight-control measure.

Experimental studies within whole-body calorimeters have shown that under highly controlled isoenergetic conditions, energy expenditure is not significantly affected by meal frequency, suggesting that it does not have a direct effect on body weight regulation. However in the free-living situation, when subjects are allowed to eat *ad libitum*, the impact of snacking on body weight may depend on its effect on subsequent appetite. This in turn may be a function of the type of snacks consumed. However a crossover study in which subjects consumed high or low fat, and savoury or sweet snacks in a $2 \times 2$ Latin square design, showed no significant difference in body weight throughout the study. Although the total fat intake varied, individuals appeared to compensate at mealtimes for differences in energy intake from snacks.

## CONCLUSIONS

Studies of the relationship between energy intake and body weight are confounded by methodological difficulties, especially in relation to the underreporting of food intake. It is clear from the energy balance equation that for any given level of energy expenditure, there is close link between energy intake and body weight. However, in the real-life situation, changes in body weight are a consequence of the precision of coupling energy intake and energy needs rather than a function of either component independently. Understanding the susceptibility of some individuals to weight gain or, less commonly, to weight loss, will require a more detailed understanding of the impact of energy expenditure on the physiological regulation of energy intake in humans, and the social and cognitive factors that modulate this innate control.

## FURTHER READING

Bellisle, F., McDevitt, R., & Prentice, A. M. (1997). Meal frequency and energy balance. *British Journal of Nutrition, 77,* S57–S70.—A review of the literature pertaining to feeding frequency and obesity.

Black, A. E., Prentice, A. M., Goldberg, G. R., Jebb, S. A., Bingham, S. A., Livingstone, M. B., & Coward, W. A. (1993). Measurements of total energy expenditure provide insights into the validity of dietary measurements of energy intake. *Journal of the American Dietetic Association, 93,* 572–579.—A review of evidence in relation to underreporting energy intake.

Blundell, J. E., & Stubbs, R. J. (1998). Diet composition and the control of food intake in humans. In G. A. Bray, C. Bouchard, & W. P. T. James (Eds.), *Handbook of obesity* (pp. 243–272). New York: Marcel Dekker.—An overview of the impact of dietary macronutrients on the control of food intake.

Bray, G. A., & Popkin, B. A. (1998). Dietary fat intake does affect obesity. *American Journal of Clinical Nutrition, 68,* 1157–1173.—A consideration of the impact of dietary fat on body weight, including an analysis of low-fat intervention studies.

Lissner, L., & Heitmann, B. L. (1995). Dietary fat and obesity: Evidence from epidemiology. *European Journal of Clinical Nutrition, 49,* 79–90.—Review of the epidemiological evidence linked the intake of fat specifically to obesity.

Prentice, A. M., Black, A. E., Murgatroyd, P. R., Goldberg, G. R., & Coward, W.A. (1989). Metabolism or appetite: Questions of energy balance with particular reference to obesity. *Journal of Human Nutrition and Dietetics, 2,* 95–104.—A review of studies demonstrating high levels of energy expenditure in obese women and highlighting problems of underreporting energy intake.

Schwartz, M. W., Baskin, D. G., Kaiyala, K. J., & Woods. S. C. (1999). Model for the regulation of energy balance and adiposity by the central nervous system. *American Journal of Clinical Nutrition, 69,* 584–596.—A review describing a model of energy homeostasis in which various signals controlling energy intake are integrated to control energy balance. Although it should be noted that this is a rapidly developing area and important new mechanisms are being identified, this paper provides a useful conceptual framework.

# 8

# A Psychobiological System Approach to Appetite and Weight Control

## JOHN E. BLUNDELL

Appetite control implies a control over energy intake. Some researchers argue that habitual addition of only 20–30 kcal per day over a number of years will lead to significant body weight increases. If human beings are the most intelligent life force on this planet, why can they not adjust their eating by the very small amounts required for weight stability? Some explanation for this may be found in an examination of the processes involved in the regulation of appetite.

## A PSYCHOBIOLOGICAL SYSTEM

The power of a systems approach is that it allows the simultaneous evaluation of a number of factors that influence the expression of appetite and the control of body weight. It permits an assessment of the *relative* strength of each factor rather than concentrating only on one domain. Research is certainly needed on specific mechanisms that control particular aspects of our physiology, biochemistry, nutrition, and behavior related to eating and weight control. Also required is a conceptualization of how these mechanisms act cohesively to influence the physiology, conscious sensations, and actions of people functioning as individuals. This can be provided by the psychobiological system.

The essence of this view is the intention to understand the control of appetite and body weight (and disorders of these phenomena) as the products of a network of interactions among elements forming part of a psychobiological system. A simplified model of the system is set out in Figure 8.1.

A consideration of anthropological, epidemiological, and experimental evidence suggests that it is easier for human beings to gain weight than to reduce weight. This implies that the control of appetite (by the psychobiological system) is asymmetrical. Figure 8.2 illustrates a simple conceptualization of how this arises. The extension of Claude Ber-

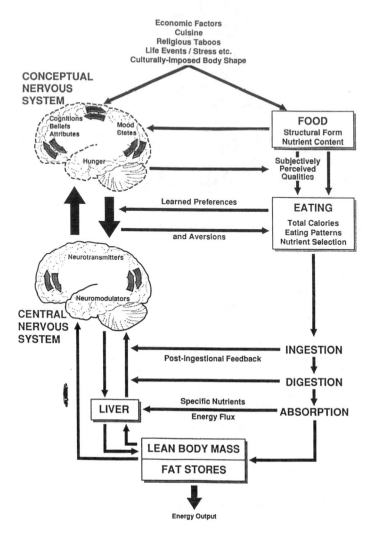

**FIGURE 8.1.** Conceptualization of certain significant aspects of the biopsychological system underlying the control of feeding behavior.

nard's principle of homeostasis to include behavior is often referred to as the behavioral regulation of internal states. Logic demands that behavior (eating) is controlled in accordance with biological states of need. This constitutes a form of biological regulation. However, the expression of behavior is also subject to environmental demands, and behavior is adapted in the face of particular circumstances. In the case of human appetite, consideration should be given to the conscious and deliberate control over eating behavior. Humans can decide to alter their eating to meet particular objectives, for example, a display of moral conviction (political hunger strike) or a demonstration of aesthetic achievement (e.g., dieting). In both of these examples, eating is curtailed, with an ensuing interruption or depletion of the nutrition supply. Regulatory mechanisms will tend to oppose this undersupply and generate a drive to eat. In many parts of the world, environmental adaptation also means adjusting to a food supply characterized by an abundance

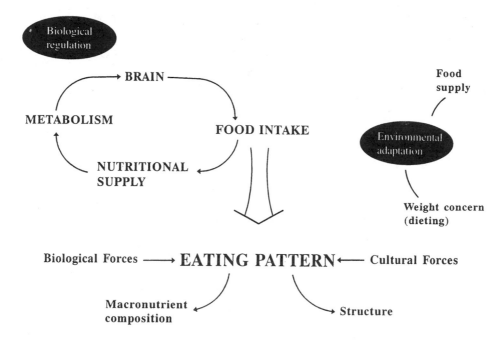

**FIGURE 8.2.** Schematic diagram to illustrate that the pattern of eating behavior arises from an interaction between biological regulation and environmental adaptation. Eating is a product of both biology and culture.

of palatable, energy-dense (mainly high-fat) foods or by a large proportion of fatty items (see Chapters 74 and 78). Exposure to these types of diets usually gives rise to an overconsumption of energy. Since this does not appear to be biologically driven (by a need state), and is not consciously intended, this phenomenon has been referred to as passive overconsumption. This, in turn, in an interaction with genetic vulnerability, leads to an increase in fat deposition.

This passive overconsumption leading to the accumulation of body fat does not appear to generate any biological drive to undereat. Obese people do not appear to get any help from their adipose tissue to reduce their appetites. Hence, the operation of the regulatory system is not symmetrical.

## LOOSE COUPLING BETWEEN APPETITE AND PHYSICAL ACTIVITY

Understanding the interaction between physical activity and appetite control has both theoretical and practical implications. More than 40 years ago, the commonsense view implied that the regulation of food intake functions with such flexibility that increased energy output due to exercise is automatically followed by an equivalent increase in caloric intake. This view supports the commonly held belief that exercise is futile as a form of weight control, since the energy expended simply increases hunger and drives up food intake to compensate for the energy lost. However, there is now much evidence to demonstrate that physical activity does not automatically increase eating. Indeed, after exercise, food intake most often remains unchanged and, in certain circumstances, declines. Moreover, when physical activity is reduced (when an individual becomes more sedentary), food intake is not down-regulated; this leads to a positive energy balance and weight gain. All of these findings suggest a rather loose coupling between physical activity and appetite control (at least in the short term). However, the degree of this coupling may be different in men and women.

## RISK FACTORS FOR APPETITE CONTROL

Just as certain metabolic variables (such as low basal metabolic rate, low energy cost of physical activity, low capacity for fat oxidation) can lead to a positive energy balance, we can envisage behaviorally mediated processes leading to hyperphagia or overconsumption. These processes may be patterns of behavior, the sensory or hedonic events that guide behavior, or sensations that accompany or follow eating. For convenience, this cluster of events can be referred to as behavioral risk factors. These events may include a preference for fatty foods, weakened satiation (end of meal signals), relatively weak satiety (postingestive inhibition over further eating), strong orosensory preferences (e.g., for sweetness combined with fattiness in foods), a binge potential, high food-induced pleasure response, or a persistent high level of hunger (see Chapter 7). These behavioral risk factors can be regarded as biological dispositions that create vulnerability for weight gain.

However, such risk factors alone would be unlikely to lead to a positive energy balance in a benign environment, that is, one in which the food supply and the cultural habits work against excessive consumption. In most of today's societies, however, the food environment exploits biologically based dispositions and this promotes the achievement of a high-energy intake. This conceptualization is set out in Table 8.1.

**TABLE 8.1. Postulated Interactions between Behavioral Risk Factors and the Obesigenic Environment, Which Generate a Tendency for Overconsumption**

| Biological vulnerability (behavioral risk factor) | Environmental influence | Potential for overconsumption |
|---|---|---|
| Preference for fatty foods | Abundance of high-fat (high energy-dense) foods | ↑ fat intake |
| Weak satiation (end of meal signals) | Large portion sizes | ↑ meal size |
| Orosensory responsiveness | Availability of high palatability foods with specific sensory–nutrient combinations | ↑ amount eaten<br>↑ frequency |
| Weak postingestive satiety | Easy accessibility to foods and presence of potent priming stimuli | ↑ frequency of eating<br>↑ tendency to reinitiate eating |
| Persistent high level of hunger | Ready availability of foods | ↑ persistent drive to seek and eat food |

## NUTRITION AND THE APPETITE CASCADE: SATIETY SIGNALING

How does the appetite control system operate to reflect these processes? One way to think about this issue is to consider how eating behavior is held in place by the interaction between the characteristics of food and the biological responses to ingestion. These biological responses are often thought of as "satiety signals." Several characteristics of ingested food must be monitored, including taste (intensity and hedonic aspects), volume and weight, energy density, osmolarity, and the proportion of macronutrients. Generated biological responses include oral afferent stimulation, stomach distension, rate of gastric emptying, release of hormones such as cholecystokinin and insulin, triggering of digestive enzymes (and cofactors), and plasma profiles of glucose, amino acids, and other metabolites. The organization of this activity can be conceptualized in the form of a cascade (Figure 8.3, lower portion). Two features are worth considering. First is the distinction between satiation and satiety. Satiation refers to the processes that bring a period of eating to an end and thus influence the size of meals and snacks. Satiety refers to the inhibition over hunger and further eating that arises as a consequence of food ingestion. These two processes therefore control events within and between meals. Second is the potency of the mediating processes of the cascade and particularly the relative strength of postabsorptive mechanisms. It is clearly the properties of food (and the act of ingesting it) that trigger the initiation of the overlapping physiological responses. The amount (quantity) and nature (quality) of the food will determine the intensity and time course of the biological processes generated. This situation reflects the idea of the different satiating power of different types of food.

## INTERRELATED LEVELS IN THE SYSTEM

The biological responses generated by food ingestion form part of a feedback circuit that influences the pattern of eating being displayed. This circuit can be seen as a network with three levels, which are displayed simply in Figure 8.3. The network includes the level of psychological events (hunger, perception, cravings, hedonic sensations) and behavioral operations (meals, snacks, energy, and macronutrient intakes); the level of peripheral physiology and metabolic events; and the level of neurotransmitter and metabolic interactions in the brain. The expression of appetite reflects the synchronous operation of events and processes in the three levels. Neural events trigger and guide behavior, but each act of behavior involves a response in the peripheral physiological system; in turn, these physiological events are translated into brain neurochemical activity. This brain activity represents the strength of motivation and the willingness to refrain from feeding.

## IMPLICATIONS OF THE SYSTEM APPROACH

Viewed in this way, the psychobiological system permits an understanding of the interrelationships among behavioral events that comprise eating, peripheral physiology and metabolism, and central neurochemical processes. The system also provides a possibility for

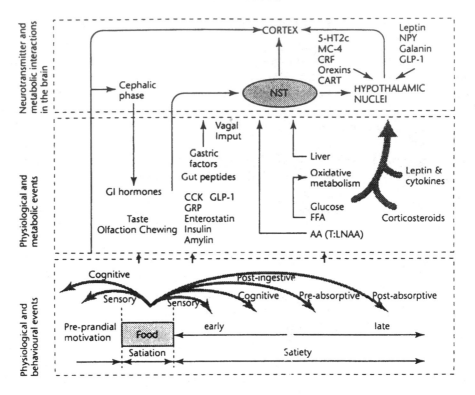

**FIGURE 8.3.** Diagram showing the expression of appetite as the relationship between three levels of operations: behavior, peripheral physiology and metabolites, and brain activity. PVN, paraventricular nucleus; NST, nucleus of the tractus solitarius; CCK, cholecystokinin; AA, amino acids; FFA, free fatty acids; T:LNAA, tryptophan: large neutral amino acids.

thinking about the way in which conscious motivations and cravings may emerge from the timing and organization of actions within the system.

## SYNCHRONY AND DESYNCHRONY

Recognizing the holistic nature of the psychobiological system also has clinical implications. In a healthy, well-functioning appetite system, it can be assumed that the three levels operate harmoniously and are well integrated. However, it has been argued that dieting is a form of behavioral control that desynchronizes the appetite system (see Chapters 15, 16, and 17). During the development of eating disorders, the bingeing, vomiting, and other drastic procedures lead to an erratic delivery of nutrients, with aberrant triggering of physiological responses. This means that the processes of the satiety cascade will be severely disorganized. This disorganization will lead to desynchrony between behavior and physiology, and between physiological processes and neurotransmitter activity. Therefore, the harmonious interplay of levels of functioning (Figure 8.3) responsible for the orderly expression of appetite will be undermined. This corruption of the processes of the biopsychological system is likely to confer an enduring legacy that will have to be corrected during treatment.

## FURTHER READING

Blundell, J. E. (1991). Pharmacological approaches to appetite suppression. *Trends in Pharmacological Sciences, 12*, 147–157.—Detailed account of the integration of biological mechanisms influencing food intake.

Blundell, J. E., & Cooling, J. (2000). Routes to obesity: Phenotypes, food choices and activity. *British Journal of Nutrition, 83*(Suppl. 1), S33–S38.—Description of differing patterns of habitual diet selection, appetite control, and risk factors.

Blundell, J. E., & King, N. A. (1998). Effects of exercise on appetite control: loose coupling between energy intake and energy expenditure. *International Journal of Obesity, 22*, S22–S29.—Evaluation of the impact of physical activity on food intake replaces myth with scientific evidence.

Blundell J. E., & Stubbs, R. J. (1998). Diet composition and the control of food intake in humans. In G. A. Bray, C. Bouchard, & W. P. T. James (Eds.), *Handbook of obesity* (pp. 243–272). New York: Marcel Dekker.—Detailed evaluation of the evidence on nutrient composition of the diet, energy density, and the control over food ingestion.

De Castro, J. M., & Elmore, D. K. (1988). Subjective hunger relationships with meal patterns in the spontaneous feeding behaviour of humans: Evidence for a causal connection. *Physiology and Behaviour, 43*, 159–165.—Careful analysis of the close relationship between the subjective motivation to eat and actual eating behavior under natural conditions.

Eaton, S. B., & Konner, M. (1985). Paleolithic nutrition—a consideration of its nature and current implications. *New England Journal of Medicine, 312*, 283–289.—Fascinating account of the evolutionary and anthropological background to current eating habits.

Prentice, A. M., Black, A. E., Murgatroyd, P. R., Goldberg, G. R., & Coward, W. A. (1989). Metabolism or appetite?: Questions of energy balance with particular reference to obesity. *Journal of Human Nutrition and Dietetics, 2*, 95–104.—Coherent description of the evidence considering appetite control in the light of energy balance.

Ravussin, E., & Swinburn, B. A. (1992). Pathophysiology of obesity. *Lancet, 340*, 404–408.—Closely argued account of the role of macronutrient (particularly fat) balance in the control of body weight.

# 9

# Taste, Taste Preferences, and Body Weight

## ADAM DREWNOWSKI

Perhaps the most critical issue in obesity research is whether the current obesity epidemic is caused by genetics or by diet (see Chapters 3 and 78). Given that obesity rates in the United States have doubled over the past two decades, while the genetic pool remained stable, the explanation must lie in reduced physical activity and altered eating habits. Though the mainstream of obesity research continues to focus on genetic, metabolic, and physiological issues, dietary choices and behaviors are more likely to be the answer. The recent *Dietary Guidelines for Americans 2000* suggests that the increase in obesity rates may be tied to the wide availability of cheap and palatable foods.

## TASTE AND PALATABILITY

Taste is the key influence on food selection. Infants seek out sweet and reject bitter and sour tastes. In 3-day-old infants, facial expressions in response to sweet involve relaxation, a slight smile, and licking of the upper lip. Young infants prefer sugar solutions to water, select sweeter sugars over less sweet ones, and selectively consume the most concentrated sugar solutions available. Infant response to sweet sucrose leads to a more rapid heartbeat, avid sucking response, and less regular breathing. In contrast, infants presented with bitter quinine or urea stick out their tongue, spit or prepare to vomit, and give every sign of rejection and disgust. Judging from facial expressions and sucking response data, infant preferences for sweet and the rejection of bitter tastes are present at birth.

The pleasure response to sweetness is also wired in. Placing a sweet substance on the tongue of a crying newborn has a remarkable calming effect. This persists for several minutes and can be used to quiet the infant between blood draws and other painful procedures. Studies have linked the sweetness response to the release of endogenous opiate peptides, or endorphins. In some animal studies, a comparable calming effect was obtained with fat emulsions in water, suggesting that taste preferences for sugar and fat may have a strong physiological basis. One role of sweet taste, the characteristic feature of mother's milk, is to maintain infant feeding behavior. In contrast, the instinctive rejection of bitter protects the infant from bitter poisons.

Children ages 3 to 5 years use only two criteria, familiarity and sweetness, in making food choices. Novel flavors find acceptance only if they are paired with a concentrated source of energy, generally fat, sugar, or starch. In general, foods that offer maximum energy per unit weight are preferred over less energy-dense foods. In practice, such energy-dense foods contain fat or sugar, or both. The more palatable foods tend to be energy-dense and vice versa. Sweetness and fat serve to introduce new foods and additional nutrients into the child's diet. However, contrary to popular belief, varying exposure to sweet stimuli in infancy and early childhood has no documented impact on preferences for sweet foods in later life. Liking for sweet taste and sugars consumption both peak by age 12 years.

In addition to the four basic tastes—sweet, sour, salty, and bitter—the concept of food "taste" includes olfaction and texture. Fat in foods is perceived through a combination of texture, mouth feel, and aroma. Higher-fat diets tend to be more varied, richer-tasting, and more palatable. The human sensory system is geared toward the selection of the most nutritive energy- dense foods. Until recently, such foods were scarce in the human diet. The traditional diet of preindustrial societies was based on complex carbohydrates, including whole grains, vegetables, and fruit. The widespread availability of cheap sugar and vegetable oils is a relatively recent phenomenon. Sensory mechanisms responsible for maintaining the supply of energy-rich foods may be ill suited to cope with the conditions of dietary excess.

## SWEET TASTE AND BODY WEIGHT

One of the more cherished concepts in the obesity literature is that body weight is regulated and that obesity represents a deviation from the norm. Genetic vulnerability, personality disorders, abnormalities in taste and smell, and aberrant food choices have all been put forward as potential explanations for excessive weight gain. Another influential concept was that taste response to sweetness predicts distance from the physiological "set point" of body weight.

The prevailing view in the 1970s was that obesity is largely a psychological problem. Overeating was said to be a maladaptive behavior that could be shaped or modified through behavioral therapy. Eliminating the reinforcing properties of palatable foods would shape the behavioral response toward other, equally rewarding, activities. Obese patients were told to become more aware of their eating habits by keeping food diaries, and were taught to become less susceptible to events that triggered eating behavior (see Chapter 94). At the time, food palatability was equated with sweet taste. Exerting behavioral control over sweet foods was the first step toward successful weight reduction.

The belief that obese persons are more susceptible to external cues, such as the taste of foods, was especially popular. The externality hypothesis held that obese humans (and rats) were "finicky" eaters, eating more of palatable but less of unpalatable foods. The research emphasis on the obese "sweet tooth" was consistent with the concurrent belief that sugars and starches are the most fattening of foods. Studies reported that obese men and women found sweet solutions difficult to resist, even after ingesting a sweet glucose solution, suggesting that they were in a state of a continuing energy need and below their physiological set point. Their taste response to sweet was said to override satiety signals, leading to overeating of sweets and other desserts.

Eventually, it became clear that taste responses of obese persons were not alike. Some obese patients liked the sweet taste of sugar, whereas others did not. Studies using sucrose solutions, sweetened Kool-Aid, and chocolate milkshakes found no relationship between sweet taste preferences and overweight. Large-scale consumer studies found no link between body weight and liking for sugar in apricot nectar, canned peaches, lemonade, or vanilla ice cream, nor was there evidence that weight loss resulted in heightened preferences for sweet taste, as predicted by the set point hypothesis.

## DIETARY FAT AND BODY WEIGHT

Noting that most studies on obesity and taste had been conducted with sugar solutions in water, researchers in the 1980s began to explore the role of dietary fat. Among the complex sensory stimuli used in sensory evaluation studies were milkshakes, soft white cheese, cake frostings, and ice cream. In a series of studies using 9-point category scales, obese and anorectic women tasted and rated 20 different mixtures of milk, cream, and sugar of varying sweetness and fat content. There was an inverse relationship between body mass and relative preferences for sugar over fat. Whereas the thinnest women liked sugar and rejected dairy fat, obese and formerly obese women preferred high-fat stimuli with a low sugar content. Later sensory studies confirmed that sensory preferences for fat in foods were linked to the respondents' own body mass index or percent body fat. Clinical studies also found that diets of obese patients tend to be richer in fat.

Sensory responses to sugar and fat among adults may also be mediated by the endogenous opiate system. One clinical study examined the effects of opiate antagonist naloxone on taste preferences and food consumption among binge eating, obese, and normal-weight women. The patients tasted and rated 20 sweetened dairy products and were offered snack foods varying in sugar and fat content. Naloxone selectively reduced the consumption of foods that were sweet, high-fat foods such as chocolate. These effects were observed only among binge eaters and were not related to body weight. While opiate blockade is not a viable strategy for weight loss, it may be useful in the clinical management of the binge eating disorder.

## ENERGY DENSITY OF FOODS

Studies on obesity and food preferences showed that the most highly preferred foods were rich in fat. Obese men selected steaks and roasts, hamburgers, french fries, pizza, and ice cream. In contrast, obese women tended to list foods that were sweet, rich in fat, or both. Among their frequent choices were ice cream, chocolate, cake, and other desserts. These foods may be liked because of either their fat content or their high-energy density. According to some current theories, energy density of the diet, as opposed to its sugar or fat content, is the main reason for overeating and the growing prevalence of overweight.

This argument is based on the premise that under *ad libitum* conditions, people tend to consume a fixed volume of food as opposed to a given amount of energy. Foods with lower-energy density, that is, fewer calories per unit weight or volume, would then deliver less energy per eating occasion than would energy-rich foods. Much research has focused on the role of energy density in promoting satiety and satiation. Current theories suggest that energy-dilute foods are more satiating than energy-dense foods. Cake, hamburgers, and fries provide from 3 to 5 kcal/g. Chocolate and peanut butter provide 5 to 6 kcal/g. In contrast, raw vegetables and fruit provide only 0.1 to 0.5 kcal/g. In the current view, it is the energy density of fat that suppresses satiety signals, leading to passive overeating of fat-rich foods.

A similar argument was used years ago to explain why sweet taste overrode satiety signals, leading to active overeating of sweet desserts. The fact is that energy density and palatability are linked. While studies have sometimes contrived to separate energy density and palatability under laboratory conditions, these factors are intertwined in real life. In general, energy-dense foods such as chocolate are more palatable and less satiating than energy dilute and more satiating foods such as spinach. While there is little evidence for specific macronutrient appetites, it is clear that humans prefer energy-dense over energy-dilute foods.

## FOOD CHOICES AND BODY WEIGHT

Several lines of evidence suggest that sensory preferences for energy-dense foods are innate and present at birth. For the most part, such foods contain dietary sugars and fats. From the evolutionary standpoint, sensory and physiological mechanisms controlling food intake were meant to protect the organism against energy depletion and so respond primarily to energy needs. A plentiful food supply, with a ready accessibility of cheap and palatable foods, is a recent phenomenon. The question is whether the existing mechanisms of taste, appetite, or satiety can also guard against the conditions of dietary excess. While researchers continue to believe that obesity is an abnormal phenomenon, due to a genetic or metabolic malfunction, the rapidly rising rates of obesity and diabetes make it a public health problem. Far from being an abnormality or a disease, obesity may represent an adaptive response to the current environmental conditions.

## FURTHER READING

Birch, L. L. (1999). Development of food preferences. *Annual Review of Nutrition, 19,* 41–62.—An authoritative account of food preferences in early childhood.

Blundell, J. E., & Macdiarmid, J. I. (1997). Fat as a risk factor for overconsumption: satiation, satiety and patterns of eating. *Journal of the American Dietetic Association, 97*(Suppl. 7), S63–S69.—Laboratory and clinical studies on the role of fat in weight gain.

Bray, G., & Popkin, B. M. (1998). Dietary fat intake does affect obesity! *American Journal of Clinical Nutrition, 68,* 1157–1173.—A persuasive response to an earlier article by Willett that had questioned the link between fat consumption and weight gain.

Cabanac, M., & Duclaux, R. (1970). Obesity: Absence of satiety aversion to sucrose. *Science, 168,* 496–497.—A classic paper revealing that obese persons show a heightened response to sweet taste regardless of energy needs

Drewnowski, A. (1986). Obesity and sweet taste. In J. Dobbing (Ed.), *Sweetness, ILSI Nutrition Foundation Symposium*. Berlin: Springer-Verlag.—A review of laboratory and clinical studies on sweet taste and weight gain.

Drewnowski, A. (1997). Taste preferences and food intake. *Annual Review of Nutrition, 17*, 237–250.—A review of the many mechanisms mediating the link between taste factors and actual food consumption.

Drewnowski, A., Brunzell, J. D., Sande, K., Iverius, P. H., & Greenwood, M. R. C. (1985). Sweet tooth reconsidered: Taste responsiveness in human obesity. *Physiology and Behavior, 35*, 617–622.—The first paper showing that obese women select fat as opposed to sugar.

Drewnowski, A., Krahn, D. D., Demitrack, M. A., Nairn, K., & Gosnell, B. A. (1985). Naloxone, an opiate blocker, reduces the consumption of sweet high-fat foods in obese and lean female binge eaters. *American Journal of Clinical Nutrition, 61*, 206–1212.—The only clinical study showing that sugar and fat preferences may involve the endogenous opiate peptide system. The majority of such studies have been done with rats.

Drewnowski, A., & Popkin, B. M. (1997). The nutrition transition: New trends in the global diet. *Nutrition Reviews, 55*, 31–43.—Analyses of global dietary trends showing that fat consumption is no longer dependent on income.

Groop, L. C., & Tuomi, T. (1997). Non-insulin dependent diabetes mellitus—a collision between thrifty genes and an affluent society. *Annals of Medicine, 29*, 37–53.—Evidence that physiological mechanisms may not be suited to deal with dietary excess.

Holt, S. H. A., Brand-Miller, J. C., Petocz, P., & Farmakalidis, E. (1995). A satiety index of common foods. *European Journal of Clinical Nutrition, 49*, 675–690.—A compelling laboratory study showing that the most satiating foods are also the least palatable.

Jeffery, R. W., & French, S. A. (1998). Epidemic obesity in the United States: Are fast foods and television viewing contributing? *American Journal of Pubic Health, 88*, 277–80.—A persuasive argument that obesity may be the outcome of environmental conditions.

Mela, D. J., & Sacchetti, D. A. (1991). Sensory preferences for fats: Relationships with diet and body composition. *American Journal of Clinical Nutrition, 53*, 908–915.—Provides the needed link between dietary fat intakes and percent body fat in a small clinical sample.

Prentice, A. M., & Poppitt, S. D. (1996). Importance of energy density and macronutrients in the regulation of food intake. *International Journal of Obesity, 20*(Suppl. 2), 651–660.—An argument that energy density of the diet, as opposed to its fat content, may influence intakes and affect body weight.

# 10

# Energy Expenditure and Body Weight

## ERIC RAVUSSIN

There has been considerable speculation concerning the reasons the human genome could harbor genes predisposing to positive energy balance and obesity in our "obesegenic" environment (see Chapters 3, 5, and 12). The most frequently stated theory is that of the "thrifty genotype." During human history, food was not very abundant and required much physical work to obtain. Survival mechanisms evolved to confer protection against periods of food scarcity. It is therefore not surprising that highly industrialized populations now struggle with the problem of obesity due to rapid environmental changes (see Chapter 78). This has led us to propose another hypothesis: that obesity in our present environment is an "essential" condition and only those with fewer obesity susceptibility genes (the former nonsurvivors) can resist our "obesigenic" environment and maintain a normal weight without conscious effort (see Chapter 4). The common thread between these two hypotheses is that what was an asset to early humans is now rapidly becoming a liability. Although the pathogenesis of obesity is not completely understood, recent studies of energy intake and expenditure in humans have shown that obesity is not simply the result of bad behavior or so-called "sloth and gluttony."

## RELEVANCE OF ENERGY EXPENDITURE COMPONENTS TO OBESITY

Obesity results from a chronic positive energy imbalance between energy intake and energy expenditure. Since food intake assessment is precise only under laboratory conditions that do not reflect everyday life, and measurement in free-living conditions is inaccurate, scientists have concentrated on the energy expenditure side of the energy–balance equation (see Chapter 24). Technological advances have made possible the use of indirect calorimetry for measures of metabolic rates over periods of hours using a ventilated hood system, or over 1 day or more using a respiratory chamber. In such chambers, all components of sedentary energy expenditure can be measured (i.e., sleeping metabolic rate, the energy cost of arousal, the thermic effect of food, and the energy cost of spontaneous physical activity or nonexercise activity thermogenesis (Figure 10.1). The doubly labeled water method provides accurate measures of total energy expenditure over periods of days and, in combination with indirect calorimetry, can be used to assess physical activity in free-living conditions.

## RESTING METABOLIC RATE

The resting metabolic rate (RMR) is the amount of energy expended when an adult organism is awake but resting, not actively digesting, and at thermal neutrality. Because work is not performed on the environment, all energy expended is released as heat. Metabolic rate decreases below RMR by approximately 10% during sleep but can decrease by as much as 30% with starvation and increase 10- to 20-fold for short periods of vigorous exercise. In most sedentary adults, RMR accounts for approximately 60–70% of daily energy expenditure. The strong relationship between RMR and body size has been known for many years and led to the development of equations still widely used to predict RMR in each sex based on height and weight. The heavier the individual, the greater the absolute RMR and, indeed, total energy expenditure. Although RMR correlates best with fat-free body mass, it is also, to a lesser extent, independently influenced by fat

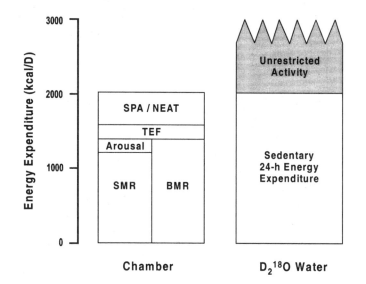

**FIGURE 10.1.** Components of daily energy expenditure in humans. Daily energy expenditure can be divided into three major components: basal metabolic rate (BMR) [sleeping metabolic rate (SMR) + energy cost of arousal], which represents 50–70% of daily expenditure; the thermic effect of food, which represents approximately 10% of energy expenditure; and the energy cost of physical activity [spontaneous physical activity (SPA) + unrestricted/voluntary physical activity], which represents 20–40% of daily energy expenditure. SPA has also been called nonexercise activity thermogenesis (NEAT). *Left*: The measure of sedentary daily energy expenditure measured over 24 hours by indirect calorimetry in a respiratory chamber. *Right*: The total energy expenditure measured over 7–10 days using the doubly labeled water method. Combinations of indirect calorimetry and doubly labeled water methods are used to assess the energy cost of unrestricted physical activity.

mass, age, and sex. Together fat-free body mass, fat mass, age, and sex explain approximately 80–85% of the variance in RMR. As shown in siblings and twins, some of the residual interindividual variability in RMR is likely to be genetically determined. Our studies and others have clearly identified that sympathetic nervous system activity is a significant determinant of the variability in resting metabolic rate. Furthermore, the variability in metabolic rate (adjusted for body weight and composition) is related to variability in body temperature. Body temperature in humans might therefore be a marker of a high or low relative metabolic rate, as previously shown in animals.

If the origin of positive energy balance lies in the chronic imbalance of energy intake and oxidation, then the absolute intake and oxidation rates of macronutrients are less important than the relationship between the two. It is important to know if obesity is caused by high intake, low expenditure, or both, and to identify the conditions that allow a long-lasting imbalance between intake and expenditure. An examination of each nutrient balance equation (carbohydrate, protein, and fat) to determine if chronic imbalance between intake and oxidation exists is only valid if each nutrient has its separate balance equation implying separate regulation. In practical terms: Is each nutrient either oxidized or stored in its own compartment (separate regulation), or does it get converted into another compartment for storage? This applies particularly to whether carbohydrate is stored as fat (de novo lipogenesis) as is commonly believed. De novo lipogenesis is very limited in humans and occurs only when very large excesses of carbohydrate are ingested. Thus, under physiological conditions, it is reasonable to consider each nutrient balance equation as a separate entity. Growing evidence indicates that alcohol balance, protein balance, and carbohydrate balance are very well controlled and unlikely to underlie significant weight gain. In marked contrast, body fat stores are large, and fat intake has no influence on fat oxidation (Table 10.1). Therefore, fat is the only nutrient that can cause a chronic imbalance between intake and oxidation, resulting in excess fat storage in the adipose tissue. As pointed out by Flatt, the use of the fat balance equation and the measurement of fat oxidation are of increasing importance in the assessment of the pathophysiology of human obesity.

## THERMOGENESIS

Thermogenesis is the increase in resting metabolic rate in response to stimuli such as food intake, cold or heat exposure, psychological influences such as fear or stress, or the administration of drugs or hormones that increase the metabolic rate. The thermic effect of food (the major form of thermogenesis in humans) accounts for approximately 10% of daily energy expenditure. Opinions differ as to whether a decreased thermic effect of food is present in obese individuals or involved in the etiology of obesity. This most difficult to measure and least reproducible component of energy expenditure is affected by many factors, such as test meal size and composition, palatability of the food, technique used for measurements, time and duration of the measurement, and the subject's genetic background, age, physical fitness, and sensitivity to insulin. Prospective studies have not identified a low thermic effect of food as a predisposing factor for body weight gain. In summary, one could safely state that any decrease in the thermic effect of food amounts to only a small number of calories and that a minimal weight gain (and thus increased RMR) would be sufficient to offset this decreased energy expenditure.

**TABLE 10.1. Comparison of Macronutrient Stores and Balance in Adult Man**

|                                    | Carbohydrate | Protein  | Alcohol | Fat   |
|------------------------------------|--------------|----------|---------|-------|
| Stored in tissues as . . .         | Glycogen     | Protein  | —       | Fat   |
| Sizes of stores                    | Tiny         | Moderate | —       | Large |
| Daily variability in size          | Large        | Small    | —       | Small |
| Potential for expansion            | Tiny         | Moderate | —       | Large |
| Stores regulated                   | Yes          | Yes      | —       | No    |
| Oxidation stimulated by intake     | Yes          | Yes      | Yes     | No    |
| Potential for long-term imbalance  | No           | Yes[a]   | No      | Yes   |

[a]Only under influence of growth stimuli (hormones, exercise, increasing fat mass, drugs, etc.).

## PHYSICAL ACTIVITY

The most variable component of daily energy expenditure is that expended during physical activity, which accounts for a large amount of calories in very active people. However, sedentary adults exhibit a range of physical activity that represents only about 20–30% of the total expenditure. Reduced physical activity, as a cause of obesity, is an obvious and attractive hypothesis that is supported by the secular increase in obesity paralleling the increase in sedentary lifestyle. However, until the recent introduction of doubly labeled water, there has been no satisfactory method to assess the impact of physical activity on daily energy expenditure (see Chapter 24). Recent reviews in which doubly labeled water data have been pooled show that the level of physical activity can vary widely between people. The energy cost of weight-bearing activities is proportional to body weight and is therefore high in obese individuals, although obesity is generally associated with lower activity levels. The net energy expenditure related to physical activity may therefore be "normal" in obese people compared to their lean counterparts despite lower levels of physical activity.

Using a respiratory chamber, significant differences between individuals in spontaneous physical activity (small, "fidgeting type" movements) have been reported. This activity could account for 100 to 700 kcal/day and is a familial trait indicating a genetic background. People less prone to weight gain during overfeeding have increased levels of spontaneous physical activity compared to those prone to weight gain. The best predictor of fat gain during 56,000 kcal overeating was the amount of activities of daily living, termed nonexercise activity thermogenesis, or NEAT. One of the potential mechanisms underlying the variability in spontaneous physical activity is the activity of the sympathetic nervous system.

## DAILY ENERGY EXPENDITURE

Measurements of energy expenditure using indirect calorimetry in respiratory chambers are very accurate and precise. Numerous studies have shown that 24-hour energy expenditure is directly proportional to fat-free body mass or body weight. The major disadvantage is the confinement of subjects to a small room and that these measurements do not indicate the level of physical activity in the subjects.

Measuring energy expenditure in unconfined subjects has obvious advantages, but the original methods (factorial and intake methods) have been tedious and unreliable. The doubly labeled water technique was first used in humans in 1982. It is a form of "indirect calorimetry" based on the differential elimination of two stable isotopes, deuterium and $^{18}$oxygen ($^{18}O$), from body water after ingestion of the two isotopes. Since $^{18}O$ exits the body as water and $CO_2$ and deuterium exit the body only as water, the difference between the two elimination rates is proportional to $CO_2$ production and, therefore, energy expenditure. With the decreasing cost of isotope ratio mass spectrometers and probably a decrease in the cost of $^{18}O$ in the future, this method will probably become one of the best tools to measure energy expenditure without limitation in activity. The method is noninvasive, can be used in pregnant women, infants, and adults, as well as elderly subjects, and has been validated repeatedly. After adjustment for RMR, total energy expenditure in free-living conditions can be used as a measure of physical activity.

Two points emerge from studies in both the respiratory chamber and in free-living conditions. The larger the body size, the higher the absolute metabolic rate and, therefore, the higher the food intake. Therefore, studies showing no or negative correlations between food intake and weight suggest that obese people underreport what they eat. The second point is that the lowest 24-hour energy expenditures, reported mostly in lean women, are of the order of 1,200–1,300 kcal/day. Therefore, energy intakes less than that will produce an energy deficit and weight loss in any obese individual (see Chapter 89).

## METABOLIC PREDICTORS OF BODY WEIGHT GAIN

In prospective studies conducted in Pima Indian subjects, four metabolic parameters known to have a familial component predict weight gain: low relative resting metabolic rate (RMR adjusted for differences in fat-free mass, fat mass, age, and sex); low level of spontaneous physical activity; a low fat oxidation (i.e., a high 24-hour respiratory quotient); and low activity of the sympathetic nervous system.

All four parameters correlate with body size: RMR positively with fat-free mass; energy cost of spontaneous physical activity positively with weight; 24-hour respiratory quotient negatively with body fat; and sympathetic nervous system activity positively with body fat. When these parameters are adjusted for differences in body size, the initial value predicts the rate of change in body weight over the subsequent years. After weight gain, the original deviation from the value predicted on the basis of population (e.g., low relative RMR, high 24-hour respiratory quotient, low energy cost of activity, low sympathetic nervous system activity) tends to diminish, suggesting a progressively decreasing physiological drive for further body weight gain (Table 10.2). Thus, the high RMR, the high-energy cost of spontaneous physical activity, the low respiratory quotient, and the high sympathetic activity seen in obesity may act to limit additional weight gain. The relationships of these metabolic factors with body weight changes are relatively weak, indicating the involvement of other factors such as total food intake, the composition of the diet, and the level of physical activity. Even if weak, the impact of these four risk factors for weight gain resembles that for socioeconomic and lifestyle risk factors. Furthermore, studies comparing obese to lean subjects yield little information on the mechanisms leading to weight gain.

**TABLE 10.2. Metabolic Characteristics of Obese and Preobese Individuals**

|                                       | Obese (factors associated with obesity) | Pre- or postobese (factors predicting weight gain) |
| ------------------------------------- | --------------------------------------- | -------------------------------------------------- |
| Relative resting metabolic rate       | High or normal                          | Low                                                |
| Energy cost of activity               | Normal                                  | Low                                                |
| Fat oxidation                         | High                                    | Low                                                |
| Sympathetic nervous system activity   | High                                    | Low                                                |

## CONCLUSIONS AND FUTURE STUDIES

The pioneering work of Flatt has redirected research in energy metabolism. Chronic imbalances between intake and oxidation of nonfat nutrients cannot lead to obesity, but fat stores are not controlled and the capacity for expansion is enormous. Obesity is therefore due to a long-lasting positive fat balance that is due simply to a high-fat diet and/or an impaired capacity for fat oxidation. The rate of fat oxidation is a genetically determined trait that seems to be related to the level of physical fitness. Studies are now designed so that researchers better understand how to change fat balance. Strategies targeting fat balance by lowering dietary fat and/or increasing fat oxidation are likely to be efficacious in the treatment of obesity.

Future studies should look at the effect of acute challenges such as short-term overfeeding or fasting on the response in RMR, thermogenesis, and physical activity. We must also know whether there are metabolic differences in adaptation to weight loss or gain between those with large weight changes versus those who will quickly reach a new equilibrium.

Another important topic is the study of the molecular mechanisms of adaptive thermogenesis. Mitochondria, the organelles that convert food to carbon dioxide, water, and adenosine triphosphate (ATP), are fundamental in mediating energy dissipation. Recent advances have been made in our understanding of the molecular regulation of energy expenditure in mitochondria and of the mechanisms of the transcriptional control of genes involved in mitochondrial respiration. Such studies will help us to understand the regulation of energy balance and, more specifically, energy expenditure and its contribution to the development of obesity.

## FURTHER READING

Black, A. E., Coward, W. A., Cole, T. J., & Prentice, A. M. (1996). Human energy expenditure in affluent societies: An analysis of 574 doubly-labeled water measurements. *European Journal of Clinical Nutrition, 50,* 72–92.—Presents the most comprehensive collection of data by doubly labeled water in free-living individuals, covering a wide range in age, body weight, and body composition.

Flatt, J. P. (1993). Dietary fat, carbohydrate balance and weight maintenance. *Annals of the New York Academy of Sciences, 683,* 122–140.—Fat balance versus energy balance. Flatt presents the idea of considering separately fat, carbohydrate, and protein balance rather than just energy balance.

Levine, J. A., Eberhardt, N. L., & Jensen, M. D. (1999). Role of nonexercise activity thermogenesis in resistance to fat gain in humans. *Science, 283*, 212–214.—Presents new evidence that the level of nonexercise activity thermogenesis (small and fidgeting type movements) is related to the variability in weight gain during an 8-week overfeeding period.

Prentice, A. M., Black, A. E., Coward, W. A., & Cole, T. J. (1996). Energy expenditure in overweight and obese adults in affluent societies: An analysis of 319 doubly-labelled water measurements. *European Journal of Clinical Nutrition, 50*, 93–97.—Provides information on the impact of obesity on free-living energy expenditure.

Ravussin, E., & Gautier, J. F. (1999). Metabolic predictors of weight gain. *International Journal of Obesity and Related Metabolic Disorders, 23*, 37–41.—This short review describes the misleading information yielded by cross-sectional studies comparing lean and obese subjects.

Ravussin, E., & Swinburn, B. A. (1992). Pathophysiology of obesity. *Lancet , 340*, 404–408.—A review of the pathogenesis and etiology of obesity in humans.

Rosenbaum, M., Leibel, R. L., & Hirsch, J. (1997). Obesity. *New England Journal of Medicine, 337*, 396–407.—A review of the pathogenesis and etiology of obesity in humans.

Weyer, C., Pratley, R. E., Salbe, A. D., Bogardus, C., Ravussin, E., & Tataranni, P. A. (2000). Energy expenditure, fat oxidation, and body weight regulation: A study of metabolic adaptation to long-term weight change. *Journal of Clinical Endocrinology and Metabolism, 85*, 1087–1094.—Energy metabolism responses to weight change among Pima Indians.

Weyer, C., Snitker, S., Rising, R., Bogardus, C., & Ravussin, E. (1999). Determinants of energy expenditure and fuel utilization in man: Effects of body composition, age, sex, ethnicity and glucose tolerance in 916 subjects. *International Journal of Obesity and Related Metabolic Disorders, 23*, 715–722.—Larger study of energy expenditure and fuel utilization in a respiratory chamber.

# 11

# Body Composition

## TIMOTHY G. LOHMAN

Recent developments in the field of body composition assessment include health-related standards based on both body mass index (BMI) and percentage of body fat; increased prevalence of obesity in the U.S. population based on BMI; multicomponent models for more accurate assessment of body composition; validation studies of dual-energy X-ray absorptiometry (DXA) as a reference method for body fat and lean as well as bone density; increased use of body composition methods in national surveys, multicenter research projects, and epidemiological investigations; search for indirect estimates of abdominal and visceral fat components and their relationship to health; and assessment of body composition changes with short- and long-term interventions. In this chapter, I review these developments to describe the advantages and limitations of various body composition models and methods.

## CHOICE OF BODY COMPOSITION MODELS AND METHODS

The development of multicomponent models has enabled more accurate assessment of body composition, particularly in populations where the two-component model does not apply, for example, children, elderly, and certain athletic groups. BMI as a prediction of body fat has a relatively large error (standard error of estimate, or SEE) for the individual (4–6%). Use of field methods such as bioelectric impedance, skinfolds, and circumferences have errors between 3 and 4.5% depending on the investigation and population. Laboratory methods such as underwater weighing, total body water, and DXA have errors between 2.5% and 3.5%. Multicomponent models can estimate percent fat with 1.0–3.0% error. The selection of a body composition method is dependent in part on the accuracy desired, the equation available, as well as the setting, sample size, and population under study (Figure 11.1). BMI works better with

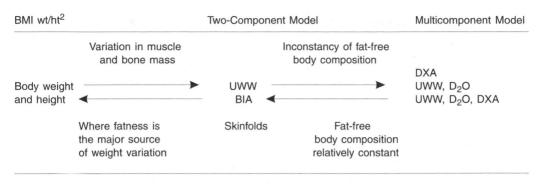

**FIGURE 11.1.** Selection of body composition method. DXA, dual-energy X-ray absorptiometry; UWW, underwater weighing; $D_2O$, total body water by deuterium dilution; BIA, bioelectric impedance.

postmenopausal women, where SEE is 4%. For most populations, SEE is 5% or greater using BMI to estimate fatness.

In large epidemiology studies within a given population, secular trends may be successfully followed using BMI, as in the National Health and Nutrition Examination Survey (NHANES). However, BMI does not track body fat changes well over time, when muscle and bone mass are changing in addition to the fat mass. Where muscle and bone mass are increasing, as in weight-training studies, changes in BMI may overestimate changes in body fatness.

Where body composition cannot be accurately estimated from BMI, the two-component models may be selected using underwater weighing, total body water, bioelectrical impedance, or skinfolds. In the two-component model, the composition of the fat-free body is assumed to be relatively constant as in young adult males and females (Figure 11.1). In general, the constancy of hydration of fat-free mass is well established. Where the assumptions of the two-component models do not hold, various multi-component models can improve on the accuracy of body composition assessment.

## BODY COMPOSITION INDICES

Indices of obesity, sarcopenia, and osteoporosis have been quantified and defined by various national and international groups (Table 11.1). General consensus has been reached for using weight/height$^2$, when only height and weight data are available. Though dimensional analyses support the use of weight/height$^3$, empirical results indicate that weight/height$^2$ is the best indicator of percent fat. For sarcopenia, a low fat-free mass (FFM/height) has been defined in the elderly as two standard deviations below the mean of the young adult reference population. Again, dimensional analysis supports FFM/height$^2$ or FFM/height$^3$. Future validation studies are needed better to define this index of sarcopenia, so that the relation of low FFM to height can be used as a marker of physiological aging. Finally, regional bone mineral density, expressed as g/cm$^2$, is now well established as a measure of osteopenia (less than one standard deviation below the young adult reference population) and osteoporosis (less bone density than $2\frac{1}{2}$ standard deviations below the young adult reference population).

**TABLE 11.1. Indices of Obesity, Sarcopenia, and Osteoporosis**

| Obesity | Sarcopenia | Osteoporosis |
|---|---|---|
| Weight (kg)/Height$^2$ | FFM (kg)/Height (cm) | BMD (g)/cm$^2$ |
| Weight/Height | FFM/Height$^2$ | BMC (g)/Height$^2$ |
| Weight/Height$^3$ | FFM/Height$^3$ | BMC (g)/Height$^3$ |

## BODY COMPOSITION AND HEALTH

Standards for BMI and percent fat have been established. A BMI greater than 25 has been defined as overweight and a BMI above 30 as obesity (see Chapter 68). In general, percent fat above 20–25% for men and above 30–35% for women are the lower limit for obesity (Table 11.2). Based on various regression equations for BMI with percent fat, the relationship varies with age of population, ethnicity, physical activity level, and investigator (Table 11.3). In our standards an upper limit of 22–25% is the lower limit of obesity for men, and 35–38% the lower limit for women.

## MULTICOMPONENT MODELS FOR ASSESSING BODY COMPOSITION

Recent advances in multicomponent models indicate increased accuracy in measuring body composition and its changes. The most often used model is the four-component model assessing body density using underwater weighing, total body water using deuterium dilution, and total bone mineral content using DXA. Multicomponent models better account for variation in the composition of the fat-free body mass, especially in children, in whom water and mineral content are not at reference mean values, and in the elderly, in whom the mineral content is decreasing. Also, in measuring body composition changes from weight loss or exercise-training interventions, variation in water, muscle, and bone density may confound estimates of body composition changes using the assumptions and methods of two-component models.

**TABLE 11.2. Percent Fat Health Standards for Men and Women**

| Age group | Sex | Not recommended | Recommended body fat levels | | | |
|---|---|---|---|---|---|---|
| | | | Low | Middle | Upper | Obesity |
| Young adult | Women | < 20 | 20 | 28 | 35 | ⟶ |
| | Men | < 8 | 8 | 13 | 22 | |
| Middle age | Women | < 25 | 25 | 32 | 38 | |
| | Men | < 10 | 10 | 18 | 25 | |
| Elderly | Women | < 25 | 25 | 30 | 35 | |
| | Men | < 10 | 10 | 16 | 23 | |

**TABLE 11.3. Screening for Body Fatness, Fat Distribution, Lean Mass, and Bone Mineral Status by Life Stage**

| Component | Pediatric (1–5) | Childhood (6–11) | Youth (12–17) | Adult (18–40) | Middle aged (40–60) | Elderly (> 60) |
|---|---|---|---|---|---|---|
| Body fatness | ✓ | ✓ | ✓ | ✓ | ✓ | |
| Fat distribution | | | ✓ | ✓ | ✓ | |
| Bone mineral status | | | ✓ | ✓ | ✓ | ✓ |
| Lean mass | | | | ✓ | ✓ | |

## DUAL-ENERGY X-RAY ABSORPTIOMETRY AS A REFERENCE METHOD

DXA has recently become a reference method for body composition assessment. Differences in software, hardware, hydration level, and subject size have been addressed and show general agreement with the four-component model. DXA is being used by Health ABC to follow changes in body composition with aging over a 7-year period in 3,000 older adults ages 70–79 years. In addition, DXA data will be gathered on a representative sample of the U.S. population in NHANES IV in the next several years. DXA is also the method of choice in the new multisite Study of Health Outcomes of Weight Loss (SHOW) trial studying long-term effects of weight loss on cardiovascular disease risk in an obese, diabetic, female population.

The use of DXA has been extended from quantitative regional and total body bone mineral density to regional and total body composition analysis including muscle and fat estimation. An important effort is to compare DXA estimates of skeletal muscle mass (using arm and leg estimates) with computed tomography (CT) scans throughout the body to obtain quantitative estimates of total muscle mass.

## FAT DISTRIBUTION AND HEALTH

The relation between fat depots and health needs additional study in large samples of subjects. Evidence indicates a relationship between abdominal circumference, abdominal subcutaneous fat, and visceral fat, and chronic disease, suggesting the importance of assessing upper body obesity (see Chapters 68, 84, and 86). The use of DXA for regional body fat will help sort out relationships with different fat depots and health.

## FURTHER READING

Baumgartner, R. N., Koehter, K. M., Romero, L. J., Lindeman, R. O., & Garry, P. J. (1998). Epidemiology of sarcopenia in elderly people in New Mexico. *American Journal of Epidemiology*, 147, 744–763.—Presents a quantitative definition of sarcopenia and its relation to disability.

Ellis, K. J. (2000). Human body composition: *In vivo* methods. *Physiological Reviews*, 80, 649–686.—An excellent review of body composition methods.

Evans, E. M., Saunders, M. J., Spano, M. A., Arngrimsson, S. A., Lewis, R. D., & Cureton, K. J.

(1999). Body composition changes with diet and exercise in obese women: A comparison of estimates from clinical methods and a 4-component model. *American Journal of Clinical Nutrition, 70*, 5–12.—An excellent article estimating body composition changes using a multicomponent model.

Heymsfield, S. B., Wang, Z. M., & Withers, R. T. (1996). Multicomponent molecular models of body composition analysis. In A. F. Roche, S. B. Heymsfield, & T. G. Lohman (Eds.), *Human body composition* (pp. 129–147). Champaign, IL: Human Kinetics.—Provides an overview of different multicomponent models.

Heyward, V. H., & Stolarczyk, L. M. (1996). *Applied body composition assessment.* Champaign, IL: Human Kinetics.—Reviews and presents some of the most valid body composition equations using field methods.

Lohman, T. G. (1993). *Advances in body composition assessment.* Champaign, IL: Human Kinetics.—A review of many issues in the field of body composition assessment.

Lohman, T. G., Going, S. B., & Houtkooper, L. B. (1997). Body fat measurement goes high-tech. *American College of Sports Medicine Health and Fitness Journal, 2*, 16–19.—Provides health standards for body fatness in adult and elderly populations.

Lohman, T. G., Harris, M., Teixeira, P. J., & Weiss, L. (2000). Assessing body composition and changes in body composition. In S. Yasumura, J. Wang, & R. N. Pierson, Jr. (Eds.), *In vivo body composition studies. Annals of the New York Academy of Sciences, 904*, 45–54.—A review of issues related to assessing body composition and its changes.

Wang, Z. M., Deurenberg, P., Wang, W., Pietrobelli, A., Baumgartner, R. N., & Heymsfield, S. B. (1999). Hydration of fat-free mass: Review and critique of a classic body composition constant. *American Journal of Clinical Nutrition, 69*, 833–841.—An excellent overview of the constancy of hydration levels in animal and human studies.

Yasumara, S., Wang, J., & Pierson, R. N., Jr. (Eds.). (2000). *In vivo* body composition studies. *Annals of the New York Academy of Science, 904*, 1–637.—Recent work on *in vivo* body composition.

# 12

# The Nature of the Regulation
# of Energy Balance

## JAMES O. HILL

## IS ENERGY BALANCE REGULATED?

This chapter begins with the assertion that there is a physiological system(s) within the body that to some extent regulates energy utilization. The strongest evidence is the relative stability of body weight within individuals over time. Granted, the population of the United States is slowly gaining weight, but for any individual, this still represents a very small error in overall energy balance regulation. Consider that an average adult might consume 1,000,000 kcal each year. If that same individual gains 1–2 pounds per year, the error in matching energy expenditure to energy intake is still less than 0.5%. This suggests an extraordinary degree of regulation of energy.

The fact that body weight is defended further suggests the existence of some regulatory process. Any dieter can attest to the difficulty in sustaining a reduction in body weight below the "usual" level, suggesting processes that oppose weight loss and maintenance of a reduced weight.

While the regulation of energy balance occurs, the process is not perfect. The gradual weight gain seen in most people over the adult years suggests that the regulatory system may not be sufficient to maintain a constant body weight under all circumstances. Furthermore, the system may not be symmetrical, with defense against body weight gain weaker than the defense against body weight loss (see Chapter 8).

## THE NATURE OF THE ENERGY BALANCE REGULATORY SYSTEM

What might a regulatory system look like and how might it function to match energy intake with energy expenditure? Many different models have been developed. My colleagues and I have suggested that the nature of energy balance regulation and the body weight maintained over time is dependent on the individual's functional phenotype, which represents his or her current behavioral and metabolic state. The functional phenotype is influenced by genetic and nongenetic factors, and determines the way in which energy balance is achieved and the resulting level of body weight and body composition that will be maintained within any given environment.

The functional phenotype is influenced by genetic factors but can be modified over time by nongenetic (environmental) factors. Body weight for an individual would remain relatively stable as long as both genetic and nongenetic influences on the functional phenotype remain relatively stable.

Part of the functional phenotype is a basic biological system for energy balance regulation. This is the physiology that links instinctive behavior (within the behavioral phenotype) with the basic metabolic pathways that generate and receive signals about the state of energy balance (within the metabolic phenotype). However, many environmental factors can modify the metabolic and/or behavioral phenotypes, and these in turn may alter the functional phenotype, with a resulting change in the level at which body weight is maintained over time. For example, a sedentary individual who becomes a regular exerciser will experience many metabolic and behavioral consequences. This can alter both the metabolic and behavioral phenotypes, and result in energy balance at a reduced body weight and body fat mass.

## THE BASIC BIOLOGICAL SYSTEM FOR REGULATING ENERGY BALANCE

The basic biological system for regulating energy balance would involve a functional phenotype consisting of both instinctual behavior and a metabolic system for assessing and modifying the state of energy balance at any given time. One view is that the basic biological system for regulation of energy balance is the system "genetically programmed" within the organism. Indeed, when the environment is strictly controlled, as in some animal models, body weight regulation is a function of this biological system.

The metabolic pathways within a basic biological system are complex and have not been fully identified. The way in which a system might function has been described by Bray. Short- and long-term signals about the state of energy intake, energy expenditure, and substrate availability arise in the periphery and are transmitted to the brain. The brain acts to integrate complex, redundant, short- and long-term signals to determine the state of energy balance and to initiate appropriate behavior (eating, physical activity) to maintain energy balance and body weight at optimum levels.

The rapid progress being made in understanding this metabolic system is described in several chapters in this book. Leibowitz (Chapter 1) and Smith and Gibbs (Chapter 2) have reviewed work clearly demonstrating peripheral and central signals (both long- and short-term) that arise as a consequence of the beginning and end of eating. Similarly, Ravussin (Chapter 10) describes how energy expenditure may be related to both body energy stores and energy intake. Leptin appears to be the long-sought signal from adipose tissue that indicates a state of energy balance and may help link energy intake and energy expenditure (see Chapter 6). Lohman (Chapter 11) reviews signals that arise as a consequence of the amount and type of energy stored in the body.

Along with metabolic pathways, the basic biological system may also involve instinctive behavior. In response to the appropriate signals, the organism begins eating (if food is available) and, in response to different signals, stops eating (see Chapter 8). However, Drewnowski (Chapter 9) has described some food preferences that appear to be inherent characteristics of individuals. An example is a preference for sweet tastes. Regardless of the signal generated through the metabolic pathway, an organism may eat when presented with sweet foods. Eating can sometimes be independent of hunger.

This basic biological system would work well to maintain a constant body weight under stable environmental conditions, as seen with many laboratory animals. It is important to study this system to understand key aspects of body weight regulation, to identify abnormalities in the system, and to develop corrective treatments. We must further understand the "normal" variation in the system that leads to differences in body weight among individuals within a similar environment. All of this may lead to treatment and prevention strategies aimed at those who vary from the "normal" regulation. Advances on these issues have been impressive.

## MODIFICATION OF THE FUNCTIONAL PHENOTYPE

Even if we completely understand the biological regulation of energy balance, we may not be able to explain much body weight variation in humans. Many factors can influence the functional phenotype, through modification of either the metabolic and/or the behavioral phenotypes.

### Metabolic Programming

The strongest evidence for metabolic programming comes from studies of the *in utero* environment and later metabolic functioning. Barker and colleagues found that low-birth-weight babies are prone to developing obesity and other characteristics of the metabolic syndrome. This suggests that the environment *in utero* can affect the metabolic phenotype as a form of metabolic programming. The *in utero* environment does not change the genes of the individual but changes the way in which the genes are expressed.

Metabolic programming early in life can have major impacts on future regulation of energy balance and body weight, but it is possible that such programming could also occur later in life. Menopause, for example, seems to be a period where altered hormonal status is associated with total and visceral body fat gain, at least in some women.

The notion of metabolic programming adds significant complexity to the concept of a basic biological system for regulation of energy balance. It argues that the biological system is not a function solely of genes but varies with how those genes are expressed.

### Social and Cultural Influences on the Behavioral Phenotype

While the metabolic phenotype may be modifiable at certain critical periods of life, the behavioral phenotype is continuously modifiable. The basic biological system would suggest that we eat when hungry (when the periphery signals negative energy balance). However, it is clear that people eat for many reasons other than physiological signals (i.e., time of day).

Many social and cultural factors can affect the behavioral phenotype and thus alter the functional phenotype and the body weight at which energy balance is achieved. We will not truly understand body weight regulation and obesity until we understand the nature of social and cultural influences on behavior and the regulation of energy balance (see Chapter 78).

Much of human behavior is noninstinctual and consists of patterns developed and repeated over time. For example, a family may eat Chinese food every Wednesday or someone may go out for pizza with friends every Friday night. This eating is not part of the basic biological system but can significantly affect energy intake. Similarly, we develop physical activity patterns. Some people exercise every morning or take a walk every day after dinner. These behaviors can influence the behavioral phenotype and alter the functional phenotype and body weight regulation.

Humans often develop strong beliefs that influence behavior. Someone may become a vegetarian because of a belief against eating meat. This may determine the amount and composition of energy ingested and have important effects on body weight regulation. Many people develop health beliefs that drive physical activity, so that some report engaging in regular physical activity even though they do not find it uniformly pleasurable.

It is also clear that eating and physical activity patterns differ by ethnicity (see Chapter 79). For example, African American women often report engaging in very little physical activity. This may be caused by ethnic differences in beliefs about the health consequences of excess body weight. African American women may see obesity as a lesser health risk than do Caucasian women.

Our life experiences certainly affect our behaviors, which in turn affect energy intake and expenditure. For example, while some food tastes (e.g., preference for sweetness) may be innate, others can be influenced by our exposure to foods.

Our behavior also varies with values. An example is physical activity. Most people list lack of time as the major barrier to regular physical activity, suggesting that they may value time or convenience over physical activity. Social roles often affect behavior. For example, a mother making meals for her family while trying to lose weight herself may struggle and fail to meet both needs.

Our behavior is greatly affected by our life stage. College seems to be a risk period for weight gain, a period where choices about food intake and physical activity patterns may greatly increase. Physical activity may decline in young adulthood, when pressures of job and family may leave little time. Finally, there are indications that the sensory experience of foods changes with aging (i.e., foods taste different).

Those with whom we have relationships influence our behavior. Many times, the diet of one spouse will change after marriage if the other spouse is the major shopper and preparer of food. Often, friendships can be formed around physical activity (e.g., a group of coworkers walk together each day during the lunch break).

If managing weight has become more a cognitive than a physiological task, education may influence behavior. Higher education may bring better understanding of relationship between weight and health and a better understanding of how to make behavior changes. This would lead to lifestyles driven by a cognitive understanding of the behaviors needed to maximize health.

Socioeconomic status (SES) is often related to obesity, although the nature of the relationship may differ in different ethnic groups and between countries in different stages of the obesity epidemic (see Chapter 75). The issues here are complex, since SES interacts with ethnicity and education. However, in many developing countries, obesity is first seen in the higher SES groups, presumably because they have access to high-energy diets combined with declining need for physical activity (see Chapter 74).

## SUMMARY

Energy utilization in the body does seem to be regulated to some extent and is influenced by both genetic and nongenetic factors. While an understanding of the basic biological system for the regulation of energy balance is essential, this alone will not lead to complete understanding of overall regulation.

Energy balance can be achieved at a range of body weights within genetically determined limits. A major question is why so many people in the United States are now achieving energy balance at obese body weights. The answer to this question will be found in understanding how social, cultural, and other environmental factors affect the basic biological system for energy balance regulation.

Most research has focused on the basic biological system for energy balance regulation. This is a high priority, but we have focused almost no effort on understanding how nongenetic factors within our environment affect this system. Humans are not laboratory animals and we cannot understand body weight solely from biology. If we are to understand and begin to manage the current epidemic of obesity, we must initiate serious research efforts to understand how the environment affects the energy balance regulatory system.

## FURTHER READING

Barker, D. J., Gluckman, P. D., Godfrey, K. M., Harding, J. E., Owens, J. A., & Robinson, J. S. (1993). Fetal nutrition and cardiovascular disease in adult life. *Lancet, 341,* 938–941.—This paper describes how the environment *in utero* can create "metabolic programming."

Bray, G. A. (1998). *Contemporary diagnosis and management of obesity.* Newtown, PA: Handbooks in Health Care.—This comprehensive book not only describes the components of a basic biological system for body weight regulation but it also deals with almost every other aspect of obesity.

Hill, J. O., Pagliassotti, M. J., & Peters, J. C. (1994). Nongenetic determinants of obesity and fat topography. In C. Bouchard (Ed.), *Genetic determinants of obesity* (pp. 35–48). Boca Raton, FL: CRC Press.—This chapter describes in more detail how nongenetic factors can influence behavioral and metabolism, and affect the level at which body weight for an individual is regulated.

Kumanyika, S., Wilson, J. F., & Guilford-Davenport, M. (1993). Weight-related attitudes and behavior of black women. *Journal of the American Dietetic Association, 93,* 416–422.—This paper describes how different ethnic groups have different attitudes about obesity and associated behaviors.

Wadden, T. A. (1993). Treatment of obesity by moderate and severe caloric restriction: Results of clinical research trials. *Annals of Internal Medicine, 119,* 699–693.—This is a good review article describing results of behavioral weight loss studies with human subjects.

World Health Organization. (1998). *Obesity: Preventing and managing the global epidemic: Report of a WHO Consultation on Obesity* (WHO/NUT/NCD/97.2). Geneva: Author.—This document presents obesity as a global public health problem, describing how the environment worldwide contributes to the obesity epidemic.

# Psychological and Social Factors, Dieting, and Body Image

# 13

# Acquisition of Food Preferences and Eating Patterns in Children

## LEANN L. BIRCH

### PARENTS PROVIDE GENES AND THE EARLY EATING ENVIRONMENT

By definition, as mammals, we all begin life on an exclusive milk diet. During the first years of life, the transition from milk to a modified adult diet takes place, and to maintain growth and health, the infant must learn to accept at least some of the foods we offer to them. Individual differences among children in the control of food intake begin to emerge during this early transition period. As children's genetic predispositions are modified by learning and their experience with food and eating, food preferences and more adult-like controls of food intake begin to emerge. Early experience with food provides opportunities for learning that are critical to this process. Parents play a central role in shaping the child's food environment and early experience with food and eating.

Parents influence the development of food acceptance patterns by structuring children's early eating environments in a variety of ways. At birth, the parents' choice to breast-feed or formula-feed has implications for subsequent food acceptance patterns. Once the transition to solid food begins, parents also have the opportunity to shape the child's food environment by offering some foods and not others, by the timing and size of meals, and by the social contexts in which children's eating occurs. For children, eating is usually a social occasion, complete with other eaters who can serve as models.

The child of overweight parents is at greater risk for becoming overweight, and this familial resemblance is the result of the interaction of genetic and environmental factors. Childhood overweight is the result of a gene–environment interaction, in which genes and environment work in concert to produce overweight, and for children, parents provide both genes and the food environment during the early years of life. We cannot alter the child's genetic predisposition but the feeding environment is modifiable and could be the target of specific interventions once we understand how environmental factors operate in concert with genetic factors to promote or discourage the development of childhood

overweight. The very rapid increases in the prevalence of obesity and overweight in recent decades (see Chapter 75) underscore the role of the feeding environment in the current epidemic of childhood overweight, since genetic changes are far too slow to produce
such dramatic increases. However, the vast majority of recent research on obesity has focused on the explication of genetic factors, and we still have relatively little research data
on environmental factors that promote childhood overweight.

## GENETIC PREDISPOSITIONS AND EARLY EXPERIENCE

Infants come into the world equipped with genetic predispositions to prefer sweet and
salty tastes, reject sour and bitter tastes, and to reject new foods. The work of Steiner first
revealed that even prior to any postnatal experience, infants respond reflexively to sweet,
sour, and bitter tastes with facial expressions that are read by parents as like, dislike, and
distaste, respectively. An additional predisposition involves the tendency to reject new
foods, which has been termed "neophobia," meaning fear of the new. This neophobia can
impede children's acceptance of new foods but can be transformed to acceptance via experience with eating new foods. These early predispositions interact with early environmental experience to shape food acceptance patterns. As a result, children learn what is
edible and disgusting within their culture, as well as what to like, how much to eat, and
when to eat. They also begin to acquire cuisine rules regarding flavors that should and
should not be combined, and the times of day when foods are eaten.

Because early learning and experience is central in the development of food acceptance patterns, the early food environment is very important in shaping these patterns. As
omnivores, humans need dietary variety to obtain adequate nutrition. However, especially for our hunter–gatherer ancestors, ingesting a potential new food for the first time
was risky and could lead to illness or even death. Probably for this reason, humans, including young children, exhibit "neophobic" reactions to new foods. In general, children
can only learn to prefer foods if the foods are made available to them. Fortunately, the
child's initial neophobic response can be reduced by eating the food, at least when eating
is followed by positive postingestive consequences such as pleasant feelings of satiety.
(When ingestion of a new food is followed by nausea or emesis, a learned aversion to the
food is likely to result.) Postingestive signals also serve to shape children's preferences for
energy-dense foods over more energy-dilute ones; because fat is very energy-dense, children learn to prefer high-fat over low-fat foods. This type of flavor–nutrient learning, in
which flavors of foods become associated with their postingestive consequences, has been
widely demonstrated among other species of omnivores and is likely to contribute to the
reduction of neophobia and children's preferences for energy-dense foods high in fat and
sugar. Learned preferences for such foods would make adaptive sense in environments
where food is scarce and energy-dense foods are not readily available, but such learning
may be a liability in Western cultures, where energy-dense foods have become inexpensive and readily available.

## THE CHALLENGE OF CHILDREN'S DIETS

Current U.S. dietary guidelines include recommendations to choose diets moderate in
sugar and salt, and low in fat, and to consume a variety of foods. In a context in which

large quantities of palatable foods high in sugar, salt, and fat are readily available, it is no coincidence that these dietary recommendations directly oppose our predispositions to prefer sweet and salt, and to learn to prefer foods high in fat and energy. Making recommendations is relatively easy, but the real challenge for parents is to find ways to have these recommendations result in healthier diets for children. The evidence suggests that we have a long way to go before children's diets are consistent with current recommendations. A recent survey in the United States (by Muñoz and colleagues) of 4,000 youth from ages 2 to 19 years revealed that 45% of children's energy intake came from discretionary sugar and fat, and the majority of children were not meeting dietary recommendations.

What is a parent to do in the face of the rising prevalence of overweight and the dietary recommendations to reduce children's sugar, fat, and salt intake to moderate levels? In the United States these days, restricting children's access to energy-dense, palatable foods is a common child feeding strategy. To parents, this seems a reasonable approach, since dietary restriction is the most common strategy used by those dieting for weight control, especially women. An additional strategy is to pressure children to eat foods that are "good for them"—the fruits, vegetables, and complex carbohydrates that should be consumed in greater quantities.

## PARENTAL USE OF DIETARY RESTRICTION

Recently, we have been investigating the effects of these child feeding practices on the development of controls over food intake. In this research, we have questioned parents about the extent to which they restrict children's access to "unhealthy" snack foods, and have related their use of restriction to children's intake of restricted foods in a setting where the foods are freely available, and parents are not around to restrict access. We have also related mothers' reported use of restriction in child feeding to other maternal and child characteristics: maternal body mass index (BMI) and maternal dieting to measures of children's intake of restricted foods and weight status. Results of several studies reveal that maternal restriction actually *increases* children's intake of the restricted foods when children are given free access to them. These effects are much stronger for girls than for boys. Mothers who report using higher levels of restriction also have higher levels of dietary restraint. Mothers also use more restriction with girls who have higher BMIs, raising the question of the direction of these findings. We have proposed that the effects of parental restriction on children's developing controls of food intake are similar to the effects of self-imposed restriction on adult dieters, with chronic restriction eventually leading to the breakdown of restraint, "out of control" overeating of restricted foods, and negative self-evaluation. (For discussion of the relationship between dieting and binge eating, see Chapters 15, 16, 17, and 18.)

In addition to learning food acceptance patterns, children are also learning about standards of beauty, and for women and girls in Western cultures, this standard involves thinness. Recent research indicates that at least in the United States and United Kingdom, by the age of 10 or so, children have also learned to be concerned about their weight and how to diet. Recent surveys in the United States among 8- to 11-year-old girls reveal that among 8-year-olds, about one-third thought they should be thinner, and slightly more than one-third reported they had already tried to lose weight. By age 11, more than three-fourths thought they should be thinner, and about two-thirds of girls reported that they had tried to lose weight. Evidence also suggests that a substantial proportion of 5-year-old girls already have ideas about diets and dieting.

## SUMMARY AND CONCLUSIONS

Children "come equipped" with genetic predispositions to prefer and reject tastes, to be neophobic, and to learn to associate foods with the contexts and consequences of ingestion. Through early experience with food and eating, these predispositions are transformed into food preferences and styles of responding to cues in the food environment that shape future control of food intake and food acceptance. In recent years, there has been a dramatic increase in the prevalence of overweight in children and the emergence of dieting and weight concerns, especially among girls. Anticipatory guidance, prevention, and treatment programs are needed to alleviate the problem of childhood overweight and the chronic health problems associated with overweight and obesity, as well as other related problems, including anorexia nervosa and bulimia nervosa (see Chapters 67 and 103). A comprehensive solution must move beyond individual and family factors to address the environment at all levels, including the social, cultural, and economic factors that shape the larger environmental context in which families are nurturing their children.

## FURTHER READING

Birch, L. L., & Fisher, J. O. (1998). Development of eating behaviors among children and adolescents. *Pediatrics, 101,* 539–549.—An overview of factors influencing the developing controls of food intake in infants and children.

Birch, L. L., & Fisher, J. O. (2000). Mothers' child feeding practices influence daughters' eating and overweight. *American Journal of Clinical Nutrition, 71,* 1054–1061.—Presents a model of how aspects of parenting influence food intake and weight status.

Fisher, J. O., & Birch, L. L. (1999a). Restricting access to foods and children's eating. *Appetite, 32,* 405–419.—Provides evidence for links between child feeding practices and individual differences among children in eating and weight status.

Fisher, J. O., & Birch, L. L. (1999b). Restricting access to palatable foods affects children's behavioral response, food selection and intake. *American Journal of Clinical Nutrition, 69,* 1264–272.—Experimental research revealing how restriction alters children's food acceptance and intake.

Gazzaniga, J. M., & Burns, T. (1993). Relationship between diet composition and body fatness with adjustment for resting energy expenditure and physical activity in preadolescent children. *American Journal of Clinical Nutrition, 58,* 21–28.—Provides evidence for links between dietary fat intake and weight status; does not include controls for energy intake.

Hill, J. O., & Peters, J. C. (1998). Environmental contributions to the obesity epidemic. *Science, 280,* 1371–1374.—Presents the case for the role of environmental factors in the current obesity epidemic.

Johnson, S. L., & Birch, L. L. (1994). Parents' and children's adiposity and eating style. *Pediatrics, 94,* 653–661.—Introduces the links between parents' feeding practices, and children's eating and weight status.

Mennella, J. A., & Beauchamp, G. K. (1996). The early development of human flavor preferences. In E. D. Capaldi (Ed.), *Why we eat what we eat* (pp. 83–112). Washington, DC: American

Psychological Association.—An excellent review of genetic predispositions regarding taste and olfaction, and how they are influenced by early experience.

Muñoz, K. A., Krebs-Smith, S. M., Ballard-Barbash, R., & Cleveland, L. E. (1997). Food intakes of U.S. children and adolescents compared with recommendations. *Pediatrics, 100*, 323–329.—This paper, based on national survey data, presents a rather dreary picture of how children's diets fail to meet recommendations.

Nguyen, V. T., Larson, D. E., Johnson, R. K., & Goran, M. I. (1996). Fat intake and adiposity in children of lean and obese parents. *American Journal of Clinical Nutrition, 63*, 507–513.—Further evidence for links between fat intake and weight status.

Steiner, J. E. (1977). Facial expressions of the neonate infant indicating the hedonics of food-related chemical stimuli. In J. M. Weiffenbach (Ed.), *Taste and development: The genesis of sweet preference* (pp. 173–188). Washington, DC: U. S. Government Printing Office.—Classic work revealing evidence for unlearned responses to the basic tastes: sweet, sour, bitter, and salty.

Troiano, R. P., & Flegal K. M. (1998). Overweight children and adolescents: Description, epidemiology, and demographics. *Pediatrics, 101*, 497–504.—Presents current demographic evidence regarding overweight and obesity among children and adolescents.

Whitaker, R. C., Wright, J. A., Pepe, M. S., Seidel, K. D., & Dietz, W. H. (1997). Predicting obesity in young adulthood from childhood and parental obesity. *New England Journal of Medicine, 337*, 869–873.—Excellent paper examining parental and child obesity as predictors of later weight status in offspring.

# 14

# Prevalence and Demographics of Dieting

## ANDREW J. HILL

In the developed world, the malnutrition of poverty has given way to the malnutrition of affluence. Externally imposed food shortage has been superseded by self-imposed food restriction. For some sections of society, dieting and body dissatisfaction appear to have become normal, even normative. This chapter considers what is meant by dieting, summarizes the research on its prevalence, identifies who is most likely to engage in dieting, and looks to the future.

## ASSESSMENT OF DIETING

Research interest in the prevalence and reasons for dieting started in the mid-1960s. This interest has increased with a flurry of surveys published during the last decade. However, comparability across studies is problematic. Prevalence estimates vary widely according to what is asked. General questions (e.g., Are you trying to lose weight?) produce higher levels of endorsement than more specific ones (Are you currently dieting to lose weight?). Epidemiological surveys of large, representative samples tend to use a limited number of general questions, since the assessment of dieting is often a subsidiary part of the overall study. In contrast, studies with smaller samples may be designed for the purpose of detailing dieting but they tend to be directed at high-risk groups.

Dieting is not uniform in its implementation. For some dieters, it signifies a simple desire to lose weight. For others it refers to the periodic use of several weight-loss behaviors. For still others, dieting represents attempts to maintain their current weight and prevent weight gain. These differences in purpose are mirrored by differences in the composition, intensity, and duration of weight-loss diets. There are also serious questions about the validity of self-reports of dieting, since memory biases, social desirability, and the brittle nature of dieting make uncertain the degree to which simple affirmations reflect consistent changes in nutritional behavior.

## PREVALENCE OF DIETING

These assessment issues notwithstanding, it is still possible to make reasonable prevalence estimates. Summarizing the many studies of Western adults shows that approximately 39% of women and 21% of men report currently trying to lose weight. Not all should be assumed to be dieting, since asking who is currently *dieting* to lose weight reduces these figures to approximately 24% of women and 8% of men. The highest rates stem from questions on dieting history, such as ever dieting to lose weight or dieting within the last 12 months. In adults, this is reported by 55% of women and 29% of men. Compared to men, therefore, women are twice as likely to have a history of dieting or to report current dieting for weight loss. This gender difference is not apparent in dieting for weight maintenance or to avoid weight gain. "Watching what I eat" is reported by 30% of women and 25% of men.

## DEMOGRAPHICS OF DIETING

Besides gender, age, geography, body weight, ethnicity, and social class influence prevalence estimates. Compared to adult women, adolescent girls report slightly higher levels of dieting, and younger adolescents report slightly lower levels. Dieting increases in girls between the ages of 11 and 16, although up to one-fourth of 11-year-olds have already made one dieting attempt. The average age of starting to diet among today's adolescent girls is around 12 and 13. Dieting is also familiar to older women, with more than 50% of women over 60 having a history of dieting to lose weight.

Comparing across continents, some, but not all, studies show the prevalence of weight-loss attempts and dieting to be lower in Europe than the United States. Around one-third of European young women are currently trying to lose weight, with almost as many watching their weight to avoid weight gain. Only 15% are currently dieting to lose weight. In Australia, adult dieting prevalence is at or below European levels. However, for adolescent girls, there is more similarity among Europe, Australia, and America. Also of note are reports from Asia. In Japan, one-fourth of adolescent girls say they are currently trying to lose weight and one-third of 12-year-old girls have already dieted. One study found that one-third of adolescent girls in Beijing (China) reported dieting sometimes, but only 2% were dieting seriously. Similarly, only 8% of young Chinese women in Hong Kong were currently dieting to lose weight.

A key factor in interpreting some of these differences is the extent of overweight and obesity in each sample. While increasing, the prevalence of overweight and obesity is still low in Chinese people. In the Hong Kong study, for example, less than 1% of the respondents were obese. Studies of Western people show that trying to lose weight and dieting are strongly related to body mass index (BMI). Overweight women are four times more likely, and obese women, six times more likely to be currently trying to lose weight. Repeated attempts at dieting are also more common in the obese. However, the relationship between BMI and dieting is not linear. Nearly 10% of women with a BMI below 20 (i.e., underweight) are currently dieting, while up to 70% of overweight and obese women are not, although the vast majority have dieted in the past. Contrary to expectation, there are more normal-weight current dieters than there are obese dieters.

A few studies have noted a positive association between dieting and socioeconomic status (SES) in adults but not adolescents. This is interesting given the inverse relationship between SES and prevalence of obesity in women. It has also been observed that weight-control and dieting attempts are twice as likely in American white adolescent girls than black girls. Dieting increases with increasing age in white girls but does not change in black girls, who, as a group, are less likely to consider themselves overweight. A general principle applicable to all groups is that dieting is more strongly related to perceived overweight than to actual weight in normal-weight females.

## DIMENSIONS OF DIETING

Uncertainty over the validity of self-reported dieting has led some researchers to specify the variety of behavior associated with intentional weight control. Such behavior includes limiting the amount eaten at meals, avoiding fats and fatty foods, avoiding eating between meals, and avoiding confectionery and sweet drinks. These behaviors are commonly endorsed and distinguish dieters from nondieters. Longitudinal research shows that most dieters use at least one of these methods over periods of a few years, although, at best, for less than 20% of the total time.

Such healthy dieting behavior may be contrasted with unhealthy weight-control practices such as skipping meals, fasting, vomiting, taking laxatives, using diet pills, and taking up smoking. Individually, the latter forms of behavior are uncommon (smoking excepted), although around 20% of young women report using at least one during the past year. They cluster, in that dieters are more likely to use extreme weight-control methods, and those who use one method are more likely to use several.

## THE FUTURE OF DIETING

Dieting is recognized and attempted by girls at younger ages than ever before. Women now in their 50s started dieting in their early 20s. Today's adolescent girls start before they are teenagers. Dieting is not a permanent state. In a rare, long-term study by Heatherton and colleagues, only 11% of a group of 30-year-old women were dieting regularly compared with 23% at age 20. This decrease mirrored a reduction in perceived overweight. However, dieting leaves a scar, marking people's past shape and weight concerns and their possible return in the future. Dieting is also being exported to developing societies. Studies of adolescent girls in Iran, Saudi Arabia, the Pacific Islands, and other locations show associations between dieting, a drive for thinness, contact with Western society, and increasing affluence. That the last two factors are associated increasing obesity in the population ensures that dieting will further rise in its acceptance and prevalence.

## FURTHER READING

Blokstra, A., Burns, C. M., & Seidell, J. C. (1999). Perception of weight status and dieting behaviour in Dutch men and women. *International Journal of Obesity, 23,* 7–17.—An excellent characterization of adult dieting, together with an analysis of the relationship between body weight and dieting.
Dwyer, J. T., Feldman, J. J., & Mayer, J. (1967). Adolescent dieters: Who are they? Physical charac-

teristics, attitudes and dieting practices of adolescent girls. *American Journal of Clinical Nutrition, 20,* 1045–1056.—One of the first studies documenting adolescent dieting, and a reminder that this is not a new phenomenon.

French, S. A., & Jeffery, R. W. (1994). Consequences of dieting to lose weight: Effects on physical and mental health. *Health Psychology, 13,* 195–212.—An excellent review of the literature (up to 1993) documenting dieting prevalence and an evaluation of the risks of dieting.

French, S. A., Jeffery, R. W., & Murray, D. (1999). Is dieting good for you?: Prevalence, duration and associated weight and behaviour changes for specific weight loss strategies over four years in US adults. *International Journal of Obesity, 23,* 320–327.—A rare longitudinal study looking at the relationship between dieting, weight-control behavior and weight change.

French, S. A., Story, M., Downes, B., Resnick, M. D., & Blum, R. W. (1995). Frequent dieting among adolescents: Psychosocial and health behavior correlates. *American Journal of Public Health, 85,* 695–701.—Epidemiology of adolescent dieting, with a description and explanation of associations with high-risk behavior.

Heatherton, T. F., Mahamedi, F., Striepe, M., Field, A. E., & Keel, P. K. (1997). A 10-year longitudinal study of body weight, dieting and eating disorder symptoms. *Journal of Abnormal Psychology, 106,* 117–125.—An even rarer study of the persistence of dieting and weight concern, with observation of an interesting gender difference.

Lee, S. (1993). How abnormal is the desire for thinness? A survey of eating attitudes and behaviour among Chinese undergraduates in Hong Kong. *Psychological Medicine, 23,* 437–451.—A good introduction to cultural differences in dieting, weight concerns, and eating disorders.

Neumark-Sztainer, D., & Hannan, P. (2000). Weight-related behaviours among adolescent girls and boys: Results from a national survey. *Archives of Paediatrics and Adolescent Medicine, 154,* 569–577.—A characterization of adolescent dieting in the 1990s evaluating effects of age, body weight, socioeconomic status, and ethnicity in girls and boys.

Wardle, J., Griffith, J., Johnson, F., & Rapoport, L. (2000). Intentional weight-control habits in a nationally representative sample of adults in the UK. *International Journal of Obesity, 24,* 534–540.—Interesting comparison between strategies applied to lose or watch weight and associated demographic variables.

# 15

# Experimental Studies of Dieting

## JANET POLIVY
## C. PETER HERMAN

The ubiquity of dieting in young women (see Chapter 14) has launched a series of experimental investigations into dieting and its effects. Various aspects of behavior and personality have been examined, ranging from the amount eaten by dieters versus nondieters in diverse situations, to their cognitive and/or emotional responses to food and nonfood stimuli, to their personalities and general temperament. Several different questionnaires for determining dieting status have been developed, including Herman and Polivy's Revised Restraint Scale (RRS), Stunkard and Messick's Three-Factor Eating Questionnaire (TFEQ, also named the Eating Inventory), and the Dutch Eating Behavior Questionnaire (DEBQ). The first of these scales identifies dieters who cycle between restricting their intake and overeating, whereas the other two scales have separate subscales for dietary restriction and disinhibition or emotional overeating, respectively. In this chapter, the various experimental studies comparing dieters and nondieters are described to determine what, if anything, we can conclude about the effects of chronic dieting. (Further discussion of dieting and its significance is included in Chapters 16 and 17.)

## EXPERIMENTAL STARVATION AND NORMAL DIETING

Experimental studies of dieting began with the work of Keys and his colleagues observing conscientious objectors to World War II who agreed to undergo experimental starvation (down to approximately 75% of their initial body weight). The changes described by these volunteers presage to a remarkable extent the subsequent literature describing the behavior of chronic dieters or restrained eaters. For example, the starving conscientious objectors were unable to concentrate, and reported being distractible and thinking more about food. Similarly, dieters are more distractible when performing a task requiring concentration, although they perform better than do nondieters if there are no competing cues. Chronic dieters also tend to think more about food, sometimes to the point of marked preoccupation. Dieters remember more weight- and food-related information (but less other information) about other people than do nondieters. On tests of cognitive bias or attention, such as the Stroop color–word-naming task, restrained eaters tend to become more disrupted by food and/or body-shape words, indicating a cognitive bias around food and body-shape issues, although the results vary (with some studies finding effects for food words, some for body-shape words, some for both, and a few finding no effects). In addition, dieters think about food differently, tending to categorize foods as either guilt-inducing or acceptable (and eating accordingly). Food stimuli also elicit more food- and weight-related thoughts in dieters.

At the emotional level, restrained eaters again resemble the conscientious objectors, who became progressively more irritable and emotionally volatile. Restrained eaters in the laboratory have been shown to be more emotionally responsive than unrestrained eaters, reacting more extremely to both positively and negatively valenced emotional cues. Studies of currently restricted dieters often find them to be irritable and emotionally labile. Moreover, in a recent study, participants who spent 4 weeks dieting for 4 days and then eating *ad libitum* for the other 3 days each week reported worsened mood, difficulty concentrating, irritability, and heightened fatigue when dieting.

## FOOD INTAKE AND BODY WEIGHT

There have been studies of dieters' food intake and body weight. In one of the earliest studies of weight loss and associated changes in taste perception, three investigators embarked on a diet designed to lower their body weight by 10%. They experienced an absence of negative alliesthesia (i.e., the normal response of finding sweet solutions less palatable following a sweet, high-calorie load). Normal dieters have also been shown to continue to find sweet solutions palatable after a glucose load, a phenomenon that may have some bearing on other aspects of their eating, as discussed below.

Studies of daily caloric intake, using the TFEQ, the DEBQ, or the RRS to identify dieters, generally find that they report eating less over a typical day than nondieters (although the recent division of TFEQ restraint into "flexible" versus "rigid" control shows that those with flexible control are more likely to report eating less). However, prospective studies of weight change in dieters generally find large fluctuations over time and little, if any, decrease in body weight. The resolution to this apparent paradox stems from the dieters' replacement of internally regulated (hunger-driven) eating with planned, cognitively determined, diet-approved eating. Unfortunately, ignoring internal hunger signals in order to adhere to a calorically reduced eating plan may result in the disruption of normal caloric regulation.

Not surprisingly, then, the eating behavior of chronic dieters or restrained eaters has been shown repeatedly to differ in important respects from the eating of nondieters. The studies of experimental starvation and prisoners of war found that periods of caloric restriction are frequently followed by bouts of overeating or even frank binge eating. More recently, laboratory investigations of eating behavior have shown that chronic dieters do not compensate for consuming a diet-breaking food high in calories by minimizing subsequent intake, as nondieters do after eating a large amount. Instead, dieters appear to become disinhibited and overeat; after being preloaded with fattening food, they eat *more* than do similarly treated nondieters or dieters who have not contravened their diets. In fact, it does not matter whether the initial food eaten was actually high in calories; as long as dieters *believe* that it was, they tend to overeat subsequently, when offered attractive food. Even simply planning to eat a diet-breaking meal later in the day unleashes consumption. This phenomenon has been called "counterregulation" (and has been viewed as an analogue of binge eating). This may reflect dieters' cognitively mediated abandonment of dieting once it is felt to be pointless, and it may be exacerbated by the absence of negative alliesthesia, so that the fattening food that breaks the diet remains highly palatable despite the prior consumption. Once dieters become disinhibited and counterregulate, they also become inaccurate at reporting their intake, underestimating consistently.

Chronically restrained eaters are susceptible to a variety of other stimuli. For example, dieters (even as young as 13 to 16 years) who are emotionally distressed, lonely, or dysphoric tend to eat more and snack more than do calm dieters or distressed nondieters, who often eat less when anxious or fearful than when calm. When confronted with an anxiety-producing threat to self-esteem, restrained eaters increase their food consumption. Two categories of explanation have been proposed to account for this heightened intake. A functional hypothesis suggests that increased eating temporarily counteracts or masks the dysphoria. Alternatively, stimulus sensitivity theories propose that distress shifts the dieter's attention to external stimulus properties (e.g., taste) and to activities stimulated by such external cues. Data supporting the former theory suggest that distressed dieters increase their intake of food regardless of taste properties and thus are relatively unaffected by the external stimulus properties of the food. This debate has yet to be resolved definitively. Furthermore, recent theorizing about self-control offers another possible explanation; ego strength depletion (such as might be entailed in facing a stressor or ego threat) causes subsequent self-regulatory failure. Placed in situations of internal conflict (such as an Asch conformity task), restrained eaters do indeed overeat relative to unrestrained eaters or conflict-free, restrained eaters.

Even watching an amusing film clip, thinking about or smelling attractive food, interacting with an attractive person, or being intoxicated (by alcohol) can stimulate overeating in dieters. When weighed on a scale doctored to indicate that they have gained weight, restrained eaters feel worse about themselves, become depressed, and in one study, also subsequently overate. In addition, chronic dieters report greater levels of cravings for foods, often those forbidden by their diet regimens. Dietary restraint thus seems to be fragile and easily disrupted. It is not so surprising, therefore, that chronically restrained eaters do not appear to be particularly successful at losing weight. While typically restricting their intake, occasional bouts of disinhibited eating cancel out the accumulated caloric deficit.

## NEGATIVE ASSOCIATIONS OF DIETING

Dieting has been shown to be associated with (other) maladaptive behaviors and states. Dieters often smoke cigarettes in an attempt to control their weight, and make fewer and shorter attempts to stop smoking, possibly because they gain more weight when they stop. Dieting has also been implicated in the etiology of both anorexia nervosa and bulimia nervosa, often beginning with an apparently normal attempt to diet (see Chapter 29).

Restrained eaters have lower self-esteem than do unrestrained eaters, and tend to report being more anxious and neurotic. They have also been shown to score higher on Ellis's irrational thoughts measure, to have unrealistic expectations about self-improvement following weight loss, to expect eating to reduce negative affect, and to have mothers who rate them as being less attractive than other girls. Finally, restrained eaters appear to be more suggestible than unrestrained eaters. Dieters seem to be insecure, uncertain of themselves and their internal state, and as a consequence, more vulnerable to social or environmental influences. Insensitivity to internal cues is a quality that dieting is likely to promote. Over time, ignoring hunger, a necessity previously discussed, may well progress to an insensitivity to other internal cues, with a correspondingly greater reliance on external/environmental cues.

## CONCLUSION

The literature on the effects of dieting suggests that while society may encourage and applaud weight loss, dieting has a variety of associations and consequences that suggest it is less than desirable for most people. Although the personality effects noted earlier are merely correlational, true experimental manipulations of dieting and correlational experiments on self-selected dieters are remarkably consistent in the picture they paint: Dieters are food-preoccupied, distractible, emotional, binge-prone, and unhappy. Longitudinal studies of children may help to identify factors that encourage them to diet and allow researchers to determine who is susceptible to dieting's more negative sequelae, as well as to separate causes from correlates.

## FURTHER READING

Heatherton, T. F., Striepe, M., & Wittenberg, L. (1998). Emotional distress and disinhibited eating: The role of self. *Personality and Social Psychology Bulletin, 24,* 301–313.—A recent experimental investigation of dieter–nondieter differences in eating in response to emotions of various types.

Keys, A., Brozek, J., Henschel, A., Mickelson, O., & Taylor, H. L. (1950). *The biology of human starvation* (2 vols.). Minneapolis: University of Minnesota Press.—This classic World War II study of normal-weight males who agreed to restrict their eating in order to lose 25% of their initial body weight, so that the effects of starvation could be studied, was the first experimental study of the effects of voluntary food restriction in order to lose weight (dieting).

Laessle, R. G., Platte, P., Schweiger, U., & Pirke, K. M. (1996). Biological and psychological correlates of intermittent dieting behavior in young women: A model for bulimia nervosa. *Physiology and Behavior, 60,* 1–5.—Study of alternating food restriction and *ad libitum* eating over a 4-week period.

Polivy, J. (1996). Psychological consequences of food restriction. *Journal of the American Dietetic Association, 96,* 589–594.—This paper reviews restraint research, concluding that food restriction, whether voluntary or involuntary, results in a tendency toward bingeing, heightened emotional responsiveness, cognitive disruptions, and higher stress levels.

Polivy, J., & Herman, C. P. (1999). The effects of resolving to diet on restrained and unrestrained eaters: The "false hope syndrome." *International Journal of Eating Disorders, 26,* 434–447.—An experimental induction of dieting behavior in chronic dieters and nondieters, identifying factors that contribute to failure to maintain self-change resolutions over the long term.

Westenhoefer, J., Stunkard, A. J., & Pudel, V. (1999). Validation of the flexible and rigid control dimensions of dietary restraint. *International Journal of Eating Disorders, 26,* 53–64.—A recent attempt to identify subgroups of restrained eaters with different dieting styles.

# 16

# Dietary Restraint and Overeating

## MICHAEL R. LOWE

Dietary restraint may be defined as a self-initiated attempt to restrict food intake for the purpose of weight control. Interest in dietary restraint has increased dramatically during the past 25 years because (1) previously observed differences in the behavior of normal-weight and overweight individuals appear to be better explained by co-occurring differences in restrained eating than by weight status; (2) there is concern about possible adverse effects of dieting among normal-weight people (and young women in particular), including the development of eating disorders; (3) the prevalence of obesity has risen rapidly in developed countries, spurring an increase in dietary efforts to counteract it.

This chapter addresses four topics: definitions of restrained eating and dieting; mechanisms of dietary restraint; dietary restraint and eating disorders; and dietary restraint and obesity. (Further discussion of dietary restraint and its significance is included in Chapters 15 and 17.)

## DEFINITIONS OF DIETARY RESTRAINT

It is important to distinguish the meaning ascribed to three interrelated terms used in this chapter: *restrained eating* (typically measured by one of three restraint scales); *dieting* (usually measured by single items assessing dieting status); and *dietary restraint* (a global term that refers to any type of attempted or actual self-imposed food restriction).

### Herman and Polivy's Restraint Scale

During the first decade of research on restrained eating, the construct was assessed with Herman and Polivy's 10-item Restraint Scale (RS). In a now-classic study, Herman and Mack found that restrained eaters increased, and unrestrained eaters decreased, their ice-cream consumption after drinking a high-calorie milkshake. The restrained eaters' response was labeled "counterregulatory eating." Subsequent studies identified similar differences between restrained and unrestrained eaters when negative affect was used in place of milkshakes. Herman and Polivy attributed these results to the disinhibitory impact of these stimuli on restrained eaters' cognitively mediated restrictions on their eating.

In the mid-1980s, investigators began to question the adequacy of the RS. It was criticized because (1) nearly all its items describe either weight fluctuations or concerns about eating and overeating; that is, despite its name, the RS does not actually contain items that describe restrained eating or dieting behaviors; (2) it is not a unitary measure (factor analyses show that, depending on the sample, it contains two or more factors); (3) it suffers from criterion confounding, since it partially measures the phenomena (overeating and overconcern about eating and weight) that it is meant to predict; (4) overweight individuals experience larger weight fluctuations than normal-weight people; thus, its inclusion of weight-fluctuation items confounds restraint with overweight; (5) it does not predict naturalistic caloric restriction; and (6) its internal consistency among overweight individuals is low. These shortcomings led to the development of two additional measures of restrained eating and to increased research on dieting.

## Other Measures of Restrained Eating

The two newer measures of restrained eating are the Eating Inventory (formerly called the Three-Factor Eating Questionnaire)—Cognitive Restraint scale (EI-CR) and Dutch Eating Behavior Questionnaire—Restrained Eating scale (DEBQ-R). Both scales measure specific behavioral and cognitive strategies for reducing food intake and have sound psychometric properties. Restrained eaters selected by these two scales tend to eat less than unrestrained eaters in the natural environment. However, they do not show the counter-regulatory eating exhibited by restrained eaters selected using the RS.

Recent research has led to further distinctions among restrained eaters selected by the EI-CR. A factor analysis of the EI-CR identified two factors, labeled "rigid control" and "flexible control." The rigid control subscale is associated with high levels of overeating and weight, whereas the opposite is true of the flexible control subscale. The second distinction involves distinguishing between restrained eaters (assessed with the EI-CR or DEBQ-R scales) who are high or low in susceptibility to failure of restraint. Research has shown that those who score high in EI-CR restraint but are susceptible to failure of restraint (i.e., who also score high on a measure of disinhibitory eating) exhibit overeating in the same context that induces overeating in restrained eaters assessed with the RS. However, those who score high in EI-CR restraint, but low in disinhibition, successfully limit the amount of food they eat. This indicates that restraint does not always undermine eating control and suggests that restraint and overeating coexist in only a subset of weight-conscious people.

## Dieting to Lose Weight

In restraint theory "restrained eating" and "dieting" are viewed synonymously. However, research has shown that these two phenomena are neither semantically nor functionally equivalent. One study found that most restrained eaters on the RS are not currently dieting to lose weight. Furthermore, the currently dieting subgroup shows an eating pattern opposite to that shown by RS restrained eaters in earlier research. That is, current dieters have been found to *reduce* their food intake significantly following a high-calorie preload. Additional evidence indicates that the appetitive responses of RS restrained eaters differ from those of actual dieters in other ways (e.g., on sweetness preferences and salivary output). Thus, a thorough understanding of the effects of dietary restraint requires that one know if someone is currently dieting (and if so, whether it is to lose, or to avoid gaining, weight). If dieting to lose weight is assessed via self-report, it is also important to determine if such reports actually reflect a reduction of intake below energy needs (thereby increasing the likelihood of physiological adjustments to the diet).

## MECHANISMS OF DIETARY RESTRAINT

Restraint theory proposes that (RS) restrained eaters impose a "diet boundary" on themselves to try to align their food intake with their weight-control aspirations. Such efforts are thought to produce frustration (because of self-denial of favored foods) and stress (from constantly trying to control a biologically based drive). Frequent past cycles of undereating and overeating are also assumed to impair normal hunger and satiety responses. Thus, when restrained eaters breach the diet boundary, they abandon restraint and continue to eat until their elevated satiety boundary is reached.

A problem with this conceptualization is that it assumes that restrained eating and disinhibitory eating go hand in hand; that is, that dietary restraint sows the seeds of its own destruction by producing overeating. While this does appear to be the case under certain circumstances (as shown in the classic Keys study of semistarvation), it is far from invariable. Furthermore, studies using other common measures of restrained eating (the EI-CR, the DEBQ-R, or self-report measures of current dieting) indicate that these scales, which measure actual dieting behavior, are not associated with disinhibitory eating.

These findings highlight two important issues for future research. The first is why some individuals high in dietary restraint are vulnerable to disinhibitory eating or other forms of overeating (e.g., binge eating), whereas others are not. The second is to determine the direction of this association. Since weight-conscious people are likely, at least temporarily, to restrict their food intake following overeating, such overeating could produce reactive dieting rather than—or in addition to—dieting producing overeating.

## DIETARY RESTRAINT AND EATING DISORDERS

Research on the relationship between dieting and the development of eating disorders is characterized by both consensus and controversy. There is consensus that strict dieting and weight loss usually constitute an early step in the development of both anorexia nervosa and bulimia nervosa (see Chapter 29), although little is known about why some individuals with an incipient eating disorder are able to maintain strict control over their eating (most of those who develop anorexia nervosa), whereas others subsequently begin to binge eat. More controversial is the extent to which dieting per se (i.e., in the absence of other risk factors) raises the chances of developing an eating disorder. One model (the continuity or dimensional viewpoint) suggests that risk of developing an eating disorder is proportional to the intensity of dieting. Many studies among college students have found an association between more intensive dieting and the likelihood of reporting eating disorder symptoms. The other model (the discontinuity or categorical viewpoint) suggests that dieting leads to the development of eating disorders only in the presence of other risk factors (see Chapter 44). A study of college females found that, contrary to the continuity model, neither (RS) restrained eaters nor self-identified current dieters engaged in clinically meaningful binge eating. Similarly, a study using the best method (taxometrics) for distinguishing whether a disorder is dimensional or categorical in nature found evidence for categorical (i.e., qualitative) differences in eating disorder symptoms between bulimic individuals and female college students.

## DIETARY RESTRAINT AND OBESITY

The development of restraint theory was based on the idea that previously observed behavioral differences between normal weight and overweight individuals were due to overweight individuals being more restrained in their eating. This reasoning was supported by the demonstration that normal-weight (RS) restrained eaters differed from unrestrained eaters in ways that paralleled previously found obese–normal differences in behavior. However, while this is true of some phenomena such as salivary output and emotional reactivity, it is now clear that it does not apply to the counterregulatory eating shown by restrained eaters (i.e., among college students, neither overweight individuals in general nor overweight restrained eaters show counterregulation in laboratory experiments). On the other hand, a study revealed that overweight clinic attendees exhibited the classical counterregulatory behavior pattern. Furthermore, extent of counterregulation was directly proportional to intensity of binge eating problems in these women. These results have two implications. First, overweight clinic attendees, but not overweight college students, may demonstrate counterregulatory eating because the former experience far more binge eating than the latter. Second, since the clinic attendees had not yet begun their diets, these findings raise additional questions about the causal role of dieting in producing counterregulatory eating.

More straightforward are findings regarding the traditional meaning of dietary restraint in overweight individuals, that is, dieting to lose weight. Research has shown that behavioral programs for obesity (which involve increased dietary restraint) do not promote overeating; rather, they result in weight loss, at least in the short-term (see Chapter 94).

## CONCLUSIONS

From its inception 25 years ago, research on dietary restraint has progressed considerably. We now know that "restraint" is not a unitary phenomenon but describes a variety of practices that have divergent effects on behavior. While the RS was successful in identifying the intriguing phenomenon of disinhibitory eating, we still lack a theoretically consistent explanation for this eating pattern. Dieting appears to be causally linked to the development of eating disorders, but whether this link is dependent on the co-occurrence of other risk factors remains unknown. The parallels originally proposed between restrained eating and obesity have been partially supported, and there is evidence that the counterregulatory eating pattern is closely related to binge-eating tendencies in overweight individuals. Future research is needed to identify why only some restrained eaters are susceptible to disinhibition and to clarify the causal direction of the relationship between dietary restraint and overeating where it exists.

## FURTHER READING

Brownell, K. D., & Rodin, J. (1994). The dieting maelstrom: Is it possible and advisable to lose weight? *American Psychologist, 49,* 781–791.—An analysis of the risks and benefits of weight-loss dieting.

French, S. A., & Jeffrey, R. W. (1994). Consequences of dieting to lose weight: Effects on physical and mental health. *Health Psychology, 13,* 195–212.—A comprehensive review of the effects of dieting to lose weight on physical and mental health.

Gleaves, D. H., Lowe, M. R., Snow, A. C., Green, B. A., & Murphy-Eberenz, K. P. (2000). Continuity and discontinuity models of bulimia nervosa: A taxometric investigation. *Journal of Abnormal Psychology, 109,* 56–68.—A review of the continuity and discontinuity models of bulimia nervosa, including the first test of these models using taxometric methods.

Herman, C. P., & Mack, D. (1975). Restrained and unrestrained eating. *Journal of Personality, 43,* 647–660.—The original, classic study demonstrating counterregulatory eating in restrained eaters.

Herman, C. P., & Polivy, J. (1984). A boundary model for the regulation of eating. In A. J. Stunkard & E. Stellar (Eds.), *Eating and its disorders* (pp. 141–156). New York: Raven Press.—A cognitive model for understanding the effects of restrained eating on hunger, satiety, and the regulation of eating.

Keys, A., Brozek, K., Henschel, A., Mickelson, O., & Taylor, H. L. (1950). *The biology of human starvation.* Minneapolis: University of Minnesota Press.—The classic study of the psychological and biological effects of extensive weight loss induced by semistarvation.

Lowe, M. R. (1993). The effects of dieting on eating behavior: A three-factor model. *Psychological Bulletin, 114,* 100–121.—A critical review of literature on restrained eating and a proposal for a new, multifactorial model of dieting.

Ruderman, A. J. (1986). Dietary restraint: A theoretical and empirical review. *Psychological Bulletin, 99,* 247–262.—A detailed review of restraint theory and the empirical literature supporting it.

Tuschl, R. J. (1990). From dietary restraint to binge eating: Some theoretical considerations. *Appetite, 14,* 105–109.—A brief overview of the evidence for and against a causal relationship between dieting and binge eating.

Westenhoefer, J., Stunkard, A. J., & Pudel, V. (1999) Validation of the flexible and rigid control dimensions of dietary restraint. *International Journal of Eating Disorders, 26,* 53–64.—A study validating the two factors (rigid and flexible restraint) of the EI-CR.

# 17

# The Controversy over Dieting

## G. TERENCE WILSON

For decades, dieting was the thing to do. The assumption that dieting would lead to the twin advantages of better health and improved looks was held as a self-evident truth. More recently, however, the effects of dieting have been called into question. Critics have charged that dieting is ineffective at best, and damaging to health at worst. These criticisms have been the rationale for such extreme recommendations as the call for a moratorium on weight loss programs. In a related fashion, dieting has been indicted as an element of societal oppression in some feminist critiques of the development of eating disorders and problems in weight regulation.

Too often lost in the controversy over dieting is the understanding of what precisely is said to be good or bad. From a scientific perspective, it is unhelpful to ask whether dieting helps or harms people. The more useful question is what are the effects of the various forms of dieting (namely, self-imposed restriction in food energy intake), in whom, and when undertaken for what purpose? (Further discussion of dieting and its significance is included in Chapters 15 and 16.)

## DIETING AND INTENTIONAL WEIGHT LOSS IN OBESE ADULTS

Scientifically based weight control programs have long eschewed "fad diets" as quick and easy solutions to losing weight. Often these diets are of dubious nutritional value, if not downright hazardous to health. Modern behavioral weight control treatments emphasize change in nutrition as one of several components of a comprehensive program aimed at lifestyle modification, including increased physical activity (see Chapter 94). The goal is a balanced but flexible diet that emphasizes reduced saturated fat and increased complex carbohydrates. Overall caloric intake is intentionally restricted to one degree or another to produce a negative energy balance. Some programs include a very-low-calorie diet (VLCD) as an interim stage in the overall program (see Chapter 96).

Comprehensive weight control programs that combine dietary modification with increased exercise and other lifestyle changes are effective in producing significant weight loss in people with mild-to-moderate obesity. This weight loss is successfully maintained by roughly two-thirds of patients in the short term, although long-term (5-year) follow-ups reveal that almost all patients revert to their baseline weights. (See Chapters 106 and 107 for discussion of maintenance of weight loss in obesity.) Extreme critics of dietary interventions have branded these sophisticated, multicomponent weight control programs as harmful to health, devastating to psychological well-being, and iatrogenic in initiating or exacerbating binge eating.

## Effects on Weight and Health

A pattern of recurrent weight gains and losses has been identified as weight cycling or what is more popularly known as "yo-yo dieting." The putative negative effects of weight cycling are alleged to include reduction in lean body mass relative to body fat; enhanced metabolic efficiency, making future weight loss even more difficult, or even leading to still greater obesity; and increased risk of cardiovascular disease. Whether the gradual weight loss produced by state-of-the-art behavioral treatment programs, followed by gradual regain, often extending over a period of a year or more, is an example of yo-yo dieting is questionable. It would appear to be markedly different from the rapid loss of relatively large amounts of weight that have been studied in animal models of weight cycling. Most research has concluded that there is no consistent evidence linking weight cycling to changes in metabolism or body composition.

The evidence on health outcomes in people, despite inconsistencies, does suggest that weight variability has a negative impact on all-cause mortality, and particularly cardiovascular mortality (see Chapter 88). However, drawing causal inferences from existing studies linking variability in weight to health outcomes is fraught with difficulties. One problem is determining whether the cycles of weight loss were voluntary or not. The possibility that weight loss reflected an existing illness is difficult to discount. In a study of the longevity of Harvard alumni, researchers found that variability in weight predicted early mortality. The data also clearly showed that the more obese the alumni, the higher their risk of mortality from all causes, and particularly from coronary heart disease.

## Psychological Effects

Behavioral weight control programs have typically resulted in favorable short-term psychological effects, including significant reductions in depression and enhanced self-esteem. At worst, no deterioration in mood has been documented. Critics have asserted that subsequent relapse, the experience of most patients who lose weight, can have negative psychological consequences. Yet studies have failed to show a significant relationship between increased psychological distress and weight regain following treatment-induced loss.

The data indicate that many instances of weight regain are accompanied by a return to baseline levels of mood and self-esteem. However, evidence from prospective research also shows that reductions in depressed mood can be maintained over follow-up despite total weight regain.

## Effects on Binge Eating

It is commonly believed that the treatment of obesity, which involves dietary restriction, will contribute to the development of binge eating. However, the evidence from treatment studies consistently demonstrates that moderate caloric restriction does not trigger binge eating in obese adults. Studies of behavioral treatment with severe caloric restriction (VLCD) have yielded similar results. Only one study has shown any indications of apparent VCLD-induced binge eating during the refeeding period. The binge-eating episodes in this study were transient.

A compelling test of the hypothesis that dieting causes or exacerbates binge eating is provided by the results of behavioral weight loss treatments for patients with binge eating disorder (BED), an eating disorder characterized by recurrent binge eating but without the compensatory behavior (e.g., purging) that defines bulimia nervosa (see Chapter 31). At least in the short term, behavioral weight loss treatment with either moderate or severe caloric restriction has proved effective in reducing binge eating and associated eating disorder psychopathology in BED patients (see Chapter 63). Longer-term studies of the impact of weight loss treatment in these patients are needed before any definitive conclusion can be reached.

## DIETING AND INTENTIONAL WEIGHT LOSS IN NORMAL-WEIGHT PERSONS

Persons of normal weight show reactions to dieting that differ markedly from those seen in overweight or obese people. The negative effects of extreme dieting were shown by Keys and colleagues' study of young men on a semistarvation diet that resulted in the loss of roughly 25% of their body weight. Extreme negative emotional reactions were common. More conventional, self-initiated dieting is also associated with adverse psychological effects in young women of normal weight. Cross-sectional studies of adolescent girls have indicated that, independent of the effect of body weight itself, dietary restraint is correlated with feelings of failure, lowered self-esteem, and depressive symptoms. Dieting has also been shown to predict stress; however, stress is not a predictor of dieting.

## DOES DIETING CAUSE EATING DISORDERS?

### Dieting as a Risk Factor

Dieting is clearly linked to the development of anorexia nervosa and bulimia nervosa in young women. Eating disorders are most common in the specific groups that are most involved in dieting and weight loss—predominantly white, middle- to upper-class women. An overall correlation exists between cultural pressure to be thin and prevalence of eating disorders both across and within different ethnic groups. More importantly, prospective studies have also linked dieting to the development of eating disorders. In a representative sample of 15-year-old schoolgirls in London, dieters were eight times more likely than nondieters to develop an eating disorder within 1 year. Similarly, in a population-based study of adolescents in Australia, Patton and colleagues showed that girls defined as severe dieters were 18 times more likely than nondieters to develop an eating disorder (broadly defined) within 6 months. Even moderate dieters were at risk compared with nondieters.

Clinical descriptions consistently indicate that patients with bulimia nervosa typically report that their binge eating began after they started to diet. However, both clinical and community-based studies have shown that in a subset of women, binge eating may precede dieting.

Dieting may not be a risk factor for obese patients with BED. These patients reliably report less dietary restraint than bulimia nervosa patients. Moreover, a large percentage report that their binge eating preceded dieting. These findings, taken in conjunction with data indicating that even severe caloric restriction does not exacerbate existing binge eating in obese patients, suggest that dieting has quite different effects in obese and normal-weight individuals.

## Dieting Alone Does Not Cause Eating Disorders

Some investigators consider dieting to be a necessary but not sufficient cause of eating disorders. Others question whether dieting is simply an antecedent with no causal significance. The available data do not provide a definitive answer to this question. In linking dieting to the development of disordered eating and eating disorders, it is important to be aware of the different types of dieting and dieters. Dieters vary both in their eating patterns and in what they eat. A subgroup of restrained eaters who appear to have achieved stable, long-term weights that are lower than their previous weights have been called "successful dieters" or "weight suppressors." They differ functionally from other restrained eaters in that they do not show counterregulation in the laboratory. It has been suggested that some forms of dietary restraint are more likely to disrupt eating habits than others, and that the more chaotic the everyday eating behavior, the higher the risk of developing an eating disorder.

It must also be noted that most adolescent and young adult women in Western countries diet (see Chapter 14), yet the lifetime prevalence for bulimia nervosa in women is estimated to be 1.5% to 2.0 % (see Chapter 41). Some other factor(s) must interact with dieting to cause eating disorders. These risk factors may range from genetic predisposition and biological vulnerability to personality and individual psychopathological factors, to familial influences (see Chapters 42, 43, and 44).

## MECHANISMS LINKING DIETING TO BULIMIA NERVOSA

Dieting has various biological, cognitive, and affective consequences that may predispose persons to binge eating. Among biological effects, short-term dieting in women produces an increase in the prolactin response to the administration of L-tryptophan, which is a marker of disturbance in brain serotonin levels. Several other lines of evidence suggest that dysfunctional serotonergic mechanisms play a role in the maintenance of eating disorders (see Chapter 49).

At the cognitive level, unrealistically rigid standards of dietary restraint coupled with a sense of deprivation may leave dieters vulnerable to loss of control after perceived or actual transgression of their diet (see Chapters 15, 16, and 18). A lapse leads to an "all-or-nothing" cognitive reaction. In this phenomenon, the person attributes the lapse to a complete inability to maintain control, abandons all attempts to regulate food intake, and temporarily overeats. Dieting can also be associated with different conditioning processes that may predispose a person to binge eating. For example, it may increase the appeal of "forbidden" or "binge" foods (typically those high in fat and sugar) directly by nutritional preference conditioning.

## FURTHER READING

Cowen, P. J., Anderson, I. M., & Fairburn, C. G. (1992). Neurochemical effects of dieting: Relevance to changes in eating and affective disorders. In G. H. Anderson & S. H. Kennedy (Eds.), *The biology of feast and famine* (pp. 269–284). New York: Academic Press.—A review of dieting's effects on serotonin in men and women.

Fairburn, C. G., Welch, S. L., Doll, H. A., Davies, B. A., & O'Connor, M. E. (1997). Risk factors for bulimia nervosa: A community-based case-control study. *Archives of General Psychiatry, 54*, 509–517.—Well-controlled epidemiological investigation of risk factors, including dieting, for bulimia nervosa.

Foster, G. D., Wadden, T. A., Kendall, P. C., Stunkard, A. J., & Vogt, R. A. (1996). Psychological effects of weight loss and regain: A prospective evaluation. *Journal of Consulting and Clinical Psychology, 64*, 752–757.—A controlled, prospective study of the effects of weight loss and subsequent weight regain on psychological functioning in obese patients.

French, S. A., & Jeffery, R. W. (1994). Consequences of dieting to lose weight: Effects on physical and mental health. *Health Psychology, 13*, 195–212.—Review of psychological effects of dieting in overweight and obese individuals.

Howard, C. E., & Porzelius, L. K. (1999). The role of dieting in binge eating disorder: Etiology and treatment implications. *Clinical Psychology Review, 19*, 25–44.—A review of the role of dieting in the development, maintenance, and modification of binge eating disorder.

Hsu, L. K. G. (1990). *Eating disorders.* New York: Guilford Press.—Thorough review of the association between dieting and eating disorders.

Keys, A., Brozek, K., Henschel, A., Mickelson, O., & Taylor, H. L. (1950). *The biology of human starvation.* Minneapolis: University of Minnesota Press.—Classic study of the psychological and biological effects of extensive weight loss induced by semistarvation.

National Task Force on the Prevention and Treatment of Obesity. (1994). Weight cycling. *Journal of the American Medical Association, 272*, 1196–1201.—Review of the literature on the effects of weight cycling in humans.

National Task Force on the Prevention and Treatment of Obesity. (2000). Dieting and the development of eating disorders in overweight and obese adults. *Archives of Internal Medicine, 160*, 2581–2589.—Critical review of dieting and the development of binge eating in obese adults.

Patton, G. C., Selzer, R., Coffey, C., Carlin, B., & Wolfe, R. (1999). Onset of adolescent eating disorders: Population-based cohort study over 3 years. *British Medical Journal, 318*, 765–768.—Prospective, population-based study of adolescents in Australia linking dieting to the onset of eating disorders.

Smaller, J. W., Wadden, T. A., & Stunkard, A. J. (1987). Dieting and depression: A critical review. *Journal of Psychosomatic Research, 31*, 429–440.—Summary of psychological effects of treatment-induced weight loss.

# 18

# The Psychology of Binge Eating

## GLENN WALLER

Binge eating is found in a range of eating disorders (bulimia nervosa, binge eating disorder, anorexia nervosa of the binge–purge subtype, atypical cases; see Chapters 28 and 30 for a discussion of the classification of eating disorders), but it is also found widely in the nonclinical female population. It is important to consider issues of definition. Objective binge eating has two components—the consumption of a large amount of food over a relatively short period of time and the sensation of loss of control during that ingestion. These components are not always linked. Many patients describe subjective "binges," which involve eating relatively small amounts of food and where loss of control is the distressing component. Others have behaviors that have been described as "grazing" (eating a large amount but over a long period of time, and with no perceived loss of control). The present review focuses on objective binges as the unit of analysis, since such eating creates the greatest level of distress and physical damage. Objective binges are also the best understood of the overeating phenomena.

In order to explain the behaviors that contribute to the onset and maintenance of binge eating, it is necessary to understand the interlinking behavioral, cognitive, affective, and interpersonal systems. The most comprehensive framework for understanding these factors from a psychological perspective is functional analysis—the explanation of behaviors in the context of their antecedents, consequences, and environmental setting. While such an approach is independent of theory, it most closely relates to a cognitive-behavioral analysis. This conclusion follows from the fact that cognitive-behavioral psychology has developed as an explanatory theory (generating models and predictions that are capable of being disproved), whereas other theoretical stances tend to be descriptive (involving post hoc rationalization of behavioral manifestations). At one end of the spectrum, cognitive-behavioral models are supported by evidence from a range of naturalistic, correlational, and experimental studies derived from theory; at the other, they are supported by impressive evidence from trials of cognitive-behavioral therapies. Finally, the cognitive-behavioral approach to understanding eating disorders is able to explain the route of effect of other influences on bulimic behaviors (e.g., social factors, trauma history).

## PSYCHOLOGICAL FACTORS IN A FUNCTIONAL
## ANALYSIS OF BINGE EATING

Understanding binge eating as a behavior in context is dependent upon identifying the role of its antecedents and consequences. However, it is critical to divide these contextual features into the proximal and the distal components. It is also important to consider mediating and moderating factors, since these can often explain the role of environmental correlates. Mediators are "carrier" mechanisms, which explain the link between an independent variable and a dependent variable (e.g., if parenting plays a causal role in the development of a child's depressed mood, it might be that this link is explained by the parenting that causes the child to experience poor self-esteem). Moderators are those factors that influence the strength of the link between independent and dependent variables (e.g., the impact of parenting upon childhood depression might be reduced if the child has a supportive peer group). Both mediators and moderators are important targets for therapeutic interventions.

### Distal Antecedents (Predisposing Factors)

Many "background" factors have been cited as relevant to the etiology of binge eating (see Chapter 44). These influences do not directly induce binge eating but are hypothesized to predispose the individual to this behavior. These factors include social (e.g., media portrayal, peer influences; see Chapter 19), familial (e.g., attachment, parenting, family interaction), interpersonal (e.g., neglect, abuse), and psychological (e.g., core beliefs, poor self-esteem, poor locus of control, perfectionism) factors. However, the supporting research suffers from a number of central flaws. First, most of the studies involved do not establish causality, since the widespread use of cross-sectional designs means that the findings can be explained as easily using correlational models. There are a few longitudinal studies that overcome this problem, and these broadly support the cross-sectional findings (e.g., an early pattern of restriction followed by more bulimic attitudes). However, far more extensive, theory-based, prospective studies are needed.

Second, the findings are not specific to binge eating. The literature on factors such as trauma and parenting style suggests that they can best be understood as general risk factors for psychopathology, and for emotional and behavioral disturbances, rather than specific risk factors (see Chapter 44). Similarly, while it is possible to argue that the social presentation of "ideal" physical shapes contributes to the dissatisfaction that is common among persons with eating disorders, it is far more likely that this is a predisposing factor for general eating psychopathology than for binge eating per se.

Finally, this literature is not clear about differentiating the range of potential antecedents. The usual assumption is that the variables studied as predisposing factors are causal agents or mediators that arise from those agents, whereas they might better be understood as moderators of any true causal links. For example, whereas particular forms of parenting have been suggested to be pathogenic, they might be seen equally well as influencing the impact of other factors. Similarly, trauma might be best understood as moderating the impact of other distal antecedents (rather than being an antecedent in its own right), "steering" the pathology toward the use of escape-blocking behaviors (such as binge eating). A number of problems arise from ignoring this moderating role. In particular, the assumption that such factors are pathogenic in their own right leads us to discount the potential positive role of moderating factors that can be protective as well as problematic (e.g., the role of positive parenting).

## Proximal Antecedents (Immediate Triggers)

There is much more convincing causal evidence for the immediate triggers and consequences of binge eating. Food restriction and negative emotional states trigger bingeing and may have their greatest impact on eating when they coincide. It has been suggested that binges are triggered more by physiological states (hunger, starvation, and cravings) early on in the course of the eating disorder, but that the triggers shift more toward the affective states later in the disorder (as the individual learns through experience the emotional "blocking" consequences of binge eating; see below). Negative social interactions have also been identified as immediate triggers for binge eating, although their mechanism of action is most likely to be mediated by emotional states.

The conventional cognitive-behavioral account of the maintenance of bulimia nervosa suggests that the most important antecedent process for binge eating (and the other parts of the bulimic cycle) is primarily cognitive. Patients set themselves complex and strict dietary rules, which they fail to achieve (often with no resulting physiological deprivation). They interpret these "lapses" as evidence of their inability to control their eating. In turn, this perceived inability leads to their temporary abandonment of control over eating, manifested in binge eating. However, this model cannot explain how all binges are triggered, and it is important to take into account the role of emotional factors (as well as the interaction of starvation and affect). Bulimia nervosa patients report that at least 50% of their binges are affect-driven rather than hunger-driven. The emotional states that have been linked to binge eating are often socially driven and include loneliness, anxiety, anger, boredom, and (to a lesser extent) depression.

## Proximal Consequences

The short-term reinforcing consequences of binge eating are best understood relative to the antecedents identified earlier. First, the eating reduces aversive hunger and starvation levels (and can be pleasurable in itself). Second, the uncontrolled nature of binge eating allows the individual to block awareness of intolerable cognitive and affective states (e.g., abandonment beliefs and loneliness). Finally, the individual can avoid considering the social and interpersonal situations (e.g., loss of relationships) that have led to those cognitive and emotional states. It is noteworthy that a large number of binge eaters find it hard to identify immediate antecedents and consequences due to the blocking of broader awareness by the focus on food. Thus, many binge eaters are unable to identify the factors that play the strongest role in initiating and maintaining the behavior.

It is doubtful whether binge eating is a unique "escape behavior." It can be argued that a range of other behaviors (e.g., self-harm, alcohol abuse, shoplifting, risky sexual behavior) serve the same cognitive–emotional blocking function, and there is strong evidence that such impulsive behaviors tend to cluster. The use of binge eating (rather than another behavior) by an individual at a specific time is likely to be explained best by experiential and situational variables. For example, food tends to be relatively easily available, and binge eating has comparatively immediate but short-term blocking effects. In contrast, alcohol may be less immediately available and getting drunk takes longer to have its effect than bingeing, but the blocking effect lasts longer. Thus, the choice of blocking behavior may depend on what was modeled during the individual's development (e.g., parents who used food to pacify their child's emotions); the individual's ability to tolerate distress (e.g., to wait until the preferred blocking behavior is available vs. using a less preferred behavior more immediately); the social and practical availability of the blocking behavior (e.g., it may be more acceptable to binge eat during the working day but to binge on alcohol socially); and the intensity and duration of effect that is desired.

## Distal Consequences and Maintenance Processes

Following its immediate consequences (reduction of aversive cognitive, emotional, and starvation states), binge eating has a number of longer-term consequences. The most obvious is that binges are commonly (but not universally) followed by efforts at purging and compensation. These behaviors themselves often serve dual functions, both reducing anxiety about weight gain and reestablishing personal and emotional control. For example, exercise can both compensate for food ingested and establish a dissociative state. However, it is also necessary to remember that the bingeing (and the purging/compensatory behaviors) become self-maintaining by adding to the unhealthy cognitions, emotions, and social situations that initially drove the binge eating. Those cognitions are present at a range of levels, including unconditional, schema-level representations (e.g., defectiveness, social isolation) and conditional-level beliefs (e.g., dysfunctional assumptions regarding food, shape, and weight). The emotions that are enhanced by the bulimic behaviors (and that enhance further blocking behaviors) include shame, loneliness, poor self-esteem, and depression. Finally, the binge eating maintains itself by encouraging purging and compensatory dietary restraint, which return the individual to attempted or actual dietary restriction and (in some cases) the starvation/hunger state.

## IMPLICATIONS FOR PSYCHOLOGICAL THEORY AND THERAPIES

These psychological models of binge eating are of the greatest use when they generate testable hypotheses regarding treatment. Our understanding of cognitive and interpersonal issues has generated treatments that can (if applied properly) reduce or halt binge eating in the majority of cases of bulimia nervosa and binge eating disorder (see Chapters 54, 57, and 63). The challenge now is to determine how to develop psychologically based treatments that add to this level of success—particularly among those patients who do not benefit from existing therapies and those who do not meet these diagnostic criteria (e.g., bulimic anorexics, atypical cases). These treatment developments will require us to extend our understanding of the range of cognitive representations and their link to affect, behavior, and interpersonal difficulties. Thus, they should also improve our understanding of the psychology of the broad range of eating behaviors. Such work will also help to determine the utility of our psychological models of binge eating across different ages and cultures, since there has been little research on the generalizability of such models to date.

## FURTHER READING

Cooper, M. (1997). Cognitive theory in anorexia nervosa and bulimia nervosa: A review. *Behavioural and Cognitive Psychotherapy*, *25*, 113–145.—Offers a critique of the empirical and conceptual base of theories regarding the eating disorders, including the need to extend our models to include a broader range of triggers to binge eating.

Fairburn, C. G. (1997). Eating disorders. In D. M. Clark & C. G. Fairburn (Eds.), *Science and practice of cognitive behaviour therapy* (pp. 209–241). Oxford, UK: Oxford University Press.—Outlines the most clearly established model of bulimia nervosa, used as the basis for most cognitive-behavioral therapy in this disorder.

Heatherton, T. F., & Baumeister, R. F. (1991). Binge eating as escape from self-awareness. *Psychological Bulletin*, *110*, 86–108.—Review article examining evidence that binge eating is a consequence of the disinhibition that follows efforts to avoid negative self-awareness (rather than being a blocking behavior per se).

McManus, F., & Waller, G. (1995). A functional analysis of binge eating. *Clinical Psychology Review*, *15*, 845–863.—This review outlines the way in which binge eating can be a result of different antecedents and consequences. It brings together starvation, blocking, and "escape from awareness" explanations to construct a model of the development and maintenance of binge eating.

Meyer, C., Waller, G., & Waters, A. (1998). Emotional states and bulimic psychopathology. In H. Hoek, M. Katzman & J. Treasure (Eds.), *The neurobiological basis of eating disorders* (pp. 271–289). Chichester, UK: Wiley.—Reviews the evidence that affect plays a role in the etiology and maintenance of bulimic behaviors and considers possible neurobiological mechanisms that might underpin this relationship.

Root, M. P. P., & Fallon, P. (1989). Treating the victimized bulimic. *Journal of Interpersonal Violence*, *4*, 90–100.—Although derived specifically from a traumatized population, this paper considers the range of functions that binge eating can serve.

Steiger, H., Gauvin, L., Jabalpurwala, S., Séguin, J. R., & Stotland, S. (1999). Hypersensitivity to social interactions in bulimic syndromes: Relationship to binge eating. *Journal of Consulting and Clinical Psychology*, *67*, 765–775.—Demonstrates the impact of negative social/interpersonal experiences on binge eating.

Vitousek, K. M. (1996). The current status of cognitive-behavioral models of anorexia nervosa and bulimia nervosa. In P. M. Salkovskis (Ed.), *Frontiers of cognitive therapy* (pp. 383–418). New York: Guilford Press.—Reviews the role of cognitive-behavioral therapy in anorexic and bulimic disorders, highlighting evidence of its impressive impact upon binge eating.

# 19

# Sociocultural Influences on Body Image and Eating Disturbance

## ERIC STICE

Sociocultural influences have long been suspected of promoting disturbances of body image and eating. These sociocultural pressures center around the idealization of thinness and physical fitness, and the disparagement of overweight, and they primarily originate from the mass media, family, and peers.

## THEORIES OF SOCIOCULTURAL INFLUENCE

Sociologists have proposed two processes by which socialization agents may promote attitudes and behavior: social reinforcement and modeling. Social reinforcement refers to the process whereby people internalize attitudes and exhibit behaviors approved of by respected others. Within the domain of body image and eating disturbance, social reinforcement could be defined as comments or actions of others that serve to support and perpetuate the thin–ideal body image for women. For example, an adolescent girl may be more likely to pursue an ultraslender physique through dieting if she perceives the mass media as glorifying slenderness. Social reinforcement of the thin–ideal might also be manifest by socialization agents who are preoccupied by their weight, engage in dieting, or criticize overweight people. Theoretically, social reinforcement of the thin–ideal promotes an internalization of this ideal and thereby body dissatisfaction. These factors in turn are thought to result in dieting and negative affect, which increase the risk for the emergence of unhealthy weight control behaviors and eating pathology.

Modeling, on the other hand, refers to the process wherein individuals directly emulate behaviors they observe. For instance, a woman may be more likely to use laxatives for weight control if she sees a peer engage in this behavior. Socialization agents may also model preoccupation with body dimensions, excessive dieting, unhealthy weight-control behaviors, and binge eating. Observing others engage in disordered eating behaviors might also give the impression that these behaviors are normative, which might make it more likely that they will be emulated.

Social psychologists have also suggested that social comparison plays an important role in the adverse effects of exposure to media-portrayed thin–ideal images. According to this account, individuals compare themselves to these idealized images of beauty and judge themselves lacking (an upward social comparison), which promotes body dissatisfaction and may motivate unhealthy weight-control behaviors.

There is considerable empirical documentation of these various sociocultural pressures and of the relation of these pressures to the development of body image disturbance and disordered eating.

## MEDIA INFLUENCES

There is mounting evidence that the mass media promote body image and eating disturbance. First, content analyses have established that the body dimensions of female models, actresses, and other female cultural icons have become thinner over the last several decades. Indeed, one-fourth of the models in some magazines satisfy the weight criteria for anorexia nervosa. That this thinning trend correlates positively with the apparent rise in eating disturbance was the initial line of evidence suggesting that the media contributes to disordered eating. Conversely, there are few overweight individuals in the media, despite the fact that one in four people in Western countries is obese. Second, data suggest that there is greater emphasis on dieting and weight management in media targeting females compared to that targeting males, which parallels the gender distribution of eating pathology. Third, there is evidence that use of media with thin–ideal content is correlated with concurrent and future body image and eating disturbance. Fourth, individuals with bulimia nervosa perceive greater pressure to be thin from the media than controls and often report that they learned unhealthy weight-control techniques from the media (e.g., self-induced vomiting). Fifth, randomized experiments have documented that acute exposure to media-portrayed thin–ideal images results in increased body dissatisfaction and negative affect (e.g., depression, shame, and anger). Interestingly, these effects are often greater among "at-risk" individuals characterized by initial body dissatisfaction and thin–ideal internalization. In the only randomized experiment that manipulated long-term exposure to thin–ideal media images, Stice and colleagues found that assignment of subjects to a fashion magazine subscription led to increased body dissatisfaction, dieting, negative affect, and bulimic symptoms, but only for vulnerable girls characterized by initial body dissatisfaction and pressure to be thin, and deficits in social support. Finally, a natural experiment (noted by Becker) found that the rates of body image and eating disturbance increased following the introduction of Western media to Fiji, a culture initially devoid of thin–ideal images.

In summary, there is considerable correlational, prospective, and experimental evidence that mass media contribute to body image and eating disturbance, although these effects are often small in magnitude. There is also evidence that the adverse effects of mass media are amplified by preexisting vulnerability factors such as heightened thin–ideal internalization.

## FAMILY INFLUENCES

There is also support for the assertion that sociocultural pressures emanating from the family promote body image and eating disturbance. First, parental pressure to lose weight, family criticism regarding weight, and maternal investment in a daughter's slenderness are positively correlated with adolescent eating disturbance. Second, relative to control mothers, mothers of girls with eating disorders show elevated restriction of their daughters' eating, encourage their daughters to diet and exercise, and perceive their daughters to be more overweight and less attractive (see Pike & Rodin). However, there appear to be few differences between controls and fathers of youths with eating disorders. Third, research indicates that bulimic individuals perceive greater pressure to be thin from their family than controls, and many patients report that they initiated bulimic behavior following family pressure to lose weight. Fourth, there is some indication that general disturbances in family functioning are related to eating pathology: Individuals with eating disorders reporting that their families are more conflicted, disorganized, critical, and less cohesive compared to controls. Fifth, there is evidence of direct modeling of abnormal eating behaviors by parents. One study found that mothers of youths with eating disorders evidenced greater dieting and eating pathology than did control mothers, although this effect has not replicated well. Sixth, perceived pressure to be thin from family members has been found to predict increased body dissatisfaction, dieting, negative affect, and bulimic behaviors. Finally, parental body dissatisfaction, internalization of the thin–ideal, dieting, and bulimic symptoms prospectively predict emergence of eating disturbance during early childhood.

Thus, there is considerable correlational and prospective evidence (although no experimental data) for the assertion that family influences contribute to body image and eating disturbance. Most of this research has focused on parents rather than siblings. It is possible that these effects reflect the processes that mediate genetic risk for eating pathology (see Chapters 42 and 43).

## PEER INFLUENCES

There is growing support for the assertion that peers contribute to body image disturbance and disordered eating. First, perceived peer interest in dieting and thin–ideal internalization have been found to correlate positively with eating pathology. Second, individuals with bulimia nervosa report perceiving greater pressure from their peers to be thin than controls, and many patients indicate they initiated bulimic behavior following pressure from a friend to lose weight. Third, peer teasing about weight prospectively predicts increases in body dissatisfaction and eating disturbance. Fourth, there is evidence of direct modeling effects: One study found a positive relation between binge eating and peer binge eating, and that the magnitude of this effect increased as the friendships became more cohesive over time. Similarly, a large number of bulimic patients report learning to vomit for weight-control purposes from a friend. Fifth, perceived pressure from peers to be thin prospectively predicts body dissatisfaction, dieting, negative affect, and bulimic pathology. There is also emerging evidence that peers may contribute to eating disturbance in a less obvious fashion. Specifically, in one study, bulimic individuals showed hypersensitivity to negative interpersonal transactions and this appeared to precipitate binge eating.

In summary, there is mounting correlational and prospective support for the claim that peer influences contribute to body image disturbance and disordered eating. As yet, this relationship has not studied experimentally. Little attention has been paid to the potential impact of romantic partners.

## CONCEPTUAL AND METHODOLOGICAL LIMITATIONS

It is important to consider the conceptual and methodological limitations of this research when interpreting the findings. Regarding conceptual shortcomings, there has been relatively little theoretical work on the factors that may render certain individuals vulnerable to sociocultural influences and others relatively resistant. Another problem is that few of the empirically tested etiological models have incorporated sociocultural influences. Furthermore, little attention has been paid to the distinction between processes involved in the development of eating disturbance and those involved in their maintenance.

The research has also had certain methodological limitations. Most importantly, there has been an overreliance on cross-sectional studies that do not provide information regarding the direction of effects. Additionally, reliance on self-report data renders it impossible to rule out the possibility that individuals with eating disturbance simply perceive greater sociocultural pressures. There has also been little experimental research on the effects of family and peer influences. Targeted prevention programs that either render youth more resilient to these pressures or actually reduce them offer an ethical vehicle by which to study these processes experimentally.

## PREVENTION AND TREATMENT IMPLICATIONS

Findings suggest that prevention programs that make individuals more resilient to the adverse effects of sociocultural influences would be beneficial. For example, there is emerging evidence that brief interventions that help women become more critical consumers of the media buffer them from the adverse effects of exposure to thin–ideal images. Results also imply that interventions that directly reduce these sociocultural pressures (e.g., family pressures to be thin) might produce consequent reductions in body image disturbance and disordered eating. Findings also suggest that treatments that help patients become more resilient to sociocultural pressures facilitate recovery and decrease relapse rates. (See Chapter 67 for discussion of the prevention of eating disorders.)

## DIRECTIONS FOR FUTURE RESEARCH

As suggested earlier, more research should be directed at understanding the processes that mitigate and potentiate the adverse effects of sociocultural influences. Increased use of prospective and experimental designs would greatly advance our understanding of these influences. Use of observational data and confederate reports would help to ensure that sociocultural pressures are not solely in the eye of the beholder. Research is needed to explore the role of interpersonal processes in the promotion of eating pathology. Finally, more research should be directed at distinguishing between those factors that influence the etiology of body image disturbance and disordered eating, and those that primarily contribute to their maintenance.

## FURTHER READING

Becker, A. E. (1995). *Body, self, and society: The view from Fiji.* Philadelphia: University of Pennsylvania Press.—An interesting anthropological analysis of the effects of introducing Western media to a culture initially free of the thin–ideal.

Fairburn, C. G., Welch, S. L., Doll, H. A., Davies, B. A., & O'Connor, M. E. (1997). Risk factors for bulimia nervosa: A community-based case-control study. *Archives of General Psychiatry, 54,* 509–517.—First in a series of three case-control studies of risk factors for developing various forms of eating disorder. Implicates family factors.

Heinberg, L. J., & Thompson, J. K. (1995). Body image and televised images of thinness and attractiveness: A controlled laboratory investigation. *Journal of Social and Clinical Psychology, 14,* 325–338.—An exemplary experiment on the effects of exposure to media-portrayed thin–ideal images.

Levine, M. P., & Smolak, L. (1996). Media as a context for the development of disordered eating. In L. Smolak, M. P. Levine, & R. Striegel-Moore (Eds.), *The developmental psychopathology of eating disorders* (pp. 183–204). Mahwah, NJ: Erlbaum.—A comprehensive overview of the media-effects literature.

Pike, K. M., & Rodin, J. (1991). Mothers, daughters, and disordered eating. *Journal of Abnormal Psychology, 100,* 198–204.—Controlled study of mothers of daughters with eating disorders.

Piran, N., Levine, M. P., & Steiner-Adair, C. (2000). *Preventing eating disorders: A handbook of interventions and special challenges.* Philadelphia: Brunner/Mazel.—Includes an interesting discussions of how to target sociocultural influences in prevention programs.

Posovac, H. D., Posovac, S. S., & Weigel, R. G. (in press). Reducing the impact of exposure to idealized media images of female attractiveness on women's body image: An investigation of three psychoeducational interventions with a high risk sample. *Journal of Social and Clinical Psychology.*—An excellent example of media literacy intervention.

Stice, E., Spangler, D., & Agras, W. S. (in press). Exposure to media-portrayed thin–ideal images adversely affects vulnerable girls: A longitudinal experiment. *Journal of Social and Clinical Psychology.*—Experiment assessing long-term effects of exposure to thin–ideal media images.

Thompson, J. K., Heinberg, L. J., Altabe, M., & Tantleff-Dunn, S. (1999). *Exacting beauty: Theory, assessment, and treatment of body image disturbance.* Washington, DC: American Psychological Association.—Comprehensive exploration of sociocultural influences on body image disturbance, focusing on media, family, and peer influences.

# 20

# Stigma, Discrimination, and Obesity

REBECCA PUHL
KELLY D. BROWNELL

Negative attitudes toward obese people constitute one of the last socially acceptable forms of discrimination. With the increased prevalence of both child and adult obesity, the number of people potentially affected by this bias is large. The literature on this topic is scattered, but when brought together, forms a clear picture of discrimination against obese persons that occurs in key areas of living.

## EMPLOYMENT DISCRIMINATION

Experimental studies point to widespread weight bias in virtually every stage of the employment process. Overweight individuals are at a disadvantage even before a job interview begins. Studies have manipulated perceived body weight of fictional employees through vignettes, photographs, or videos, while holding credentials constant, and then asked participants to evaluate applicants' hiring potential. Overweight employees are evaluated more negatively than average-weight employees and rated as being less likely to be hired. This bias is especially pronounced for sales positions in which overweight applicants are perceived as unfit employees and more appropriate for jobs involving little face-to-face contact.

Discrimination appears to continue once an overweight person is employed. Overweight employees are perceived to be lazy, sloppy, less competent, lacking in self-discipline, disagreeable, less conscientious, and poor role models. Such negative attitudes likely contribute to additional weight-based discriminatory practices such as unequal wages, denied promotions, and wrongful termination.

Some evidence shows that overweight women, for the same work, receive less pay than average-weight women. Overweight women are also more likely than thinner counterparts to hold low-paying jobs. Obese men are underrepresented in higher paying managerial and professional positions and are more likely to hold lower-paying jobs. Obese employees are perceived to have lower promotion potential, and are less likely to be recommended for promotion when compared to average-weight employees with identical qualifications.

Both self-report studies and legal case documentation demonstrate the firing of obese employees due to their weight. Termination may be the result of prejudiced employers or arbitrary weight standards. Case reports show that terminated employees have held positions as teachers, office managers, and computer analysts, in which body weight has little or no bearing on job-related duties, and some have been terminated despite formal recognition for fine job performance.

## MEDICAL AND HEALTH CARE DISCRIMINATION

Antifat attitudes have been documented among physicians, nurses, and medical students. Common attributions include perceptions of obese patients as unintelligent, unsuccessful, weak-willed, unpleasant, overindulgent, and lazy. Bias in these groups may stem from perceived causes of obesity, which have included assertions that obesity arises from emotional problems, that it can be prevented by self-control, and that patient noncompliance is the reason for lack of success in weight loss.

Prejudice may lead to poor medical care for obese patients. Studies show that physicians admit not intervening as much as they should with obese patients, claiming that weight loss counseling is inconvenient. Physicians also report low rates of discussion of weight issues with their patients. One study with nurses reported that 12% were reluctant to touch obese persons and 24% found obese patients to be "repulsive."

Negative attitudes may lead obese individuals to avoid seeking treatment. Some research demonstrates a delay in seeking medical care by obese women for pelvic examinations and preventative health care services such as breast and gynecological exams. Body mass index (BMI) is positively related to appointment cancellations. Obese patients have attributed this to embarrassment about weight and previous negative experiences in discussing weight with physicians.

Discrimination within the medical arena can extend to poor access to beneficial treatment. Inconsistent and absent medical coverage are common despite evidence of cost-effectiveness with treatments such as drugs and surgery, and recognition that small weight losses can improve comorbid conditions. Societal perceptions that obesity is a problem of willful behavior (i.e., obese people get what they deserve and deserve what they get) may be a central reason why treatment is excluded from medical coverage.

## EDUCATIONAL DISCRIMINATION

There is a large literature indicating that obese students face multiple forms of weight discrimination. Perhaps most harmful to children is peer rejection in educational settings. Research shows that peers are the most frequent critics of obese children and that school is the most frequent venue. Experimental studies showing photographs of children with various weights and physical disabilities demonstrate that obese children are rated as the least desirable friends and playmates by peers. These negative stereotypes may be formed as early as preschool age. Self-reports of overweight children also indicate that they, too, attribute their exclusion in social activities and lack of friends to their weight. Many studies have shown enduring negative effects of teasing in childhood.

At the college level, educational discrimination may act in different ways. Lawsuits have been filed by obese students dismissed from college because of their weight. Obese students are less likely to be accepted to college than average-weight students, despite having equivalent application rates and academic performance. This seems especially true for overweight females.

Crandall and colleagues found a reliable relationship between body mass index (BMI) and financial support for education. Average-weight students received more financial support from parents than did overweight students, who depended more on financial aid and jobs. This effect was strong for overweight females, and differences in parental support remained despite controlling for education, income, ethnicity, and family size. Politically conservative attitudes of parents were positively correlated with BMI of students and predicted who paid for college, suggesting that parents with certain ideological beliefs may be less likely to give financial support to their overweight children.

## UNEXPLORED AREAS OF DISCRIMINATION

The literature has hinted at additional forms of discrimination, though there is inadequate information to make confident conclusions. Claims have been made of denied accommodation to obese persons in public services, biased jury selection (obese jurors may be dismissed on the basis of weight), and denial of the right to adopt a child because of weight-based adoption criteria or outright bias.

Anecdotal evidence also suggests that obese people are more likely to be charged more than thin persons for apartment rentals and health club memberships. Obese persons may face other subtle forms of prejudice in daily life, such as waiting longer for assistance from store clerks or being the recipients of negative body language in interpersonal interactions. These unexplored avenues provide another lens with which to empirically investigate weight discrimination.

## LEGAL CHALLENGES TO WEIGHT DISCRIMINATION

No federal laws in the United States prohibit weight discrimination, and only a few states include weight as a protected category. Victims of weight discrimination have depended primarily on the American Disabilities Act for protection and compensation.

The number of successful cases pursued under this legislation has varied, and courts have been inconsistent on whether obesity meets disability criteria. Many courts have adopted views of obesity as a voluntary and mutable condition and in turn rarely accept it as a disability unless other medical conditions result in impairment. Inconsistent rulings will likely continue until conceptualizations of disability, impairment, and obesity are clarified.

It is also questionable whether it is desirable for obese persons to be considered disabled. Obesity is disabling in only a small percentage of cases, so it may be preferable to create new statutes that directly prohibit discrimination based on weight. This may provide broader and more uniform coverage to obese persons who otherwise face unequal employment and educational opportunities.

## COMPONENTS UNDERLYING STIGMA

A priority for research is to understand better why and how such negative attitudes arise toward obese people. One theoretical model with accumulating empirical support is Crandall's social ideology perspective, which proposes that traditional, conservative North American values of self-determination, individualism, and self-discipline represent the core of antifat attitudes. These values are at the heart of blame, resulting in the tendency to attribute outcomes of others to internal, controllable causes. Such attributions probably lead to stigmatization toward people who are perceived to be responsible for their fates, such as obese persons, who are viewed to be personally responsible for their weight.

Other research addressing stigma suggests that perceived causes of obesity and the perceived stability of being overweight are central components in attributions about obese people. Although current information provides a starting point from which to address stigmatization toward obese individuals, many theoretical issues have yet to be studied.

## CONCLUSIONS

There is a clear and consistent pattern of discrimination against obese persons in major life areas of employment, medical care, and education. Negative attributions are being made about the core human traits and values of obese persons despite no evidence that such traits are associated with increased weight.

Methodological limitations in the literature include an overreliance on student samples and self-report methods, use of nonrandom designs, and assessment measures with questionable reliability. While many research questions have not yet been addressed and the literature is not sufficiently mature to generalize across all areas of living, there is enough information to know that weight discrimination is a major problem.

As research better documents weight discrimination and refines conceptual frameworks for understanding this phenomenon, stigma reduction strategies and interventions to eliminate obesity discrimination can be developed. Preliminary studies have reported a reduction in antifat attitudes through emphasizing the complex etiology of obesity. Further studies of stigma reduction strategies are needed to address this important social problem.

### ACKNOWLEDGMENT

This work was supported by the Rudd Foundation. We are grateful for input from the Rudd Scholars, Steven Blair, James Early, and James Hill, and from the Foundation staff.

### FURTHER READING

Adamitis, E. M. (2000). Appearance matters: A proposal to prohibit appearance discrimination in employment. *Washington Law Review, 75,* 195–223.—A detailed review of the legal status of weight-based employment discrimination in the United States that addresses the major obstacles in current legislation.

Adams, C. H., Smith, N. J., Wilbur, D. C., & Grady, K. E. (1993). The relationship of obesity to the frequency of pelvic examinations: Do physician and patient attitudes make a difference? *Women and Health, 20,* 45–57.—A study documenting the negative impact of patient obesity on physician practices.

Crandall, C. S. (1995). Do parents discriminate against their heavyweight daughters? *Personality and Social Psychology Bulletin, 21,* 724–735.—A fascinating study examining parental attitudes toward obesity and their implications for the educational disadvantages of overweight students.

Crandall, C. S., & Martinez, R. (1996). Culture, ideology, and antifat attitudes. *Personality and Social Psychology Bulletin, 22,* 1165–1176.—A cultural comparison of attitudes toward obesity, highlighting ideological components of stigmatizing attitudes.

Neumark-Sztainer, D., Story, M., & Faibisch, L. (1998). Perceived stigmatization among overweight African-American and Caucasian adolescent girls. *Journal of Adolescent Health, 23,* 264–270.—A good description of weight prejudice experienced by adolescents, with implications for clinicians and educators.

Price, J. H., Desmond, S. M., Krol, R. A., Snyder, F. F., & O'Connell, J. K. (1987). Family practice physicians' beliefs, attitudes, and practices regarding obesity. *American Journal of Preventive Medicine, 3,* 339–345.—A study demonstrating questionable practices and biased attitudes among physicians.

Puhl, R., & Brownell, K. D. (in press). Obesity and discrimination. *Obesity Research.*—A comprehensive literature review documenting weight discrimination in employment, education, and medical settings.

Roehling, M. V. (1999). Weight-based discrimination in employment: Psychological and legal aspects. *Personnel Psychology, 52,* 969–1017.—An excellent review of empirical research assessing employment discrimination against obese individuals.

Solovay, S. (2000). *Tipping the scales of justice: Fighting weight-based discrimination.* Amherst, NY: Prometheus Books.—An informative and up-to-date account of weight-based discrimination in the United States, with a focus on legal issues and weight prejudice in multiple areas of living.

Wiese, H. J. C., Wilson, J. F., Jones, R. A., & Neises, M. (1993). Obesity stigma reduction in medical students. *International Journal of Obesity, 16,* 859–868.—A study testing the effectiveness of an intervention to reduce antifat attitudes among medical students.

# 21

# Body Image and Body Dysmorphic Disorder

## KATHARINE A. PHILLIPS

Body dysmorphic disorder (BDD), also known as dysmorphophobia, is an intriguing disorder that has been described around the world for more than a century. BDD appears to be relatively common in the general population and in psychiatric, dermatologic, and cosmetic surgery settings. However, it remains underrecognized and has received relatively little investigation.

BDD consists of a preoccupation with an imagined defect in appearance; if a slight physical anomaly is present, the person's concern is markedly excessive. The preoccupation causes clinically significant distress or impairment, and it cannot be better accounted for by another mental disorder (such as anorexia nervosa). In the fourth edition of the American Psychiatric Association's *Diagnostic and Statistical Manual of Mental Disorders* (DSM-IV), BDD is classified as a somatoform disorder, whereas its delusional variant is classified as a psychotic disorder—a type of delusional disorder, somatic type.

## CLINICAL FEATURES

### Appearance Preoccupations

Individuals with BDD are preoccupied with the idea that some aspect of their appearance is unattractive, deformed, or "not right" in some way, when, in reality, the perceived flaw is minimal or nonexistent. Preoccupations commonly involve the face or head, most often the skin, hair, or nose (e.g., acne, scarring, thinning hair, or a large or crooked nose). However, any body part can be the focus of concern.

BDD preoccupations are distressing, time-consuming, and usually difficult to resist or control. Clinical observations and research findings suggest that these preoccupations are typically associated with low self-esteem, shame, embarrassment, and fear of rejection. Most patients have poor insight or are delusional, not recognizing that the flaw they perceive is actually minimal or nonexistent. A majority have ideas or delusions of reference, thinking that others take special notice of the supposed defect and perhaps talk about or mock it.

## Compulsive Behaviors

Nearly all patients perform repetitive compulsive behaviors, such as excessive checking of the perceived flaw in mirrors or directly, excessive grooming, camouflaging the perceived deformity (e.g., with hair, makeup, body position, or clothing), reassurance seeking, comparing with others, and skin picking.

## Complications

BDD often causes severe distress and markedly impaired social and occupational functioning. In one case series more than 25% of patients had been completely housebound for at least 1 week, more than 50% had been psychiatrically hospitalized, and nearly 30% had attempted suicide. A study of dermatology patients who committed suicide found that most had acne or BDD. Quality of life is notably poor.

## Comorbidity

Most patients seen in psychiatric settings have other mental disorders, most commonly, major depression, social phobia, and obsessive–compulsive disorder. A majority of patients have a personality disorder, most often avoidant personality disorder.

## Demographic Features and Course of Illness

The gender distribution varies between series: In the largest published case series 51% were men. The majority of patients have never been married. BDD usually begins during adolescence, although it can occur in childhood. It usually appears to be chronic, although prospective studies of its course are needed.

## THE NATURE OF BODY IMAGE DISTURBANCE

Little is known about body image disturbance in BDD. One study found that, compared to normal controls, patients with BDD were less satisfied with their body image and more likely to feel that their body was unacceptable, as has been found for obese patients and those with eating disorders. Regarding body image distortion, it is not known whether patients' views of their appearance have a basis in abnormal sensory (perceptual) processing or in attitudinal/cognitive–evaluative dissatisfaction. Clinical observations suggest that at least some patients with BDD have abnormal sensory processing, and perhaps experience a visual illusion or hallucination. However, preliminary empirical reports suggest that these patients may not have a primary sensory processing deficit, and, to the contrary, may have even better discriminatory ability than normal controls. In one report,

BDD patients were more accurate than normal controls or cosmetic surgery patients in their assessments of facial proportions. Another pilot study similarly found that BDD patients had a more accurate perception of nose size and shape than a normal control group. These findings are discordant with many studies showing size-estimation inaccuracy (overestimation of body size) in patients with eating disorders.

Compared to normal controls, patients with BDD have been shown to have deficits in verbal and nonverbal memory that appear due to organizational (i.e., executive) dysfunction. These consist of overfocusing on minor and irrelevant stimuli. This finding raises the question of whether these patients' appearance-related beliefs arise from overfocusing on minimal appearance flaws (isolated details rather than their overall appearance), causing a visual attention bias.

## PATHOPHYSIOLOGY AND ETIOLOGY

The etiology of BDD has received little attention. Family history data, while limited, indicate that BDD occurs in 6–10% of first-degree family members, which is almost certainly higher than the rate in the general population, suggesting that BDD is familial. The neuropsychological studies implicating impaired executive dysfunction suggest frontal–striatal pathology. Available treatment data (see below), while providing only indirect evidence about etiology, suggest a role for serotonin (and in several case reports BDD symptoms have been worsened by serotonin antagonists). Perceptual abnormalities may be present, the neuroanatomical and neurochemical bases of which require elucidation.

BDD's etiology is likely to be multifactorial, with evolutionary, sociocultural, and psychological factors playing a role. One study found that BDD patients reported receiving poorer parental care than normal controls. It seems plausible that frequent criticism of or teasing about one's appearance would be a risk factor for BDD, but such potential risk factors have not been studied.

## THE RELATIONSHIP BETWEEN BDD AND EATING DISORDERS

The literature on BDD contains little investigation, discussion, or theorizing about its relationship to the eating disorders. Most of the focus has been on obsessive–compulsive disorder, depression, schizophrenia, and social phobia. BDD and eating disorders have some obvious similarities, for example, a preoccupation with perceived appearance flaws, a disturbance in body image, and a sense that one's body is unacceptable (see Chapters 29 and 54 for further description of these features with respect to eating disorders); performance of repetitive behaviors such as mirror checking and body measuring; and a similar age of onset and course of illness. However, there are some differences, including a focus on body shape and weight versus more specific body parts (although this distinction can break down, in that BDD patients may be concerned with overall appearance, such as general ugliness or overall body build, and patients with eating disorders may focus on specific body parts, such as their stomach or hips). BDD and eating disorders also differ in terms of gender distribution and are not as highly comorbid with each other as with many other disorders. Family history and treatment data, while limited, also do not strongly support the hypothesis that these disorders are closely related.

There is a diagnostic gray area between these disorders, where symptoms overlap to the point that the correct diagnosis is sometimes unclear. An example of this "fuzzy boundary" is muscle dysmorphia, a newly recognized condition in which individuals (usually men) are preoccupied with their "small" and "puny" body build, which in reality is often large and muscular. Individuals with this condition also typically focus excessively on body fat, diet, and exercise. Muscle dysmorphia is currently conceptualized as a form of BDD, but it does have similarities to the eating disorders, as reflected by its previous name, "reverse anorexia."

Another unanswered question is whether the DSM-IV diagnostic hierarchy is correct: Should BDD be diagnosed only if body image concerns are not better accounted for by an eating disorder? Might the eating disorders actually be a form of BDD given their important feature of disturbed body image? While this seems unlikely given the disorders' apparent differences, the hierarchy needs to be empirically examined.

## TREATMENT

### Pharmacotherapy

Case reports, case series, open-label trials, and a controlled crossover study indicate that serotonin reuptake inhibitors (SRIs) are often effective for BDD, and more effective than other psychotropic medications. Although fluvoxamine and clomipramine are the best studied SRIs in BDD, clinical experience suggests that all of them may be effective. Of note, available data suggest that patients with delusional BDD are as likely as those with nondelusional BDD to respond to these drugs. Although other psychotropic medications have been less well studied, available data suggest that they are generally ineffective when used as single agents, but that certain ones may be useful as adjunctive agents in combination with a SRI.

### Cognitive-Behavioral Therapy

Cognitive-behavioral therapy also appears effective for BDD. Exposure (e.g., to avoided social situations) and response prevention (e.g., not seeking reassurance), as well as other cognitive-behavioral techniques, have been used in most studies. (See Chapters 54 and 55 for accounts of cognitive-behavioral therapy for eating disorders.)

### Other Treatments

The efficacy of other types of therapy for BDD has not been well studied, although available data suggest that supportive psychotherapy and insight-oriented psychotherapy are generally ineffective (although clinical experience suggests that they may have a useful adjunctive role). A majority of BDD patients seen in a psychiatric setting have sought and received nonpsychiatric treatment, most commonly dermatologic treatment and cosmetic surgery. Although the efficacy of these treatments has not been studied prospectively, available data suggest that they are usually ineffective and may even worsen appearance concerns.

## RESEARCH

Although research on BDD is rapidly increasing, it is still limited and at an early stage. Investigation of virtually all aspects of this disorder is needed. Placebo-controlled pharmacotherapy studies, psychotherapy studies using attention-control groups or alternative treatments, and studies of the combination of psychotherapy and pharmacotherapy are greatly needed. Nearly all treatment studies have been short term; continuation and maintenance studies are needed to elucidate longer-term outcome.

Because body image disturbance is likely central to BDD's development and maintenance, this is an important area for future research. Neuroimaging studies are needed, as are other approaches to investigating the temporal and occipital lobes, which process facial images and (along with the parietal lobes) are involved in neurological disorders involving disturbed body image. Psychological and sociocultural contributions to BDD also require elucidation, since knowledge of the mechanisms that underlie this disorder may ultimately inform much-needed treatment and prevention strategies.

## FURTHER READING

Hardy, G. E. (1982). Body image disturbance in dysmorphophobia. *British Journal of Psychiatry, 141,* 181–185.—One of the few studies on body image disturbance in BDD.

Hollander, E., Allen, A., Kwon, J., Aronowitz, B., Schmeidler, J., Wong, C., & Simeon, D. (1999). Clomipramine vs desipramine crossover trial in body dysmorphic disorder: Selective efficacy of a serotonin reuptake inhibitor in imagined ugliness. *Archives of General Psychiatry, 56,* 1033–1039.—The first controlled pharmacotherapy study of BDD.

Phillips, K. A. (1991). Body dysmorphic disorder: The distress of imagined ugliness. *American Journal of Psychiatry, 148,* 1138–1149.—The most comprehensive review of BDD.

Phillips, K. A. (1996). *The broken mirror: Recognizing and treating body dysmorphic disorder.* New York: Oxford University Press. The most comprehensive source of information on BDD for both professionals and lay readers.

Phillips, K. A., McElroy, S. L., Keck, P. E., Jr., Pope, H. G., Jr., & Hudson, J. I. (1993). Body dysmorphic disorder: 30 cases of imagined ugliness. *American Journal of Psychiatry, 150,* 302–308.—The first descriptive series of BDD using modern assessment methods.

Pope, H. G., Phillips, K. A., & Olivardia, R. (2000). *The Adonis Complex: The secret crisis of male body obsession.* New York: Free Press.—An overview of BDD, muscle dysmorphia, and eating disorders in men.

Rosen, J. C., & Ramirez, E. (1998). A comparison of eating disorders and body dysmorphic disorder on body image and psychological adjustment. *Journal of Psychosomatic Research, 44,* 1–9.—The only published comparison study of BDD and eating disorders.

Thomas, C. S., & Goldberg, D. P. (1995). Appearance, body image and distress in facial dysmorphophobia. *Acta Psychiatrica Scandinavica, 92,* 231–236.—One of the few studies on body image distortion in BDD.

Veale, D., Boocock, A., Gournay, K., Dryden, W., Shah, F., Willson, R., & Walburn, J. (1996). Body dysmorphic disorder: A survey of fifty cases. *British Journal of Psychiatry, 169,* 196–201.—A descriptive series of patients with BDD.

Veale, D., Gournay, K., Dryden, W., Boocock, A., Shah, F., Willson, R., & Walburn, J. (1996). Body dysmorphic disorder: A cognitive behavioural model and pilot randomized controlled trial. *Behaviour Research and Therapy, 34,* 717–729.—One of the two controlled psychotherapy studies of BDD.

# Measurement Methods

# 22

## Measurement of Total Energy Stores

STEVEN B. HEYMSFIELD
STANLEY HESHKA

Total body energy stores are distributed into a number of body composition compartments or components. Figure 22.1 shows the traditional energy stores at the molecular level as three components: lipid, proteins, and glycogen (i.e., carbohydrate). The corresponding tissue systems are adipose tissue, skeletal muscle, and other organs and tissues. With weight gain or loss, there may be changes in the size of compartments at all levels of body composition analysis.

The aim of this chapter is to review the main methods of quantifying each of the major body compartments related to total body energy stores. Two major groups of methods are presented: laboratory methods and clinical or field methods.

## LABORATORY METHODS

### Imaging Methods

Simple radiographs were used in the 1950s to quantify soft tissue composition and bone. By the mid-1970s, computerized tomography (CT) was introduced and subsequently became a major method of evaluating human body composition. The method produced high tissue contrast, allowing clear separation of anatomic components including adipose tissue, skeletal muscle, bone, and visceral organs. The cross-sectional imaging procedure allows three-dimensional reconstruction of body compartments and examination of components not previously evaluated such as visceral adipose tissue. Unlike computerized tomography, magnetic resonance imaging (MRI) uses nonionizing radiation. Images of compartments created with MRI are almost equivalent to those of CT. The one exception is visceral adipose tissue, which is less highly resolved by MRI than CT because of peristaltic movement through the gastrointestinal tract. Once images are created by CT and MRI, they are analyzed slice-by-slice and combined to determine the volume of each

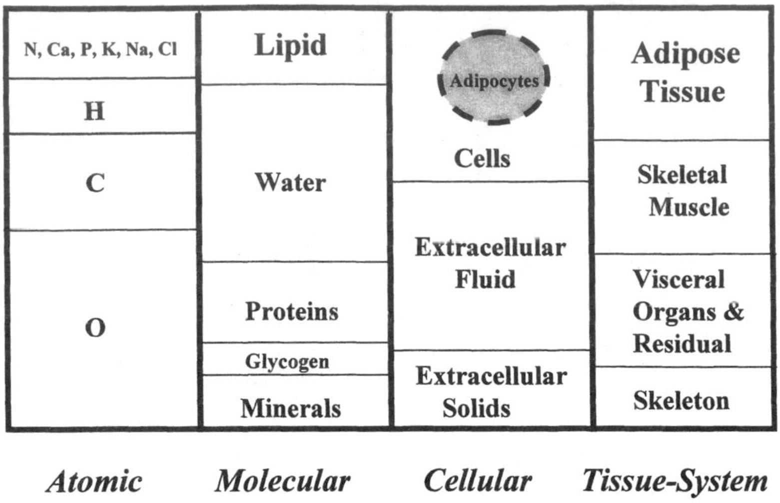

| N, Ca, P, K, Na, Cl | Lipid | Adipocytes | Adipose Tissue |
| --- | --- | --- | --- |
| H | | | |
| C | Water | Cells | Skeletal Muscle |
| O | | Extracellular Fluid | Visceral Organs & Residual |
| | Proteins | | |
| | Glycogen | Extracellular Solids | Skeleton |
| | Minerals | | |

| *Atomic* | *Molecular* | *Cellular* | *Tissue-System* |

**FIGURE 22.1.** Major components at the first four levels of body composition.

compartment. Reconstruction algorithms vary from automated to technician-oriented reconstruction.

CT and MRI are widely used for evaluating tissue system compartments including adipose tissue, skeletal muscle, bone, and visceral organs. Imaging methods are currently the reference for quantifying the visceral adipose tissue compartment using either a single slice or reconstructing the entire compartment. Of the body composition reference methods, they are among the most costly. Additionally, CT produces ionizing radiation and is therefore not applicable in young children and women in their childbearing years.

## Isotope Dilution

The classical method for evaluating total body fat at the molecular level is isotope dilution of total body water. One of three isotopes is used, oxygen-18, deuterium, and tritium. Fat-free mass can then be calculated, as healthy adults typically have a mean hydration of 73%.

Isotope dilution for total body water has the advantage of being simple, inexpensive, portable, and relatively simple to carry out. A known quantity of isotope is ingested, and after allowing for equilibration, a sample of body fluids, usually serum, is taken. The concentration of the isotope is then measured by mass spectroscopy or infrared methods. Isotope dilution methods serve as not only a reference for body composition, particularly body fat, but also as a potential field method in remote settings. The three isotopes vary in cost and complexity of analysis. Deuterium and tritium are the least expensive, and deuterium has the advantage of not being a radioactive isotope.

## Photon Absorptiometry

Dual-photon absorptiometry was introduced as a method of quantifying bone mineral mass in regions with overlying soft tissue. The method also provides an estimate of fat and lean soft tissue in regions in which bone is not present. The subsequent introduction of dual-energy X-ray absorptiometry (DXA) has permitted more stable and faster scans with higher resolution. It also has the capability of providing total body and regional soft tissue estimates for fat and lean components. Both methods have been validated for use in animals and humans. Although a number of technical issues remain, DXA is widely considered a reference method for subjects of all ages. Radiation exposure is very low, thus allowing studies of children and women in the childbearing years. A limitation of DXA is that very large subjects cannot be accommodated on the imaging table. The upper limit in weight for most scanners is in the range of 250 pounds (or a body mass index [BMI] greater than 35). One solution is to carry out half-body or partial-body scans and compensate for "missing" portions during image analysis.

## Densitometry

Body density is linearly related to the fraction of body weight as fat. This observation has been formulated into the two-compartment densitometry model. The model assumes that the body consists of two compartments: one has fat, with a density of 0.90 g/cc; and the other is fat-free mass, with a density of 1.10 g/cc. Assuming these two compartment densities and knowing the subject's measured density then allows estimation of the fraction of body weight as fat and fat-free mass.

Body density can be measured using one of two main methods, underwater weighing and air plethysmography. The former is a widely available and accepted method. Systems are inexpensive and relatively simple to operate, although subjects are required to hold their breath for several seconds while under water. More recently introduced, the air plethysmography method is based upon classical gas laws of physics. Body volume is estimated while the subject rests quietly inside a sealed chamber. Validation studies show that it is comparable to underwater weighing and other reference body composition methods in adults, although data from studies of children remain limited.

Underwater weighing systems have been installed and used throughout the world, including developing countries. They are less costly than an air plethysmography system. However, the air plethysmography system is relatively portable and can be operated even in remote settings.

## Multicomponent Models

Multicomponent models provide body composition estimates of three or more compartments. Evaluations may combine several methods, including DXA, densitometry, and isotope dilution. As most multicomponent models rely on fewer assumptions than the two-component model, these methods are often considered the reference for body fat when evaluating subjects varying widely in characteristics such as age, ethnicity, and body habitus.

## *In Vivo* Neutron Activation Analysis

The group of methods referred to as *in vivo* neutron activation analysis allow estimation of all major elements at the atomic level. These are then used to reconstruct various body compartments based on assumed element molecular component relationships. Two approaches for measuring total body fat are recognized, one based on total body carbon, and the other on the measurement of other elements, including total body nitrogen. *In vivo* neutron activation analysis, combined with whole-body counting, provides an important reference method for measuring total body fat. However, systems are limited in availability and radiation exposure tends to be relatively high. Use is therefore limited to research centers.

## $^{40}$K Counting

The element potassium, measured by whole-body counting of the naturally occurring potassium-40 isotope, has been used for many years as a means of estimating fat-free mass and fat using a two-compartment model. Again, whole-body counters are of limited availability. There are also questions regarding the validity of the two-compartment total-body potassium model.

# CLINICAL AND FIELD METHODS

## Anthropometry

Anthropometric measurements include body weight, height, various diameters, circumferences, and skin fold thickness. Combinations of these variables have been used in many studies to provide prediction formulae for estimating total body fat. These formulae are particularly useful in field settings or in clinical trials where other, more complex, reference methods are not feasible. BMI (weight in kg/height in m$^2$) is often used as a surrogate measure of adiposity, and formulae are available for converting BMI to percent body fat.

An important consideration when applying anthropometric methods is that technicians should be trained according to established, previously described protocols and retrained at periodic intervals. Anthropometric methods that require measurement of skin folds or circumferences tend to be less accurate in subjects with a high BMI.

## Bioimpedance Analysis

There is less resistance to an alternating electrical current passing through tissues that contain fluid and electrolytes than through those containing high relative amounts of lipid. This phenomenon is utilized by bioimpedance analysis (BIA). Systems vary from simple single-frequency BIA analyzers to complex, multifrequency systems. The measured impedance is directly related to body fluid and water content, and thus fat-free mass. Body fat can then be calculated as the difference between body weight and fat-free mass.

BIA is simple, safe, portable, and relatively inexpensive. A critical aspect is controlling for extraneous factors: Temperature, subject position, hydration status, and diet all influence impedance and thus affect body-fat estimates. Optimum results are provided by carefully controlling these variables prior to measurement. The method has been widely applied in clinical settings and in field studies. As with most other body composition methods, BIA estimates of body fat are not reliable for evaluating short-term changes in adiposity, although the method provides reliable information over the long term, even with weight gain and weight loss interventions. BIA methods are particularly suitable for studying group changes as opposed to individual differences, since there may be sizable errors in any single individual's result.

## CONCLUSIONS

A wide array of methods is thus available for quantifying adiposity in individuals and populations. The selection of a method depends on the purpose of the assessment. Laboratory methods are used to estimate total body fat in individual patients and, potentially, to evaluate relatively short-term or small changes in fatness. Cost, availability, and potential radiation exposure are all considerations. With respect to the field methods, the choice of method depends upon the availability of trained technicians for anthropometry and suitable measurement conditions for BIA. Additionally, for both field methods, appropriate body-fat prediction formulae for the specific population under study should be available.

## FURTHER READING

Chumlea, W., & Guo, S. (1994). Bioelectrical impedance and body composition: Present status and future directions. *Nutrition Reviews, 52*, 123–131.—A good overview of the BIA method.

Heymsfield, S. B., Wang, Z. M., Baumgartner, R. N., & Ross, R. (1997). Human body composition: Advances in models and methods. *Annual Review of Nutrition, 17*, 527–558.—An in-depth review of available body composition methods.

Lohman, T. G., Roche, A. F., & Martorell, R. (Eds.). (1988). *Anthropometric standardization reference manual.* Champaign, IL: Human Kinetics Books.—An invaluable treatise on anthropometry for serious students of the subject.

Lukaski, H. C. (1987). Methods for the assessment of human body composition: Traditional and new. *American Journal of Clinical Nutrition, 46*, 537–556.—A good review of the various available body composition methods.

Wang, Z. M., Pierson, R. N., Jr., & Heymsfield, S. B. (1992). The five level model: A new approach to organizing body composition research. *American Journal of Clinical Nutrition, 56*, 19–28.—An overview of the major body compartments and their organization.

# 23

## Measurement of Food Intake

### SACHIKO T. ST. JEOR

The assessment of food intake is challenging since food choices, quantity of foods eaten, and eating patterns are highly variable. Furthermore, complex interactions between what is eaten and physiological cues, psychological status, behavioral factors, and environmental opportunities are subtle and not well understood. However, understanding why, when, what, and how we eat is critical to identifying the etiology, diagnosis, and most effective treatment for eating disorders and obesity. Thus, this chapter outlines the basic methods for measuring food intake and provides information relevant to data collection, analysis, and interpretation.

### METHODS FOR MEASURING FOOD INTAKE

There are five basic methods for assessing dietary intake.

   1. *Diet histories*. These usually take the form of questionnaires of varying length and detail, and provide general information regarding usual dietary intake, food preferences, and associated behavior. A 24-hour recall is often included (see below). Diet histories are usually directed at specific issues of interest and can include questions regarding the use of dietary supplements, dieting history, food cravings, food aversions or allergies, and so on. They are generally self-administered and therefore easy and economical to use. There is a tendency to ask open-ended questions for hypothesis generation, but when closed questions are used, data analysis is much easier. Diet histories often serve as the basis on which dietary interventions are formulated.
   2. *Food records*. These are prospective food diaries. Although they may be kept for varying lengths of time, a minimum of 7 days is viewed as generally representative of usual intake. Records of 3–4 days are popular and useful when at least one weekend day is included. To improve accuracy, food models, food weighing scales, and measuring cups may be used. Detailed instructions are essential. Continuous or periodic food records

have been utilized to increase adherence to dietary interventions in clinical and research settings. Because food records are tedious to keep over long periods of time, abbreviated versions are of value.

3. *24-hour dietary recall*. This involves the retrospective reporting of intake to a trained interviewer. It is the most widely used method and generally covers the preceding 24 hours. Recalls may be obtained either in person or by prescheduled or random telephone interviews. Problems of memory, difficulties estimating portion size, and describing how food was prepared all complicate the method. Various techniques have been used to enhance the accuracy of recall, including utilizing food models and multiple pass techniques to facilitate memory retrieval. Underreporting is a common problem, especially in obese individuals. To be more representative of an individual's usual intake, multiple recalls are needed for at least three random, nonconsecutive days. Dietary recalls are used in clinical and research settings. In the clinical setting, it is helpful to ask patients how their eating differed from that on an "typical" day, and how special events affect their eating. Importantly, because the assessment is done after eating has taken place, this method is less likely than others to affect the participant's behavior. The interview usually takes about 20 minutes.

4. *Food frequency questionnaires (FFQs)*. These are self-administered questionnaires designed to elicit information about usual food consumption over a specified period of time, ranging from 1 week to 1 year. They consist of a list of foods in defined categories and portion sizes. The most widely used FFQ in the United States is the Health Habits and History Questionnaire (HHHQ), also known as the Block questionnaire. This is a 100-item FFQ developed at the National Cancer Institute. FFQs are primarily designed for use in large-scale epidemiological studies.

5. *Food lists*. These questionnaires target groups of foods with a common nutrient or content. They have become popular for the quick assessment of deficiencies or excesses. Food lists that have targeted the intake of calcium, folate, fat, and carbohydrate, regardless of other nutrients, have been useful in the assessment of risk for certain disease states.

All these methods facilitate the quantitative assessment of food and nutrient intake. Most are affected by the accuracy with which portion sizes are estimated or weighed, how food preparation procedures are described, and the specificity with which the food is characterized.

## DATA COLLECTION

In free-living situations, validation against what is actually eaten is almost impossible. Correlations between different methods have been made, generally by comparing them with food records, since these are thought to reflect variability in individual intake more accurately than recall methods. Although the exact number of recording days needed is debated, a period of 7 days is generally recommended, since differences between weekdays and weekend days are included and day-to-day variation can be captured. However, both 3- and 4-day records are commonly used and provide useful data.

Long-term studies have shown that the number of days of monitoring needed to bring accuracy to within 10% of usual intake varies among and also within individuals for different nutrients. These studies have found that 3 days is the mean length of time required to estimate the true average intake for energy (kilocalories), whereas to estimate the average intake of vitamin A (which is concentrated in certain foods) requires more than 40 days. An estimate of total energy intake is important when assessing the intake of many nutrients. Four days of monitoring ensures that 95% of the observed values of calorie-adjusted total fat intake lie within 20% of the true mean, and within 40% when not calorie-adjusted. Studies have shown that day-to-day variations in intake account for 37% of the variance. This is why at least three recalls of nonconsecutive days are recommended.

In general, the energy-adjusted coefficients that correlate nutrient intake, assessed by FFQs and food records, are in the range of $r = .40–.70$. Correlations between a FFQ and a 4-day diet record (FDDR) in the Women's Health Trial were lower for energy $(r = .30)$ and fat $(r = .29)$ than for fat as percent energy $(r = .40)$. However, when comparisons of responsiveness to intervention were compared after 1 year, the FDDR was only slightly more sensitive than the FFQ to changes made by participants, and a fat-related dietary habits questionnaire was most responsive. These data suggest that shorter, inexpensive measures can be as useful as multiple-day diet records, especially when specific nutrients or foods are targeted.

The major sources of error in data collection include bias by the respondent (recalls) or recorder (records), the interviewer (recalls), the interpreter, or the reviewer (records). In addition, the process of collecting the data may affect eating patterns and introduce inaccuracy. Errors introduced by the interviewer include behavioral factors, such as the manner of asking questions and nonverbal body language that may distract the subject or even encourage certain responses.

## DATA ANALYSIS

Data analysis is complicated by the constant introduction of new foods, the overwhelming number and types of food available, the difficulties estimating portion size, and problems detailing how food is prepared and eaten. The method of choice depends on the food, food component, or nutrient under study. Dietary intake is most often defined in terms of nutrient composition and its contribution to nutritional adequacy. Databases and computer software programs for quantifying self-reports have greatly facilitated the assessment of nutrient intake for both research and clinical purposes. These differ in their requirements for specificity and accuracy, and their practical utility.

Although there are a number of sources of information, the publications and programs of the U.S. Department of Agriculture (USDA) provide the most comprehensive and up-to-date information in the United States. Their National Nutrient Databank System (NDBS) is the repository of several types of food information, including food names, descriptors, formulations, and recipes, and it contains data on over 6,200 foods and up to 82 nutrients. An online database search program is available: *www.nal.usda.gov/fnic/foodcomp*.

There are two well-established analysis systems for researchers. The first is the Nutrition Data System for Research (NDS-R) available from the Nutrition Coordinating Center of the University of Minnesota—(612) 626–9450; *www.ncc.umn.edu*. The second is the Food Intake Analysis System available from the University of Texas School of Public Health—(713) 500–9775; *www.sph.uth.tmc.edu:8052/hnc/software/soft.htm*. Both these contractors also provide support for data entry and analysis of food frequencies, recalls, records, and recipes.

Three less expensive computerized databases and interactive programs are available for use with personal computers. All three are widely used. The first is Food Processor, Nutrition Analysis and Fitness software (Esha Research, Inc., Salem, OR; (800) 659–3742; *www.esha.com*). The second is Nutritionist Pro (First DataBank, San Bruno, CA; (800) 633–3453; *www.firstdatabank.com*.) The third is Nutritional Software Library (Computrition, Inc., Chadsworth, CA; (818) 701–5544; *www.computrition.com*).

Finally, for quick analysis of specific foods, the Pennington's popular handbook is recommended. This book has served as the classic and essential guide to the nutritional value of foods since 1937, and currently lists for more than 8,100 common foods.

## ASSESSMENT OF EATING BEHAVIOR

The assessment of eating behavior is even more difficult than that of dietary intake. It is complicated by difficulties defining even such apparently simple concepts such as a meal, a snack, and picking. The assessment of overeating and binge eating is even more challenging. Chapter 26 addresses the assessment of eating disorder psychopathology, and Chapters 15 and 16 discuss the assessment of dietary restraint. The clinical assessment of patients with eating disorders and obesity is discussed in Chapters 53 and 92, respectively.

## FURTHER READING

Basiotis, P. P., Welsh, S. O., Cronin, F. J., Kelsay, L., & Mertz, W. (1987). Number of days of food intake records required to estimate individual and group nutrient intakes with defined confidence. *Journal of Nutrition, 117*, 1638–1641.—Addresses usual food intake and day-to-day variability using food intake records collected over 1 year and analyzed for energy content and 18 nutrients.

Buzzard, I. M., & Willett, W. C. (Eds.). (1994). First International Conference on Dietary Assessment Methods: Assessing diets to improve world health. *American Journal of Clinical Nutrition, 59*, 143S–306S.—Proceedings of a conference in which gaps in dietary intake methodology and guidelines for selecting appropriate assessment methods are presented.

Dwyer, J. T. (1994). Dietary assessment. In M. E. Shils, J. A. Olson, & M. Shike (Eds.), *Modern nutrition in health and disease* (pp. 842–860). Philadelphia: Lea & Febiger.—Good review of dietary assessment methods, along with their strengths, limitations, and applications.

Kristal, A. R., Beresford, S. A., & Lazovich, D. (1994). Assessing change in diet-intervention research. *American Journal of Clinical Nutrition, 59*, 185S–189S.—Introduces "responsiveness" (an index of an instrument's sensitivity in measuring change), along with concepts applicable to the improvement of food intake assessment among persons with eating disorders.

National Heart, Lung, and Blood Institute and National Institute of Diabetes and Digestive and Kidney Diseases. (1998). *Clincal guidelines on the identification, evaluation and treatment of overweight and obesity in adults: The Evidence Report* (NIH Publication No. 98-4083). Bethesda, MD: National Institutes of Health.—Current treatment guidelines for adult obesity, together with recommendations for assessing dietary intake.

Pennington, J. A. T. (1998). *Food values of portions commonly used* (17th ed.). New York:

Lippincott/Williams & Wilkins.—This handbook provides essential data on the nutritional content of more than 8,100 common foods.

St. Jeor, S. T. (Ed.). (1997). *Obesity assessment: Tools, methods, interpretations.* New York: Chapman & Hall.—Currently available from Aspen Publishers, Frederick, MD (800–638–8437).—Includes two detailed sections on the assessment of dietary intake and related behaviors.

St. Jeor, S. T., & Feldman E. (Eds.). (in press). Nutrition assessment. In C. Berndanier (Ed.), *Handbook of foods and nutrition.* Boca Raton, FL: CRC Press.—This section of this new handbook contains several useful chapters on the assessment of dietary intake. Of particular importance is the chapter by Ashley and Grossbauer on computerized nutrient analysis. Other chapters discuss methods of dietary intake assessment in children, adults, and various ethnic groups.

St. Jeor, S. T., Guthrie, H. A., & Jones, M. B. (1983). Variability in nutrient intake in a 28-day period. *Journal of the American Dietetic Association, 83,* 155–162.—Outlines relationships between food records of 3-, 4-, and 7-day duration compared with 28 days and addresses variability of intake of energy and seven selected nutrients.

Tarasuk, V., & Beaton, G. H. (1991). The nature and individuality of within-subject variation in energy intake. *American Journal of Clinical Nutrition, 54,* 464–470.—Discussion of within-subject variation among 29 adults participating in the Beltsville One-Year Dietary Intake Study. Environmental and biological determinants, as well as methodological errors, are noted.

Willett, W. (1990). *Nutritional epidemiology.* New York: Oxford University Press.—A comprehensive account of all aspects of dietary intake methodology.

# 24

## Measurement of Energy Expenditure

### ANDREW M. PRENTICE

Human energy expenditure can be estimated using a wide range of techniques of differing sophistication and cost. It is a general truism that the more complicated and expensive methods provide the most accurate and precise estimates. With the exception of the relatively new doubly labeled water method (DLW), it is also true that the most accurate methods are least representative of real life because they require the subject to be restrained or encumbered. Thus, compromises must generally be made, and it is most important to match the technique selected to the question at hand.

### DIRECT CALORIMETRY

Direct calorimetry measures heat loss (as opposed to indirect calorimetry, which measures heat production; see below). The difference between these is simply one of time: Heat loss must follow heat production, and the delay is proportional to the specific heat capacity of the body. Thus, over periods of more than 1 or 2 hours, the two methods should give identical results. This prediction was shown to be true over a century ago and has since been confirmed. Indirect calorimetry, technically much easier and cheaper, provides additional estimates of substrate utilization. Therefore, except in a few basic studies of heat physiology, it is the method of choice. There are virtually no direct human calorimeters still in use.

### INDIRECT CALORIMETRY

Indirect calorimetry calculates energy expenditure from measurements of a person's oxygen consumption and carbon dioxide production, which are proportional to the rate at which energy-yielding substrates are burned. The technique requires some means of collecting expired breath and channeling it to accurate gas meters to measure the rate of air-

131

flow and the concentration difference compared to the fresh in-breathed air. Breath collection techniques vary according to the conditions under which the measurement is made.

Short-term studies of exercise physiology use a mouthpiece (and noseclip) that provides a very fast response time but is uncomfortable and unnatural. Medium-term studies (e.g., of basal metabolic rate [BMR] or diet-induced thermogenesis [DIT]) often use a ventilated hood placed over the patient's head while he or she sits or reclines. Commercially built exercise monitors and ventilated hood systems are available. The most widely used application is for the measurement of BMR.

Long-term studies must use whole-body calorimeters in which the subject can reside indefinitely. These consist of room-size chambers that can be comfortably furnished to meet the subject's needs and may include a cycle ergometer and/or treadmill. Food and other daily needs are passed into the chamber, and waste products leave, through air locks. Whole-body calorimeters used to be limited by their inherently slow response time due to the dilution of the subject's expired air in the large volume of the chamber, but modern software has overcome this problem. The numerous advantages of whole-body calorimeters have contributed greatly to our understanding of human energy metabolism. Their disadvantages are that they are expensive to build and run, and experiments are very time-consuming. There are approximately 15 functioning whole-body calorimeters worldwide and each has been individually constructed as a "home build."

The calculations of energy expenditure are basically the same regardless of the method of gas collection. The energy equivalence of each liter of oxygen consumed varies somewhat according to the mix of fuels being oxidized, but in most normal circumstances, this introduces minimal error, especially if carbon dioxide production and urinary nitrogen are assessed simultaneously, as is usually the case.

An added bonus of indirect calorimetry is that it can provide an estimate of substrate utilization based on the ratio of carbon dioxide produced to oxygen consumed (known as the respiratory quotient [RQ] or respiratory exchange ratio [RER]). It is first necessary to estimate protein oxidation based on the rate of appearance of nitrogen in the urine. This is used to adjust the RQ to the nonprotein RQ, which can then be used to differentiate fat and carbohydrate oxidation on the basis of their different RQs (0.70 and 1.00, respectively). If alcohol is also consumed, then its rate of oxidation can be assessed from the rate of decrease in blood concentration; thus, the rate of oxidation of all four energy-giving macronutrients can be calculated. With careful calibration, the best systems are capable of accuracy of better than 1% for energy expenditure, and better than 5% for the individual substrates.

## THE DOUBLY LABELED WATER ($^2H_2{}^{18}O$) METHOD

The main constraint of whole-body calorimetry is that subjects are confined within an artificial environment and unable to live their normal life. In the 1940s, the DLW method was invented for measuring energy expenditure in free-living animals. In the 1980s, it was first adapted for human applications. Subjects drink an oral loading dose of water labeled with the stable nonradioactive isotopes deuterium and oxygen-18. They collect baseline and serial daily urine samples for the next 10–14 days and the concentration of the isotopes is measured by isotope ratio mass spectrometry. The initial dilution of the dose gives a measure of total body water (and hence of body composition—see Chapter 22). The difference in the rate of decline of the two isotopes over the ensuing days is proportional to the rate of carbon dioxide production, and hence to energy expenditure. The calculation of results is complex and dependent on a number of assumptions, but detailed validation studies and theoretical computations have shown it to be accurate to within a few percentage points.

The great advantage of the DLW method is that it provides the first and only method for assessing total energy expenditure (TEE) in genuinely free-living subjects, and, as such, has had a major impact on our understanding of energy metabolism in obesity. The method must be applied over at least 7 days. This is both an advantage (in providing a good estimate of habitual TEE) and a disadvantage (in providing no short-term discrimination). When combined with a separate estimate of BMR by indirect calorimetry, DLW provides an estimate of the energy cost of activity and thermogenesis (A&T = TEE − BMR), and since thermogenesis is generally a rather small and constant proportion of A&T, this figure equates closely to activity energy expenditure (AEE).

The disadvantages of the DLW method are that it is very expensive, both in terms of isotope and the capital costs of mass spectrometers, and that the technical complexity has restricted its use to a very small number of centers worldwide. New workers in the field are advised to start through collaborations with existing centers.

## THE LABELED BICARBONATE ($^{13}CO_2$) METHOD

The lack of short-term discrimination of the DLW method can be overcome by using a continuous infusion of bicarbonate labeled with $^{13}$C (stable isotope) or $^{14}$C (radioactive isotope). The rate at which this is diluted is proportional to the rate of endogenous carbon dioxide production and, hence, energy expenditure. The optimal duration of measurements varies upwards from about 6 hours to several days.

The labeled bicarbonate technique has been applied in a few short-term clinical investigations but so far has not been widely adopted. Its main disadvantage is the requirement for subjects to wear an infusion minipump.

## HEART RATE AND ACTIVITY MONITORS

Energy expenditure can be estimated approximately by means of continuous ambulatory monitoring of heart rate or movement. With the advent of microelectronics and silicon chip data storage, there have been great advances in the basic methodology in the past few years and it is now possible to store minute-by-minute records of heart rate monitors or triple-axis motion sensors over several days (see Chapter 25). In order to convert these data into energy expenditure, each subject needs to be individually calibrated by indirect calorimetry and even then, the level of precision is not as good as whole-body calorimetry or the DLW method. However, these techniques can be applied in large-scale epidemiological studies.

Heart rate and activity monitors can also be used to obtain excellent quantitative comparisons of physical activity between different subjects, without the need to convert the output into true energy expenditure.

## ACTIVITY DIARIES AND PHYSICAL ACTIVITY QUESTIONNAIRES

The most basic methods of calculating energy expenditure are by means of activity diaries or questionnaires (see Chapter 25). For the diaries, a subject's different activities are regularly recorded over the period of interest (e.g., every 15 minutes) and the duration is multiplied by standard estimates of the energy cost of each activity (available in tables). Diaries can be completed by the subject themselves or by an observer. With physical activity questionnaires, the duration of specific activities is estimated through subject recall, and then the same method is applied.

The great advantage of these methods is their relative simplicity and low cost, which make them feasible for very large-scale studies, and they can even be administered by post or through a remote computer terminal. Their disadvantages are the element of subjectivity and a very low level of precision. They are also vulnerable to observer effects, whereby subjects are tempted to misrepresent their true activity, usually by exaggerating how active they are.

## METHODS OF EXPRESSING RESULTS

Energy expenditure can be expressed as kilocalories (kcal), kilojoules (kJ) or megajoules (MJ), where 1 kcal equals 4.184 kJ. The latter International System of Units (SI) are now favored by most journals and should be used in preference. Expenditure can be expressed per subject (generally as $kJ/min^{-1}$ or $MJ/day^{-1}$) or using some component of body weight as a denominator. In general, TEE can be expressed per kilogram body weight and BMR per kilogram lean body mass. However, there are complex issues surrounding the choice of appropriate denominators and their interpretation. These are beyond the scope of this chapter, but need to be understood by anyone working in the field.

### FURTHER READING

Blaxter, K. (1989). *Energy metabolism in animals and man*. Cambridge, UK: Cambridge University Press.—A general textbook on basic energy metabolism.

James, W. P. T., & Schofield, E. C. (1990). *Human energy requirements: A manual for planners and nutritionists*. Oxford, UK: Oxford University Press.—Includes information on how to use the less sophisticated methods.

International Dietary Energy Consultancy Group. (1990). *The doubly-labelled water method for measuring energy expenditure: Technical recommendations for use in humans* (A. M. Prentice, Ed.). Vienna: Author.—The technical bible on DLW applications in man. Available free on request to the International Atomic Energy Agency in Vienna but only necessary for users of the method.

Murgatroyd, P. R., Shetty, P. S., & Prentice, A. M. (1993). Techniques for the measurement of human energy expenditure. *International Journal of Obesity, 17*, 549–568.—This is the best overall guide to the different DLW techniques and contains illustrative examples.

Prentice, A. M., Diaz, E. O., Murgatroyd, P. R., Goldberg, G. R., Sonko, B. J., Black, A. E., & Coward, W. A. (1991). Doubly-labelled water measurements and calorimetry in practice. In R. G. Whitehead & A. Prentice (Eds.), *New techniques in nutritional research* (pp. 177–206). New York: Academic Press.—This chapter presents the pros and cons of state-of-the-art methods with examples.

Schoeller, D. A. (1999). Recent advances from application of doubly labeled water to measurement of human energy expenditure. *Journal of Nutrition, 129*, 1765–1768.—A recent update on applications of the DLW method.

Speakman, J. R. (1997). *Doubly labelled water: Theory and practice*. London: Chapman & Hall.— Provides plenty of background on the DLW method and discusses applications. It is the only textbook available on the method.

# 25

# Measurement of Physical Activity

JAMES F. SALLIS
MARION F. ZABINSKI

It is necessary to assess physical activity to understand the etiology, prevention, and treatment of obesity. This chapter highlights some of the best available self-report and objective measures.

## SELF-REPORT MEASURES

Self-reports are self- or interviewer-administered recalls, activity logs, and proxy reports. They are widely used because of ease of administration, low cost, and adaptability to fit a variety of research questions. Self-reports can assess all dimensions of physical activity: intensity, frequency, duration, and type. However, they cannot be used with young children or persons with limited cognitive abilities. Absolute estimates of activity duration seem to be biased, particularly with subjects' overreporting of vigorous physical activity.

In general, interviews seem to have better validity than self-administered questionnaires. Importantly, the age range of the population under investigation will influence type of activity and possibly also response to phraseology. Questionnaires with the best psychometric properties are described for children and adolescents, adults, and older adults.

### Child and Adolescent Measures

There are seventeen self-report measures with some evidence of validity in youth aged 10–18 years; however, reliability and validity are strongly related to age. The Seven Day Physical Activity Recall interview takes 15–20 minutes and assesses the past 7 days. It has strong test–retest reliability ($r = .77$) and adequate validity ($r = .53$) compared to heart rate monitoring. The Self-Administered Physical Activity Checklist takes approximately 35 minutes for group administration and assesses activity during the previous day because children have difficulty with longer-term recall. Test–retest reliability is good ($r$ = .65), as is validity compared to heart rate monitoring ($r$ = .60).

## Adult Measures

Most of the nine frequently used self-report measures for young to middle-age adults have been validated in multiple studies. The Minnesota Leisure Time Physical Activity Questionnaire consists of a lengthy list of activities, including sports, recreation, and garden/household chores. This interviewer-based assessment covers the past 12 months and codes frequency and duration. It has high test–retest reliability over 1 month ($r$ = .89), although its validity as compared to Caltrac monitors (see below) and energy intake is low ($r$ = .21 and .17, respectively). The Modifiable Activity Questionnaire, which assesses occupational and leisure activities, as well as sedentary time for the past year, can be tailored for particular populations. Test–retest reliability over 1 to 3 weeks is high ($r$ = .82), and validity coefficients range from .59 for the Caltrac criterion to .74 when compared to the doubly labeled water method (see Chapter 24 for information on the doubly labeled water method). The Seven-Day Physical Activity Recall interview is also well validated for adults ($r$ = .86; validity = .53, compared to accelerometers).

## Older Adult Measures

Four measures have been specially designed for older adults. The Physical Activity Scale for the Elderly is self-administered and assesses the past 7 days for leisure, household, and work-related activities. The test–retest reliability for 3 to 7 weeks is .75 and validity compared to the doubly labeled water method is .58. The Zutphen Physical Activity Questionnaire is self-completed in 15 minutes. It calculates total weekly minutes of activity and includes coding for intensity. Test–retest reliability for 3 months is high ($r$ = .93), and validity compared to the doubly labeled water method is .62.

## OBJECTIVE MEASURES

The primary objective measures are heart rate monitors and accelerometers. Monitors can be used with all ages to assess intensity, frequency, and duration. The principal limitation is cost.

## Heart Rate

The rationale for using this physiological measure is that heart rate is linearly related to oxygen consumption (exercise intensity) during dynamic exercise. Heart rate monitors consist of a chest strap transmitter and a watch with a receiver and display. They cost between $200 to $500 (U.S. dollars). Data can be sampled between 15 and 60 seconds for several days and stored in memory. Some monitors can be worn during water activities. Validity is affected by temperature and humidity, hydration level, type of exercise, and emotional stress. Limitations have been documented with elderly participants and persons with obesity or anorexia nervosa. There are practical limitations in assessing heart rate over multiple days.

Because emotional stress can produce heart rate elevations in the same range as moderate exercise (e.g., brisk walking), heart rate is best used as a measure of vigorous activity. There is no consensus as to the best method for scoring heart rate data. One method determines the number of minutes above a specified percentage of maximal heart rate (calculated as 220 − age in years). A second method subtracts resting heart rate from each active heart rate, allowing for comparison of people with different fitness levels. A third method, preferred by many, monitors heart rate and oxygen consumption simultaneously while the subject performs a variety of activities. Calculation of each individual's heart rate/oxygen consumption calibration curve may provide a more precise estimate of exercise intensity.

## Motion Sensors

Motion sensors worn on the waist reflect movement of the trunk, so they are generally valid for common activities such as walking, running, dancing, and many games. They cannot be used for water activities and underestimate activities that do not involve substantial vertical motion of the trunk, such as household chores, bicycling, and weight lifting.

The oldest device is the pedometer, which assesses steps taken. Its advantages are small size and low cost. The validated Yamax Digiwalker sells for about $20. Disadvantages include insensitivity to intensity and a single cumulative score.

The Caltrac (Muscle Dynamics, Torrance, CA), a single-plane accelerometer that assesses vertical motion, sells for under $100. This device has been widely used and is supported by high interinstrument reliability ($r = .89–.94$) and validity compared to direct observation ($r = .40–.86$) and heart rate recording ($r = .42–.54$). Specific limitations include controls that allow tampering and a single cumulative score.

The Tritrac, now called RT3 (*www.stayhealthy.com*), measures acceleration in all three planes and provides a summary score. Data can be collected over several days, stored in intervals ranging from 1 second to 1 minute, and downloaded directly to a computer. The newest model costs about $300 and is the size of a pager. Correlations with energy expenditure during walking ($r = .89$) are higher than when a variety of activities are performed ($r = .62$).

The CSA 7164 monitor (Computer Science and Applications, Inc.; *csaincmfg@fwb.gulf.net*) records vertical accelerations only, but otherwise has characteristics similar to the Tritrac. It costs about $350 and is the size of a watch face. Validity of measured walking is similar to that of the Tritrac.

Both the CSA and Tritrac have been used with children and adults. A major advantage of these and similar devices is their ability to assess specific activity patterns over several days. Monitor output has been calibrated against activity intensity, making it possible to determine such relevant variables as minutes per day in moderate and vigorous physical activity.

## RECOMMENDATIONS AND FUTURE RESEARCH

There are many validated self-report measures for all ages, but results across them are not comparable. Self-reports are particularly useful for assessing type of physical activity. Because of the apparent overreporting of physical activity, particularly among persons with obesity, objective measures are recommended for both clinical and research purposes. Although pedometers have limitations as research instruments, they can be useful clinically. Accelerometers that record moment-by-moment data are recommended for research. The combined use of heart rate and activity monitors might have advantages because each partially compensates for the shortcomings of the other.

No self-report or objective measures have been validated for the assessment of strengthening, flexibility, or weight-bearing activities, which are important for selected health outcomes. Of special relevance to the obesity field is the fact that there are no validated measures of sedentary behavior, although accelerometers may be of use for this purpose.

A validated physical activity assessment should be used in virtually every study of obesity. Excellent objective instruments that can be worn for several days are available. It is feasible to include pedometers and low-cost accelerometers in treatments for obesity; however, their contribution to outcome needs to be evaluated.

## FURTHER READING

Ainsworth, B. E. (2000). Issues in the assessment of physical activity in women. *Research Quarterly for Exercise and Sport, 71,* S37–S42.—Discusses why most self-report measures of leisure-time physical activity underestimate women's activity levels.

Baranowski, T., & de Moor, C. (2000). How many days was that? Intra-individual variability and physical activity assessment. *Research Quarterly for Exercise and Sport, 71,* S74–S78.—Discusses the problem of determining how many days of assessment are needed to characterize habitual activity level. Number of days varies by population and measurement method.

Freedson, P. S., & Miller, K. (2000). Objective monitoring of physical activity using motion sensors and heart rate. *Research Quarterly for Exercise and Sport, 71,* S21–S29.—A thorough review of all available activity monitors, including reliability and validity data.

Kriska, A. M. (2000). Ethnic and cultural issues in assessing physical activity. *Research Quarterly for Exercise and Sport, 71,* S47–S53.—Explains the challenges of assessing physical activity in various cultural groups and reviews effective approaches.

Kriska, A. M., & Caspersen, C. J. (Eds.). (1997). A collection of physical activity questionnaires for health-related research. *Medicine and Science in Sports and Exercise, 29,* S1–S205.—A valuable reference that includes over 30 actual questionnaires and summaries of reliability and validity data.

Montoye, H. J., Kemper, H. C. G., Saris, W. H. M., & Washburn, R. A. (1996). *Measuring physical activity and energy expenditure.* Champaign, IL: Human Kinetics.—The definitive book on physical activity measurement. Covers all measures and provides extensive data on reliability and validity.

Nichols, J. F., Morgan, C. G., Chabot, L. E., Sallis, J. F., & Calfas, K. J. (2000). Assessment of physical activity with the Computer Science and Applications, Inc. accelerometer: Laboratory versus field validation. *Research Quarterly for Exercise and Sport, 71,* 36–43.—Provides empirically based guidelines for translating the activity counts from the CSA monitor to activity intensity.

Sallis, J. F., & Saelens, B. E. (2000). Assessment of physical activity by self-report: Status, limitations, and future directions. *Research Quarterly for Exercise and Sport, 71,* S1–S14.—Reports summaries of reliability and validity data for the most widely used self-report measures for each age group and discusses their limitations and research needs.

Washburn, R. A. (2000). Assessment of physical activity in older adults. *Research Quarterly for Exercise and Sport*, 71, S79–S88.—Reviews the assessment options for older adults and includes reliability and validity data.

Welk, G. J., Corbin, C. B., & Dale, D. (2000). Measurement issues in the assessment of physical activity in children. *Research Quarterly for Exercise and Sport*, 71, S59–S73.—Reviews the various methods of assessing children's activity levels and summarizes reliability and validity data.

# 26

# Measurement of Eating Disorder Psychopathology

## DAVID M. GARNER

The general clinical features and psychopathology associated with anorexia nervosa and bulimia nervosa are well documented and widely accepted (see Chapter 29). Less is known about psychopathology associated with binge eating disorder and other eating disorders. While there is no universally accepted assessment protocol for eating disorders, there is a consensus on the value of utilizing different assessment methods to tap the broad range of associated symptoms and traits.

The targets for assessment of patients with eating disorders can be divided into two main areas: (1) psychological features and behavioral patterns that define the core features of eating disorders ("specific psychopathology"), and (2) psychopathology, not specific to patients with eating disorders, but that has particular theoretical or clinical relevance ("general psychopathology").

## SPECIFIC PSYCHOPATHOLOGY

### Body Weight and Body Weight History

The patient's current body weight and weight history provide essential diagnostic information and allow the clinician to explore the meaning that body weight and shape has for the patient. Since amenorrhea is required to make the diagnosis of anorexia nervosa (see Chapter 28), the clinician should determine the patient's menstrual history within the context of the weight history.

In the case of anorexia nervosa, it is usually advisable for the clinician to weigh the patient as part of the clinical interview. This should be done in a sensitive but straightforward manner, emphasizing physical and psychological implications of changes in body weight. However, even if body weight is not dangerously low, weight changes are critical

141

in evaluating motivation and cognitive processes. For example, the meaning and the approach taken in a particular treatment session may be entirely different for the patient who reports improved mood and successful completion of all homework assignments but has lost 2 pounds in the past week, as compared with the same report within the context of gaining 2 pounds. Explaining the need to carefully monitor weight in a matter-of-fact manner in the initial session is usually sufficient to overcome resistance to subsequent regular weighing.

Some clinicians prefer having the patient's weight checked by a family doctor, nurse, or other medical practitioner. However, not weighing the patient represents a missed opportunity, since the act of weighing often generates valuable in-session cognitive, affective, and behavioral data.

## Binge Eating

Binge eating is a key symptom in bulimia nervosa and binge eating disorder. It occurs in about 50% of cases presenting with anorexia nervosa. Thus, its assessment is critical to diagnosis and treatment planning. DSM-IV defines binge eating as having two main characteristics: (1) consumption of a large amount of food and (2) the experience of loss of control at the time. However, research has revealed that a significant minority of patients with eating disorder describe binges involving relatively small amounts of food. Moreover, in some cases there is no real loss of control. Thus, until there is agreement on the significance of size of binge episodes, it is recommended that assessments follow the system proposed in the Eating Disorder Examination (below) for dividing episodes of overeating into four types based on amount of food eaten (large or small) and loss of control (present or absent). It is also important to determine age of onset, frequency, and duration of binge-eating episodes. Likewise, circumstances surrounding individual binge episodes (settings, times of day, social context, thoughts and emotions) should be ascertained.

## Self-Induced Vomiting and Laxative Abuse

Self-induced vomiting and laxative abuse are two common symptoms that have both diagnostic as well as prognostic significance; they are common in bulimia nervosa and occur in approximately 50% of anorexia nervosa patients. Diagnostic criteria commonly call for assessment of the frequency of these behaviors in the past 1–3 months; however, it is important to remember that these symptoms fluctuate, and that some patients' history of these behaviors falls outside the diagnostic time-frame.

## Other Extreme Weight Control Behavior

In addition to vomiting and laxative abuse, information should be gathered about onset and course of severe restrictive dieting and other extreme weight-control behavior including diuretic abuse, use of diet pills or other drugs to control appetite, use of emetics, the chewing and spitting out of food before swallowing, prolonged fasting, and excessive exercise. Diabetic patients may manipulate their insulin dose to influence their weight, as may patients taking thyroid replacement hormone. Establishing the frequency (as well as the number of symptom-free days) for vomiting, laxative abuse, and other extreme weight-control behavior is part of assessment of the severity of the eating disorder and the need for medical consultation.

## Psychopathology Related to Weight or Shape

The psychopathology related to weight or shape has been described in various ways over the years, including a drive for thinness, fear of fatness, shape and weight dissatisfaction, body size misperception, body image disturbance, and fears associated with physical maturity. Dissatisfaction with overall body shape and disparagement directed toward specific bodily regions are common among patients with eating disorders and should be a focus of assessment. Although this is not unique to patients with eating disorder, some patients' overestimation of their body size may have clinical importance, particularly for emaciated patients. A critical psychopathological feature in anorexia nervosa and bulimia nervosa is that patients must be more than merely dissatisfied with their bodies; they rely on weight and shape as the predominant or even the sole criterion for judging their self-worth. This criterion is mandatory for a diagnosis of the two main eating disorders according to DSM-IV. In anorexia nervosa, there is often a denial of the seriousness of the current low weight, as well as an intense fear of weight gain.

## GENERAL PSYCHOPATHOLOGY

Patients with eating disorder have been described as suffering from low self-esteem, feelings of ineffectiveness, lack of autonomy, obsessionality, interpersonal sensitivity, introversion, poor relationship skills, social anxiety, dependence, perfectionism, fears of psychobiological maturity, poor impulse control, external locus of control, conflict avoidance, developmental pathology, failure in separation–individuation, vulnerability to substance abuse, interoceptive deficits, and idiosyncratic or dysfunctional thinking patterns (see Chapters 29, 34, 35, and 36). Complete psychological assessment should include these areas, as well as evaluation for personality disorders, stable personality features, overall psychological distress, depression, anxiety, family functioning, history of sexual abuse, and social and vocational adaptation, all of which may be relevant to the development and maintenance of these syndromes.

Some of the clinical features of anorexia nervosa are secondary to patients' poor eating habits and low body weight. For example, poor concentration, lability of mood, depressive features, obsessional thinking, irritability, difficulties with decision making, impulsivity, and social withdrawal have been identified in normal subjects undergoing semistarvation.

## ASSESSMENT METHODS

Various assessment methods have been developed for evaluating features of eating disorders including clinical interviews, self-report measures, self-monitoring, direct behavioral observation, symptom checklists, clinical rating scales, the Stroop test, and standardized test meals. The most commonly used methods are semistructured clinical interviews, self-monitoring, and self-report measures. The most well formulated of these methods, along with their respective strengths and weaknesses, are briefly described. Other measures and methods are covered by the reviews noted at the end of this chapter. (Measures of dietary restraint are discussed in Chapters 15 and 16.)

## Clinical Interviews

Clinical interviews have been the primary method for gathering information on eating disorders. The development of standardized, semistructured clinical interviews designed to evaluate the psychopathology of eating disorders represents a major advance in the field. Several interviews have been described in sufficient detail to warrant their use. The Eating Disorder Examination (EDE), the best-validated interview, has generated a large body of research. It is an investigator-based, semistructured interview for assessing psychopathology specific to eating disorders and is the current interview method of choice. Responses are organized on four subscales (Restraint, Eating Concern, Shape Concern, and Weight Concern). The EDE can be used to arrive at a diagnosis; it has proven sensitive to treatment effects and defines different forms of overeating based upon amount of food eaten (large vs. small) and presence or absence of loss of control. The EDE has the advantages of allowing a fine-grained appraisal of the specific psychopathology of eating disorders and permitting investigator probes to clarify the meaning behind responses to questions. One study comparing the EDE with a parallel self-report measure found the interview to be more accurate in identifying ambiguous symptoms such as binge eating. Disadvantages of the interview include the fact that it takes an hour or more to administer, it requires a trained interviewer, and it is not suitable when anonymity or group administration are required.

The Yale–Brown–Cornell Eating Disorder Scale is another well-validated interview measure, consisting of a 65-item, interview-based checklist as well as 19 questions covering 18 general categories of rituals and preoccupations common among patients with eating disorders. It requires less than 15 minutes to complete.

## Self-Monitoring

Self-monitoring requires patients to record in diaries their food intake, extreme weight-control behavior, thoughts, and feelings. Self-monitoring is a valuable assessment tool and probably yields more accurate information regarding eating behavior and eating disorder symptoms than methods requiring retrospective reports or generalizations about behavior. The disadvantages are that it may be unacceptable to certain patients and may influence the frequency of the very behaviors being monitored. (Self-monitoring is central to the cognitive-behavioral treatment of eating disorders; see Chapters 54 and 55.)

## Self-Report Measures

Various self-report instruments have been introduced to measure eating disorder symptoms. The two most widely used in clinical and research settings are the Eating Attitudes Test (EAT) and the Eating Disorder Inventory (EDI). The EAT, a widely used, standardized, self-report measure of eating disorder symptoms, has been translated into many languages and norms have been reported for different cultures. In the United States, the EAT has been adopted by the National Eating Disorders Screening Program for the purpose of "case-finding." A factor analysis of the original, 40-item version resulted in a brief, 26-item measure of global eating disorder symptoms. The EDI, a standardized, multiscale instrument with a much broader focus, comprising three subscales tapping attitudes and behavior concerning eating, weight, and shape (Drive for Thinness, Bulimia, Body Dissatisfaction) plus subscales assessing more general psychological traits or organizing constructs clinically relevant to eating disorders (Ineffectiveness, Perfection, Interpersonal Distrust, Interoceptive Awareness, Maturity Fears). The EDI-2 added three new subscales to the original instrument (Asceticism, Impulse Regulation, and Social Insecurity). The EAT and EDI have good psychometric properties and are sensitive to treatment effects. The EDI provides a psychological profile that can be useful in clinical situations.

The Bulimia Test—Revised (BULIT-R) is a 28-item, multiple choice, self-report measure based on the DSM-III-R criteria for bulimia nervosa. It has generated considerable research and is a reliable psychometric measure for bulimia nervosa. The EDE-Q4, a self-report version of the EDE, is designed for situations in which an interview is not practical. It has been validated against the EDE interview. The Questionnaire on Eating and Weight Patterns—Revised (QEWP-R) measures the nature and the quantity of binge eating and has been designed for assessing binge eating disorder. Finally, the Eating Disorders Questionnaire (EDQ) is a self-report measure that covers symptom domains as well as demographic information relevant to eating disorders.

Self-report measures have the advantages of being relatively economical, brief, easily administered, and objectively scored. They are not susceptible to bias from interviewer–subject interactions and can be administered anonymously. Their major disadvantage is that they are less accurate than interview methods, particularly when assessing complex behavior such as binge eating. They need to be supplemented by symptom frequency data derived by interview or symptom checklist.

## CONCLUSION

The different methods for assessing psychopathology in eating disorders have different aims, strengths, and weaknesses. The strategy adopted should be guided by the purpose of the assessment and, whenever possible, clinicians should employ convergent methods.

## FURTHER READING

American Psychiatric Association. (2000). Practice guideline for the treatment of patients with eating disorders (Rev.). *American Journal of Psychiatry* (Suppl.), *157*, 1–39.—Practice guidelines, including assessment of patients with eating disorders.

Crowther, J. H., & Sherwood, N. E. (1997). Assessment. In D. M. Garner & P. E. Garfinkel (Eds.), *Handbook of treatment for eating disorders* (pp. 34–49). New York: Guilford Press.—An excellent review of assessment methods for eating disorders.

Fairburn, C. G., & Belgin, S. J. (1994). The assessment of eating disorders: Interview or self-report questionnaire? *International Journal of Eating Disorders, 16*, 363–370.—A detailed comparison of an investigator-based interview and a self-report measure based on that interview, showing that both measures perform similarly when assessing unambiguous behavior and favoring the interview in assessing more complex behavior.

Fairburn, C. G., & Cooper, Z. (1993). The Eating Disorder Examination (12th ed.). In C. G.

Fairburn & G. T. Wilson (Eds.), *Binge eating: Nature, assessment, and treatment* (pp. 317–360). New York: Guilford Press.—The primary reference for the EDE.

Garner, D. M. (1991). *Eating Disorder Inventory-2 professional manual*. Odessa, FL: Psychological Assessment Resources.—A comprehensive reference source for the EDI.

Garner, D. M., Olmsted, M. P., Bohr, Y., & Garfinkel, P. E. (1982). The Eating Attitudes Test: Psychometric features and clinical correlates. *Psychological Medicine, 12*, 871–878.—The primary reference for the EAT. The EAT-26, norms, and scoring instructions can also be obtained on the internet site: river-centre.org.

King, M. B. (1991). The natural history of eating pathology in attenders to primary medical care. *International Journal of Eating Disorders, 10*, 379–387.—An excellent study of the application of the EAT in a "two-stage" method of assessing eating disorders using self-report and interview methodology.

Mitchell, J. E., Hatsukami, D., Eckert, E., & Pyle, R. L. (1985). The Eating Disorders Questionnaire. *Psychopharmacology Bulletin, 21*, 1025–1043.—The primary reference for the EDQ.

Nasser, M. (1997). The EAT speaks many languages: Review of the use of the EAT in eating disorders research. *Eating and Weight Disorders, 2*, 174–181.—A review of the use of the EAT in different cultures.

Pike, K. M., Woll, S. L., Gluck, M., & Walsh, B. T. (2000). Eating disorders measures. In *American Psychiatric Association handbook of psychiatric measures* (pp. 647–671). Washington, DC: American Psychiatric Association.—An excellent overview of assessment methods for eating disorders.

Sunday, S. R., Halmi, K. A., & Einhorn, A. N. (1995). The Yale–Brown–Cornell Eating Disorder Scale: A new scale to assess eating disorder symptomatology. *International Journal of Eating Disorders, 18*, 237–245.—The primary reference for this measure.

Thelen, M. H., Farmer, J., Wonderlich, S., & Smith, M. (1991). A revision of the Bulimia Test: The BULIT-R. *Psychological Assessment: A Journal of Consulting and Clinical Psychology, 3*, 119–124.—The primary reference for the BULIT-R.

Wilson, G. T., & Vitousek, K. M. (1999). Self-monitoring in the assessment of eating disorders. *Psychological Assessment, 11*, 480–489.—Detailed discussion of the strengths and limitations of self-monitoring in assessment and treatment.

# PART II

# EATING DISORDERS

# Clinical Characteristics
# of Eating Disorders

# 27

# History of Anorexia Nervosa and Bulimia Nervosa

## WALTER VANDEREYCKEN

Throughout history we can recognize the heterogeneous manifestation of disturbed eating behavior. Whereas the terms "bulimia" and "anorexia" have been employed for ages, their nosological status has continuously been challenged. Traditionally, in medicine, both food avoidance and overeating were almost invariably looked upon as symptoms of a diversity of illnesses, predominantly gastrointestinal disorders. Preoccupations with body weight and shape, and the application of weight-control strategies such as dieting and purging have acquired popular and medical attention only in the last part of the 20th century (and only in Western or westernized countries). Hence, the specific syndromes anorexia nervosa and bulimia nervosa appear to be relatively "modern" clinical entities.

### ANOREXIA NERVOSA

Until the 19th century, "anorexia" (the medical term for loss of appetite) was considered a symptom of several physical and emotional disorders. But for centuries, voluntary abstention from food was not primarily a pathological phenomenon; extreme fasting was part of the penitential or ascetic practice of many pious Christians. Later on, forms of long-lasting food refusal, not accompanied by symptoms of well-known diseases such as tuberculosis, were more likely to stir up speculations about supernatural powers or demonic influences. Ultimately, extreme or unusual forms of food abstinence were looked upon as signs of a mental disorder. Food avoidance and emaciation were common symptoms of well-known diseases such as hysteria, mania, melancholy, chlorosis, and all kinds of psychotic disorders. At the end of the 17th century, the English physician Richard Morton described the occurrence of "nervous consumption"—a wasting different from tuberculosis and due to emotional turmoil. This is often quoted as the first medical report of anorexia nervosa, but Morton's interesting case studies (of both a girl and a boy) did not attract any attention and fell into oblivion, until rediscovered three centuries later.

Morbid self-starvation only became recognized as a distinct clinical entity in the second half of the 19th century. The Parisian clinician Ernest-Charles Lasègue and the London physician Sir William Withey Gull must be awarded "joint parenthood" for the first explicit description of anorexia nervosa. In April 1873, Lasègue published his article on "anorexie hystérique," which appeared in English translation shortly before Gull presented his paper on "anorexia hysterica" in October of the same year. His lecture was published in 1874, employing the term "anorexia nervosa." According to both clinicians, it was a psychogenic affliction that occurred predominantly in girls and young women. The characteristics described by Gull and Lasègue are still valid today: severe weight loss, amenorrhea, constipation, restlessness, and no evidence of underlying organic pathology. Although the French and British medical press showed some interest in the new syndrome, in many other countries (e.g., the United States, Germany, and Italy), anorexia nervosa remained largely a marginal phenomenon until well into the 20th century.

Initially, anorexia nervosa was generally looked upon as a mental disorder. However, when in 1914 the German pathologist Morris Simmonds found lesions of the pituitary gland in some emaciated patients, anorexia nervosa became inextricably associated with this "Simmonds' disease" or "pituitary cachexia." It took more than two decades for this erroneous idea to be clearly refuted. After World War II, the endocrinological view of anorexia nervosa made a rapid and smooth demise. Physicians' minimization of the psychological component then made room for psychiatric dramatization. In the period 1945–1960, psychiatry was strongly dominated by psychoanalytic views, and traces thereof can be found in contemporary theories on anorexia nervosa; for example, fear of food intake was linked to unconscious fears of oral impregnation. But interest in anorexia nervosa was not particularly great. After 1960, this changed drastically due to the pioneering work of (German-born) American psychiatrist Hilde Bruch, who focused attention on the lack of self-esteem and the distorted body image of these patients. This led to the addition of two features to the original clinical picture, as described by Lasègue and Gull: the relentless pursuit of thinness and the characteristic disturbance of the body image (see Chapter 29). As such, anorexia nervosa evolved in the late 20th century from a rare and little known clinical entity to a "fashionable" disorder of great interest to the general public.

## BULIMIA NERVOSA

Although the term "bulimia nervosa" is of recent origin, reports on morbid hunger may be found under a multitude of different labels as far back as medical records exist. According to Plutarch, *bulimos* referred to an evil demon and originally would have meant a great famine, but philologists later claimed that it was taken from the Greek *bous* (ox) and *limos* (hunger), denoting hunger of such intensity that a man had the capacity to eat an entire ox. This morbid hunger also implied weakness and fainting, and was supposed to be closely connected with digestive dysfunctions.

In view of the modern clinical picture of bulimia nervosa, historical accounts of gorging combined with vomiting need special attention. In medicine, this eating abnormality was generally known under the label "kynorexia" or *fames canina* (i.e., a dog-like insatiable voracity followed by spontaneous vomiting). Again, dysfunctions and abnormalities of the stomach were considered to be the cause. Some 18th-century clinicians distinguished several forms of bulimia, some of which were viewed as being primary, or "idiopathic," bulimia, including bulimia helluonum (excessive hunger), bulimia syncopalis (fainting from hunger) and bulimia emetica (overeating with vomiting). Although emotional factors were taken into consideration well into the 20th century, internists (especially those from French- and German-speaking countries) considered bulimia primarily a sign of gastric dysfunction. In 19th-century accounts of hysteria, overeating and vomiting had been frequently mentioned symptoms, sometimes labeled as "hysterical vomiting," but they were not looked upon as a specific eating disorder.

It was in the context of anorexia nervosa that the modern notion of bulimia nervosa emerged. Sporadic reports appeared on patients with compulsive overeating followed by self-induced vomiting, but these symptoms were regarded as a neurotic condition or a variation in the eating pattern of anorectic patients. The most carefully documented case report (although the case was [mis]diagnosed as schizophrenia) was published by the Swiss psychiatrist Ludwig Binswanger in 1944. It is a moving account of Ellen West's relentless pursuit of thinness and her struggle with bulimia, leading to violent vomiting and excessive abuse of laxatives. From the early 1970s on, a discrete cluster of symptoms was identified, distinguishable from anorexia nervosa and obesity. Clinicians increasingly reported on women who binged on copious quantities of food but maintained their weight within the normal range by inducing vomiting or abusing laxatives and by constant dieting. A multitude of different names for this syndrome were coined, including "dysorexia," "bulimarexia," "thin–fat syndrome," "binge–purge syndrome," and "dietary chaos syndrome." In 1979, the British psychiatrist Gerald Russell coined the term "bulimia nervosa," referring to "powerful and intractable urges to overeat" in combination with "a morbid fear of becoming fat" and the avoidance "of the fattening effects of food by inducing vomiting or abusing purgatives or both" in women with a normal body weight. Initially, only the term "bulimia" found its way into international classification systems of mental disorders such as DSM-III (1980). However, the (mainly American) use of the term was confusing and overinclusive, unlike Russell's notion of bulimia nervosa, which he considered an "ominous variant of anorexia nervosa." In the 1987 revised version of DSM-III, the diagnosis was brought into line with British terminology and renamed "bulimia nervosa."

## NEW DISORDERS?

Considering the multifaceted continuum of eating abnormalities, the history of eating disorders is age-old. Undoubtedly, disturbed patterns of eating, such as food avoidance and gorging followed by spontaneous vomiting, have always been with us. But clear-cut and explicit descriptions closely matching modern anorexia nervosa were not discovered prior to about 1850. And only in the last decades of the 20th century did a specific form of bulimia achieve the status of a widely accepted psychiatric diagnosis. The individual behaviors were not new, but their basic psychological meaning certainly was, probably because of a new cultural context.

At the heart of both anorexia nervosa and bulimia nervosa lies an intense fear of becoming overweight. Does the history of eating disorders reflect the history of a changed ideal of beauty? Are these disorders a sign of a deranged obsession for thinness, the product of a new body culture, a morbid epiphenomenon of a consumer society? From the 15th century onward, Western society has idealized three types of female figures. Until the 17th century, the tummy-centered and—by present-day standards—rather plump woman was admired. This "reproductive" type was then replaced by the "hour-glass" model, with a narrow waist, full bosom, and round bottom. Since the late 19th century, the idealized shape for women has been the lean, almost "tubular" body type, deprived of any symbolism of fertility and motherhood. The thinness of the "new women" expressed sexual liberation and rejection of the traditional female role.

Parallel to this has been increasing aversion to overweight or corpulency. For men in particular, the preservation of health has been used as a justification and placed within the evolutionism of the "survival of the fittest": Progress did not benefit from fat people and gluttons. For women—particularly in the late 19th-century upper classes—a new ideal of slenderness gradually arose. Here, health concerns played only a minor role. Although a certain plumpness still continued to be desirable, by the turn of the 20th century, the modern ideal of slenderness had come into being. The "battle against fatness" had started: Obesity was the "enemy" and physicians provided the "weapons." Modern diet-culture emerged, and it is going to be with us for many years to come, probably together with eating disorders, "old" or "new.". . .

## FURTHER READING

Brumberg, J. J. (1988). *Fasting girls: The emergence of anorexia nervosa as a modern disease*. Cambridge, MA: Harvard University Press.—The first book on the history of anorexia nervosa, written from a feminist perspective.

Parry-Jones, B., & Parry-Jones, W. L. (1991). Bulimia: An archival review of its history in psychosomatic medicine. *International Journal of Eating Disorders, 10*, 129–143.—Detailed analysis of medical reports on "pathological voracity" from the 15th to the 18th century.

Russell, G. F. M. (1979). Bulimia nervosa: An ominous variant of anorexia nervosa. *Psychological Medicine, 9*, 429–448.—The classic description of bulimia nervosa by the clinician who coined the term.

Stein, D. M., & Laakso, W. (1988). Bulimia: A historical perspective. *International Journal of Eating Disorders, 7*, 201–210.—A short overview of the history of bulimia (nervosa) over the last three centuries.

Vandereycken, W. (1994). Emergence of bulimia nervosa as a separate diagnostic entity: Review of the literature from 1960 to 1979. *International Journal of Eating Disorders, 16*, 105–116.—A detailed reconstruction of how bulimia nervosa became a well-established clinical concept in modern medical literature.

Vandereycken, W., & Van Deth, R. (1994). *From fasting saints to anorexic girls: The history of self-starvation*. New York: New York University Press. (Also published in Dutch, German, Italian, and Japanese.)—Richly documented account of the history of self-starvation as a wonder, a spectacle, and an illness.

Van Deth, R., & Vandereycken, W. (1994). Continuity and discontinuity in the history of self-starvation. *Eating Disorders Review, 2*, 47–55.—Discussion of whether a "modern" diagnosis such as anorexia nervosa is applicable to food abstinence in previous centuries.

Van Deth, R., & Vandereycken, W. (1997). The striking age-old minority of fasting males in the history of anorexia nervosa. *Food and Foodways, 7*, 119–130.—An overview of the history of anorexia nervosa in males.

van 't Hof, S. (1994). *Anorexia nervosa: The historical and cultural specificity. Fallacious theories and tenacious "facts."* Amsterdam: Swets & Zeitlinger.—Detailed discussion of whether anorexia nervosa is historically and culturally specific or universal and for all times.

# 28

# Classification and Diagnosis of Eating Disorders

## PAUL E. GARFINKEL

There has been rapid evolution in the classification and understanding of eating disorders in a relatively brief period of time. Anorexia nervosa was the first eating disorder to be classified, with specific diagnostic criteria developed in the 1970s. In 1979, bulimia nervosa was described. In the 1980s, the existence of atypical eating disorders (that is, eating disorders other than anorexia nervosa and bulimia nervosa—see Chapter 30) was recognized. Most recently, two new eating disorders have been demarcated—namely, "binge eating disorder" and the "night eating syndrome" (see Chapters 31 and 32, respectively)—although their diagnostic status remains the subject of debate.

The focus of this chapter is on the classification and diagnosis of the two best established eating disorders, anorexia nervosa and bulimia nervosa.

## DIAGNOSTIC CRITERIA FOR ANOREXIA NERVOSA

Since 1969, a variety of operational criteria for anorexia nervosa that emphasize signs and symptoms have been developed. The first such criteria were proposed by Gerald Russell in 1970. Russell emphasized (1) a behavioral disturbance, (2) a characteristic psychopathology, and (3) an endocrine disorder. The behavioral disturbance leads to a marked loss of body weight; the psychopathology is characterized by a morbid fear of getting fat; and the endocrine disorder manifests itself clinically by amenorrhea in females and loss of sexual potency and sexual interest in males. These criteria have evolved into the current DSM-IV and ICD-10 criteria (shown in Tables 28.1 and 28.2, respectively).

**TABLE 28.1. DSM-IV Diagnostic Criteria for Anorexia Nervosa**

A. Refusal to maintain body weight at or above a minimally normal weight for age and height (e.g., weight loss leading to maintenance of body weight less than 85% of that expected; or failure to make expected weight gain during period of growth, leading to body weight less than 85% of that expected).

B. Intense fear of gaining weight or becoming fat, even though underweight.

C. Disturbance in the way in which one's body weight or shape is experienced, undue influence of body weight or shape on self-evaluation, or denial of the seriousness of the current low body weight.

D. In postmenarcheal females, amenorrhea, i.e., the absence of at least three consecutive menstrual cycles. (A woman is considered to have amenorrhea if her periods occur only following hormone, e.g., estrogen, administration.)

*Specify* type:

   **Restricting Type:** during the current episode of Anorexia Nervosa, the person has not regularly engaged in binge eating or purging behavior (i.e., self-induced vomiting or the misuse of laxatives, diuretics, or enemas)

   **Binge-Eating/Purging Type:** during the current episode of Anorexia Nervosa, the person has regularly engaged in binge-eating or purging behavior (i.e., self-induced vomiting or the misuse of laxatives, diuretics, or enemas)

*Note.* From American Psychiatric Association. (1994). *Diagnostic and statistical manual of mental disorders* (4th ed.). Washington, DC: Author. Copyright 1994 by the American Psychiatric Association. Reprinted by permission.

## Behavior Designed to Produce Weight Loss

An exaggerated drive for thinness has been recognized by many as central to anorexia nervosa; this is what Bruch referred to as the "relentless pursuit of thinness." In DSM-IV (criterion A), it is specified as "Refusal to maintain body weight at or above a minimally normal weight for age and height (e.g., weight loss leading to maintenance of body weight less than 85% of that expected; or failure to make expected weight gain during period of growth, leading to body weight less than 85% of that expected)." The latter is directed at younger patients who would be expected to continue growing.

While there is agreement on the need for this criterion, views on the weight threshold necessary for the diagnosis have varied and the optimal level is not known. In principle, this depends on the point at which either starvation symptoms supervene or physiological consequences are first evident.

## Psychopathology Characterized by a Morbid Fear of Becoming Fat

This involves both an intense fear of becoming fat and basing self-worth on weight and shape (DSM-IV criteria B and C). These disturbances in feelings and attitudes have been demonstrated in empirical studies and they distinguish anorexia nervosa (and bulimia nervosa) from other psychiatric syndromes.

The earlier DSM-III criteria defined this feature in terms of "body image distur-bance." Many studies of body image in patients with anorexia nervosa have focused on visual self-perception. The results show that many patients do not overestimate their size, and that overestimation is not unique to those with the disorder. Given these findings, it was appropriate to change this criterion to focus on the distinctive attitudinal and affec-

**TABLE 28.2. ICD-10 Diagnostic Criteria for Anorexia Nervosa**

A. There is weight loss or, in children, a lack of weight gain, leading to a body weight at least 15% below the normal or expected weight for age and height.

B. The weight loss is self-induced by avoidance of "fattening foods."

C. There is self-perception of being too fat, with an intrusive dread of fatness, which leads to a self-imposed low weight threshold.

D. A widespread endocrine disorder involving the hypothalamic–pituitary–gonadal axis is manifested in women as amenorrhea and in men as a loss of sexual interest and potency. (An apparent exception is the persistence of vaginal bleeds in anorexic women who are on replacement hormonal therapy, most commonly taken as a contraceptive pill.)

E. The disorder does not meet criteria A and B for bulimia nervosa.

*Note.* From World Health Organization. (1993). *ICD-10 classification of mental and behavioural disorders: Diagnostic criteria for research.* Geneva, Switzerland: Author. Copyright 1993 by the World Health Organization. Reprinted by permission.

tive dimensions of body image. As well, it is important that criterion C acknowledges these patients' characteristic denial of the serious consequences of their low weight.

## Evidence of an Endocrine Disorder: Amenorrhea in Females and Loss of Sexual Potency and Interest in Males

Amenorrhea is a common feature of anorexia nervosa that in part stems from the loss of body weight and fat. But the presence of amenorrhea is not well understood (see Chapters 48 and 50); it occurs in a significant minority of women before there is any significant weight loss and may persist after weight regain. Studies in the community have shown that women who have continued to menstruate while displaying all the other features of anorexia nervosa are as ill as those who meet full syndrome criteria. This calls into question the value of this criterion.

## Subtypes of Anorexia Nervosa

Attempts at distinguishing subtypes of anorexia nervosa date back to Janet, early in the last century, who recognized hysterical and obsessional types. This was ignored until Dally utilized it in the late 1960s. Shortly after, Beumont began to subtype anorexia nervosa by the presence or absence of vomiting. This was refined a few years later to distinguish subtypes on the basis of the presence or absence of binge eating or purging (the collective term for vomiting or laxative misuse; see Table 28.1). Major differences between these groups have been described. In comparison with those who do not regularly binge eat, those with regular binge eating have weighed more in childhood and have more frequently been obese; have often come from heavier families, with more frequent familial obesity; and more commonly use extreme methods of weight control. In addition, they more frequently display other impulsive behavior, such as alcohol and drug abuse, stealing, and self-mutilation. They also display different personality types: frequently borderline, narcissistic, or antisocial, a group that discharges impulses through action. A minority of patients with anorexia nervosa purge but do not binge. They are classified in the same way as those who binge since they share many features.

## DIAGNOSTIC CRITERIA FOR BULIMIA NERVOSA

When Russell described bulimia nervosa, he defined the syndrome by (1) powerful and irresistible urges to overeat, (2) consequent compensatory behavior, and (3) the underlying psychopathology of a morbid fear of fat. These criteria have undergone various modifications. The DSM-IV and ICD-10 criteria are shown in Table 28.3 and Table 28.4, respectively.

### Powerful and Irresistible Urges to Overeat (Resulting in Binge Eating)

This corresponds to DSM-IV criteria A and C. DSM-IV defines what constitutes a "binge" in terms of the quantity of food eaten, the subjective state (a sense of loss of control) at the time, and the discrete nature of the eating episode. With regard to the amount eaten, what is most relevant is that the person is eating more than is usual given the circumstances.

Far less clear is the frequency of binge eating needed to make the diagnosis. In DSM-III-R, a minimum average of twice a week was specified. There is value in setting a minimum frequency, but there is a problem with the arbitrary nature of this threshold, since there is no evidence that it is a meaningful level (based on studies of coexisting psycho-

---

**TABLE 28.3. DSM-IV Diagnostic Criteria for Bulimia Nervosa**

A. Recurrent episodes of binge eating. An episode of binge eating is characterized by both of the following:
   (1) eating, in a discrete period of time (e.g., within any 2-hour period), an amount of food that is definitely larger than most people would eat during a similar period of time and under similar circumstances
   (2) a sense of lack of control over eating during the episode (e.g., a feeling that one cannot stop eating or control what or how much one is eating)

B. Recurrent inappropriate compensatory behavior in order to prevent weight gain, such as self-induced vomiting; misuse of laxatives, diuretics, enemas, or other medications; fasting; or excessive exercise.

C. The binge eating and inappropriate compensatory behaviors both occur, on average, at least twice a week for 3 months.

D. Self-evaluation is unduly influenced by body shape and weight.

E. The disturbance does not occur exclusively during episodes of Anorexia Nervosa.

*Specify* type:
   **Purging Type:** during the current episode of Bulimia Nervosa, the person has regularly engaged in self-induced vomiting or the misuse of laxatives, diuretics, or enemas

   **Nonpurging Type:** during the current episode of Bulimia Nervosa, the person has used other inappropriate compensatory behaviors, such as fasting or excessive exercise, but has not regularly engaged in self-induced vomiting or the misuse of laxatives, diuretics, or enemas

*Note.* From American Psychiatric Association. (1994). *Diagnostic and statistical manual of mental disorders* (4th ed.). Washington, DC: Author. Copyright 1994 by the American Psychiatric Association. Reprinted by permission.

**TABLE 28.4. ICD-10 Diagnostic Criteria for Bulimia Nervosa**

A. There are recurrent episodes of overeating (at least twice a week over a period of 3 months) in which large amounts of food are consumed in short periods of time.

B. There is persistent preoccupation with eating, and a strong desire or sense of compulsion to eat (craving).

C. The patient attempts to counteract the "fattening" effects of food by one or more of the following:
   (1) self-induced vomiting;
   (2) self-induced purging;
   (3) alternating periods of starvation;
   (4) use of drugs such as appetite suppressants, thyroid preparations, or diuretics; when bulimia occurs in diabetic patients they may choose to neglect their insulin treatment.

D. There is self-perception of being too fat, with an intrusive dread of fatness (usually leading to underweight).

*Note.* From World Health Organization. (1993). *ICD-10 classification of mental and behavioural disorders: Diagnostic criteria for research.* Geneva, Switzerland: Author. Copyright 1993 by the World Health Organization. Reprinted by permission.

pathology or clinical outcome). Indeed, there is evidence that those with once-weekly binge eating are no different than those who binge eat more often.

## Avoidance of the Fattening Effects of Food by Inducing Vomiting, Abusing Purgatives, or Both

This corresponds to DSM-IV criterion B and is useful, since (1) the presence of purging is often an indication of the intensity of the person's concern about weight and shape; (2) while dieting and vigorous exercise are not considered especially unusual, purging is thought to be pathological in our society; (3) purging is easily defined and is quantifiable; and (4) serious physiological complications may arise as a result of purging (see Chapter 50).

## A Morbid Fear of Becoming Fat

This fear of fat corresponds to criterion D in DSM-IV. The earlier DSM-III criteria did not include such concerns about weight and shape. The advantages of this criterion include (1) it covers what many view to be the "core psychopathology" of bulimia nervosa (and anorexia nervosa); (2) it makes the diagnosis more restrictive; and (3) it draws the syndrome closer to the related disorder, anorexia nervosa.

## Subtypes of Bulimia Nervosa

DSM-IV has recently subtyped bulimia nervosa into purging and nonpurging types. The purging type corresponds to Russell's original bulimia nervosa category. In comparison with nonpurging patients, those who purge have elevated rates of psychopathology, for example, greater body image disturbance, more anxiety concerning eating, and more self-injurious behavior. They also have exceptionally high rates of comorbidity for depression, anxiety disorders, and alcohol abuse.

## PROBLEMS THAT REMAIN

### Problems Due to Current Levels of Understanding

With regard to anorexia nervosa, the optimal weight threshold is not known and the need for amenorrhea as a criterion is questionable. Second, for bulimia nervosa, the optimal thresholds for the frequency of binge eating and purging are not clear. Third, the relationship between the nonpurging form of bulimia nervosa and binge eating disorder requires clarification (see Chapters 30 and 31). They may be phases of the same disorder or closely related conditions, although recent studies of their development and course suggest that this is not the case (see Chapter 31).

### Problems Due to the Nature of the Eating Disorders

Other problems relate to the nature of the eating disorders themselves. For example, eating disorders are heterogeneous in character. While a core psychopathology has been identified (the overevaluation of shape and weight—see Chapter 29), this is variable in its severity and form. Eating disorders are also sensitive to cultural influences that affect their expression and change over time (see Chapters 27 and 47). They also exist on a continuum that ranges from innocuous but persistent dieting, through subthreshold states of uncertain clinical significance, to full cases of anorexia nervosa or bulimia nervosa. While this continuum is beginning to be better defined, problems with categorization remain and probably always will. Yet another problem is that the presence of comorbid states can affect the clinical picture, for example, the use of insulin for weight control in insulin-dependent diabetes mellitus (see Chapter 51).

### Problems Due to Overemphasis on Diagnosis

Another problem relates to the risk of overemphasizing diagnosis at the expense of understanding people. Diagnosis, imperative for clinical practice, represents a form of communication that permits detailed examination, investigation of approaches to treatment, and delineation of prognosis. Used in a concrete or thoughtless manner, however, it may detract from, rather than enhance, care. One may make a diagnosis while knowing little about the patient as a person. Awareness of psychological theories of development, unconscious conflict, or the therapeutic process is not needed to make a diagnosis. This absence of meaning must be addressed if we are to retain a humanistic orientation, for it is impossible to treat suffering individuals if we are devoid of an awareness of history, symbolic meaning, conflict, ambivalence, social context, and the primacy of existential concerns.

### FURTHER READING

Bulik, C. M., Sullivan, P. F., & Kendler, K. S. (2000). An empirical study of the classification of eating disorders. *American Journal of Psychiatry, 157*, 886–895.—An attempt to identify natural clusters of eating disorder features using a community sample.

Garfinkel, P. E., Kennedy, S., & Kaplan, A. S. (1995). Views on classification and diagnosis of eating disorders. *Canadian Journal of Psychiatry, 40*, 445–456.—A thorough analysis of the empirical and clinical standing of the DSM-IV scheme for clarifying disorders.

Garfinkel, P. E., Lin, B., Goering, P., Spegg, C., Goldbloom, D., Kennedy, S., Kaplan, A., & Woodside, B. (1995). Bulimia nervosa in a Canadian community sample: Prevalence and comparison of subgroups. *American Journal of Psychiatry, 152,* 1052–1058.—Large-scale interview-based study of the prevalence of bulimia nervosa and its association with other psychiatric disorders.

Garfinkel, P. E., Lin, B., Goering, P., Spegg, C., Goldbloom, D., Kennedy, S., Kaplan, A., & Woodside, B. (1996). Purging and non-purging forms of bulimia nervosa in a community sample. *International Journal of Eating Disorders, 20,* 231–238.—A comparison of the purging and nonpurging types of bulimia nervosa using data from a large community survey.

Garfinkel, P. E., Lin, B., Goering, P., Spegg, C., Goldbloom, D., Kennedy, S., Kaplan, A., & Woodside, D. B. (1996). Should amenorrhea be necessary for the diagnosis of anorexia nervosa? Evidence from a Canadian community sample. *British Journal of Psychiatry, 168,* 500–506.—A comparison of cases of "anorexia nervosa" with and without amenorrhea.

Hay, P., Fairburn, C., & Doll, H. (1996). The classification of bulimic eating disorders: A community-based cluster analytic study. *Psychological Medicine, 26,* 801–812.—An attempt to identify natural clusters of eating disorder features among a community sample of women with recurrent binge eating.

# 29

# Clinical Presentation of Anorexia Nervosa and Bulimia Nervosa

## PIERRE J. V. BEUMONT

## ANOREXIA NERVOSA

Anorexia nervosa is a condition of self-engendered weight loss, usually seen in adolescent girls and young women, and less commonly in prepubertal children and middle-age women or men. It has been recognized in medicine for more than 150 years, but for much of that time was largely confined to affluent societies that espouse Western cultural ideals (see Chapter 27 for a discussion of the history of anorexia nervosa and bulimia nervosa). It now occurs at all socioeconomic levels, and there are increasing reports of anorexia-like illnesses from non-Western societies (see Chapter 47). The criteria that have been proposed for its diagnosis point to three sets of related features: (1) an intense preoccupation with weight and shape; (2) behaviors directed at the relentless pursuit of thinness; and (3) the physical consequences of these behaviors, such as emaciation, disturbed endocrine function, and other nutritional abnormalities. (The diagnostic criteria for anorexia nervosa and bulimia nervosa are discussed in Chapter 28.)

### Psychiatric Presentation

The objective psychopathology is difficult to label. It has been termed hysterical, a phobia of weight gain, an obsession, or even a delusion, but perhaps an overvalued idea is best. Patients are overwhelmed by concerns about their bodies and protest that they feel themselves to be fat even when they are actually emaciated. They are preoccupied with ways to reduce their weight further or, at the least, to prevent any gain. Patients appear genuinely terrified at the prospect of being overweight, and some state openly that they would rather be dead than fat. Although so extreme as to be pathological, such beliefs represent an exaggeration of the widespread concern about weight control that has been engendered in our community.

Onto this core concern are imposed other psychological symptoms, many of which are known to be common to semistarvation irrespective of cause. These include depressed mood, irritability, social withdrawal, loss of sexual libido, preoccupation with food, obsessional ruminations and rituals, and, eventually, reduced alertness and concentration. Dysphoria, an integral feature of the illness, is particularly important. This intimate association is not understood by many clinicians, who make an inappropriate second diagnosis of a mood disorder. (See Chapter 34 for a discussion of the relationships between eating disorders and mood and anxiety disorders.) Similarly, severe obsessional symptoms, usually relating to eating and food but sometimes of a more general nature, are common in anorexia nervosa patients. Often, but not invariably, these symptoms also improve with weight gain.

The illness is associated with premorbid perfectionism, introversion, poor peer relations, and low self-esteem (see Chapter 36). The patient is described as having been a biddable and helpful child, whose current obstinate refusal to eat is all the more extraordinary because of her previous compliance. In the early stages, as the patient becomes increasingly preoccupied with dieting, she withdraws from peer relationships, concentrating on study or work to the exclusion of all other interests. However, these features are not found in all patients, some of whom are more extroverted and interactive, with outgoing personality profiles and a history of behavioral disturbance.

Patients react to efforts to alter their behavior with anger, deception, and manipulation, often inconsistent with their previous behavioral standards. With chronicity, they become absorbed by their illness, dependent on family or therapists, and restricted in their interests. The serious long-term effects of regression, invalidism, and social isolation come to dominate the clinical picture.

Many patients' emotional problems arise from separation anxiety and difficulties with identity. There is sometimes a "pathogenic secret," such as sexual abuse, which results in intense feelings of shame. Starving is a means of assuaging the pain and gaining control over the course of sexual development. The patient holds on to her emaciation as a form of self-realization and identifies with her wasted body.

Although this pattern of disturbance imparts a conformity to the psychiatric presentation, the underlying phenomenology (see below) and psychodynamic psychopathology are varied. Each patient needs to be understood as an individual.

## Dieting (Restricting) and Purging Forms of Anorexia Nervosa

Anorexic behaviors, although all directed at either decreasing energy intake or increasing energy expenditure, are not uniform. Some patients employ only the restrictive behaviors commonly associated with "normal" dieting, such as undereating, refusal of high-energy foods, and strenuous exercise. This is the "dieting" or "restricting" form of the illness. These patients differ from healthy girls mainly in the extent of these behaviors and their inability to desist. Others also use vomiting and laxative or diuretic abuse. The presentation then is that of the "purging" form of anorexia nervosa. The distinctions between the two forms of the illness are important, particularly in respect to prognosis (worse for purging). Unfortunately, the advent of the concept of the less serious illness of bulimia nervosa has obscured the difference between restricting and purging anorexics, the latter often being misdiagnosed as "bulimia."

## Restricting Behaviors

Food choices are determined by misconceptions acquired from dubious sources such as popular magazines. As fads have changed over the years, so have the foods that are rejected. In the 1960s, patients selectively avoided simple sugars and other carbohydrates (sweets and potatoes). In the 1980s and 1990s, fatty foods and red meat were considered "unhealthy," and vegetarianism has become the most common dietary perversion. Energy-reduced dietary products, foods with a high fiber content, and supplementary vitamins are preferred. Further changes in the next decade may include an avoidance of genetically modified foods.

At the table, patients cut their food into minute portions, choose inappropriate utensils (a teaspoon for dessert), eat painfully slowly, add excessive condiments, adopt a bizarre sequence of dishes, drink too much (or too little) fluid, dispose of food secretly, and count calories. These forms of behavior result in conflict with the family that, together with the patient's increasing anxiety related to food, lead her to avoid eating in the company of others. She takes different meals and eats at different times, often late at night, after hours of procrastination. Patients become overinvolved in reading recipe books, cooking, and may take over the responsibility of preparing the family meals, although they will eat hardly anything themselves. Other family members, including pets, put on weight while the patient becomes thinner. Less commonly, the patient imposes her Spartan diet on the whole family. In small children, one of the reasons for failure to thrive is an anorexic mother. (See Chapter 39 for a discussion of the childrearing of patients with eating disorders.)

## Overactivity

Most anorexia nervosa patients are overactive. It is almost as characteristic as the dietary restriction and just as difficult to modify. There are two kinds of presentation.

First, many patients exercise deliberately to burn calories and induce weight loss. Activity may be surreptitious, such as going up and down stairs frequently on various pretexts, or getting off public transport several stops before the destination and walking the rest of the way. Some quote this phrase: "Never sit if you can stand, never stand if you can walk, never walk if you can run." For others, the activity is strenuous physical exercise, usually in the form of aerobic classes or running. Typically, the exercise is solitary. It has a strongly obsessive character and is performed in a regular and rigid sequence. Patients feel guilty if they do not do the exercise. Exercise and eating are linked by "debting": the patient "earns" the right to eat by undertaking prescribed activities or, conversely, she "pays" for self-indulgence with an extra exercise session.

The second presentation is a persistent restlessness that occurs late in the illness. Beyond voluntary control, it is associated with sleep disturbance and is similar to the ceaseless overactivity seen in laboratory animals when they are deprived of food. Restlessness persists until the patient's physical condition has deteriorated to weakness and lassitude. The overactivity may be related to the fall in core body temperature seen in severely ill patients. A passage in an early paper by Gull emphasizes that rewarming is as essential as refeeding in treating anorexia nervosa. The need to raise core body temperature may also account for the paradoxical increase in diet-induced thermogenesis noted during refeeding.

## Purging Behaviors

In addition to food restriction, many patients use vomiting, laxatives, and diuretic abuse to induce further weight loss. This purging form of illness is particularly malignant, since the behaviors in themselves are injurious to health. Serious physical complications arise in patients who maintain a persistently low weight and in whom purging is prominent (see Chapter 50).

At first, some physical maneuver is necessary to bring on retching, but patients soon learn to vomit at will. Strong cathartics or herbal laxatives are also taken, ostensibly to combat constipation, but really to induce diarrhea. Although patients believe the diarrhea will prevent them from absorbing calories, the weight loss produced is simply the result of dehydration. Oral diuretics have a similar effect.

Compared with "restricting-only" patients, purging anorexics are more likely to have problems with impulse control and substance abuse. There is confusion between the serious purging form of anorexia nervosa and bulimia nervosa. Patients with anorexia nervosa often say they are also bulimic. They mean that they eat more than they wish: subjective rather than objective binges. The experience of having lost control of eating is important psychopathologically, but it is different from true or objective gorging. Only a small minority of these patients have objective binges. Because being undernourished is more important clinically than having binges, the diagnosis of anorexia nervosa trumps that of bulimia nervosa.

## Physical Consequences

The undernutrition of anorexia nervosa differs from that of protein calorie malnutrition in a Third World setting in that patients are unlikely to have their illness compounded by parasitical infestation, but, like the victims of starvation, they are malnourished as well as undernourished—lacking in vitamins and other essential nutrients, and deficient in protein. On nutritional restoration, they regain protein as well as fat tissue, unlike patients with diseases such as cystic fibrosis, in whom protein depletion is difficult to correct. The change in the typical anorexic diet, which was mentioned earlier, results in a microcytic and iron deficient diet rather than macrocytic anemia as in the past. Patients are also likely to be dehydrated.

There is no ideal way of determining the extent of malnutrition. Measurement of body composition does not give a complete picture. The proportion of body fat in total body composition is reduced to under 10%, but this does not indicate the severity of protein loss. In contrast, a patient who has exercised strenuously may have replaced fat with muscle, and her low body fat may exaggerate the extent of undernutrition. Measuring body weight is similarly inaccurate because it makes no allowance for changes in body composition! Weight is only meaningful if related to the range of peers, that is, expressed as a percentage of ideal weight, a body mass index (BMI), or a BMI percentile. The difficulty is compounded in children: Age-corrected weight and height tables are consulted, and the discrepancy between them noted. But this may underestimate the nutritional problem, because the child's growth may have been stunted by the illness.

Because current diagnostic criteria include subjects with a BMI of 17.5 or even higher, some patients are thin rather than emaciated. Others, however, have lost 50% or more of normal body weight (BMI of 10 or less). Fortunately, the degree of malnutrition is usually less severe than that of undernutrition in patients with anorexia nervosa. Malnutrition in the earlier phases of the disease may be relatively mild and manifest only in signs such as the overgrowth of lanugo hair, alopecia, and dry skin. However, some patients do show more serious evidence of vitamin deficiency and significant protein depletion.

In the early phase of illness, the patient with anorexia nervosa chooses a diet low in energy-dense foods. This type of diet, together with the characteristically high level of activity, exerts a nitrogen-sparing effect, so that the initial weight reduction is due mainly to loss of fat. With severe weight loss, the glucose stored in glycogen deposits in the liver is soon exhausted and fat reserves are mobilized, leading to the formation of ketone bodies. These ketone bodies account for a sweet smell of acetone on patients' breath. As the body accommodates to semistarvation, gluconeogenesis is stimulated and protein tissue is broken down, leading to protein depletion, water loss from the intracellular compartment, electrolyte imbalance, and metabolic complications.

The medical manifestations of anorexia nervosa are discussed in Chapters 48 and 50. Some manifestations (e.g., altered thyroid metabolism and anovular infertility with amenorrhea) may best be considered physiological adaptations to starvation. More serious manifestations, requiring specific intervention, are usually found in chronic, severely emaciated patients who abuse laxatives and induce vomiting. They may go unnoticed until initial refeeding upsets the patient's precarious equilibrium. Other manifestations, such as osteoporosis and stunting of growth, develop insidiously during the course of a chronic illness.

Although almost invariable, the prominence assigned to amenorrhea in the diagnostic criteria is unwarranted. It is merely one aspect of widespread endocrine dysfunction. Menstrual disorder often precedes severe weight loss and may persist for months after weight restoration. Ultrasound studies confirm ovarian regression. Depressed sexual libido and low testosterone levels are the equivalent in male patients. (Eating disorders in men are discussed in Chapter 33.)

## Staging

Diagnostic criteria of anorexia nervosa inadequately denote the patient's clinical condition. At one extreme, anorexic thoughts and behavior merge with those of the peer population. At most, these are incipient cases. When the criteria are met, the patient has a recognizable illness but is not particularly ill. As it progresses, she reaches a stage at which the physical effects of emaciation, and the behaviors used to induce it, are such as to cause severe physical morbidity and threaten life. The psychiatric presentation also changes, so that anorexic cognitions are replaced by more profound mental disturbances. The course is typically one of remission and relapse until recovery or chronicity intervene (see Chapter 40). For these reasons, anorexia nervosa requires staging, like neoplasia. This is a task for the future.

## BULIMIA NERVOSA

Bulimia nervosa is not a variant of anorexia nervosa, nor is it particularly ominous. However, the illnesses share many clinical and demographic features. One essential distinction is that patients with bulimia nervosa maintain an apparently normal weight. Another is that, by definition, patients always have episodes of bulimia, "eating like an ox," or objective binges. Unlike anorexia nervosa, bulimia nervosa has come to medical attention only in recent years, but it is even more common (see Chapter 41).

It has been claimed that bulimia nervosa often arises from prior anorexia nervosa, and reports of bulimia nervosa patients in the literature often refer to a large proportion who were previously anorexic. Detailed and careful follow-up studies that have been undertaken on severely ill anorexia nervosa sufferers show that only a small proportion actually go on to bulimia nervosa. This discrepancy is probably due to a loose usage of terminology. (The course of anorexia nervosa and bulimia nervosa are discussed in Chapter 40.)

The development of bulimia nervosa is essentially similar to that of anorexia nervosa, and originates from long-continued attempts to restrain eating. But few patients have actually have fulfilled the diagnostic criteria of anorexia nervosa. The persistent dietary restriction is eventually interrupted by episodes of reactive hyperphagia (binge eating, or bulimia) and compensatory behaviors that usually include vomiting and laxative abuse. The patient's weight fluctuates, usually within the normal range, despite overeating. The behaviors become the focus of intense guilt feelings but often serve to reduce tension.

The history is distinctive. Restricted eating comes first, motivated by the supreme importance of being slender. All patients attempt to control their weight by dieting and abstaining from high-energy foods, at least in the early stage. They are constantly preoccupied with thoughts of food as a reaction to their long-continued restriction. The pattern of eating that develops is one of semistarvation on the one hand and episodes of gorging on the other. Self-induced vomiting and laxative abuse follow. Some patients recall their delight at discovering that they could eat as much as they craved without gaining weight.

Initially, patients are secretive about their bulimic episodes, concealing their behavior for years. Others leave such obvious signs of their disturbed behavior (stacks of empty food containers or plastic bags filled with vomitus) that one may only conclude that they wish to be discovered.

Bulimic episodes are frequently planned. Food is stored to be consumed at a time when the patient will be able to gorge without interruption. Binge foods are selected because they are easy to swallow and regurgitate. Typically, they are fatty, sweet, high-energy foods that patients deny themselves at other times. Some patients may eat as much as 30 times the recommended daily allowance of calories in one binge, but the amount of food ingested is usually more moderate. However, it is important that the clinician ascertain that the amount of food eaten in an alleged binge is in fact excessive. Much confusion is caused by patients with anorexia nervosa or restricted eaters who label any break in their dieting, or any meal in which they eat more than they would have liked, as an episode of binge eating (a "subjective" binge). A useful strategy for the clinician is to refer to "gorging" rather than to "bingeing," since the former term seems to elicit a more accurate response.

People with bulimia nervosa have a tendency to eat rapidly during a binge, stuffing in a large amount of food within minutes. Chronic patients, however, will binge at a slower rate, particularly if there is little risk of discovery. Others report "picking" behavior, taking small quantities at a time (e.g., a teaspoon of ice cream or a portion of cheese) for hours, until they have ingested thousands of calories. Bulimic episodes may be precipitated by anxiety, tension, or boredom; being reminded about food; drinking alcohol or smoking cannabis; being anxious about a date; or being tired from working hard. Only rarely do patients admit that hunger led them to binge, even though they may have fasted for 24 hours before an episode of gorging. Patients may attempt to resist the urge to eat by taking appetite suppressants or other stimulants. They may also avoid situations in which they are likely to be exposed to food, such as going out to dinner with friends or to a party. This avoidance behavior adds to the problems patients already have with social relations and establishes a vicious cycle of increasing binge eating, purging, and social withdrawal. Patients may also have problems with activity, either exercising frenetically to compensate for overindulgence, or going through phases of restricting eating and regularly exercising, or binge eating and being slothful.

Some patients chew food and then spit it out (regurgitation), but most induce vomiting; at first, they need to activate the gag reflex by inserting a finger down the throat but later learn to vomit at will. Others use emetics, take massive amounts of purgatives to bring on diarrhea, or abuse diuretics to lose fluid. They feel disgusted with themselves for having overeaten but are relieved by the purging behavior, are no longer uncomfortable because of abdominal distension, and are gratified to feel that they will not gain weight as a result of the binge.

Mood disturbance is so common in patients with bulimia nervosa that it has been suggested the condition is a form of depressive illness (see Chapter 34). However, careful analysis of the history usually reveals that the eating disturbance preceded the depression, and the patient herself usually relates her unhappiness to her eating problems. The mental state is characterized by feelings of anxiety, tension, helplessness, failure, and self-deprecatory thoughts. Some patients report past sexual and physical abuse that contributes to their low self-esteem. Self-mutilation is common, as are thoughts of suicide. On the other hand, because the bulimic episodes and the consequent purgation often have an anxiety-relieving effect, other patients admit they resort to binge eating at times when they are experiencing difficulty in coping with stress. A significant proportion of patients have personality disorders, disturbed interpersonal relations, and difficulties with impulse control and substance abuse. In these premorbid features they tend to differ from patients with anorexia nervosa, who are usually more introverted, inhibited, and obsessional.

The medical complications of bulimia nervosa, described in Chapter 50, are less severe than those found in anorexia nervosa.

## ATYPICAL EATING DISORDERS

One-third or more of patients considered for treatment at eating disorder clinics do not fulfill the diagnostic criteria of either anorexia or bulimia nervosa and are classified as atypical. These states, discussed in Chapter 30, include partial cases of anorexia nervosa (not thin enough), bulimia nervosa (relatively infrequent binge episodes), obese patients with a disturbed eating pattern resembling that of bulimia nervosa but without the compensatory weight-losing behaviors ("binge eating disorder"; see Chapter 31), and cases of food refusal and undernutrition secondary to hypochondriasis, abnormal illness behavior, or psychotic ideation.

## PHENOMENOLOGY

Although the objective psychopathology is similar, the core experiences (phenomenology) of patients with anorexia nervosa and bulimia nervosa are different. Both accord an unduly high salience to weight and shape, are preoccupied with eating and not eating, relate low self-esteem to their view of their own bodies, and tend either to deny their thinness or overestimate their size, but none of these features is unique to these illnesses. Obese girls, binge eaters, and even many healthy young women have essentially similar cognitions, and what distinguishes bulimia and anorexia nervosa is their intensity, not their quality. However, in bulimia nervosa, these concerns are the essence of the disorder. The bulimic patient seeks slenderness but wants it in order to be healthy and happy. It may be foolish, but it is not irrational. In the anorexia nervosa patient, this is true only in the early phase of the disease. These patients come to believe that they are not worthy of life and do not deserve any form of gratification; they must punish themselves by unrelenting exercise. They are not like other people, in that what is acceptable in others is not acceptable in them. If they let up on their anorexic behaviors, they are filled with self-loathing and guilt. Being emaciated is a goal in itself, not a means of achieving happiness. Work is an obsession and patients are driven by fear of failure rather than hope of success. It is not that they are closed to reason about their physical condition, but rather that it is irrelevant because the sole purpose of their lives is their illness. The extent of their divorce from the reality that most of us recognize is so great that they are incapable of being responsible for their decisions in relation to their illness. (Compulsory treatment of anorexia nervosa is discussed in Chapter 61.)

## FURTHER READING

Abraham, S. F., & Beumont, P. J. V. (1982). How patients describe bulimia or binge eating. *Psychological Medicine, 12*, 625–635.—An objective description of how bulimic patients describe their own disorder in the context of a detailed clinical examination.

Al-Alami, M., Beumont, P. J. V., & Touyz, S. (1987). The further development of the concept of anorexia nervosa. In P. J. V. Beumont, G. D. Burrows, & R. Casper (Eds.), *The handbook of eating disorders: Part 1. Anorexia and bulimia nervosa* (pp. 117–141). Amsterdam: Elsevier/North-Holland.—The authors review the various clinical features of anorexia nervosa on which attention has been focused for the last century and longer.

Beumont, P. J. V. (1998). The behavioural disturbance, psychopathology, and phenomenology of eating disorders. In H. W. Hoek, J. L. Treasure, & M. A. Katzman (Eds.), *Neurobiology in the treatment of eating disorders* (pp. 27–46). Chichester, UK: Wiley.—How phenomenology differs from psychopathology.

Beumont, P. J. V., Arthur, B., Russell, J. D., & Touyz, S. W. (1994). Excessive physical activity in dieting disorder patients: Proposals for a supervised exercise programme. *International Journal of Eating Disorders, 15*, 21–36.—Overactivity, which is frequently overlooked as a major feature of the clinical presentation of dieting disorders, is examined from a clinical viewpoint.

Beumont, P. J. V., George, G. C. W., & Smart, D. E. (1976). "Dieters" and "vomiters and purgers" in anorexia nervosa. *Psychological Medicine, 6*, 617–622.—The separation between restrictive and purging forms of anorexia nervosa antedates the description of bulimia. The purging variety of anorexia is indeed an ominous variant of the illness, with distinct clinical features.

Russell, G. F. M. (1979). Bulimia nervosa: An ominous variant of anorexia nervosa. *Psychological*

*Medicine, 9*, 429–448.—This seminal paper established the intimate relationship that exists between bulimia nervosa and anorexia nervosa, particularly the purging form of the latter illness. However, it overstated the case. Anorexia and bulimia nervosa are different illnesses, their phenomenology and course is different, and bulimia nervosa is certainly the less ominous of the two.

Touyz, S. W., Beumont, P. J. V., Collins, J. K., McCabe, M., & Jupp, J. (1984). Body shape perception and its disturbance in anorexia nervosa. *British Journal of Psychiatry, 144*, 167–171.—Rather than being evidence of a core disturbance of perception, the apparent body image distortion reported in patients with anorexia nervosa relates to affective changes and to a misconception of what constitutes normality.

Vandereycken, W., & van Deth, R. (1990). A tribute to Lasègue's description of anorexia nervosa (1873), with completion of its English translation. *British Journal of Psychiatry, 157*, 902–908.—The patients with anorexia nervosa described in France and in England between 1850 and 1890 closely resemble the patients with anorexia nervosa we see today.

# 30

# Atypical Eating Disorders (Eating Disorder Not Otherwise Specified)

CHRISTOPHER G. FAIRBURN
B. TIMOTHY WALSH

The leading classificatory systems in psychiatry both recognize two main eating disorders, anorexia nervosa and bulimia nervosa. Anorexia nervosa was characterized in the late 19th century, and bulimia nervosa was first described in 1979. (See Chapter 27 for an account of the histories of anorexia nervosa and bulimia nervosa.) These "typical" eating disorders have been the focus of much clinical and research attention, and there is a tendency to equate the concept of an "eating disorder" with these two diagnoses. This is not appropriate, for it appears that the relatively neglected "atypical" eating disorders are at least as common as anorexia nervosa and bulimia nervosa in clinical practice, and are a substantial source of morbidity. These atypical eating disorders are the subject of this chapter. (Certain atypical eating disorders seen in children differ from those seen in adults. These are discussed in Chapter 37.)

## DEFINITION AND CLASSIFICATION OF ATYPICAL EATING DISORDERS

To start with, it is necessary to define an eating disorder. There have been surprisingly few attempts to do this. We suggest that an "eating disorder" be defined as *a persistent disturbance of eating behavior or behavior intended to control weight, which significantly impairs physical health or psychosocial functioning. This disturbance should not be secondary to any recognized general medical disorder (e.g., a hypothalamic tumor) or any other psychiatric disorder (e.g., an anxiety disorder).* Clearly, anorexia nervosa and bulimia nervosa fulfill this definition. (See Chapter 28 for discussion of the diagnostic criteria for anorexia nervosa and bulimia nervosa.) The term "atypical eating disorders" denotes the remaining eating disorders; that is, *those conditions that meet the definition of an eating disorder but not the criteria for anorexia nervosa or bulimia nervosa.*

Some investigators have defined "atypical eating disorders"with reference to anorexia nervosa and bulimia nervosa by simply broadening their diagnostic boundaries. However, restricting the definition of atypical eating disorders to clinical states that are clear extensions of these two disorders does not appear sufficient to cover the wide range of clinical problems encountered. It is also important to stress that atypical eating disorders should not be viewed as mild or "subclinical" in severity (in fact, a misuse of this particular term), since by definition they are associated with a clinical level of impairment.

Both the tenth edition of the *International Classification of Diseases* (ICD-10) and the fourth edition of the American Psychiatric Association's *Diagnostic and Statistical Manual of Mental Disorders* (DSM-IV) recognize the existence of atypical eating disorders. In ICD-10, six different codes are allocated to them (see Table 30.1). In DSM-IV, they are placed together within the single residual category of "eating disorder not otherwise specified" (commonly referred to as EDNOS) (see Table 30.2).

## TABLE 30.1. Atypical Eating Disorders in ICD-10

*F50.1 Atypical anorexia nervosa*

This term should be used for those individuals in whom one or more of the key features of anorexia nervosa (F50.0), such as amenorrhea or significant weight loss, is absent, but who otherwise present a fairly typical clinical picture. Patients who have all the key symptoms but to only a mild degree may also be best described by this term. This term should not be used for eating disorders that resemble anorexia nervosa but that are due to known physical illness.

*F50.3 Atypical bulimia nervosa*

This term should be used for those individuals in whom one or more of the key features listed for bulimia nervosa (F50.2) is absent, but who otherwise present a fairly typical clinical picture. Most commonly this applies to people with normal or even excessive weight but with typical periods of overeating followed by vomiting or purging. Partial syndromes together with depressive symptoms are also not uncommon. Includes normal-weight bulimia.

*F50.4 Overeating associated with other psychological disturbances*

Overeating that has led to obesity as a reaction to distressing events should be coded here. Includes psychogenic overeating.

*F50.5 Vomiting associated with other psychological disturbances*

Apart from the self-induced vomiting of bulimia nervosa, repeated vomiting may occur in dissociative disorders (F44.-), in hypochondriacal disorder (F45.2), when vomiting may be one of several bodily symptoms, and in pregnancy, when emotional factors may contribute to recurrent nausea and vomiting. Includes psychogenic hyperemesis gravidarum and psychogenic vomiting.

*F50.8 Other eating disorders*

Includes pica of nonorganic origin in adults and psychogenic loss of appetite.

*F50.9 Eating disorder, unspecified*

*Note.* From World Health Organization. (1992). *ICD-10 classification of mental and behavioural disorders: Clinical descriptions and diagnostic guidelines.* Geneva, Switzerland: Author. Copyright 1992 by the World Health Association. Adapted by permission.

**TABLE 30.2. Atypical Eating Disorders in DSM-IV**

*307.50 Eating Disorder Not Otherwise Specified*

The Eating Disorder Not Otherwise Specified category is for disorders of eating that do not meet the criteria for any specific Eating Disorder. Examples include

1. For females, all of the criteria for Anorexia Nervosa are met except that the individual has regular menses.
2. All of the criteria for Anorexia Nervosa are met except that, despite significant weight loss, the individual's current weight is in the normal range.
3. All of the criteria for Bulimia Nervosa are met except that the binge eating and inappropriate compensatory mechanisms occur at a frequency of less than twice a week or for a duration of less than 3 months.
4. The regular use of inappropriate compensatory behavior by an individual of normal body weight after eating small amounts of food (e.g., self-induced vomiting after the consumption of two cookies).
5. Repeatedly chewing and spitting out, but not swallowing, large amounts of food.
6. Binge-eating disorder: recurrent episodes of binge eating in the absence of the regular use of inappropriate compensatory behaviors characteristic of Bulimia Nervosa.

*Note.* From American Psychiatric Association. (1994). *Diagnostic and statistical manual of mental disorders* (4th ed.). Washington, DC: Author. Copyright 1994 by the American Psychiatric Association. Reprinted by permission.

# CLINICAL CHARACTERISTICS

Systematic research into the clinical features of atypical eating disorders is needed. To our knowledge, there have been no formal descriptive studies in which their psychopathology has been well assessed. Clinical experience and case descriptions indicate that they vary considerably in form. Some resemble anorexia nervosa or bulimia nervosa but do not quite meet their diagnostic criteria, either because one of the essential diagnostic features is missing (sometimes the term "partial syndrome" is used) or, more commonly, because one or more features is not sufficiently serve to reach the specified threshold (a "subthreshold disorder"). Often, this distinction is not clear-cut. Examples of the former are disorders with all the features of anorexia nervosa except that menstruation is normal, and disorders with all the features of bulimia nervosa except that the overeating does not fulfill the definition of a "binge" (e.g., the amount eaten is not truly large). Examples of the latter are otherwise typical cases of anorexia nervosa in which body weight is not sufficiently low, and disorders resembling bulimia nervosa in which the frequency of binge eating is not sufficiently high.

Other atypical eating disorders less closely resemble anorexia nervosa or bulimia nervosa. The best known example is "binge eating disorder." This is the term used in DSM-IV to denote an eating disorder characterized by recurrent episodes of binge eating in the absence of the extreme weight-control behavior seen in bulimia nervosa (e.g., recurrent, self-induced vomiting). Binge eating disorder is discussed in Chapter 31. Other forms of atypical eating disorder also exist. Many involve chronic dietary restriction, sometimes accompanied by overexercising or laxative misuse, and in most there is the overevaluation of eating, shape, and weight that is characteristic of patients with anorexia nervosa or bulimia nervosa (see Chapters 29 and 54).

There have been several attempts using multivariate statistical techniques to subdivide the atypical eating disorders on the basis of their current clinical features. None has been entirely satisfactory, either because their measures or definitions have been problematic or because the samples have been unrepresentative. The one consistent finding is that there appears to be a subgroup of people with recurrent episodes of binge eating accompanied by low levels of vomiting and laxative misuse. This eating pattern does not fit the currently formulated description of binge eating disorder. Rather, it highlights the problematic boundary between purging bulimia nervosa, nonpurging bulimia nervosa, and binge eating disorder.

## DIFFERENTIAL DIAGNOSIS

Disturbances of eating occur in association with other disorders. Anorexia and hypophagia are seen in many physical disorders as well as in depression and dementia. Food refusal in the form of a hunger strike sometimes occurs in the context of severe personality disturbance. Hyperphagia is characteristic of certain organic disorders, including hypothalamic tumors and the Kleine–Levin and Prader–Willi syndromes. It is also seen in some cases of depression, mania, and dementia. Anxiety about eating with others may be an expression of social phobia, and repeated, spontaneous vomiting may also be anxiety-related. Given the definition of an eating disorder specified above, such disturbances of eating are not "eating disorders" as such, since they are secondary either to a general medical disorder or to another psychiatric condition. This perspective is consistent with that of DSM-IV. However, ICD-10 diverges from DSM-IV in this regard in allowing eating disturbances associated with other disorders to be classified in the eating disorders section (F50), where they receive codes F50.4, F50.5, or F50.8 (see Table 30.1).

## DISTRIBUTION

Little is known about the distribution of atypical eating disorders. The community-based studies of the prevalence and incidence of eating disorders have focused on the rates of anorexia nervosa and bulimia nervosa, at least in part because there has been no simple definition of what constitutes an atypical eating disorder. Therefore, current prevalence and incidence figures must underestimate the true number of eating disorder cases. The few studies of the prevalence of binge eating disorder (see Chapter 31) suggest that the disorder affects a broader and older age group than that vulnerable to typical eating disorders. The gender ratio also seem less uneven.

There have been several reports of the rates of atypical eating disorders among patients seeking treatment for an eating disorder. For example, Millar reported on the diagnostic composition of the first 531 patients seen at a new outpatient eating disorder service in northern Scotland. Fourteen percent had anorexia nervosa, 40% had bulimia nervosa, and the remaining 47% had an atypical eating disorder. Across the various reports, the proportion of patients with an atypical eating disorder ranges from 20% to 61%. Much of this variation is as likely due to differences in diagnostic practice as to differences in the samples themselves. What is abundantly clear is that a substantial proportion of cases is "atypical."

## DETERMINANTS

The research on the etiology of eating disorders has mostly focused on the two typical disorders—or at least it has appeared to do so. In practice, this has not always been the case, since such broad case definitions have been applied that many apparently typical cases will have been atypical. This is especially true of the twin studies (see Chapter 42). As a result, much of what we have learned from twin research on eating disorders applies to a spectrum of eating disorders, including subthreshold anorexia nervosa and bulimia nervosa, rather than to typical forms of these disorders. Thus, it seems that there is a significant heritable component to the etiology of broad forms of anorexia nervosa and bulimia nervosa. This conclusion extends the findings of family–genetic studies of eating disorders, which have found that there is a raised rate of atypical eating disorders among the female family members of probands with anorexia nervosa or bulimia nervosa. On the basis of these and other findings, it has been argued that there may be a continuum of liability to develop an eating disorder.

Less is known about the contribution of other classes of risk factor since the retrospective risk factor studies have tended to recruit true cases of anorexia nervosa and bulimia nervosa rather than broader, atypical cases (see Chapter 44). An exception, a case-control study of risk factors for the development of binge eating disorder, found that the risk factors identified were fewer in number and weaker in strength than those for anorexia nervosa and bulimia nervosa (see Chapter 31).

Recently, there have been two prospective studies of the development of eating disorders among adolescents. Both have focused on partial syndromes and have therefore been studies of atypical eating disorders. The first found that, on multivariate analysis, a measure of concern about weight was the only significant predictor of developing a partial syndrome. The second study found that dieting and psychiatric morbidity independently predicted onset. It is a moot point whether dieting and weight concerns should be viewed as risk factors of possible etiological significance or as mere precursors of an incipient eating disorder.

## COURSE AND OUTCOME

The research on the course and outcome of eating disorders has illuminated the relationship between typical and atypical eating disorders and has revealed that there is considerable fluidity over time, an important point that is missed when a cross-sectional perspective is taken. In the absence of recovery, anorexia nervosa and bulimia nervosa both tend to evolve into atypical eating disorders. There have been few studies of the course of atypical eating disorders themselves. One study of participants with subthreshold forms of anorexia nervosa or bulimia nervosa found that, over a mean follow-up period of 41 months, few participants recovered and almost half went on to develop typical anorexia nervosa or bulimia nervosa. The authors described the participants' course as "persistent and highly variable."

There are beginning to be studies of the course of binge eating disorder. These are obtaining rather different findings than those described earlier. First, it seems that there is a high remission rate, even in the absence of treatment; and second, there appears to be no tendency for the disorder to evolve into any other eating disorder.

## TREATMENT

The research on the treatment of eating disorders has focused on anorexia nervosa and the purging form of bulimia nervosa. There has been no research on the treatment of atypical eating disorders other than the emerging work on binge eating disorder (see Chapters 63 and 64). This research suggests that the disorder responds well to a variety of treatments. Indeed, the studies of pharmacological and psychological treatments reinforce the findings of naturalistic follow-up studies in suggesting that there is a marked tendency for the disorder to remit. This is evident in the high rate of response to placebo and the identical response to cognitive-behavioral therapy and interpersonal psychotherapy (see Chapter 57), findings quite unlike those obtained with bulimia nervosa.

## IMPLICATIONS FOR CLINICAL PRACTICE AND RESEARCH

The neglect of the atypical eating disorders is a source of concern for two main reasons. First, by focusing exclusively on anorexia nervosa and bulimia nervosa, researchers (and, to a lesser extent, clinicians) have failed to view eating disorders in their entirety. Second, by developing treatments exclusively for anorexia nervosa and bulimia nervosa, the needs of a large population of patients have been ignored. The recent interest in binge eating disorder represents progess in this regard, but much remains to be done.

## ACKNOWLEDGMENTS

The first author is grateful to the Wellcome Trust for their support (Grant No. 046386).

## FURTHER READING

Clinton, D. N., & Glant, R. (1992). The eating disorders spectrum of DSM-III-R. *Journal of Nervous and Mental Disease, 180,* 244–250.—A description of the diagnostic composition of 86 consecutive eating disorder cases from a defined urban catchment area in Sweden.

Fairburn, C. G., Cooper, Z., Doll, H. A., Norman, P., & O'Connor, M. (2000). The natural course of bulimia nervosa and binge eating disorder in young women. *Archives of General Psychiatry, 57,* 659–665.—A prospective, community-based study of the course of bulimia nervosa, showing that atypical eating disorders are a common outcome, whereas full recovery is the norm among those with binge eating disorder.

Fairburn, C. G., Doll, H. A., Welch, S. L., Hay, P. J., Davies, B. A., & O'Connor, M. E. (1998). Risk factors for binge eating disorder: A community-based, case-control study. *Archives of General Psychiatry, 55,* 425–432.—Well-controlled, retrospective risk-factor study contrasting BED, bulimia nervosa, psychiatric, and non-eating disordered controls.

Herzog, D. B., Hopkins, J. D., & Burns, C. D. (1993). A follow-up study of 33 subdiagnostic eating disordered women. *International Journal of Eating Disorders, 14,* 261–267.—A study of the course of atypical eating disorders that revealed considerable movement between typical and atypical eating disorders, and high levels of continuing morbidity.

Lilenfeld, L. R., Kaye, W. H., Greeno, C. G., Merikangas, K. R., Plotnicov, K., Pollice, C., Rao, R., Strober, M., Bulik, C. M., & Nagy, L. (1998). A controlled family study of anorexia nervosa and bulimia nervosa: Psychiatric disorders in first-degree relatives and effects of proband comorbidity. *Archives of General Psychiatry, 55,* 603–610.—A family history study revealing high rates of atypical eating disorders among the first-degree relatives of probands with anorexia nervosa or bulimia nervosa.

Millar, H. R. (1998). New eating disorder service. *Psychiatric Bulletin, 22,* 751–754.—Gives ICD-10 diagnostic breakdown of referrals to a new eating disorder service, revealing a high rate of atypical eating disorders.

Mitchell, J. E., Pyle, R. L., Hatsukami, D., & Eckert, E. D. (1986). What are atypical eating disorders? *Psychosomatics, 27,* 21–28.—A description of 25 cases.

Mizes, J. S., & Sloan, D. M. (1998). An empirical analysis of Eating Disorder, Not Otherwise Specified: Preliminary support for a distinct subgroup. *International Journal of Eating Disorders, 23,* 233–242.—One of the studies that has attempted to identify subgroups within the atypical eating disorders using cluster analysis.

Patton, G. C., Selzer, R., Coffey, C., Carlin, B., & Wolfe, R. (1999). Onset of adolescent eating disorders: Population-based cohort study over 3 years. *British Medical Journal, 318,* 765–768.—One of the two prospective studies of the development of atypical (partial) eating disorders.

Strober, M., Freeman, R., Lampert, C., Diamond, C., & Kaye, W. (2000). Controlled family study of anorexia nervosa and bulimia nervosa: Evidence of shared liability and transmission of partial phenotypes. *American Journal of Psychiatry, 157,* 393–401.—Large family–genetic study of eating disorders. Findings suggest shared familial diathesis for anorexia nervosa, bulimia nervosa, and atypical eating disorders.

Strober, M., Freeman, R., & Morrell, W. (1999). Atypical anorexia nervosa: Separation from typical cases in course and outcome in a long-term prospective study. *International Journal of Eating Disorders, 25,* 135–142.—Naturalistic study of the long-term clinical course of atypical cases of anorexia nervosa.

Walsh, B. T., & Garner, D. M. (1997). Diagnostic issues. In D. M. Garner & P. E. Garfinkel (Eds.), *Handbook of treatment for eating disorders* (2nd ed., pp. 25–33). New York: Guilford Press.—Good discussion of the concept, clinical features, and importance of atypical eating disorders.

# 31

# Binge Eating Disorder

## CARLOS M. GRILO

Binge eating disorder (BED) is one example of the eating disorder not otherwise specified (EDNOS) category in the fourth edition of the *Diagnostic and Statistical Manual of Mental Disorders* (DSM-IV) of the American Psychiatric Association. (The category of EDNOS is discussed further in Chapter 30.) There it is defined as follows: *"Recurrent episodes of binge eating in the absence of the regular use of inappropriate compensatory behaviors characteristic of bulimia nervosa."*

BED is also included in Appendix B of DSM-IV, which is reserved for possible new diagnostic categories that were not included in DSM-IV since there were insufficient data to warrant their inclusion. Tentative research criteria are provided in this appendix based on the findings of two initial field trials. This chapter reviews the accumulating research regarding the clinical features of BED and major issues pertaining to the validity of the concept and the provisional diagnostic criteria.

## DIAGNOSTIC CRITERIA FOR BINGE EATING DISORDER

The general descriptive definition of BED is shown above (in italics), and the tentative research criteria are shown in Table 31.1.

The research criteria are noteworthy in several respects when compared with those for bulimia nervosa, the well-established eating disorder that is also characterized by the presence of regular binge eating. (See Chapters 28 and 29 for a discussion of diagnostic criteria and clinical features of bulimia nervosa.) First, the BED requirement that binge episodes occur 2 days per week is different than the requirement of two episodes per week for bulimia nervosa. Unlike in bulimia nervosa, where the binge eating is usually clearly terminated by some form of purging or the reestablishment of strict dietary restraint, the eating habits of patients with BED are more amorphous and sometimes difficult to separate into discrete episodes. Thus, the current practice is simply to determine the number of days on which binge eating occurred. Recent findings, however, suggest

**TABLE 31.1. Research Criteria for Binge Eating Disorder**

A. Recurrent episodes of binge eating. An episode of binge eating is characterized by both of the following:
   (1) eating, in a discrete period of time (e.g., within any 2-hour period), an amount of food that is definitely larger than most people would eat in a similar period of time under similar circumstances
   (2) a sense of lack of control over eating during the episode (e.g., a feeling that one cannot stop eating or control what or how much one is eating)

B. The binge-eating episodes are associated with three (or more) of the following:
   (1) eating much more rapidly than normal
   (2) eating until feeling uncomfortably full
   (3) eating large amounts of food when not feeling physically hungry
   (4) eating alone because of being embarrassed by how much one is eating
   (5) feeling disgusted with oneself, depressed, or very guilty after overeating

C. Marked distress regarding binge eating is present.

D. The binge eating occurs, on average, at least 2 days a week for 6 months.
   *Note*: The method of determining frequency differs from that used for Bulimia Nervosa; future research should address whether the preferred method of setting a frequency threshold is counting the number of days on which binges occur or counting the number of episodes of binge eating.

E. The binge eating is not associated with the regular use of inappropriate compensatory behaviors (e.g., purging, fasting, excessive exercise) and does not occur exclusively during the course of Anorexia Nervosa or Bulimia Nervosa.

*Note.* From American Psychiatric Association. (1994). *Diagnostic and statistical manual of mental disorders* (4th ed.). Washington, DC: Author. Copyright 1994 by the American Psychiatric Association. Reprinted by permission.

that it may be possible to reliably obtain reports of the frequency of binge-eating episodes. Difficulties in measurement notwithstanding, logic would dictate the importance of assessing how many times a person eats an unusually large amount of food rather than just the number of days on which this happens. Finer-grained assessments are needed. This may eventually help to resolve various important issues, including the consistent, but surprising, finding from treatment trials that significant reductions in the frequency of binge eating (days) are associated with little or no reductions in weight (see Chapters 63 and 64). A related point worth noting is the lack of basis for the twice-weekly threshold. Not unlike the case for bulimia nervosa, the little available evidence suggests that persons who binge just once a week are no different than those who meet the DSM-IV twice-weekly threshold criterion.

The second noteworthy variation concerns the use of a diagnostic time frame of 6 months rather than the 3-month time frame used for bulimia nervosa (and anorexia nervosa). A recent report using data from a national sample of over 3,000 women noted that the 6-month requirement resulted in a 1.0% prevalence estimate, whereas a 3-month requirement would have increased the rate to 1.6%. The value of the 6-month criterion is uncertain. As it stands, it results in many potential patients being excluded from clinical trials.

A third diagnostic variation concerns the absence of an attitudinal or cognitive criterion. The research criteria require significant distress over the binge eating, yet this appears no different than the universal requirement for psychiatric diagnoses that the syndrome must have some negative impact. There is no specific attitudinal criterion, unlike those for bulimia nervosa and anorexia nervosa (see Chapter 28), despite the fact that there is some evidence that BED is characterized by similar cognitive features.

A final diagnostic issue concerns the exclusionary criterion "regular use of inappropriate compensatory behaviors." To date, studies have varied in how this has been operationalized. Some have excluded persons who report any use of any of the compensatory behaviors, whereas others have included persons who report the behaviors up to the bulimia nervosa twice-weekly threshold. A French study found that roughly one-third of their "BED" patients regularly used extreme weight-control practices. This issue merits continued research.

## CLINICAL FEATURES

### Distribution

Community-based studies have generated prevalence figures for BED in the region of 2 to 3% of the adult population and 8% of the obese population. In contrast, and possibly reflecting both the association between severity of binge eating and obesity, and treatment-seeking patterns, higher rates of BED have been reported in obese patients seeking treatment at university weight loss clinics. Indeed, some studies have reported figures as high as 20–40%, although the studies that have used more rigorous interview-based assessment methods have obtained much lower figures (5–10%). Unlike anorexia nervosa and bulimia nervosa, BED is not uncommon in men (approximately 1.5 female-to-male ratio) or minority groups (e.g., African American, Hispanic American). (See Chapter 33 for further discussion of eating disorders in men.) Most BED patients are between 30 and 50 years old at presentation.

### Eating Behaviors

Naturalistic self-monitoring and laboratory feeding studies of persons who binge-eat have noted considerable variability in eating behaviors both during and between binge episodes. Persons with BED generally have chaotic eating behavior that differs from that of persons with bulimia nervosa (and from persons with obesity who do not binge eat). They have low levels of dietary restraint, whereas in bulimia nervosa the binge eating alternates with high levels of dietary restriction. Their episodes of overeating also vary in form: Sometimes there is overeating without loss of control, overeating with loss of control, and loss of control without the consumption of a large amount of food.

### Obesity

BED is associated with obesity and is a not uncommon problem among obese persons who seek treatment (see Chapter 73). The association is not invariable, however. Studies that do not select BED participants with coexisting obesity readily find persons with lower body mass index (BMI) values. Many questions remain regarding the relationship. For example, its direction is uncertain. Evidence suggests that in a substantial proportion (35–55%) of patients with BED, binge eating precedes their first dieting and that these patients become overweight at an earlier age than those who diet before binge eating. Interestingly, a controlled risk factor study found that while obesity risk (childhood obesity and parental obesity) was a specific risk factor for BED, it was a stronger risk factor for bulimia nervosa.

## Attitudinal Features

BED is characterized by high levels of dysfunctional attitudes regarding weight and shape. There is some evidence that these attitudes are comparable to those found in bulimia nervosa and higher than those found in overweight persons who do not binge eat. The degree of such psychopathology is not related to the degree of obesity. These findings suggest that such cognitive features are important in BED and do not simply reflect the impact of obesity (if present). BED is also characterized by a generally higher level of body image dissatisfaction than that among persons with obesity who do not binge eat, and more comparable to that found in bulimia nervosa.

## Psychological Functioning

BED is associated with a wide range of psychological problems (e.g., negative self-esteem, impaired social functioning) and, by definition, with distress. Most studies have reported higher rates of psychological problems in persons with BED than in nonpatient controls and persons with obesity who do not binge eat, but slightly lower rates than observed for persons with bulimia nervosa. There are higher rates of lifetime psychiatric disorders and personality disorders than in control groups in both community and clinical (treatment-seeking) BED samples, although the rates are higher in the clinical samples. Major depressive disorder is consistently found to be the most common comorbid diagnosis (lifetime rates generally 50–60%), but the rates of alcohol use disorders and anxiety disorders are also elevated. One study with treatment-seeking BED patients found only one gender difference in the prevalence rate of lifetime psychiatric disorders: Males had a higher rate of substance use disorders than females (57% vs. 28%). Another study found that the presence of personality disorder, but not psychiatric disorder, was associated with more severe eating disorder psychopathology at baseline, but neither predicted response to treatment.

## VALIDITY OF BINGE EATING DISORDER

Continued research is clearly needed to address many unanswered questions regarding the nature and definition of BED, as well as the validity of the construct. Overall, the first decade of research suggests that persons with BED differ from those who do not binge eat and that BED has important similarities to, and differences from, bulimia nervosa.

Three recent major studies have produced data generally supportive of the validity of the BED diagnosis. First, Fairburn and colleagues' community-based, case-control study of risk factors for the development of eating disorders found that women with BED differed from healthy controls (in terms of greater exposure to risk factors for general psychiatric disturbance and obesity) and from women with bulimia nervosa (where the exposure rates were higher and more varied) . Second, a related, naturalistic 5-year prospective study by the same group found that BED and bulimia nervosa were characterized by different courses and outcomes and that few persons moved across the two diagnostic categories. In most participants, BED appeared to be a self-limiting state. Third, Bulik and colleagues' latent class analysis produced categories that resembled anorexia nervosa, bulimia nervosa, and BED.

## FURTHER READING

Bulik, C. M., Sullivan, P. F., & Kendler, K. S. (2000). An empirical study of the classification of eating disorders. *American Journal of Psychiatry, 157,* 886–895.—Latent class analysis applied to nine eating disorder symptoms of 2,163 female twins (Virginia Twin Registry) produced classes of eating-related pathology broadly resembling anorexia nervosa, bulimia nervosa, and BED.

Fairburn, C. G., Cooper, Z., Doll, H. A., Norman, P., & O'Connor, M. (2000). The natural course of bulimia nervosa and binge eating disorder in young women. *Archives of General Psychiatry, 57,* 659–665.—The first study of its kind, this 5-year prospective, naturalistic study of two-community cohorts found that bulimia nervosa and BED have different course and outcome and that few persons switch between diagnostic categories.

Fairburn, C. G., Doll, H. A., Welch, S. L., Hay, P. J., Davies, B. A., & O'Connor, M. E. (1998). Risk factors for binge eating disorder: A community-based, case-control study. *Archives of General Psychiatry, 55,* 425–432.—Well-controlled, retrospective risk-factor study contrasting BED, bulimia nervosa, psychiatric, and non-eating disordered controls.

Grilo, C. M. (1998). The assessment and treatment of binge eating disorder. *Journal of Practical Psychiatry and Behavioral Health, 4,* 191–201.—Recent critical review of assessment and treatment for BED.

Spitzer, R. L., Devlin, M., Walsh, B. T., Hasin, D., Wing, R., Marcus, M., Stunkard, A., Wadden, T., Yanovski, S., Agras, S., Mitchell, J., & Nonas, C. (1992). Binge eating disorder: A multisite field trial of the diagnostic criteria. *International Journal of Eating Disorders, 11,* 191–203.—Initial multisite field trial of diagnostic criteria for BED.

Spitzer, R. L., Yanovski, S., Wadden, T. A., & Wing, R. (1993). Binge eating disorder: Its further validation in a multisite study. *International Journal of Eating Disorders, 13,* 137–153.—Second multisite field trial of diagnostic criteria for BED.

Striegel-Moore, R. H., Dohm, F. A., Solomon, E. E., Fairburn, C. G., Pike, K. M., & Wilfley, D. E. (2000). Subthreshold binge eating disorder. *International Journal of Eating Disorders, 27,* 270–278.—Forty-four females with subthreshold BED compared with 44 females with DSM-IV-defined BED and 44 "healthy" controls. Subthreshold and threshold BED patient groups were similar on most measures.

Widiger, T. A., Frances, A. J., Pincus, H. A., Ross, R., First, M. B., Davis, W., & Kline, M. (1998). *DSM-IV sourcebook* (Vol. 4). Washington, DC: American Psychiatric Press.—Contains a report by Dansky and colleagues pertaining to BED in a U.S. national sample and a study by Flament and colleagues in a French multisite sample.

Wilfley, D. E., Friedman, M. A., Dounchis, J. Z., Stein, R. I., Welch, R. R., & Ball, S. A. (2000). Comorbid psychopathology in binge eating disorder: Relation to eating disorder severity at baseline and following treatment. *Journal of Consulting and Clinical Psychology, 68,* 641–649.—Description of comorbid features of BED and their relationship to severity of the disturbance of eating.

Wilfley, D. E., Schwartz, M. B., Spurrell, E. B., & Fairburn, C. G. (2000). Using the Eating Disorder Examination to identify the specific psychopathology of binge eating disorder. *International Journal of Eating Disorders, 27,* 259–269.—Three groups of patients (BED, anorexia nervosa, bulimia nervosa) and two control groups (normal weight and overweight) compared using the Eating Disorder Examination. Findings support the BED diagnosis and highlight the importance of dysfunctional cognitions regarding eating, weight, and shape that are not attributable to weight status.

# 32

# Night Eating Syndrome

## ALBERT J. STUNKARD

Recent years have seen a renewal of interest in the relationship between eating disorders and obesity. Such an interest goes back a long way, to a time when all obesity was believed to be due to an eating disorder. People became obese by eating too much, the argument went: What better evidence was there that their eating was disordered? This simplistic view is no longer held and, as a result, for some time little attention was paid to the possibility that disturbed eating might contribute to obesity. This situation is changing, and two eating disorders have now been linked to obesity. The first is binge eating disorder (see Chapter 31), and the second is the night eating syndrome.

The night eating syndrome was first described by the author in 1955 as a disorder comprising the triad of morning anorexia, evening or nocturnal hyperphagia (in full consciousness), and insomnia. Clinical investigation revealed that it occurred (1) disproportionately among obese persons, (2) during periods of life stress, and (3) responded to alleviation of the stress. The night eating syndrome appeared to be a special circadian stress response characteristic of some obese persons.

Studies using the above criteria estimate that the prevalence of the night eating syndrome in the general population is approximately 1.5% and that prevalence increases with increasing weight, from about 10% of persons enrolling in obesity clinics to as high as 25% of patients undergoing surgical treatment for obesity. Among persons identifying themselves as binge eaters, binge eating disorder (see Chapter 31) is somewhat more prevalent (20%) than the night eating syndrome (15%). It occurs among about 5% of those presenting for the treatment of insomnia (although other sleep-related eating disturbances are also seen in which patients are either partially or totally unconscious).

## BEHAVIORAL FEATURES

Much of what we know about the night eating syndrome is derived from a study by Birketvedt and colleagues. It revealed that the food intake of obese night eaters was somewhat greater than that of obese control subjects (2,930 kcal vs. 2,334 kcal). The more striking difference between the two groups was in the temporal pattern of their food intake. Figure 32.1 shows that the cumulative caloric intake of the night eaters lagged behind that of the control subjects so that, by 6:00 P.M., they had consumed only 37% of their daily intake compared to 74% by the controls. The food intake of the controls slowed during the evening, while that of the night eaters continued at a rapid pace until after midnight. During the period from 8:00 P.M. to 6:00 A.M., the night eaters consumed 56% of their caloric intake, compared to 15% for the control subjects.

Changes in the mood of the night eaters were also distinctive. Their average mood, measured on a 10-cm visual analogue scale, was 5.1 out of the possible 10.0, significantly lower than the 7.8 of controls. They also showed a striking difference in the diurnal pattern of mood: In contrast to the usual improvement in the mood of depressed persons during the evening, that of the night eaters fell.

The night eaters suffered from both sleep onset insomnia and sleep maintenance insomnia, awakening 3.6 times per night compared to 0.3 times for the controls. Half of the awakenings of the night eaters were associated with food intake; none of the controls ate when they awoke. This food intake did not constitute a "binge." In fact, it was of only moderate size, averaging 271 kcal. The carbohydrate content of these "snacks" was

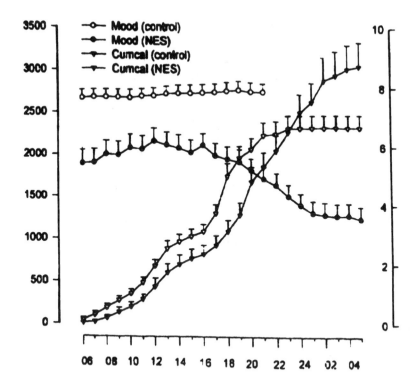

**FIGURE 32.1.** Twenty-four-hour pattern of cumulative food intake and mood. The cumulative food intake of the night eaters lags behind that of the control subjects until 11:00 P.M. and then greatly exceeds it. Daytime mood of the night eaters is lower than that of the controls and falls during the evening. Error bars represent standard deviations.

high (70% compared to 47% for their food intake during the rest of the day) and the carbohydrate-to-protein ratio of the nighttime snacks was also elevated, at 7:1. This nutrient pattern (a high carbohydrate-to-protein ratio) increases the availability of tryptophan for transport into the brain, and its conversion into serotonin with its sleep-promoting properties.

## NEUROENDOCRINE FEATURES

The neuroendocrinology of the night eating syndrome was also investigated by Birketvedt and colleagues. They found highly significant differences between night eaters and control subjects in plasma levels of melatonin, leptin, and cortisol. As shown in Figure 32.2, plasma melatonin levels at night in the night eaters were significantly lower than those of controls, and there was no difference between the melatonin levels of overweight and normal-weight night eaters. As expected, plasma leptin levels were considerably higher among overweight subjects than among normal-weight ones, both for night eaters and controls. The big difference between the night eaters and control subjects lay in their nighttime responses. The nighttime plasma leptin concentrations of the night eaters did not rise in contrast to the expected rise among the control subjects. The 24-hour plasma cortisol levels of the night eaters were higher than those of the controls. It is worthy of

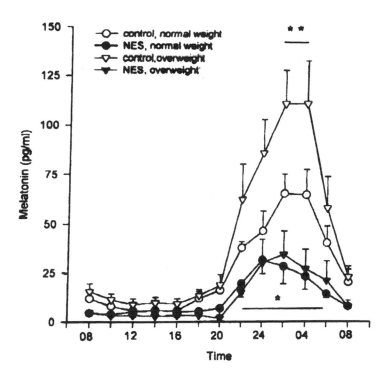

FIGURE 32.2. Twenty-four-hour plasma melatonin levels in night eaters (7 overweight, 5 normal weight) and control subjects (10 overweight, 7 normal weight). Asterisks indicate significant differences between the two groups.

note that the timing of the peaks and nadirs of these three neuroendocrine measures did not differ between night eaters and controls. Apparently, there was no displacement of the neuroendocrine circadian rhythms of the night eaters in contrast to the apparent phase delay in their eating behavior.

Thus, night eating syndrome appears to be a unique combination of eating disorder, sleep disorder, and mood disorder. A distinctive neuroendocrine pattern helps to link these three dimensions. The blunting of the nighttime rise in melatonin may contribute to the sleep maintenance insomnia of the night eaters. Lowered levels of melatonin have been reported in depression and may contribute to the generally lowered mood of the night eaters. The failure of leptin to rise at night must limit its expected nighttime suppression of appetite and may permit the breakthrough of hunger impulses, further disrupting sleep. The finding of elevated serum cortisol levels in the night eaters supports the clinical observation, derived from long-term psychotherapy and reported in 1955, that persons with the night eating syndrome may be manifesting a specific type of response to stress.

## TREATMENT

Treatment of the night eating syndrome has not been considered since the author's original 1955 report. In that report, it was noted that long-term psychodynamic psychotherapy was associated with improvement in the night eating behavior of some patients. Anecdotal reports to the author from night eaters who have explored treatment options suggest that selective serotonin reuptake inhibitors have been helpful, as might be expected from their favorable effects on disturbances in mood and sleep. In view of the lack of rise in nighttime melatonin, provision of such agents at bedtime would seem a rational option.

Further research on the night eating syndrome is needed. It will be important to assess the validity of the diagnostic criteria and the robustness of the neuroendocrine findings to date. Studies of treatment are also needed.

## FURTHER READING

Birketvedt, G., Florholmen, J., Sundsfjord, J., Osterud, B., Dinges, D., Bilker, W., & Stunkard, A. J. (1999). Behavioral and neuroendocrine characteristics of the night-eating syndrome. *Journal of the American Medical Association, 282,* 657–663.—A detailed account of the night eating syndrome, including its behavioral and neuroendocrine aspects.

Manni, R., Ratti, M. T., & Tartara, A. (1997). Nocturnal eating: Prevalence and features in 120 insomniac referrals. *Sleep, 20,* 734–738.—This study revealed that about 5% of referrals with insomnia manifest the night eating syndrome.

Rand, C. S. W., Macgregor, M. D., & Stunkard, A. J. (1997). The night eating syndrome in the general population and among post-operative obesity surgery patients. *International Journal of Eating Disorders, 22,* 65–69.—One of the few studies of the prevalence of the night eating syndrome.

Schenk, C. H., & Mahowald, M. W. (1994). Review of nocturnal sleep-related eating disorders. *International Journal of Eating Disorders, 15,* 343–356.—Includes a description of an eating disorder that differs from the night eating syndrome in that subjects are not fully conscious when eating.

Stunkard, A., Berkowitz, R., Wadden, T., Tanrikut, C., Reiss, E., & Young, L.(1996). Binge eating disorder and the night eating syndrome. *International Journal of Obesity, 20,* 1–6.—A comparison of the prevalence of binge eaters and night eaters based on recruitment of a large number of subjects for a study on binge eating.

Stunkard, A. J., Grace, W. J., & Wolff, H. G. (1955). The night-eating syndrome: A pattern of food intake among certain obese patients. *American Journal of Medicine, 19,* 78–86.—The first and, until recently, the only paper describing the night eating syndrome. It is based upon long-term psychotherapy of 20 obese persons with the disorder.

# 33

# Eating Disorders in Males

## ARNOLD E. ANDERSEN

Despite being mentioned among the first case presentations in the English language 300 years ago, males with eating disorders have at times been ignored, neglected, dismissed because of statistical infrequence, or legislated out of existence by theoretical dogma. In this chapter, the basic body of information concerning males with eating disorders is presented in two overlapping but relatively distinct categories: (1) well-established facts based on sound scientific studies; and (2) highly probable information based on less complete studies or clinical experience.

## WELL-ESTABLISHED FACTS

### Diagnosis and Clinical Features

The diagnostic criteria for males with anorexia nervosa are similar to those for females (see Chapter 28), but the symptomatic marker of reproductive hormone abnormality (viz., loss of sexual appetite secondary to lowered testosterone) develops in a gradual manner unlike the more abrupt cessation of menses among females. Doctors are less likely to think of the diagnosis of anorexia nervosa in males. The diagnosis of bulimia nervosa is probably not gender-biased.

Males are affected by similar comorbid psychiatric conditions to those affecting females, especially mood and personality disorders. Contrary to previous assumptions, males are more severely afflicted by osteopenia and osteoporosis, with lower bone mineral density than equivalent female patients.

The notion of "reverse anorexia nervosa," sometimes called "muscle dysmorphia," has become well-established. It occurs almost exclusively in males and is characterized by the subjective thinness even when highly muscular. It is often associated with the abuse of anabolic steroids.

## Epidemiology and Etiology

Males with eating disorders have been reported since 1689. The findings from recent community-based epidemiological studies of anorexia nervosa and bulimia nervosa suggest a ratio of one male case to about six female cases. In clinic samples, the ratio is somewhat lower with 10 to 20% of cases of anorexia nervosa being male. Male cases of bulimia nervosa are uncommon. In contrast, in binge eating disorder the gender ratio appears to approach one-to-one. In preadolescent cases (of anorexia nervosa), about one-fourth of cases are males (see Chapter 37).

In Western societies, men are clearly exposed to less general sociocultural pressure to be slim and to diet, with only 10% as many articles and advertisements promoting dieting in magazines read by young males compared to young females. (See Chapter 19 for a discussion of media influences on body image and dieting.) Beginning in elementary school, boys are less likely to consider themselves in need of dieting but are equally dissatisfied with their body image. As many boys want to become bigger as want weight loss, and all want to be more muscular. Dieting in males is more likely to be related to participation in sports, past obesity, gender identity conflicts, and fear of future medical illness, than sociocultural endorsement of dieting. Adult males describe themselves as overweight at weights 15% higher than females (with reference to ideal body weights). Women feel thin, generally, only when below 90% of ideal body weight, whereas men rate themselves as thin when as high as 105% of ideal weight.

The idealized body image for males is increasingly that of a V-shaped upper body—muscular, moderate in weight, with virtually no fat—as evidenced by changes in action toys and media ideals. More and more skin exposure is apparent in advertisements directed toward males, with particular emphasis on well-defined abdominal and chest muscles ("six-packs" and "pecs," respectively). Desire for decreased weight is concentrated among specific subgroups of men, for example, those who wrestle. With regard to the influence of sexual orientation, desire for weight loss among men is ranked in the following order: heterosexual females > gay males = lesbian females >> heterosexual males. While the frequency of homosexual orientation among males with eating disorders is high at approximately 20%, it should be noted that this still applies to only a minority of cases. Nevertheless, homosexual orientation is an established risk factor. Another established risk factor is premorbid obesity, which is present in about 50% of cases.

## Treatment

The basic principles of treatment in males and females are similar: restoring normal weight; interrupting abnormal behaviors; treating comorbid conditions; helping patients think differently about the value of weight loss or shape change; and preparing them for reintegration into their sociocultural, gender-specific roles. Restoration of a healthy weight in males leads to increased testosterone, but 10–20% are left with some testicular abnormality.

Indications for hospitalization are independent of gender. There has been increasing recognition of bias against the treatment of males, with many programs refusing to admit males or lacking gender-specific components. Males with eating disorders appreciate working with clinicians who are sensitive to male concerns. Anorexia nervosa is more ego-alien to males than to females. Women with eating disorders may stigmatize males with eating disorders, who often feel isolated in therapeutic groups of women.

## Outcome

Being male is not an adverse prognostic factor. Men respond well to competent treatment, with short- and long-term outcome being equal to that of females. Pre-illness sexual fantasy or behavior improves prognosis.

## PROBABLE FACTS

### Diagnosis and Clinical Features

Males with eating disorders score lower on the Eating Attitudes Test (EAT) and in the Drive for Thinness score on the Eating Disorder Inventory (EDI), but are equally distressed on the Beck Depression Inventory and the Minnesota Multiphasic Personality Inventory (MMPI), suggesting that screening questionnaires may not be asking the pertinent questions of males. Compared to females, males with eating disorders are more likely to have substance abuse as a comorbid condition. Recent pilot studies have reported that males with anorexia nervosa also suffer from decreased brain size secondary to self-starvation. Binge eating disorder may go unrecognized because overeating in males is less likely to provoke attention.

### Epidemiology and Etiology

There appears to be a rough correlation between the prevalence of anorexia nervosa and the degree of social reinforcement for slimming, suggesting a dose–response curve independent of gender. (See Chapters 19, 45, and 47 for further discussion of sociocultural influences on eating disorders.) The two genders probably experienced parallel increases in the incidence of eating disorders until the mid-1980s. About this time, however, the distressed, cachetic appearance of the first males with AIDS decreased the value of slimness in men and returned the idealized image in males to one of more muscularity. Testosterone may have some protective effect on the development of eating disorders by creating a mesomorphic, athletic appearance that is incompatible with severe starvation.

Changes in secondary sexual characteristics and social functioning during puberty cause less distress in males, who are therefore less likely to use eating disorders as a defense against maturation. The decreasing age of puberty may have affected boys less than girls.

### Treatment

More than one male patient in a treatment program yields benefits such as the possibility of male-only patient groups, thereby allowing greater openness and confidence. It also helps patients to explore gender-specific aspects of etiology. Gender has less influence on treatment in severe cases. With increasing weight, male manifestations of increased testosterone include flirting, masturbation, and sexual comments. Males are more likely to benefit from weight training during treatment, since many develop prominent abdominal fatness on weight restoration and, as a result, quickly return to dieting.

## Outcome

As with females, males have a worse prognosis when they have a very low weight or a long-established low weight, marked comorbidity, or an unsupportive family. Negative prognostic features also include failure to achieve a truly normal weight and lack of follow-up treatment.

## CONCLUSIONS

There are many similarities in the clinical features, epidemiology, etiology, treatment, and outcome for males and females with eating disorders, sufficient similarities to allow the clinician to identify cases and undertake the essentials of treatment. It is clear, however, that the experience of being male in our society, from conception on, differs from that of being female. These differences include the effect of a steady state of gonadotropin, the percent of body fat needed for pubertal onset, the psychosocial experience of puberty, the genomic influence on body shape, as well as possible differences in how precursor amino acids for neurotransmitter synthesis are metabolized in the brain. In addition, the sociocultural environment differs from birth on in its reinforcement for dieting and weight loss, and these differences are evident even in elementary school.

Clinicians may be confident in diagnosing males with eating disorders, certain that early comprehensive treatment and good follow-up not only reduce mortality and morbidity but also increase quality of life. In both genders, the goal of complete cure, defined by return to gender-specific cultural normality (not perfection), is achievable.

## FURTHER READING

Andersen, A. E., Watson, T., & Schlechte, J. (2000). Osteoporosis and osteopenia in men with eating disorders. *Lancet, 355,* 1967–1968.—The first documentation of severe bone mineral deficiency in males with eating disorders.

Braun, D., Sunday, S., Huang, A., & Halmi, K. (1999). More males seek treatment for eating disorders. *International Journal of Eating Disorders, 25,* 415–424.—The best documentation of increasing prevalence of eating disorders in males.

Carlat, D., Camargo, C. A., & Herzog, D. (1997). Eating disorders in males: A report on 135 patients. *American Journal of Psychiatry, 154,* 1127–1132.—A large, comprehensive study of a 135 males, emphasizing the psychosexual vulnerabilities and comorbidity of males with eating disorders.

Drewnowski, A., & Yee, D. (1987). Men and body image: Are males satisfied with their body weight? *Psychosomatic Medicine, 49,* 626–634.—A population-based study of males versus females in regard to body dissatisfaction, showing equal dissatisfaction but of a different type.

Holbrook, T. (2000). Walking in the woods. In A. Andersen, L. Cohn, & T. Holbrook (Eds.), *Making weight: Men's conflicts with food, weight, shape and appearance* (pp. 117–134). Carlsbad, CA: Gürze Books.—A most poignant, clinically sophisticated, and detailed personal account of anorexia nervosa in a male.

Maloney, M. J., McGuire, J., Daniels, S. R., Specker, B. (1989). Dieting behavior and eating attitudes in children. *Pediatrics, 84,* 482–489.—A study of 318 girls and boys, noting the high prevalence of body-weight dissatisfaction and gender differences in young children.

Pope, H., Olivardia, R., Gruber, A., & Borowiecki, J. (1999). Evolving ideals of male body image as seen through action toys. *International Journal of Eating Disorders, 26,* 65–72.—The psychosocial image of the ideal male, which has changed drastically over the last 30 years, is documented in this innovative study.

Schmit, G., & Rouam, F. (1984). L'anorexie mentale chez l'adolescent de sexe masculin. *Neuropsychiatrie de l'Enfance, 32,* 245–257.—Classical analytic reasoning for anorexia nervosa among adolescent boys, as well as a continental viewpoint.

Siever, M. (1994). Sexual orientation and gender as factors in socioculturally acquired vulnerability to body dissatsifaction and eating disorders. *Journal of Consulting and Clinical Psychology, 62,* 252–260.—A detailed study of the effect of gender and sexual orientation on eating disorders.

Van Deth, R., & Vandereycken, W. (1997). The striking age-old minority of fasting males in the history of anorexia nervosa. *Food and Foodways, 7,* 119–130.—A historical examination of cultural and biological explanations for the lower prevalence of eating disorders in males.

# 34

# Anxiety, Depression, and Eating Disorders

## CYNTHIA M. BULIK

The earliest clinical descriptions of anorexia nervosa and bulimia nervosa noted the frequent presence of both depression and anxiety. Subsequent investigations using structured diagnostic methodology in clinical and epidemiological samples and in family studies have verified those early observations. Of the many possible models of comorbidity, five are particularly plausible to explain the relation among eating, affective, and anxiety disorders. Each of these models yields a unique set of predictions.

Model One posits that depression and anxiety are sequelae of eating disorders. It predicts that depression and anxiety would not be apparent in individuals with anorexia nervosa and bulimia nervosa prior to the development of an eating disorder. Moreover, unless one posits a permanent scarring effect, this model predicts the alleviation of anxiety or depressive symptoms with recovery from the eating disorder.

Model Two, the converse of Model One, posits that eating disorders are sequelae of affective or anxiety disorders. It predicts a pattern of onset in which depression or anxiety manifest prior to the onset of eating disorders.

Model Three, the *forme fruste* model, posits that eating disorders are expressions of an underlying depressive or anxiety disorder. Eating disorders may be age- and gender-specific manifestations of depression or anxiety, with etiological factors completely shared among the classes of disorders.

Model Four posits that eating, anxiety, and affective disorders are different expressions of the same underlying causal factor (e.g., neuroticism or neuroendocrine disturbance).

Model Five posits that whereas eating, affective, and anxiety disorders are unique sets of conditions, they may share some etiological factors. It makes no predictions about whether the eating, depressive, or anxiety disorders manifest first but predicts the existence of both shared and independent etiological factors across the disorders.

Given these five models of comorbidity, how can extant data assist with illuminating the nature of the relationship among these three disorders?

## ANOREXIA NERVOSA AND ANXIETY DISORDERS

### Clinical Manifestations

Anxiety in anorexia nervosa manifests in several forms. During the acute phase of the illness, women with anorexia nervosa are pervasively anxious about issues related to shape, weight, and food. Slight increases in weight or transgressions of rigidly prescribed dietary rules result in severe anxiety. Parallels have also been drawn with obsessive–compulsive disorder, because individuals with anorexia nervosa display preoccupation with food, eating, weight, and exercise. Retrospective clinical information suggests that women with anorexia nervosa have premorbid obsessional traits that become exaggerated during the acute phase of the illness, possibly secondary to starvation. Outcome studies indicate that those who remain ill retain high scores on obsessionality indices, whereas the scores of those who recover approach those of healthy controls. (See Chapter 40 for a discussion of the course and outcome of eating disorders.)

### Nature of the Comorbid Relationship

Both clinical and epidemiological data support substantial comorbidity between anorexia nervosa and anxiety disorders. Clinical studies have consistently noted elevated rates of anxiety disorders in women with anorexia nervosa. The most methodologically sophisticated studies suggest that well over half of women with anorexia nervosa report the lifetime presence of an anxiety disorder—most commonly generalized anxiety disorder, obsessive–compulsive disorder, and social phobia. Moreover, most studies indicate that the onset of anxiety disorders usually precedes the onset of anorexia nervosa. Whereas this pattern of onset may simply reflect the natural course of the two disorders (i.e., the average age of onset of some anxiety disorders is younger than the average age of onset of anorexia nervosa), it may also indicate that childhood anxiety represents one significant pathway toward the development of anorexia nervosa.

Clinical samples may artifactually identify significant associations that do not exist in the community because of differential referral. Epidemiological studies provide estimates of comorbidity that are not confounded by treatment seeking. In a population-based sample of over 2,000 female twins, odds ratios for generalized anxiety disorder, phobias, and panic disorder were significantly elevated in women with varyingly stringent definitions of anorexia nervosa. Thus, the presence of anorexia nervosa significantly increases patients' risk of also suffering from a comorbid anxiety disorder.

## ANOREXIA NERVOSA AND MAJOR DEPRESSION

### Clinical Manifestations

Clinical observation of women with anorexia nervosa commonly reveals depressed or flat affect, feelings of hopelessness and guilt, a sense of worthlessness, paralyzingly low self-esteem, irritability, insomnia, and suicidal ideation and attempts. Retrospective reports indicate that both patterns of onset occur—depression before anorexia nervosa and vice versa. Although depressed mood can occasionally improve with refeeding, several medium- and long-term outcome studies suggest that depression may persist even after recovery. In addition to the frequent comorbid pattern, family history studies have shown that relatives of individuals with anorexia nervosa are at significantly greater risk for major depression than relatives of healthy controls.

## Nature of the Comorbid Relationship

Studies on clinical samples of women with anorexia nervosa that have used structured psychiatric diagnostic instruments have suggested a wide range of estimates (20–80%) for the percentage of women who report at least one episode of lifetime major depression. Epidemiological data are somewhat scarce due to the relative rarity of the condition; however, extant studies suggest that major depression is the most commonly observed comorbid psychiatric disorder in women with anorexia nervosa.

The nature of this comorbid relation has been explored directly using twin studies. This approach allows one to determine the extent to which shared genetic and shared environmental factors contribute to the development of each disorder. The results suggest not only the presence of unique sets of genes that contribute independently to anorexia nervosa and to depression, but also a shared genetic component indicating the existence of some genes that contribute to both anorexia nervosa and depression. Thus, the two disorders may be influenced by shared genetic factors.

## BULIMIA NERVOSA AND ANXIETY DISORDERS

### Clinical Manifestations

The high prevalence of anxiety disorders in women with bulimia nervosa has fueled several etiological theories in which anxiety is the central feature. These include the anxiety reduction model, which focuses on the potential anxiolytic effects of both bingeing and purging behavior, models that liken bingeing and purging to obsessive–compulsive behaviors, and models that focus on the role of heightened social anxiety in fueling body dissatisfaction and bulimic eating behaviors and attitudes. Clinically, the most commonly observed comorbid anxiety disorders in women with bulimia nervosa are social phobia and generalized anxiety disorder.

### Nature of the Comorbid Relationship

The most rigorous studies using structured diagnostic tools suggest the presence of lifetime anxiety disorders in well over half of women with bulimia nervosa in both clinical and community samples. Anxiety disorders predate the emergence of an eating disorder in the majority of cases. Such findings across studies have led researchers to suggest that early-onset anxiety disorders may be an etiological factor for bulimia nervosa. Genetic epidemiological studies have further explored the nature of this association by examining the multivariate structure of the genetic relationship among bulimia nervosa, phobias, generalized anxiety disorder, panic disorder, major depression, and alcoholism. These analyses have identified shared genetic factors across bulimia nervosa, phobias, and panic disorder, thus siting bulimia within the genetic "family" of these anxiety disorders.

## BULIMIA NERVOSA AND MAJOR DEPRESSION

### Clinical Manifestation

Depression is common in women with bulimia nervosa. On the basis of psychometric data, it has been suggested that the nature of the depressive features differs somewhat between individuals with major depression only and those with depression associated with bulimia nervosa. Like anorexia nervosa, both orders of presentation occur—bulimia nervosa prior to depression and vice versa. Individuals with bulimia nervosa may continue to experience depression even after recovering from the eating disorder. In addition, relatives of women with bulimia nervosa are at significantly greater risk for depression than relatives of healthy controls. Further associations between bulimia nervosa and depression have been suggested based on the observation that women with bulimia nervosa respond to antidepressant medication (see Chapter 58). Although important, drawing conclusions regarding etiology based on treatment response is ill-advised.

### Nature of the Comorbid Relationship

Clinical samples of women with bulimia nervosa have routinely reported high prevalences of lifetime comorbid affective disorders. These high rates have been demonstrated, in part, to be an artifact of Berkson's bias—that individuals with more than one diagnosis are more likely to seek clinical care, thereby artificially inflating comorbidity rates observed in clinical samples. An excellent study from New Zealand by Bushnell and colleagues found the prevalence of affective disorders to be significantly higher in a clinically ascertained sample of women with bulimia nervosa than in a randomly selected population sample of women with the disorder. However, the prevalence of depression in the community sample of bulimic women was still significantly higher than the rates of depression in population-based controls. Other population-based studies have consistently shown that major depression is the most commonly observed comorbid condition in women with bulimia nervosa.

The nature of this comorbid relationship with major depression has also been explored directly using the twin design. Similar to the study of depression and anorexia nervosa, the results revealed a moderate genetic correlation between bulimia nervosa and major depression—suggesting either the presence of some genes that predispose to both disorders or a shared genetic effect. The result also suggests that the two disorders are not the result of the same environmental risk factors predisposing to both disorders.

## CONCLUSIONS

Returning to the models of comorbidity, the data reviewed enable tentative conclusions to be drawn regarding the nature of the comorbid relationship among eating, affective, and anxiety disorders. There is little evidence to support the theory that depression and anxiety are simply sequelae of eating disorders (Model One). The strongest counterevidence to this argument is the frequent observation that depression and anxiety disorders predate the onset of both anorexia nervosa and bulimia nervosa. Especially for the relation between eating and anxiety disorders, there is reasonable support for the notion that anxiety may represent a pathway of risk for the development of eating disorders in a substantial number of cases (Model Two). There is little support for the notion that anorexia nervosa or bulimia nervosa represent a *forme fruste* of depression or anxiety (Model Three). These disorders are not universally comorbid and information from genetic epidemiological studies disconfirms the notion of a single, shared etiological factor. Support for Model Four is less clear. Additional studies are required at the neurocognitive and neurohormonal level to determine whether single underlying causal mechanisms may predispose to each of these sets of disorders. At this stage, the most compelling model allows for the existence of both shared and specific etiological factors (Model Five). Indeed, there is some suggestion of shared genetic factors among these classes of disorders. As we progress further in our understanding of comorbidity, we may be able to identify more precisely the nature of the common as well as specific etiological factors.

## FURTHER READING

Braun, D. L., Sunday, S. R., & Halmi, K. A. (1994). Psychiatric comorbidity in patients with eating disorders. *Psychological Medicine, 24*, 859–867.—Structured interview-based study of comorbidity among consecutively admitted inpatients to an eating disorders facility that carefully breaks down diagnostic subgroups of eating disorders.

Brewerton, T., Lydiard, R., Herzog, D., Brotman, A., O'Neil, P., & Ballenger, J. (1995). Comorbidity of Axis I psychiatric disorders in bulimia nervosa. *Journal of Clinical Psychiatry, 56*, 77–80.—Clinical study explores rates of affective, anxiety, and substance use disorder in women with bulimia nervosa and highlights common patterns of onset of affective disorder relative to bulimia nervosa.

Bulik, C., Sullivan, P., Fear, J., & Joyce, P. (1997). Eating disorders and antecedent anxiety disorders: A controlled study. *Acta Psychiatrica Scandinavica, 96*, 101–107.—Examines comorbidity of anxiety disorders in women with bulimia and anorexia nervosa as well as the timing and pattern of onset using structured diagnostic methodology.

Bushnell, J. A., Wells, E., McKenzie, J. M., Hornblow, A. R., Oakley-Browne, M. A., & Joyce, P. R. (1994). Bulimia comorbidity in the general population and in the clinic. *Psychological Medicine, 24*, 605–611.—Methodologically sound study examining differences in comorbidity between treatment-seeking and population-ascertained women with bulimia nervosa.

Herzog, D. B., Keller, M. B., Sacks, N. R., Yeh, C. J., & Lavori, P. W. (1992). Psychiatric comorbidity in treatment-seeking anorexics and bulimics. *Journal of the American Academy of Child and Adolescent Psychiatry, 31*, 810–818.—Examines (via structured psychiatric interview) rates and patterns of comorbidity in 229 patients with anorexia nervosa, bulimia nervosa, and mixed eating disorder pathology.

Kendler, K. S., Walters, E. E., Neale, M. C., Kessler, R. C., Heath, A. C., & Eaves, L. J. (1995). The structure of the genetic and environmental risk factors for six major psychiatric disorders in women: Phobia, generalized anxiety disorder, panic disorder, bulimia, major depression and alcoholism. *Archives of General Psychiatry, 52*, 374–383.—Comprehensive, multivariate twin study that explores the genetic and environmental relation among six common psychiatric disorders in women.

Lilenfeld, L., Kaye, W., Greeno, C., Merikangas, K., Plotnikov, K., Pollice, C., Rao, R., Strober, M., Bulik, C., & Nagy, L. (1998). A controlled family study of restricting anorexia and bulimia nervosa: Comorbidity in probands and disorders in first-degree relatives. *Archives of General Psychiatry, 55*, 603–610.—Explores issue of comorbidity in eating disorders in the context of a large family study.

Mitchell, J., Specker, S., & De Zwaan, M. (1991). Comorbidity and medical complications of

bulimia nervosa. *Journal of Clinical Psychiatry, 52,* 13–20.—Review and overview of psychiatric and medical comorbidity in bulimia nervosa.
Wade, T. D., Bulik, C. M., Neale, M., & Kendler, K. S. (2000). Anorexia nervosa and major depression: Shared genetic and environmental risk factors. *American Journal of Psychiatry, 157,*
   469–471.—Bivariate twin analysis exploring the extent to which anorexia nervosa and major
   depression share genetic and environmental risk factors.
Walters, E. E., Neale, M. C., Eaves, L. J., Heath, A. C., Kessler, R. C., & Kendler, K. S. (1992).
   Bulimia nervosa and major depression: A study of common genetic and environmental factors. *Psychological Medicine, 22,* 617–622.—Bivariate twin analysis exploring the extent to
   which bulimia nervosa and major depression share genetic and environmental risk factors.

# 35

# Eating Disorders
# and Addictive Disorders

## G. TERENCE WILSON

The binge eating that is a prominent feature of many eating disorders shares many similarities with substance abuse. People with binge eating and substance abuse report cravings to consume the substance. Both groups experience a sense of loss of control and report using the substance to regulate their emotional state and cope with stress. Both become preoccupied with their problem, make repeated attempts to stop, and seek to keep it secret. Many experience both eating and alcohol or drug problems, sometimes simultaneously. Accordingly, binge eating (and, by extension, eating disorders) have been viewed as addictive disorders.

## THE ADDICTION MODEL OF EATING DISORDERS

The addiction model of binge eating (and eating disorders) assumes that particular individuals are biologically vulnerable to certain foods that can cause chemical dependence; that patients must abstain from these toxic foods (chemicals); and that since eating disorders and addictive disorders are essentially different expressions of the same underlying problem, the treatment of eating disorders should not differ fundamentally from that of substance abuse.

The similarities between binge eating and substance abuse may seem obvious, but they obscure fundamentally important differences. Addiction or chemical dependency is characterized by the phenomena of tolerance, physical dependence, and withdrawal reactions. No credible scientific evidence shows that these phenomena apply to eating disorders. The biological consequences of food hardly make it an addictive substance, just as the biological effects of activities such as sex, sleep, and exercise do not make these behaviors physiologically addictive. Starvation, or the withdrawal of food, produces a specific constellation of physiological and psychological symptoms, including irritability and distractibility, preoccupation with food and weight, and binge eating. But these starvation symptoms are not equivalent to drug withdrawal effects. A key assumption of the addiction model of eating disorders is that food is a drug, and that it can therefore have psychoactive effects on mood and behavior. However, the evidence indicates that the effects of food are different from those of psychoactive substances, and foods have little, if any, pharmacological effect.

Selective cravings for particular foods are often cited as evidence that individuals who crave them are addicted to food. "Carbohydrate craving" is often viewed as a contributing cause of eating disorders. The notion of carbohydrate craving is based on the premise that carbohydrates increase the transport into the brain of tryptophan relative to other, large neutral amino acids. This increase enhances serotonin synthesis, which in turn is thought to reduce negative mood. Although tryptophan depletion may be a trigger for increased eating in patients with bulimia nervosa (see Chapter 49 for a discussion of the role of serotonin in eating disorders), there is no evidence that carbohydrate consumption or tryptophan repletion relieve negative mood.

Several well-controlled studies show that patients with bulimia nervosa do not preferentially consume simple carbohydrates during binge eating. When the eating of bulimia nervosa patients and that of normal controls is studied directly in the laboratory, macronutrient selection is found to be similar for both groups. The essential appetitive abnormality in bulimia nervosa lies in the control of quantity of food consumed, not in the consumption of a specific macronutrient. The same holds true for patients with binge eating disorder.

Loss of control characterizes binge eating. But this phenomenon differs from the concept of loss of control as used in the addiction-as-disease theory of alcoholism. The notion there is that the ingestion of alcohol triggers an uncontrollable biochemical reaction to continue drinking that overrides all reason or choice. Bulimia nervosa patients do not invariably lose control and binge despite violating their dietary restraint by ingesting a "forbidden" food, especially if they know they cannot subsequently purge. Uncontrolled binge eating in bulimia nervosa is explained by a combination of nutritional deprivation and psychological mechanisms (see also Chapter 18).

The addiction model of eating disorders focuses too narrowly on binge eating, the symptom most closely resembling psychoactive substance abuse. But binge eating is but one facet of bulimia nervosa (and is not even present in many eating disorders—see Chapters 28, 29, and 30). The cognitive-behavioral model of the processess that maintain bulimia nervosa details how binge eating is largely a product of rigid and unhealthy dietary restraint. The latter is driven by the desire to restrict eating in order to lose weight, which is a function of negative self-evaluation and dysfunctional concerns about body weight and shape (see Chapter 54). There are no comparable mechanisms operating in substance abuse disorders: The substance abuse is not a product of sobriety.

## Therapeutic Implications of the Addiction Model

The addiction model of treatment prescribes unremitting dietary restraint, featuring absolute avoidance of particular foods and a highly structured eating pattern, resulting in a sense of powerlessness over food. In contrast to the addiction model, cognitive-behavioral therapy is designed to reduce dietary restraint and modify abnormal attitudes about the importance of body weight and shape (see Chapter 54). In cognitive-behavioral therapy, both the physiological sequelae of caloric deprivation and the psychological costs of self-denial are addressed by the establishment of regular, nutritionally balanced meals and the introduction of previously avoided foods into a flexible diet.

Evidence supporting the effectiveness of the leading addiction-based treatment for eating disorders (the 12-step approach) is lacking. Unlike the 12-step approach, cognitive-behavioral therapy has been extensively evaluated in controlled clinical trials (see Chapter 54). It produces broad and lasting reductions in binge eating and the other hallmark symptoms of bulimia nervosa, and has a similar effect in binge eating disorder (see Chapter 63). The consistent success of methods derived from a model that is so at odds with the addiction approach challenges the fundamental premises of the latter.

## COMORBIDITY OF EATING AND SUBSTANCE ABUSE DISORDERS

Eating disorders may not be a form of psychoactive substance abuse, but the two disorders co-occur at a rate that is greater than chance. Rates of lifetime substance abuse are significantly higher in both clinical and community samples of individuals with anorexia nervosa and bulimia nervosa, but not among those with binge eating disorder. However, the association between eating disorders and substance abuse disorders is not a specific one. Rates of substance abuse tend to be elevated among patients with psychiatric disorders in general, indicating that patients with psychological problems are more likely to abuse alcohol or drugs. Moreover, there are data showing that the comorbidity of anxiety and mood disorders with anorexia nervosa and bulimia nervosa is higher than that of substance abuse disorder and eating disorders (see Chapter 34).

Evidence regarding whether individuals with both an eating disorder and a substance abuse disorder are a distinctive subgroup is mixed. Some studies show overlapping psychopathology, whereas others indicate that patients with both disorders differ in degree of psychiatric disturbance from those with an eating disorder only. It does not appear that a history of substance abuse is a negative prognostic indicator for success in treating bulimia nervosa.

Alcohol-dependent patients with an eating disorder are younger than those without an eating disorder. Eating disorders generally precede the development of substance abuse, leading some investigators to conclude that an eating disorder is a risk factor for alcohol dependence.

### Mechanisms Linking Eating Disorders and Substance Abuse Disorders

The addiction model is a prototypical example of the shared etiology view of the comorbidity between eating and substance abuse disorders. The shared etiology hypothesis is that eating and substance abuse disorders are different expressions of the same underlying vulnerability. However, several lines of evidence fail to provide empirical support for this hypothesis.

First, the association is not a specific one. Whereas there is good evidence of a reciprocal causal link between alcohol dependence and anxiety disorders, no such connection has been established between substance use disorders and eating disorders. Second, the pattern of familial transmission of the two sets of disorders is inconsistent with the notion of a common causal factor. The data do show that first-degree relatives of patients with eating disorders have higher rates of substance abuse disorder than community controls, and in a case-control study of the development of bulimia nervosa, alcohol problems in parents were a specific risk factor for bulimia nervosa. But the familial aggregation of substance abuse in probands with bulimia nervosa is independent of bulimia nervosa, and the findings of a twin study of the association between the disorders suggested that their genetic risk factors were different. If a common underlying mechanism is responsible for both sets of disorders, there should be a reciprocal relationship in familial transmission, with higher rates of eating disorders in the first-degree relatives of alcoholics. Yet the available evidence does not show familial crossover between eating disorders and alcohol dependence. The rate of eating disorders among the relatives of alcoholics is no higher than the rate among the relatives of controls.

## CLINICAL RECOMMENDATIONS

Given the association between eating disorders and psychoactive substance abuse, women seeking treatment for eating disorders should be routinely screened for the presence of substance abuse. Similarly, women in treatment primarily for substance abuse problems should be assessed for disturbances in eating. In cases where eating and substance abuse disorders co-occur, the latter should generally be treated first. Once the substance abuse problem is under control, attention can then be directed to the eating problem. If the alcohol or drug abuse is not severe, it may be possible to treat the two problems simultaneously.

## CONCLUSION

Despite the absence of empirical support and its conceptual weaknesses, the addiction model of eating disorders remains influential in some countries (particularly the United States). Haddock and Dill point out that the adherence to the addiction model of eating disorders is a specific instance of a more general societal belief in the putative psychoactive properties of food. This more general notion has similarly proved resistant to the accumulation of unsupportive scientific findings. Fundamental to belief in the addiction model of food is the well-documented finding that explaining unwanted or puzzling behavior in terms of some unknown disease state enjoys popular appeal. But simply relabeling a problem does not advance our understanding of it, nor in this case has it led to a treatment that has been shown to be effective.

### FURTHER READING

Dansky, B. S., Brewerton, T. D., & Kilpatrick, D. G. (2000). National women's study. *International Journal of Eating Disorders, 27,* 180–190.—A study of the comorbidity of bulimia nervosa and alcohol use disorders in a large national sample of women in the United States.

Haddock, C. K., & Dill, P. L. (2000). The effects of food on mood and behavior: Implications for the addictions model of obesity and eating disorders. *Drugs and Society, 15,* 17–47.—An incisive analysis of the alleged psychoactive effects of food on behavior.

Holderness, C. C., Brooks-Gunn, J., & Warren, M. P. (1994). Co-morbidity of eating disorders and substance abuse: Review of the literature. *International Journal of Eating Disorders, 16*, 1–34.—A review of the research on the comorbidity of eating and substance abuse disorders.

Johnson, C. L., & Sansone, R. A. (1993). Integrating the twelve-step approach with traditional psychotherapy for the treatment of eating disorders. *International Journal of Eating Disorders, 14*, 121–134.—A conceptual analysis that seeks to combine the principles of a 12-step treatment approach with conventional psychotherapy for eating disorders.

Kendler, K. S., Walters, E. E., Neale, M. C., Kessler, R. C., Heath, A. C., & Eaves, L. J. (1995). The structure of the genetic and environmental risk factors for six major psychiatric disorders in women: Phobia, generalized anxiety disorder, panic disorder, bulimia, major depression and alcoholism. *Archives of General Psychiatry, 52*, 374–383.—An examination of the relationship between alcoholism and various other psychiatric disorders (including bulimia nervosa) using data from the Virginia Twin Registry.

Kushner, M. T., Abrams, K., & Borchardt, C. (2000). The relationship between anxiety disorders and alcohol use disorders. *Clinical Psychology Review, 20*, 149–171.—A comprehensive review of the well-documented comorbidity between anxiety disorders and substance use disorders.

Vandereycken, W. (1990). The addiction model in eating disorders: Some critical remarks and a selected bibliography. *International Journal of Eating Disorders, 9*, 95–101.—A scholarly analysis of the problems inherent in drawing analogies between eating disorders and substance abuse disorders.

Walsh, B. T. (1993). Binge eating in bulimia nervosa. In C. G. Fairburn & G. T. Wilson (Eds.), *Binge eating: Nature, assessment, and treatment* (pp. 37–49). New York: Guilford Press.—A review of laboratory studies of the eating behavior of patients with bulimia nervosa.

Wilson, G. T., & Fairburn, C. G. (1998). Treatment of eating disorders. In P. E. Nathan & J. M. Gorman (Eds.), *A guide to treatments that work* (pp. 501–530). New York: Oxford University Press.—A comprehensive analysis of the research on pharmacological and psychological treatments for eating disorders.

Wolfe, W. L., & Maisto, S. A. (2000). The relationship between eating disorders and substance use: Moving beyond co-prevalence research. *Clinical Psychology Review, 20*, 617–631.—A summary of the evidence relevant to the different hypotheses proposed to account for the comorbidity between eating and substance use disorders.

# 36

# Personality and Eating Disorders

## STEPHEN A. WONDERLICH

Clinicians, theorists, and researchers have a long-standing interest in the relationship between personality and eating disorders. While early clinical descriptions emphasized the predispositional risk of personality traits for eating disorders, more recent conceptualization and research have examined how eating disorders may modify personality traits, whether certain mechanisms increase the risk of both eating disorders and certain personality characteristics, as well as the effect of personality on clinical presentation, course, and treatment of anorexia nervosa and bulimia nervosa. However, this literature continues to be plagued by conceptual and methodological problems, and debates about the nature and measurement of personality.

## CONCEPTUAL AND METHODOLOGICAL DEBATE

The categorical approach to understanding personality, represented by the *Diagnostic and Statistical Manual of Mental Disorders* (DSM) and the *International Classification of Diseases* (ICD), has come under increasing attack as a model of personality disturbance. The main criticisms include: (1) Most empirical data suggest that personality traits and disorders are continuously distributed as dimensions rather than bimodal categories; (2) cutoff points for "diagnoses" are arbitrary; (3) inadequate agreement between different personality measures (i.e., poor convergent validity); (4) poor discriminant validity between categories, resulting in marked comorbidity; (5) personality disorder categories typically do not show stability over time; and (6) extreme heterogeneity within polythetic diagnostic concepts (e.g., the 93 possible expressions of borderline personality disorder in DSM-III-R).

Although the debate continues, there is an increasing call for different approaches to the conceptualization and measurement of personality and its disorders. The most common recommendation is to move to a dimensional trait perspective. This offers numerous advantages: (1) The dimensional model is more consistent with empirical evidence suggesting that personality disorders represent exaggerations of underlying normal personality traits; (2) assessment of basic personality traits, rather than the diagnosis of a personality category, helps to diminish problems associated with determining the diagnostic threshold for a category, avoids diagnostic overlap with other personality disorders, and also allows the assessment of adaptive personality traits; and (3) dimensional models enhance statistical reliability and validity. Although there continues to be uncertainty about which model of normal personality best represents the underlying foundation for personality disorders, the Five-Factor Model continues to receive empirical support and several new measures, consistent with the Five-Factor Model, are increasingly in use.

## PERSONALITY AND EATING DISORDERS: DIRECTION OF ASSOCIATION

The potential relationships between eating disorders and personality have been frequently discussed in the literature: (1) Personality predisposes to, or increases the risk of, developing eating disorders; (2) elevations in personality traits or disorders are a simple complication, consequence, or scar of the eating disorder; and (3) eating disorders and personality share no causal relationship and both are either influenced by a third variable or, perhaps, rest on the same spectrum of disturbance. However, only rarely have empirical studies explicitly tested any of these models. Furthermore, it is possible that any personality trait may be a precipitant, scar, or correlate of a given eating disorder. This relationship has been demonstrated previously in the mood disorder literature, where neuroticism has been shown to be a vulnerability factor for the development of depression, a predictor of chronic course, a marker for the acute influence of state effects of depression, as well as a residual scar of the depressive state.

## ANOREXIA NERVOSA, PERFECTIONISM, AND OBSESSIVE–COMPULSIVE PERSONALITY DISORDER

Numerous clinical and empirical reports converge to describe the personality style of the patient with the restricting type of anorexia nervosa (see Chapter 29) as obsessional, socially inhibited, compliant, and emotionally restrained. Individuals with the bulimic type of anorexia nervosa tend to exhibit a more impulsive and extroverted personality style more similar to that seen in bulimia nervosa. However, many of these studies have been limited by the fact that they assessed patients in a state of starvation, which may significantly affect personality measurement. Some evidence suggests that many of these traits endure after recovery. While some researchers consider personality characteristics after recovery as indicative of premorbid personality vulnerability, this view is controversial because these characteristics may also reflect the scarring effect of the eating disorder. Thus, in spite of the impressive clinical convergence over the personality traits characteristic of patients with anorexia nervosa, it has proven difficult to determine if such a constellation reflects a cause or effect of the eating disorder.

The trait of perfectionism, which refers to a tendency to expect a greater performance from oneself or others than is required for a given situation, has recently received increased attention in studies of patients with anorexia nervosa. Evidence suggests that perfectionism is high among malnourished patients and appears to persist even after long-term recovery. A community-based case-control study by Fairburn and colleagues found perfectionism to be a specific antecedent risk factor. Such finding are intriguing because of the overlap between perfectionism and obsessive–compulsive personality disorder (OCPD), both of which have been shown to be elevated in samples of patients with restricting anorexia nervosa. Furthermore, blind retrospective chart reviews indicate that patients with anorexia nervosa are much more likely to show evidence of premorbid OCPD than are control subjects, and a 10-year follow-up of adolescent patients found higher than expected levels of OCPD, in spite of weight restoration.

In an effort to overcome the limitations associated with studying patients with anorexia nervosa, a recent family study by Lilenfeld and colleagues provided additional information suggesting that perfectionistic, obsessive–compulsive personality styles may be a risk factor for the development of anorexia nervosa. In this study, anorexic individuals were stratified into those who showed a concurrent OCPD and those who did not. Importantly, OCPD was elevated in the relatives of probands with anorexia nervosa, regardless of whether the proband displayed OCPD. This finding may be interpreted as supporting the idea that OCPD is part of the same phenotypic spectrum as anorexia nervosa and the two may be expressions of a similar genotype.

## ANOREXIA NERVOSA, PERSONALITY, AND CLINICAL COURSE

Although difficult to obtain, there is a small amount of data on personality predictors of outcome in patients with anorexia nervosa. For example, prospective studies of adolescent patients suggest that maturity fears, social isolation, neurotic problems, and obsessive–compulsive patterns of behavior predict a negative outcome. Similarly, in one study, the temperament dimension of high persistence and the character dimensions of low self-directedness and high self-transcendence (from Cloninger's Temperament and Character Inventory) were significant predictors of suicidal behavior in adult patients. Additionally, adolescent patients who have unremitting obsessive–compulsive personality traits have a particularly poor 10-year outcome.

## BULIMIA NERVOSA, IMPULSIVE AND NARCISSISTIC PERSONALITY

Empirical studies have historically depicted patients with bulimia nervosa as impulsive, interpersonally sensitive, and low in self-esteem. Studies of personality disorders show that these patients have elevated rates of DSM Cluster B and Cluster C personality disorders. Although there has been considerable debate about the influence of the bulimic state (especially the mood and nutritional disturbance) on Cluster B measurement, one recent family study indicates that substance use disorders, certain anxiety disorders, and Cluster B personality disorders are more prevalent among the *relatives* of probands with bulimia nervosa who also display concurrent substance use disorders than in the relatives of other probands with bulimia nervosa and normal controls. This suggests that a possible familial risk factor for bulimia nervosa and substance use is expressed in the dramatic–erratic personality style.

Trait narcissism has also received increased empirical attention. Data suggest that this trait, elevated in patients with bulimia nervosa compared with both normal and psychiatric control subjects, also remains elevated after recovery. In these studies, narcissism was defined as inflated self-importance and a need for attention and admiration. A recent study by Steiger and colleagues used daily diary methodologies to assess interpersonal transactions, self-concept, and mood, and its findings provide further support for narcissistic vulnerability in these patients. Both active and remitted patients showed greater increases in self-criticism and deterioration in mood following a stressful interpersonal transition than normal controls suggesting a hypersensitivity to interpersonal experiences that is consistent with trait narcissism. These same diary methods have also been used to study trait impulsivity. The findings from two studies converge to suggest that patients with bulimia nervosa and high levels of trait impulsivity tend to have binges that are less influenced by dietary restriction and more influenced by negative mood than less impulsive bulimic patients. In other words, trait impulsivity may be a personality continuum that helps to clarify the contributions to binge eating of dietary restraint and affective disregulation (see also Chapter 18).

The findings of another family study by Lilenfeld and colleagues highlight the complexity of the relationship between personality and eating disorders. Interestingly, this study included non-eating-disordered family members of both probands with bulimia nervosa and control subjects. It was reasoned that significant elevations in personality traits for never-ill family members of probands with bulimia nervosa may reflect an underlying personality vulnerability factor that runs in their families. The design also included recovered and acutely ill probands with bulimia nervosa, which allowed the examination of possible scarring and state effects of personality traits. The results suggested that (1) perfectionism, and the subconstructs of concern over mistakes and parental criticism, represent vulnerability factors for bulimic behavior that run in families; (2) elevations in interceptive awareness and stress reaction represent residual scar effects; and (3) elevations in alienation and absorption are accounted for by the immediate state effects of bulimia nervosa.

## BULIMIA NERVOSA, PERSONALITY, AND CLINICAL COURSE

Cluster B personality disorder has generally predicted a negative course for bulimia nervosa at 1-, 3-, and 5-year outcome assessments. Also, Cluster B pathology has been a negative predictor for treatment outcome, although one recent, large multicenter study of cognitive-behavioral therapy and interpersonal therapy failed to confirm this finding. Several personality traits have also predicted course and treatment outcome. For example, as with anorexia nervosa, high persistence, low self-directedness, and high self-transcendence are associated with suicidal behavior, whereas low self-directedness and high impulsivity predict negative outcome to cognitive-behavioral therapy.

## FUTURE DIRECTIONS

With the incorporation of new and more elaborate research designs, the role of personality in the eating disorders continues to be clarified. Future studies may benefit from examining variability in personality styles within eating disorder diagnostic categories rather than searching for correspondence between a given trait and a particular disorder. Research is also needed on personality functioning in individuals with binge eating disorder (see Chapter 31).

## FURTHER READING

Fairburn, C. G., Cooper, Z., Doll, H. A., & Welch, S. L. (1999). Risk factors for anorexia nervosa: Three integrated case-control comparisons. *Archives of General Psychiatry, 56,* 468–476.—Implicates perfectionism as a risk factor for the development of anorexia nervosa (and bulimia nervosa).

Favaro, A., & Santonastaso, P. (1998). Impulsive and compulsive self-injurious behavior in bulimia nervosa: Prevalence and psychological correlates. *Journal of Nervous and Mental Disease, 186,* 157–165.—Attempts to organize self-injurious behavior in bulimia nervosa through factor-analytic exploration. The findings reveal two large super factors: impulsive and compulsive, self-destructive behavior.

Goldner, E. M., Srikameswaran, S., Schroeder, M. L., Livesley, W. J., & Birmingham, C. L. (1999). Dimensional assessment of personality pathology in patients with eating disorders. *Psychiatry Research, 85,* 151–159.—Cluster-analytic examination of the marked variability in personality functioning within eating disorder diagnostic categories.

Lilenfeld, L. R., Kaye, W. H., Greeno, C. G., Merikangas, K. R., Plotnicov, K., Pollice, C., Rao, R., Strober, M., Bulik, C. M., & Nagy, L. (1998). A controlled family study of anorexia nervosa and bulimia nervosa: Psychiatric disorders in first-degree relatives and effects of proband comorbidity. *Archives of General Psychiatry, 55,* 603–610.—A family history study suggesting shared familial transmission of anorexia nervosa and obsessive–compulsive personality disorder.

Lilenfeld, L. R., Stein, D., Devlin, B., Bulik, C., Strober, M., Plotnicov, K., Pollice, C., Rao, R., Merikangas, K. R., Nagy, L., & Kaye, W. H. (2000). Personality traits among currently eating disordered, recovered, and never-ill first-degree female relatives of bulimic and control women. *Psychological Medicine, 30,* 1399–1410.—Family history study suggesting that perfectionist personality traits are a familial risk factor for bulimia nervosa.

Nilsson, E. W., Gillberg, C., Gillberg, I. C., & Rastam, M. (1999). Ten-year follow-up of adolescent-onset anorexia nervosa: Personality disorders. *Journal of the American Academy of Child and Adolescent Psychiatry, 38,* 1389–1395.—Longitudinal study of recovered anorexic adolescents that suggests that obsessive–compulsive personality disorder and "autistic spectrum disorder" share a strong association with anorexia nervosa even after recovery.

Special Feature: Critical issues in the classification of personality disorder—Part I and Part II. (2000). *Journal of Personality Disorders, 14*(1, 2), 1–187.—Important and thorough series of review papers examining the theoretical and methodological issues in contemporary personality research.

Steiger, H., Jabalpurwala, S., Gauvin, L., Séguin, J. R., & Stotland, S. (1999). Hypersensitivity to social interactions in bulimic syndromes: Relationship to binge eating. *Journal of Consulting and Clinical Psychology, 67,* 765–775.—An ecological momentary assessment study suggesting that bulimia nervosa is associated with particular sensitivity to negative interpersonal transactions even after recovery.

Steiger, H., Lehoux, P. M., & Gauvin, L. (1999). Impulsivity, dietary control and the urge to binge in bulimic syndromes. *International Journal of Eating Disorders, 26,* 261–274.—Ecological momentary assessment study suggesting that bulimic individuals with high levels of trait impulsivity are less likely to binge following dietary restraint than are less impulsive bulimic individuals.

Vitousek, K., & Manke, F. (1994). Personality variables and diagnoses in anorexia nervosa and bulimia nervosa. *Journal of Abnormal Psychology, 103,* 137–148.—A comprehensive overview of personality traits and disorders in anorexia nervosa and bulimia nervosa.

Wonderlich, S. A., & Mitchell, J. E. (1997). Eating disorders and comorbidity: Empirical, conceptual, and clinical implications. *Psychopharmacology Bulletin, 33,* 381–390.—A review of the association between eating disorders and personality, with particular emphasis on conceptual models of comorbidity.

# 37

# Childhood-Onset Eating Disorders

## RACHEL BRYANT-WAUGH
## BRYAN LASK

"Childhood-onset eating disorders" refers here to eating disorders with an onset before the age of 14. The term "early onset" is also sometimes used but the usage has led to confusion, since some authors refer to onset in adolescence (i.e., up to 18 years) as "early" to differentiate it from onset in adulthood. We prefer to use the term "childhood-onset" and make a plea for its consistent use for individuals between the ages of 7 and 13 years. (In our experience, 7 years is the youngest age of presentation for patients with anorexia nervosa, and incidence peaks just before 13 years.) Childhood-onset eating disorders are sometimes further grouped according to developmental markers, for example, prepubertal, pubertal, or premenarchal onset.

The eating disorders of childhood include anorexia nervosa, a discussion of which forms the main part of this chapter; bulimia nervosa, rarely seen in clinics in patients under the age of 14 years; food avoidance emotional disorder; selective eating; and pervasive refusal syndrome. (Childhood obesity is discussed in Chapter 77.)

## ANOREXIA NERVOSA

### Diagnostic Issues

Until relatively recently and despite evidence to the contrary, there has been dispute as to whether "true" anorexia nervosa occurs in childhood. This uncertainty may arise partly from difficulties applying the currently accepted diagnostic criteria for anorexia nervosa. For example, criterion D of the DSM-IV specifies "the absence of at least three consecutive menstrual cycles." Clearly, in younger girls, it is often inappropriate to consider absence of menses as pathological, since these may not yet have commenced. Furthermore, it is difficult to ascertain whether menstruation might "otherwise have occurred" in girls below the age of 14 years. Also, it is difficult to calculate accurately the expected weight of children who have been failing to grow, since expected weight is usually determined on the basis of height and age.

ICD-10 acknowledges the existence of prepubertal anorexia nervosa, and the diagnostic criteria make some allowance for it (see Chapter 28). However, these criteria still do not take into consideration children who are some years away from their growth spurt and pubertal development. Our clinical experience and research evidence leaves us in no doubt that childhood-onset anorexia nervosa does occur and is a potentially serious illness that can have a poor outcome.

## Epidemiology

The incidence of childhood-onset anorexia nervosa is not known. Although it is likely to be lower than in late adolescence and early adult life, referrals to our clinics have gradually increased over the years with no evidence of abatement. Our impression is that anorexia nervosa is truly becoming more common in this age group.

In adults with anorexia nervosa, men are thought to account for 5–10% of cases (see Chapter 33), whereas in children, boys have been reported to represent between 20% and 25% of referrals. It is not yet possible to state whether there is a true age-related difference in the gender ratio, or whether these younger boys are simply more likely to come to medical attention. The limited epidemiological data concerning younger individuals suggest that the gender ratio may indeed be different, but this tentative finding needs further study.

## Clinical Features

Common presenting features of childhood-onset anorexia nervosa include weight loss, determined food avoidance, preoccupation with weight and calories, dread of fatness, overexercising, self-induced vomiting, and laxative abuse. Obsessive–compulsive features, often including extreme conscientiousness about schoolwork, anxiety, and depression are also common. When initially seen in the clinic, a number of children report physical symptoms such as nausea, abdominal pain, feeling full, or being unable to swallow. Rarely is any physical cause found for these features other than poor nutrition.

Premorbidly, children with anorexia nervosa are often described as perfectionist, conscientious, hardworking, pleasant, and "no problem" until the onset of the eating problem (see also Chapter 36). Early feeding problems and childhood obesity are not generally features in their histories, and very few have had any previous psychiatric disorder.

Although weight loss is not an essential diagnostic feature in this age group (static weight during a period of growth is equivalent to loss of weight), all the children we have seen have indeed lost significant amounts of weight. Weight loss in children can be rapid and dramatic, and many are referred in an emaciated state. Accompanying dehydration is not uncommon and is potentially dangerous. Other physical changes include the development of lanugo hair, hypotension, bradycardia, poor peripheral circulation with skin discoloration, cold peripheries, and delayed or arrested growth (also see Chapter 50).

Determined food avoidance is invariably present, although sometimes heavily disguised. Children often manage to conceal their food avoidance either by taking meals separately from the family or by pretending to eat while furtively disposing of their food. There is typically extreme concern about weight and energy intake. An interesting difference occurs between the sexes. Girls tend to say they are dieting to be thin for aesthetic reasons, whereas boys often give health and fitness as their explanation. The dread of fatness is often concealed or denied, although it frequently emerges during treatment.

Exercising is a popular means of weight control among these patients. Athletic activities such as running and swimming are commonly used as a socially acceptable means of controlling weight. When restrictions are placed on such activities, children frequently resort to climbing stairs and press-ups. It is not uncommon for some children to do several hundred press-ups daily.

Self-induced vomiting and the abuse of laxatives and diuretics are less common than in adults but they nonetheless occur in a significant minority of children. Almost invariably, they are carried out secretively, and their incidence may therefore be underestimated. A number of children suffer esophageal bleeding from repeated vomiting.

Investigations may reveal a number of abnormalities. Ultrasound shows uterine and ovarian regression to an infantile state and hepatic steatosis (fatty deposits in the liver). Investigation of the bones commonly demonstrates reduced bone density (osteopenia) and sometimes osteoporosis. Bone age may be delayed. Biochemical investigations often reveal vitamin and mineral deficiencies, particularly hypokalemia (potassium deficiency). Electrocardiogram (ECG) abnormalities commonly accompany marked weight loss, and brain scans may show a reduction of regional cerebral blood flow in the limbic system.

## Prognosis

The prognosis in this age group is less than satisfactory. Between one-half and two-thirds make a full and sustained recovery, with the remainder experiencing persistent and often severe difficulties. Persistent amenorrhea occurs in about 30%. Complications may include delayed growth, polycystic ovaries, impaired fertility, and osteoporosis.

The illness can be conceptualized as having three stages. The first stage is characterized by the predominance of eating problems. In the second stage, there is a gradual improvement in nutritional intake and the start of a phase of intense negativism, manifested by extreme rudeness, overassertiveness, and oppositional behavior. The third stage consists of more appropriate eating and more socially acceptable ways of expressing feelings. Children who successfully pass from the second to the third stage seem to have the best chance of recovery.

## BULIMIA NERVOSA

There are no satisfactory data regarding the incidence of bulimia nervosa in children under the age of 14 years. The number of clinical referrals is low, and most of these children are at the top end of the 7- to 13-year age range. The clinical features are the same as those seen in older age groups.

## FOOD-AVOIDANCE EMOTIONAL DISORDER

This eating disorder appears to be restricted to childhood. Its main feature is one of determined food avoidance. There is often a previous history of food restriction and, usually, associated symptoms of emotional disturbance such as phobias, obsessional behavior, refusal to attend school, and depression. The food avoidance is considerably more marked than is the case with pure emotional disorders and tends to be of the same intensity as that seen in children with anorexia nervosa. However, the distorted body image and the fear of gaining weight seen in anorexia nervosa are absent. Weight loss and the accompanying physical complications are as severe as, or more severe than, anorexia nervosa. This disorder might constitute a "partial syndrome" of anorexia nervosa, generally with a better prognosis, or it might be conceptualized as intermediate between anorexia nervosa and emotional disorder of childhood.

## SELECTIVE EATING

This condition, which in some children seems to be an extension of the normal food faddiness of preschool life (see Chapter 13), is manifested by the child's consumption of an extremely narrow range of foods. This is often limited to as few as four or five foods, ones usually high in carbohydrate. Despite this restricted intake, most of these children do not suffer from impaired growth or low weight, indicating that their energy intake is probably sufficient. Rarely are there any accompanying problems other than those resulting from social restrictions. There is no overconcern about weight or shape and no distorted perception of body size. The incidence of this type of eating disorder is not known, but it is possibly more common than previously realized. Boys seem to be affected more than girls. Any attempt to increase the repertoire of foods eaten is usually met with extreme resistance. Commonly, the parents are far more distressed by the condition than the children.

## PERVASIVE REFUSAL SYNDROME

This life-threatening condition consists of a profound and pervasive refusal to eat, drink, walk, talk, or engage in any form of self-care. Usually, a child with pervasive refusal shows the characteristic features of anorexia nervosa, but as treatment is initiated, the child rapidly manifests an increasing number of avoidant behaviors. Typically, the child adopts a fetal position and quietly moans or remains totally mute except when attempts are made to feed or in some way care for her or him. Such efforts are met with either terror or anger, along with intense avoidance. There is no evidence of organic disease. These symptoms do not fit comfortably into any one diagnostic category. Our experience leads us to believe that these children have often been severely traumatized, either in the form of sexual abuse or other severe violence, and subsequently silenced. Pervasive refusal syndrome may eventually be conceptualized as a form of post-traumatic stress disorder.

## TREATMENT

Given the potential seriousness of some of childhood-onset eating disorders, a rapidly initiated, intensive, and comprehensive treatment program is usually indicated. Essential components of treatment include providing information and education for the parents and child; ensuring that adults are in charge of issues concerning the child's health and safety; making a decision about the need for hospitalization; drawing up clear plans for refeeding, when required; and monitoring regularly the child's physical state.

In most instances, family therapy or parental counseling forms the mainstay of therapeutic input. Individual therapy (motivational enhancement, psychodynamic or cognitive therapy) may be a useful adjunct, while group therapy and other therapies (e.g., physiotherapy) may be offered on an inpatient basis. Medication is required in a minority of cases and usually takes the form of antidepressants for children with a concurrent depressive disorder.

## FURTHER READING

Bryant-Waugh R., & Lask B. (1995). Annotation: Eating disorders in children. *Journal of Child Psychology and Psychiatry, 36,* 191–202.—A review of research in this area.

Chowdhury, U., & Lask, B. (2000). Neurological correlates of eating disorders. *European Eating Disorders Review, 8,* 126–133.—An overview of the relationship between eating disorders and the brain.

Higgs, J., Goodyer, I., & Birch, J. (1989). Anorexia nervosa and food avoidance emotional disorder. *Archives of Diseases in Childhood, 64,* 346–351.—An important article that highlights the variability in types of eating disturbance in childhood.

Hoek, H. (1993). Review of the epidemiological studies of eating disorders. *International Review of Psychiatry, 5,* 61–74.—A useful overview of the epidemiology of eating disorders (see also Chapter 41).

Lask, B., Britten, C., Kroll, L., Magagna, J., & Tranter, M. (1991). Pervasive refusal in children. *Archives of Diseases in Childhood, 66,* 866–869.—The first paper to describe an extreme and pervasive form of childhood refusal, which often first appears to be anorexia nervosa.

Lask, B., & Bryant-Waugh, R. (1997). Prepubertal eating disorders. In D. M. Garner & P. E. Garfinkel (Eds.), *Handbook of treatment for eating disorders* (2nd ed., pp. 476–483). New York: Guilford Press.—A detailed description of a comprehensive approach to the management of eating disorders in children.

Lask, B., & Bryant-Waugh, R. (Eds.). (2000). *Anorexia nervosa and related eating disorders in childhood and adolescence* (2nd ed.). Hove, UK: Psychology Press.—Detailed overview of eating disorders in children, with an emphasis on clinical management.

Nicholls, D., & Stanhope, R. (2000). Medical complications of anorexia nervosa in children and young adolescents. *European Eating Disorders Review, 8,* 170–180.—An overview of medical issues.

# 38

# Families of Patients with Eating Disorders

## WALTER VANDEREYCKEN

Early family theories and studies of eating disorders overemphasized mother–child interactions, reflecting the myth that "parenting means mothering." Later, the "absent father" gradually came into the picture. Then, the importance of the whole family was stressed by the systems theory approach. The interaction between the parental subsystem and the children was usually analyzed in terms of communication, problem solving, boundary setting, and so on. More recently researchers have started to focus on the specific educational role of parents. Siblings of patients with eating disorders, however, may still be considered a "forgotten" group, and interest in married patients—their choice of partners, their marital interactions, and their offspring—is still marginal. Most of these topics are reviewed in this chapter. Other chapters address the related topics of family–genetic studies of eating disorders (Chapter 42), risk factors for eating disorders, including intrafamilial traumatic experiences (Chapter 44) and the impact of maternal psychopathology on childrearing (Chapter 39).

## FAMILY SIZE AND BIRTH ORDER

It has been suggested by some clinicians that patients with anorexia nervosa are more often than expected only children, while others have claimed the opposite. Systematic comparative studies of large clinical samples, however, have failed to reveal any significant relation between family size and the presence of an eating disorder. Similarly, it has been suggested that anorexic patients are more often firstborns or lastborns rather than middle children, but again, in controlled studies, no significant differences in birth order have been observed. Furthermore, follow-up studies of patients with anorexia nervosa have shown that neither sibship position nor family size has prognostic significance. This finding does not exclude the possibility, however, that in some cases, a child's occupation of a "special" position within the family may be linked to the development of an eating disorder.

## SIBLINGS

In the bulk of the literature on the families of patients with eating disorders, siblings oc-cupy a strikingly marginal position, although some special attention has been paid to twins in attempts to explore possible hereditary aspects of eating disorders (see Chapter 42), and preliminary work on sisters discordant for anorexia nervosa has been designed to identify important environmental influences.

Compared with those in "normal" families, siblings of patients with eating disorders seem to show a somewhat greater likelihood of developing eating and weight problems themselves, as well as other psychiatric disorders, especially mood and substance abuse disorder. Little systematic research has been done on these patient's identification with, overattachment to, and rivalry with a sibling. As noted earlier, comparison of sister pairs may reveal differential environmental factors of etiological importance: Sisters with an-orexia nervosa perceive more maternal control and experience more antagonism toward, and jealousy of, their sisters than do unaffected sisters. The potentially positive role brothers and sisters can play in either protecting their sibs from developing an eating dis-order or in facilitating their recovery has been neglected.

## FAMILY STRUCTURE AND INTERACTION

In self-report studies that reveal the "insider's perspective" on family life, patients are more critical of the family's functioning than are parents. Generally speaking, patients with eating disorders are more likely to perceive their families as having excessive appear-ance and achievement concerns. Furthermore, it has been reported that bulimic patients view their families as conflicted, badly organized, uncohesive, and lacking in nurturance or caring. Patients with anorexia nervosa perceive their families as stable, nonconflictual, cohesive, and not lacking in nurturance. Although parents in general report similar per-ceptions, they tend to be less extreme in their reports than their daughters with eating dis-orders.

Observational studies relying on the "outsider's view" of how the family interacts seem to yield a picture that only partially corresponds to the self-reported findings (the similarity is greater for patients with bulimia nervosa than for those with anorexia nervosa). Compared with "normals," anorexic families show more rigidity in their family organization, have less clear interpersonal boundaries, and tend to avoid open discussion of disagreements between parents and children. As such, the anorexic family may be characterized as "consensus-sensitive," whereas the bulimic family appears more "dis-tance-sensitive." The latter implies stronger interpersonal boundaries, a less stable family organization, and less avoidance of disagreements. Observers tend to see patients with bulimia nervosa as angrily submissive to rather hostile and neglectful parents.

## CHILDREARING

In the literature on the families of patients with eating disorders, the educational role of the parents and their parenting style have been neglected to a great extent. Little system-atic research has been focused on this aspect. From a clinical viewpoint, the most commonly observed feature is the lack of adequate, joint parental authority. This means that the parents have problems finding a balance between adequate (i.e., rational and flexible) control of their child and allowing age-appropriate autonomy. In many cases, these problems appear to be related to the parents' failure to reach a basic agreement about child-rearing issues. Of course, these shortcomings in conjoint parental functioning may reflect problems in the marital relationship.

Compared to normal adolescents, only small differences are observed in the perception of parental rearing practices as expressed by anorexia nervosa patients. They often report high-concern parenting in infancy, thus showing that, in many cases, parental overprotection has preceded rather than accompanied anorexia nervosa. Compared with parents of bulimic patients and normal controls, parents of anorexics are viewed as giving a "double message" of nurturant affection combined with neglect of their daughters' need to express themselves. Bulimia nervosa patients tend to report more troubled childhood experiences than anorexics and normal controls. Bulimics recall their rearing in childhood as characterized by a lack of care, especially by their mothers. These mothers, however, are not perceived as overprotective. Thus, a picture emerges—in the eyes of the patients—of rather "neglectful parenting" by their mothers. Since fathers are more often seen as overprotective, their rearing practices are viewed by bulimic patients as being closer to a pattern of "affectionless control."

## MARRIED PATIENTS

Anorexia nervosa and bulimia nervosa are typically considered to affect adolescent girls. Nevertheless, these disorders are often observed in adult women, either as a continuation of an eating disorder that originated during adolescence or as one that developed de novo during adulthood. Since many of these older patients are married or live with a partner, questions arise as to the impact of an eating disorder on marital relationships and how marital relationships influence the course of an eating disorder. If a significant connection exists between the occurrence of an eating disorder and the properties of the patient's marriage, it is evident that the latter must be taken into account in treatment.

Surprisingly, the marital relationships of adult patients with eating disorders have received little research attention. In fact, the literature about this patient group consists almost exclusively of descriptive case reports offering at best a variety of clinical speculations about these patients' marital characteristics. The lack of empirical data is particularly striking in view of the widely accepted role that family variables play in the development of eating disorders during adolescence. It seems reasonable to assume that the quality of these patients' marital relationships also influences the course of their eating disorders. One of the major observations emphasized in the clinical literature is that married patients and their partners often report significant dissatisfaction with their relationship. While the subjects themselves usually consider their marital problems to be the result of the patient's eating disorder, clinicians often assume the opposite, although their views are based on subjective impressions rather than solid research data.

In the only controlled study in which both self-report findings and data from coded videotaped interactions were used, Van den Broucke and colleagues found that couples in which one partner had an eating disorder appeared to lack some of "nondistressed" couples' skills of constructive communication but managed to avoid the destructive communication style of "maritally distressed" couples. As suggested in the clinical literature, their overall level of intimacy was lower than that of normal couples but higher than that of maritally distressed couples. Whereas this quantitative difference may reflect couples' different levels of marital satisfaction, an additional qualitative discrimination might be made between eating disorder couples and the two control groups on account of the former group's relatively low level of openness and intimacy. This important combination of (probably interrelated) interactional problems—a lack of openness, a low level of marital intimacy, and deficient communication skills—may represent an important obstacle to the constructive evolution of the marriage and recovery from the eating disorder.

## DISCUSSION

The reports on the characteristics of families of patients with eating disorders are difficult to compare because of differences in the assessment methods used (e.g., self-report measures, interview, and direct observation) and great variation in the sociocultural and demographic characteristics of the subjects. The assessment of patients' and relatives' perceptions of the family may be colored by the nature of the crisis that brought the patient into treatment. Having an eating disorder distorts perceptions of one's family (e.g., unusual sensitivity to family attitudes concerning weight, shape, and achievement). The perceived relationship with family members may also be influenced by the subject's actual degree of attachment to or emotional separation from the family. Since separation–individuation is a core issue for many anorexics and bulimics, it should be taken into account when analyzing patients' family perceptions. Patients' ages and, perhaps more important, their actual stage in the family lifecycle (e.g., the "leaving home" phase), are also relevant to the evaluation of family interactions.

An important methodological stumbling block concerns the attitude of patients with eating disorders and their families toward psychological assessment. In the acute stage, or before entering into treatment, anorexic patients in particular often deny any problems. They also have a tendency to try to please clinicians and researchers, with the result that their answering patterns may be distorted in the direction of social desirability. Anorexia nervosa families of middle- and upper-socioeconomic classes are known to idealize the family picture, or at least to present themselves as if nothing were wrong except for the eating disorder.

It is also important to note that the perception of family interactions may be linked to particular communication patterns. It has been found, for example, that the levels of critical comments ("Expressed Emotion" or EE) from parents toward bulimic offspring were significantly higher than those toward anorexic offspring. A dysfunctional family interaction, or its description by a family member, may be seen, therefore, as an expression of a more generally negative atmosphere within the families of bulimic patients. However, it must also be noted that in distressed parent–child relationships, chronic negative emotion may be both a cause and a consequence of interactions that undermine parents' concerns and children's development. An emotionally overinvolved response style may represent an understandable reaction by parents to the occurrence of a serious illness in their child!

These remarks highlight a most important point concerning the families of patients with an eating disorder, namely, that even if a particular family interaction pattern is

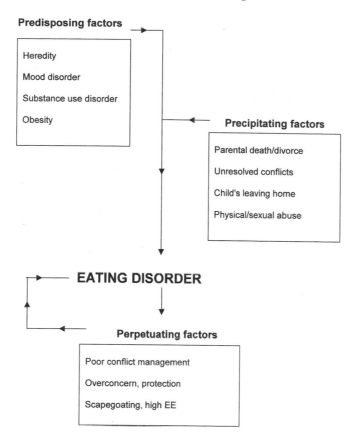

**FIGURE 38.1.** Family factors that influence the development of an eating disorder.

found to be (cor)related with the presence of an eating disorder, its specificity and causal significance remain to be demonstrated. The influence of family factors on the development of an eating disorder is manyfold, with a complex interaction between predisposing, precipitating, and perpetuating factors (see Figure 38.1). Although it may be difficult to prove that family factors have played a specific role in the development of an eating disorder, the assessment of family characteristics is of great relevance in planning family-oriented treatments (see Chapter 56). From a transgenerational perspective, it is also important to search for the transmission of interactional patterns, attitudes, or beliefs (e.g., attachment style: dismissing vs. preoccupied). If present, they provide a potential opportunity for preventive work, especially since it is known that patients with eating disorders can themselves have serious difficulties parenting their own children (see Chapter 39).

## FURTHER READING

Van den Broucke, S., Vandereycken, W., & Norré, J. (1997). *Eating disorders and marital relationships*. London and New York: Routledge.—A detailed overview of the research on marital issues and their practical implications for the management of eating disorders.

Van den Broucke, S., Vandereycken, W., & Vertommen, H. (1995). Marital communication in eating disorder patients: A controlled observational study. *International Journal of Eating Disorders*, *17*, 1–22.—The only controlled study of patients with eating disorders in which both self-report and observational data on marital interaction have been used.

Vandereycken, W. (1994). Parental rearing behavior and eating disorders. In C. Perris, W. A. Arrindell, & M. Eisemann (Eds.), *Parenting and psychopathology* (pp. 218–234). Chichester, UK, and New York: Wiley.—An overview of studies on the relationship between child rearing and the occurrence of an eating disorder later in life.

Vandereycken, W., Kog, E., & Vanderlinden, J. (1989). *The family approach to eating disorders: Assessment and treatment of anorexia nervosa and bulimia*. New York: PMA Publishing.— A detailed review and discussion from both a clinical and a research viewpoint of all family-related topics in eating disorders.

Vandereycken, W., & Van Vreckem, E. (1992). Siblings of patients with an eating disorder. *International Journal of Eating Disorders*, *12*, 273–280.—A review of the research literature on family size, birth order, eating and other disorders in siblings, as well as sibling rivalry and incest.

Ward, A., Ramsay, R., & Treasure, J. (2000). Attachment research in eating disorders. *British Journal of Medical Psychology*, *73*, 35–51.—Overview of studies on the possible association between attachment style (in parent–child and other interpersonal relations) and eating disorder diagnostic subtypes.

Wearden, A. J., Tarrier, N., Barrowclough, C., Zastowny, T. R., & Armstrong Rahill, A. (2000). A review of expressed emotion research in health care. *Clinical Psychology Review*, *20*, 633–666.—Discussion of an issue that is best known in studies of schizophrenic patients but might have important prognostic meaning for patients with eating disorders.

# 39

# Eating Disorders and Childrearing

## ALAN STEIN

There is now good evidence that psychiatric disorders among parents have the potential to interfere with their childrearing capacities and hence the development of their children. Eating disorders are an important source of psychiatric morbidity among women of childbearing age. They are of particular concern for at least two reasons. First, the core symptoms are extremely pervasive and disruptive of daily living, and thus may conflict with sensitive parenting. These symptoms include a preoccupation with body shape, weight, and food, as well as extreme behaviors both to limit food intake and to compensate for overeating, all of which may draw parental attention away from the needs of the child. Second, parents with eating disorders commonly have difficulties in their interpersonal relationships that may extend to their relationships with their children.

Infancy and adolescence are likely to be the times when children are particularly vulnerable to the influence of parental eating disorder psychopathology. Parents spend much time during the first months and years feeding their young infants, and feeding is one of the ways in which much communication occurs between parents and their children. The attitudes, preoccupations, and behaviors manifested by people with eating disorders may interfere with their ability to sit patiently feeding their infants, while responding appropriately to their hunger needs and cues. Adolescence, also an important time, is when children become increasingly aware of social pressures to conform and develop increased interest in body shape and attractiveness.

Surprisingly little research has been conducted on the childrearing practices of parents with eating disorders. Most of the reports have consisted of case reports and case series, although, recently, a few controlled studies have been conducted on the young children of mothers with eating disorders. There have also been a few studies of eating disorder psychopathology among mothers and their adolescent daughters.

## STUDIES OF YOUNG CHILDREN

The case reports and series have raised concern that the children of mothers with eating disorders may be at risk of adverse sequelae. Most of the work has concentrated exclusively on mothers with eating disorders, with little reference to fathers. Some studies have found that such mothers are overconcerned about their children's weight and are trying to slim their children down. In other studies, extreme concerns about feeding have been noted, with a general disruption of parenting.

Two reports have suggested that children's growth might be affected by parental eating disorders. Most notably, in Brinch and colleagues' long-term follow-up study of a group of mothers with a history of anorexia nervosa, 17% of the infants failed to thrive in the year following childbirth. However, this finding should be interpreted with caution, because it relied largely on maternal report and used a loose definition of "failure to thrive." Also, the study was retrospective, with children's age at follow-up ranging from 1 year to 38 years.

In a controlled study by the author and his colleagues that employed direct observation of 1-year-old children, mothers and infants were assessed at home during both mealtimes and play. The main findings were that, compared with controls, the index mothers were more intrusive with their infants during both mealtimes and play, and expressed more negative emotion (critical and derogatory remarks) during mealtimes but not during play. The most common precipitant of such negative emotion was the mothers' concern that their infants were making a "mess." There were no differences between the groups in the extent of the positive emotion expressed toward their infants but there was considerably more conflict between index infants and their mothers during mealtimes, with index mothers showing much reluctance to allow their infants to self-feed. Mess avoidance and the need to keep control of food intake seemed particularly important to these mothers. This in turn seemed to make the mothers less likely to respond to their infants' signals. The index infants weighed less than the control infants, and infant weight was found to be inversely related to the amount of conflict during mealtimes. It was also found, however, that such problems were not invariable. Some mothers were coping well with their babies, who were growing and developing healthily. In another, smaller study that also included direct observation of mother–child interaction (the offspring ranged in age from 1 to 4 years), mothers with eating disorders were observed to make fewer positive comments than control mothers about food and eating during meals.

In a 5-year prospective study, Agras and colleagues found that female infants of mothers with eating disorders sucked faster and were weaned later than the offspring of mothers without eating disorders. Starting when their children were 2 years of age, the index mothers fed them on a less regular schedule and were more likely to use food for non-nutritive purposes. They also exhibited significantly higher concern about their daughters' weight. When the children were 5 years of age, the index mothers rated them as exhibiting greater negative affect on a measure of child temperament.

To establish whether growth faltering among the children of mothers with eating disorders is specific, Stein and colleagues extended the study reported earlier. The infants of the mothers with eating disorders were compared with infants of mothers with postnatal depression and those of a large comparison group. It was found that the infants of mothers with eating disorders were smaller, both in terms of weight and length for age, than either the normal comparison group or the infants of mothers with postnatal depression, whereas the latter two groups did not differ from each other. However, compared with the depressed mothers and the healthy comparison group, the mothers with eating disorders neither preferred thinner babies nor misperceived their children's size. On the contrary, they were highly aware of their children's shape and, compared to the other two groups, were significantly more accurate at judging their children's size. These findings suggest that these mothers did not deliberately limit their children's food intake to restrain their growth.

The strength and specificity of the association between maternal eating disorder psychopathology and children's feeding have also been examined in a controlled study of the mothers of young children referred with feeding disorders. Only the children with feeding disorders had mothers with significantly disturbed eating habits and attitudes indicating that their feeding disorders were specifically linked to the mothers' eating habits and attitudes. These findings have since been confirmed in a recent community-based study. The association has also been investigated prospectively by Agras and colleagues in their study of parents and children from birth to 5 years of age. The emergence of childhood eating disturbances, such as inhibited or secretive eating, overeating, and vomiting, was related to both parental and child factors—specifically to maternal body dissatisfaction, dieting, and bulimic symptoms; maternal and paternal body mass; and infant body mass and feeding behavior during the first month of life.

## STUDIES OF ADOLESCENT DAUGHTERS

The object of three other studies was to consider if mothers' eating disorder psychopathology was related to the presence of eating disorder features in their daughters. In the first study, Pike and Rodin compared two groups: mothers whose daughters had high levels of eating disorder psychopathology and those whose daughters had low levels of such psychopathology. The comparison showed that mothers whose daughters had high levels of eating disorder psychopathology had higher levels of such psychopathology themselves. A second study, however, did not confirm these findings, while a third, small study of 10 year-old girls found that mothers' and daughters' dietary restraint scores were correlated but that their levels of eating disorder psychopathology were not. Thus, the relationship between adolescent daughters' eating disorder psychopathology and equivalent maternal concerns remains unclear.

## POSSIBLE ENVIRONMENTAL MECHANISMS OF TRANSMISSION

From the limited number of studies to date, it is possible to delineate four broad environmental mechanisms through which parental eating disorder psychopathology may influence childrearing and child development. First, extreme attitudes toward eating, shape, and weight may have direct effects on the child. For example, parents' fear of fatness may cause them to underfeed their children; and their overconcern about shape, weight, and food intake may lead to mealtime conflict with their younger children and to their becoming critical of their adolescent children's eating habits and appearance. Second, eating disorders may interfere generally with parenting. For example, these parents' preoccupation with food, eating, shape, and weight may impair their concentration in such a way as to interfere with their sensitivity and responsiveness to their children's needs. Third, parents' disturbed eating behavior and attitudes may function as a role model for their children. Fourth, parental eating disorders may be associated with discordant marital and family relationships that may have their own adverse effects on child development.

## CLINICAL IMPLICATIONS

Only general guidelines can be proposed on the basis of the available literature. It is important that clinicians be aware that parental eating disorders may have adverse effects on young children. If such an effect is suspected, the quality of the interactions between the parents and their children should be assessed, as should the child's growth and nutritional status. As part of this assessment, it is helpful to observe mealtimes at home, if possible. If difficulties are noted, support might be directed to the parents to help them recognize the child's hunger and satiety cues, and prepare and pace their child's meals. Parents should be encouraged through support and education to allow their infants to experiment with and learn about self-feeding. Involving a partner or friend to support and share the feeding of a young child can be invaluable, especially if significant conflict is prevalent. If older children are involved, it might help to work with parents to lessen the attention and criticism they direct at their children's shape and weight. Parents should be encouraged to widen the focus of their interactions with their children. It is always essential to treat the parents' eating disorder itself and to focus on the cognitions that impinge on their parenting.

Finally, it must be stressed that the adverse effects discussed in this chapter are not invariable. Many parents with eating disorders manage well, and their children develop normally.

## FURTHER READING

Agras, S., Hammer, L., & McNicholas, F. (1999). A prospective study of the influence of eating-disordered mothers on their children. *International Journal of Eating Disorders, 25,* 253–262.—A prospective study of the children of mothers with a lifetime history of an eating disorder.

Attie, I., & Brooks-Gunn, J. (1989). Development of eating problems in adolescent girls: A longitudinal study. *Developmental Psychology, 25,* 70–79.—A study that did not find the association between mothers' and daughters' eating disorder psychopathology reported by Pike and colleagues.

Brinch, M., Isager, T., & Tostrup, K. (1988). Anorexia nervosa and motherhood: Reproduction pattern and mothering behaviour of 50 women. *Acta Psychiatrica Scandinavica, 77,* 611–617.—A follow-up study into motherhood of a large case series of women who had had anorexia nervosa.

Hill, A. J., Weaver, C., & Blundell, J. E. (1990). Dieting concerns of 10 year old girls and their mothers. *British Journal of Clinical Psychology, 29,* 346–348.—A study of the relationship between mothers' and daughters' levels of dietary restraint and eating disorder psychopathology.

Pike, K. M., & Rodin, J. (1991). Mothers, daughters, and disordered eating. *Journal of Abnormal Psychology, 100,* 198–204.—A report examining the relationship between eating disorder psychopathology in mothers and their adolescent daughters.

Rutter, M. (1989). Psychiatric disorder in parents as a risk factor for children. In D. Schaffer, I. Philips, & N. B. Enger (Eds.), *Prevention of mental disorders, alcohol, and other drug use in children and adolescents* (pp. 157–189). Rockville, MD: Office for Substance Abuse Prevention, U.S. Department of Health and Human Services.—A review of the mechanisms by which parental psychiatric disorder may influence child development.

Stein, A., Murray, L., Cooper, P., & Fairburn, C. G. (1996). Infant growth in the context of maternal eating disorders and maternal depression: A comparative study. *Psychological Medicine,*

26, 569–574.—A controlled study comparing the growth of infants of mothers with eating disorders and infants of mothers with postnatal depression.

Stein, A., Stein, J., Walters, E. A., & Fairburn, C. G. (1995). Eating habits and attitudes among mothers of children with feeding disorders. *British Medical Journal, 310,* 228.—A study of the specificity of the association between maternal eating disorder psychopathology and childhood feeding disorders.

Stein, A., Woolley, H., Cooper, S. D., & Fairburn, C. G. (1994). An observational study of mothers with eating disorders and their infants. *Journal of Child Psychology and Psychiatry, 35,* 733–748.—The first controlled observational study of the childrearing of mothers with eating disorders.

Stice, E., Agras, W. S., & Hammer, L. D. (1999). Risk factors for the emergence of childhood eating disturbances: A five-year prospective study. *International Journal of Eating Disorders, 25,* 375–387.—A longitudinal study of the etiology and evolution of eating disturbances in early childhood.

Waugh, E., & Bulik, C. M. (1999). Offspring of women with eating disorders. *International Journal of Eating Disorders, 25,* 123–133.—A controlled study of the children of mothers with a current or past eating disorder, including observation of mealtime interaction.

Whelan, E., & Cooper, P. J. (2000). The association between childhood feeding problems and maternal eating disorder: A community study. *Psychological Medicine, 30,* 69–77.—A community-based study of the relationship between childhood feeding problems and maternal eating disorder psychopathology.

# 40

# Course and Outcome of Anorexia Nervosa and Bulimia Nervosa

## PATRICK F. SULLIVAN

Accurate depiction of the course and outcome of a disorder is fundamental to its characterization. These are critical data for clinicians and researchers alike. "Course" refers to the temporal pattern of an illness from onset to subsequent recovery, partial recovery, nonrecovery, or death. "Outcome" describes the state of affected individuals at some specified time after the development of a disorder. Both can be assessed in multiple ways. The temporal dimension is integral to both course and outcome.

Imbedded within these basic definitions, however, are a number of vexing complexities, particularly when applied to anorexia nervosa and bulimia nervosa. First, there are fundamental uncertainties about whether the *International Classification of Diseases* (ICD-10) and *Diagnostic and Statistical Manual of Mental Disorders* (DSM-IV) nosologies accurately characterize anorexia nervosa and bulimia nervosa. The experience in many eating disorder services is that a substantial proportion of individuals presenting for care have "subthreshold eating disorders" that do not quite fit the ICD-10 or DSM-IV criteria for anorexia nervosa or bulimia nervosa. (Chapter 30 discusses atypical eating disorders, including subthreshold and partial syndromes.) Second, the potential diagnostic overlap between anorexia nervosa and bulimia nervosa remains incompletely understood, thereby adding a further level of complexity. Third, "outcome" for anorexia nervosa and bulimia nervosa has to be defined across a number of relevant domains. Fourth, the extant literature complicates the task of characterizing course and outcome by often neglecting the temporal dimension and by relying on clinical samples (particularly since there is ample evidence of profound referral bias for both disorders).

To clarify the concepts "course and outcome," Figure 40.1 schematically presents a partial set of possibilities. At some "premorbid" time, no one has anorexia nervosa or bulimia nervosa. At the "postonset" time, all cases of anorexia nervosa and bulimia nervosa have developed (depicted by the arrows from the premorbid "well" box to the postonset anorexia nervosa and bulimia nervosa boxes). Subsequently, at "follow-up,"

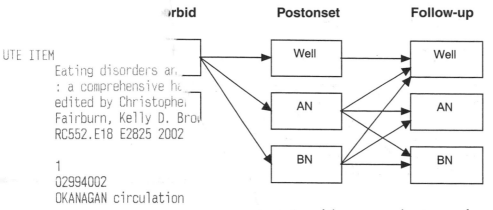

᛫sentation of the course and outcome of anorexia nervosa

limia nervosa have recovered, continue to have
᛫ed the other eating disorder (i.e., have "crossed
temporal patterns of transitions from postonset
to subjects' status at a specific follow-up point.
᛫w outcomes and time points are shown. Includ-
᛫ld disorders and death) and a greater number of
time points is desiraᴜᴵᴄ.

Table 40.1 provides a qualitative summary of the literature on the course and outcome of anorexia nervosa and bulimia nervosa, with columns for anorexia nervosa and
bulimia nervosa, and rows for a set of outcome domains. The data on which these summaries are based largely derive from clinically referred samples; because clinical samples
contain individuals with more severe, chronic, and comorbid illnesses, these estimates
may be unduly pessimistic even if somewhat more relevant for clinicians. An intermediate-
to long-term perspective (i.e., ≤ 10 years after referral) was chosen to increase the number
of applicable studies.

**TABLE 40.1. Summary of the Outcome of Anorexia Nervosa and Bulimia Nervosa**

| Domain | Intermediate- to long-term outcome of index disorder ( ≤ 10 years) after clinical referral | |
|---|---|---|
| | Anorexia nervosa | Bulimia nervosa |
| Death | 10% | ~1% |
| Persisting index disorder | 10% | 10% |
| Subthreshold eating disorder | 15% | 20% |
| "Crossover" (i.e., anorexia nervosa to bulimia nervosa or vice versa) | 15%[a] | ~1% |
| No clinical eating disorder at follow-up | 50% | 70% |

*Note.* Estimates are qualitative approximations from the accumulated literature.

[a] About half would have met criteria for bulimia nervosa at some point.

## MORTALITY

The risk of mortality in follow-up samples of individuals with anorexia nervosa is substantial (approximately 6% per decade) and grossly elevated in comparison to individuals without anorexia nervosa. Mortality results from complications of a chronic eating disorder (e.g., inanition or overwhelming infection) or suicide. Over the past 25 years, risk of mortality has probably declined in association with improved recognition and treatment of anorexia nervosa. There are fewer data about bulimia nervosa because of its relatively recent recognition. The mortality risk associated with bulimia nervosa is likely to be elevated, but death is a most unusual complication.

## RECOVERY

Over intermediate periods of follow-up, the majority of individuals with anorexia nervosa recover from the index illness. Approximately one-fourth continue to be symptomatic, and a sizable minority develops chronic anorexia nervosa. About half cross over to normal-weight bulimia nervosa. A potent risk factor for the development of bulimia nervosa is apparent "recovery" from anorexia nervosa. This process typically occurs within 2 years of onset of anorexia nervosa and is unusual more than 5 years after onset. In some respects, this can be viewed as moving from a visible (anorexia nervosa) to an invisible eating disorder (bulimia nervosa) whose the cardinal behaviors are easier to shield from relatives, friends, and health care professionals.

Although the data are fewer, a similar pattern appears to hold for bulimia nervosa, in which the majority of individuals recover but a sizable minority continues to have full syndromic or subthreshold symptoms. Crossover from bulimia nervosa to anorexia nervosa is most unusual.

### Extent of "Recovery"

Many individuals who evidence recovery from all symptoms of anorexia nervosa are nonetheless distinctive. Several features are notable. The first is the relatively slim habitus found in individuals who have recovered from anorexia nervosa. Maintaining the "anorectic stance" over time is very difficult and a common pathway in recovery may be for an individual's eating to normalize somewhat with body weight returning to the low-normal or normal range. Accommodating to a weight in the normal range might allow the individual to retain the perceived benefits of a relatively low weight, without the enormous difficulties of maintaining a weight in the anorectic range. Second, even with recovery, measures of cardinal attitudes related to anorexia nervosa (e.g., drive for thinness, cognitive restraint, and perfectionism) remain elevated. Thus, many individuals who clearly no longer meet the diagnostic criteria for anorexia nervosa continue to express "shadows" of prior psychological characteristics of the disorder. Third, even after controlling for obvious covariates, individuals with a prior history of anorexia nervosa evidence worse social and occupational functioning than controls.

Much the same can be said of bulimia nervosa. Many individuals who recover have residual features of the disorder, including overconcern about shape and weight, a tendency to restrict dietary intake, vulnerability to overeat (and then purge) in response to negative mood states, and low self-esteem. On average, body weight tends to increase slightly, although there is considerable variability in this regard.

## PRESENCE OF ASSOCIATED PSYCHOPATHOLOGY

In comparison to control groups, individuals with a history of anorexia nervosa or bulimia nervosa have higher prevalences of major depression and several anxiety disorders (particularly obsessive–compulsive and generalized anxiety disorder). Individuals with a past history of bulimia nervosa have more psychoactive substance use disorders.

These observations seem fairly well supported by the literature. The main problem of interpretation is the nature of the relationship with the eating disorder. Is the increased prevalence of mood, anxiety, and substance use disorders a direct result of the eating disorder? Or, rather, are these features directly or indirectly involved in the etiology of anorexia nervosa or bulimia nervosa? Whereas the former is relevant to the concept of outcome, the latter is more a confounding feature. There is as yet no consensus on this point. (These issues are also discussed in Chapters 34 and 35.)

## SUMMARY

The outcome of anorexia nervosa and bulimia nervosa for clinical samples is generally favorable. The more general outcome for incident cases in the community who never seek or are compelled to seek treatment is probably even better. Although not considered here in detail, certain treatments for bulimia nervosa (and perhaps for anorexia nervosa as well) clearly improve outcome (see Chapters 54, 55, 56, 57, and 58). However, a sizable minority of patients develop chronic eating disorders that are refractory to treatment.

The course of anorexia nervosa and bulimia nervosa is much less well understood. In particular, the existence of a single pathway is very unlikely. Knowledge of the manner in which genes, environment, and individual choices interact to influence course and outcome is not known. Characterization of the mechanisms leading to the significant psychiatric comorbidities would be critically informative.

## FURTHER READING

Bulik, C. M., Sullivan, P. F., Fear, J. L., & Pickering, A. (1997). Predictors of the development of bulimia nervosa in women with anorexia nervosa. *Journal of Nervous and Mental Disease*, *185*, 704–707.—Analysis of the factors that predict "crossover" from anorexia nervosa to bulimia nervosa, taking into account the temporal dimension.

Cohen, P., & Cohen, J. (1984). The clinician's illusion. *Archives of General Psychiatry*, *41*, 1178–1182.—Cogent description of the perils of research on clinically referred samples.

Fairburn, C. G., Cooper, Z., Doll, H. A., Norman, P., & O'Connor, M. (2000). The natural course of bulimia nervosa and binge eating disorder in young women. *Archives of General Psychiatry*, *57*, 659–665.—A rare community study illustrating the longitudinal course of bulimia nervosa.

Fairburn, C. G., Norman, P. A., Welch, S. L., O'Connor, M. E., Doll, H. A., & Peveler, R. C. (1995). A prospective study of outcome in bulimia nervosa and the long-term effects of three psychological treatments. *Archives of General Psychiatry, 52,* 304–312.—Large study of the outcome of a treated sample with bulimia nervosa.

Keel, P. K., Mitchell, J. E., Miller, K. B., Davis, T. L., & Crow, S. J. (1999). Long-term outcome of bulimia nervosa. *Archives of General Psychiatry, 56,* 63–69.—Large study of the outcome of a treated sample with bulimia nervosa.

Sullivan, P. F. (1995). Mortality in anorexia nervosa. *American Journal of Psychiatry, 152,* 1073–1074.—Meta-analysis of mortality studies for anorexia nervosa.

Sullivan, P. F., Bulik, C. M., Fear, J. L., & Pickering, A. (1998). The outcome of anorexia nervosa: A case-control study. *American Journal of Psychiatry, 115,* 939–946.—Large, controlled study of the outcomes of anorexia nervosa.

# Epidemiology and Etiology
# of Eating Disorders

# 41

# Distribution of Eating Disorders

## HANS WIJBRAND HOEK

Epidemiological studies show that eating disorders are not distributed randomly among the population. Young females constitute the most vulnerable group. In clinical samples, only 5–10% of patients with an eating disorder are males. Eating disorders seem to be "Western" illnesses: They occur predominantly in industrialized, developed countries. One epidemiological study in Curaçao, with a mainly black population, did find an incidence rate of anorexia nervosa within the lower range of rates reported in Western countries. Most reports of eating disorders outside the Western World tend to be of an anecdotal nature and show that eating disorders are uncommon in non-Western countries. Immigrants (e.g., Arab college students in London and Greek girls in Germany) are more likely to develop an eating disorder than their peers in their country of origin. This type of evidence demonstrates that sociocultural factors play an important role in the distribution of eating disorders (see Chapters 45 and 47).

People in some professions seem to be particularly at risk; fashion models and ballet dancers, for instance, seem to be at greater risk for the development of an eating disorder than many other professional groups. However, what is not known is whether "pre-anorectic" persons are more readily attracted to the ballet world, or whether *being* a ballet dancer is the source of increased risk. In some countries, eating disorders are overrepresented among the middle and upper socioeconomic classes, but this social class bias might be connected with the structures, norms, and thresholds of the local health care system. In European countries such as the Netherlands, which has a rather generous state health insurance system, class differences seem to have less impact on the presentation and recognition of eating disorders.

Anorexia nervosa and bulimia nervosa are also widely regarded as relatively "modern" disorders. But, as discussed in Chapter 27, eating disorders similar to those seen today have existed for centuries. In recent years, there has been such an increase in the number of patients receiving treatment for an eating disorder that some people are suggesting there is an "epidemic." Epidemiological data are not confirming that there has indeed been an equivalent increase in the number of cases in the general population.

## PREVALENCE OF ANOREXIA NERVOSA AND BULIMIA NERVOSA

Researchers in epidemiology study the occurrence of disorders and try to determine the factors associated with vulnerability to their development. Incidence and prevalence are the two principal measures of the distribution of a disorder. The (point) prevalence rate is the *actual* number of cases in a population at a certain point in time. The incidence rate is defined as the number of *new* cases in the population per year. Prevalence and incidence rates for eating disorders are commonly expressed as the rate per 100,000 population (male and female persons of all ages).

In the epidemiological research on eating disorders, prevalence studies vastly outnumber incidence studies. Prevalence studies of eating disorders are often conducted in high-risk populations such as schoolgirls or female college students. A two-stage screening strategy is now widely used. The first stage involves screening a large number of individuals for suspected cases by means of an easily administered questionnaire. The second stage involves (semistructured) interviews with the persons who, based on their answers to the questionnaire, are believed likely to have an eating disorder. Also interviewed are a number of randomly selected persons who, according to the questionnaires, do not suffer from such a disorder, to confirm that they are not cases. Two-stage surveys using strict diagnostic criteria reveal much lower prevalence rates than earlier surveys that relied exclusively on questionnaires. The average figure for the point prevalence of anorexia nervosa thus determined is 280 per 100,000 young females (i.e., 0.28%). The average point prevalence of bulimia nervosa among young females, using strict diagnostic criteria, is about 1,000 per 100,000 (i.e., 1.0%).

The prevalence of binge eating disorder and the night eating syndrome are discussed in Chapters 31 and 32, respectively.

## INCIDENCE OF ANOREXIA NERVOSA

Because the incidence of eating disorders is relatively low, no studies have been conducted on their incidence in the general population. It is impossible to screen a sufficiently large population, for instance, 100,000 people, for several years. Therefore, incidence rates have been based on detected cases in health care systems, including general hospital records and case registers of inpatients and outpatients in mental health care facilities. Although different strategies have been used in these studies, the results suggest an increase in the incidence of anorexia nervosa between 1930 and 1970. Since the 1970s, the incidence of anorexia nervosa in mental health care facilities in the Netherlands has been stable at around 5 per 100,000 population per year.

Researchers in Rochester, Minnesota, have screened not only the records of patients with a diagnosis of anorexia nervosa but also those of patients with amenorrhea, oligomenorrhea, starvation, weight loss, and other related diagnostic features. Between 1935 and 1989, the overall incidence of anorexia nervosa in the community of Rochester did not significantly increase. However, for 15- through 24-year-old females, a significant increase was found. The rates for older women remained relatively constant. As for the small number of males with anorexia nervosa, there was no change in their incidence over time.

It is unclear whether the increase in cases reported in health care facilities reflects a true increase in the incidence in the community, since it might also be due to changes in diagnostic criteria, improved methods of case detection, or wider availability of services. Studies of clinical samples will always underestimate the incidence of these disorders in the community, because only a minority of those with eating disorders come to medical attention.

The incidence of anorexia nervosa has also been studied in primary care facilities. General practitioners in the United Kingdom and the Netherlands, using criteria based on DSM-III-R, have studied the incidence of eating disorders in large representative samples. The figures obtained per 100,000 population per year were 4.2 in the United Kingdom and 8.1 in the Netherlands.

## INCIDENCE OF BULIMIA NERVOSA

Since 1979 (when bulimia nervosa was first described—see Chapter 27), an apparent "epidemic" of the disorder has appeared in Western countries. Surveys using questionnaires have revealed that up to 19% of female students report bulimic symptoms. Up until now, the incidence of bulimia nervosa has hardly been examined, in part, because most hospitals and case registers have been using the *International Classification of Diseases* (version 8 or 9), which does not provide a separate code for bulimia nervosa. General practitioners in the Netherlands, using DSM-III-R-based criteria, have studied the incidence of bulimia nervosa in a large representative sample of the Dutch population. They found the incidence of bulimia nervosa in primary care settings to be 11.4 per 100,000 population per year during the period 1985–1989. A little over half of these patients were referred for mental health care, which yields an incidence in mental health care of 6 per 100,000 population per year. Screening medical records for bulimia nervosa or related symptoms, researchers in Minnesota found an incidence of 13.5 per 100,000 population per year during 1980–1990.

These incidence rates can serve only as a minimum estimate of the true incidence rate in the community because of the secrecy that accompanies bulimia nervosa and its effect on treatment seeking and the greater difficulty detecting cases compared with anorexia nervosa cases.

## ONE-YEAR PERIOD PREVALENCE RATES

One-year period prevalence rates are useful measures for describing morbidity at different levels of health care. The 1-year period prevalence is calculated by adding together the point prevalence and the annual incidence rate. Table 41.1 presents estimates of the 1-year period prevalence rates per 100,000 young females at three levels of health care. Level Zero represents the number of young females with an eating disorder in the community, whether or not they are receiving treatment. Level 1 consists of those patients whom primary care physicians consider to have an "eating disorder." Level 2 represents patients with eating disorders who are receiving treatment from outpatient or inpatient mental health care services. The data are based on the findings of the two-stage surveys of the point prevalence of eating disorders, case register studies, and the results of the Dutch study of general practitioners' patients.

**TABLE 41.1. One-Year-Period Prevalence Rates per 100,000 Young Females**

| Level of health care | Anorexia nervosa | Bulimia nervosa |
|---|---|---|
| Zero–Community | 370 | 1,500 |
| One–Primary care | 160 | 170 |
| Two–Mental health care | 127 | 87 |

The number of individuals who pass from Level Zero to Level One depends on the "illness behavior" of the patient and the ability of the general practitioner to detect the disorder. With regard to illness behavior, we know that many patients deny or hide their eating disorder. We do not know how many people with eating disorders consult their primary care physician for help with an eating problem or for some other reason. Results of several studies have shown that general practitioners have difficulty detecting eating disorders, particularly cases of bulimia nervosa. In countries such as the Netherlands and the United Kingdom, the primary care physician occupies a critical position in determining who will be referred for psychiatric care; indeed, the general practitioner can be regarded as a filter.

On the basis of the data presented in Table 41.1, it seems that over 40% of the community cases of anorexia nervosa are detected by general practitioners and most of these patients (79%) are referred on for mental health care. In contrast, only a small proportion (11%) of the community cases of bulimia nervosa are detected, and of these, only half are referred on for specialist treatment.

## FUTURE DIRECTIONS

To date, most of the epidemiological research on eating disorders has been descriptive in character. There is a need for analytic epidemiological studies focused on their determinants. Such research is beginning, as shown by the recent publication of genetic–epidemiological studies (see Chapter 42) and risk factor research (see Chapter 44).

## FURTHER READING

Fairburn, C. G., Cooper, Z., Doll, H. A., & Welch, S. L. (1999). Risk factors for anorexia nervosa: Three integrated case-control comparisons. *Archives of General Psychiatry, 56,* 468–476.— Example of a community-based study of risk factors.

Fombonne, E. (1995). Anorexia nervosa: No evidence of an increase. *British Journal of Psychiatry, 166,* 464–471.—A review of epidemiological research of eating disorders.

Hoek, H. W. (1993). Review of the epidemiological studies of eating disorders. *International Review of Psychiatry, 5,* 61–74.—A discussion of methodological problems in epidemiological research on eating disorders.

Hoek, H. W., Bartelds, A. I. M., Bosveld, J. J. F., Graaf, Y., Van der Limpens, V. E. L., Maiwald M., & Spaaij, C. J. K. (1995). Impact of urbanization on detection rates of eating disorders. *American Journal of Psychiatry, 152,* 1272–1278.—Study of the epidemiology of eating disorders in primary care.

Hoek, H. W., Harten, P. N., Van Hoeken, D., & Susser, E. (1998). Lack of relation between culture and anorexia nervosa: Results of an incidence study on Curaçao. *New England Journal of Medicine*, *338*, 1231–1232.—This study challenges the idea that anorexia nervosa only occurs in Western societies.

Hsu, L. K. G. (1996). Epidemiology of the eating disorders. *Psychiatric Clinics of North America*, *19*, 681–700.—A review of epidemiological research on eating disorders.

Lucas, A. R., Crowson, C. S., O'Fallon, W. M., & Melton, L. J. (1999). The ups and downs of anorexia nervosa. *International Journal of Eating Disorders*, *26*, 397–405.—Important study of trends in the incidence of anorexia nervosa.

Van Hoeken, D., Lucas, A. R., & Hoek, H. W. (1998). Epidemiology. In H. W. Hoek, J. L. Treasure, & M. A. Katzman (Eds.), *Neurobiology in the treatment of eating disorders* (pp. 97–126). Chichester, UK, and New York: Wiley.—A recent review of epidemiological research of eating disorders.

# 42

# Genetic Epidemiology of Eating Disorders

## MICHAEL STROBER
## CYNTHIA M. BULIK

It has long been known that eating disorders tend to run in families. This chapter and Chapter 43 consider the possible genetic basis for this familiality. In this chapter, we consider genetic–epidemiological studies, the focus being on family and twin studies: There have been no adoption studies of eating disorders to date. Chapter 43 focuses on molecular–genetic studies of eating disorders.

## FAMILY STUDIES

The tendency for a particular illness to cluster among relatives is the hallmark of intergenerational family transmission. This phenomenon has been demonstrated, with remarkable consistency, for all major categories of psychiatric disorder. With regard to eating disorders, interest in the possible role of hereditary predisposition is not without historical precedent. As early as 1860, Louis Victor Marce noted that inherited psychopathologies were prominent in families of young women with anorexia nervosa, and that the rearing environment was often disturbed as well. Other, more contemporary, reports hint at the clustering of eating disorders or peculiar feeding habits in families. However, as these reports were derived without the benefit of specified diagnostic criteria, blind examination of relatives, and the use of appropriate control subjects, their validity is questionable.

Recently, a handful of studies has been published in which the researchers have attempted a more rigorous appraisal of family diagnostic patterns associated with anorexia nervosa and bulimia nervosa. The majority have found evidence for familial aggregation. Those studies that obtained negative findings were disadvantaged by small sample sizes and reliance on indirect, and therefore less precise, family diagnostic information. Overall, anorexia nervosa and bulimia nervosa appear to be several times more common among the biological relatives of anorexic and bulimic probands than in the general population, a finding that implicates the existence of some mechanism of transmissibility of illness within families. Of particular note, a recent study by the first author also found evidence of cross-transmission of anorexia nervosa and bulimia nervosa in families (i.e., elevated rates of anorexia nervosa among relatives of probands with bulimia nervosa, and vice versa), suggesting a shared liability bridging these disorders. In common with an earlier family study, this study also showed that familial aggregation and cross-transmission extended to the atypical eating disorders ("partial syndromes"; see Chapter 30), suggesting that these states occupy part of a continuum of familial liability.

## TWIN STUDIES

Because separate genetic and environmental components of transmission cannot be readily inferred in the classic family study, the study of twin pairs has become an increasingly important focus of research in psychiatric genetics. The key advantage of this paradigm is that statistical analyses of differences in concordance between monozygotic (MZ) and dizygotic (DZ) twins can decompose the variance in liability to illness into independent genetic and environmental sources and give estimates of their relative magnitudes. Extensions of the twin paradigm have been used recently to elucidate the contributions made by common and unique genetic and environmental factors to syndrome comorbidities.

Several reports have examined differential concordance for eating disorders in MZ and DZ twin pairs. Early reports concerned principally with the genetics of anorexia nervosa contained analyses apparently conducted on overlapping samples of twins recruited by advertisement, and on twins seeking treatment. The concordance rates were substantially greater for MZ than for DZ twins, implicating a strong etiological role for genetic factors, with heritability estimates in the range of 0.5 to 0.9. By contrast, an analysis given in one of these reports on a subset of twins ascertained as having bulimia nervosa assigned a more prominent causal role to environmental factors, with negligible genetic involvement. Caution is advised in the interpretation of these findings, however, given the biases that may arise from the use of this type of sample. A more recent analysis by Wade and colleagues of twin data from a large population-based twin sample, using a broad definition of anorexia nervosa, has suggested that there are genetic and environmental effects unique to anorexia nervosa, in addition to additive genetic effects shared in common with depressive illness.

Results of recent twin studies of bulimia nervosa also yield evidence of a genetic contribution to familial liability. In a series of studies from the Virginia Twin Registry by Kendler and, more recently, the second author, many of the problems that marred the earlier research have been overcome. These studies have shown that concordance is significantly higher in MZ than DZ twin pairs; and model fitting suggests that familial resemblance for bulimia nervosa is due mainly to additive gene action, with heritability and individual–specific environmental influences each accounting for approximately 50% of the variance in liability. Rates of bulimia nervosa have also been found to be higher in later birth cohorts, suggesting a greater likelihood of expressing the disorder in more recently born individuals. However, artifactual explanations of this phenomenon are also plausible (e.g., memory effects and increased recognition of bulimia nervosa as a disorder among younger individuals).

Attempts have also been made to quantify the contribution of genes and environment to continuous measures of disordered eating and related attitudes. One such effort, again using data from the Virginia Twin Registry, generated heritability estimates for binge eating and vomiting of 46% and 70%, respectively. In four other studies examining continuous measures of disturbed eating behavior and attitudes, the contribution of additive genetic effects ranged from modest to substantial, with the remaining variance attributed to individual–specific environmental effects.

## STUDIES OF COMORBIDITY

In clinical samples, eating disorders are strongly associated with various other categories of psychopathological disturbance. This covariation among disorders has several potential sources, including genetic factors with behaviorally diverse expressions, a common family environmental influence predisposing to multiple disorders, and individual–specific environmental events predisposing to multiple disorders.

Evidence supporting the coaggregation of various psychiatric disorders among relatives of patients with anorexia nervosa and bulimia nervosa is now available. While these studies vary appreciably in their methodological rigor, and inconsistencies in the diagnostic methods used are notable, they show, with rare exception, that the lifetime rates of certain diagnoses, mood disorders in particular, are significantly higher in relatives of patients with eating disorders than in relatives of control subjects. For unipolar and bipolar affective illness combined, relative risks are in the range of 2.0 to 3.5, indicating that affective disorders are several times more likely to develop in the biological kin of individuals with eating disorders than in people drawn at random from the general population.

Less clear is whether or not these data unambiguously support the assumption that eating disorders and mood disorders are linked to a common liability that is familially transmitted. Data relevant to this question are rather limited and contradictory. While some studies show that the increased aggregation of mood disorders in the relatives of anorexic or bulimic probands is strongly predicted by affective comorbidity in the probands, in other studies, increased risk is found even among relatives of nondepressed anorexic and bulimic probands. The former observation implies independent, hence etiologically distinct, familial transmission of these conditions, while the latter is consistent with the presence of a single, shared diathesis, with variability of expression perhaps determined by unique environmental and/or genetic factors. However, in the largest of the family studies of eating disorders conducted to date, the first author found that the cross-prevalence of eating disorders among relatives of control subjects with affective illness was zero, suggesting that the shared comorbidity of mood and eating disorders in individuals and their coaggregation in families are not likely to result from a single causal factor predisposing to both.

The possibility exists, nevertheless, of some degree of overlap in familial liability to bulimia nervosa and major depression. This overlap is suggested by an analysis of the data on comorbidity from the Virginia Twin Registry. The best-fitting model applied to the observed lifetime comorbidity of bulimia nervosa and major depression yielded a genetic correlation of 0.46, suggesting a modest sharing of predisposing genes. In other words, certain genetic factors may influence the risk of both major depression and bulimia nervosa. At the same time, the two clearly are not identical conditions, as substantial variance in the liability was found to result from genetic and environmental risk factors specific to each disorder.

Another line of inquiry concerns possible linkages between eating disorders and substance abuse. Clinically, there is considerable support for the greater prevalence of substance use and abuse among the subgroup of patients with eating disorders who binge eat (see Chapter 35). Theoretically intriguing is the notion that this greater prevalence of abuse is paralleled by analogous differences at the level of personality structure and in the domain of family environment. Specifically, whereas restricting anorexics and their parents commonly express extremes of emotional constraint, conscientiousness, and avoidance of intense or novel experiences, the contrasting pattern of affective liability, increased sociability, and stimulus seeking, coupled with family transactions marked by rancor and discord, is usually found with greater frequency in the backgrounds of patients with binge eating.

One implication of these broad generalizations is that divergent phenotypic patterns of emotionality and constraint may reflect familial temperamental traits that strongly correlate with other disinhibitory behavioral syndromes. Indeed, with respect to alcoholism, evidence from studies recently completed by the first author supports a substantial familial link with binge eating. Specifically, relatives of patients with bulimia nervosa, as well as relatives of those patients with anorexia nervosa who binge, had a three- to four-fold higher lifetime risk of substance use disorders than relatives of normal control subjects and relatives of restricting anorexics. Moreover, increased risk of substance abuse occurred even among relatives of non-substance-abusing patients, suggesting a common liability influencing the risk of both types of psychopathology.

## CONCLUSION

The research described in this chapter highlights the potential contribution of heritable factors to the pathogenesis of eating disorders. (In Chapter 43, their possible molecular basis is discussed.) The search for etiological processes must, however, retain its broad perspective, because the pathways to symptom formation are multiple and interactive. The exact manner in which genes contribute to familial aggregation of eating disorders remains speculative, but their influence on personality traits and possible biological processes underlying certain components of behavior regulation offers suggestive hypotheses. It is likely that the clinical features of anorexia nervosa and bulimia nervosa are not isolated, discrete events but rather pathological exaggerations of heritable personality and biological propensities.

## FURTHER READING

Bulik, C. M., Sullivan, P. F., Wade, T. D., & Kendler, K. S. (2000). Twin studies of eating Disorders: A review. *International Journal of Eating Disorders, 27*, 1–20.—This article reviews results from twin studies of eating disorders and examines methodological and interpretive issues in this area.

Kaye, W. H., Lilenfeld, L. R., Berrettini, W. H., Strober, M., Devlin, B., Klume, K. L., Goldman, D.,

Bulik, C. M., Halmi, K. A., Fichter, M. M., Kaplan, A., Woodside, D. B., Treasure, J., Plotnicov, K. H., Pollice, C., Rao, R., & McConaha, C. W. (2000). A search for susceptibility loci for anorexia nervosa: Methods and sample description. *Biological Psychiatry, 47*, 794–803.—A description of the background, design, and implementation of the first comprehensive molecular–genetic study of eating disorders.

Kendler, K. S., MacLean, C., Neale, M., Kessler, R., Heath, A., & Eaves, L. (1991). The genetic epidemiology of bulimia nervosa. *American Journal of Psychiatry, 148*, 1627–1637.—This article presents results from a population-based Virginia Twin Registry study of the genetics of bulimia nervosa. Both genetic and environmental risk factors are identified as contributing to the liability to develop this disorder.

Lilenfeld, L. R., Kaye, W. H., Greeno, C. G., Merikangas, K. R., Plotnicov, K., Pollice, C., Rao, R., Strober, M., Bulik, C. M., & Nagy, L. (1998). A controlled family study of anorexia nervosa and bulimia nervosa: Psychiatric disorders in first-degree relatives and effects of proband comorbidity. *Archives of General Psychiatry, 55*, 603–610.—A family history study suggesting common familial vulnerability for anorexia nervosa and bulimia nervosa.

Lilenfeld, L. R., Stein, D., Devlin, B., Bulik, C., Strober, M., Plotnicov, K., Pollice, C., Rao, R., Merikangas, K. R., Nagy, L., & Kaye, W. H. (2000). Personality traits among currently eating disordered, recovered, and never-ill first-degree female relatives of bulimic and control women. *Psychological Medicine, 30*, 1399–1410.—Family history study suggesting that perfectionist personality traits are a familial risk factor for bulimia nervosa.

Strober, M. (1992). Family-genetic studies. In K. Halmi (Ed.), *Psychobiology and treatment of anorexia nervosa and bulimia nervosa* (pp. 61–76). Washington, DC: American Psychiatric Press.—A detailed review and critique of family and twin studies of anorexia nervosa and bulimia nervosa.

Strober, M., Freeman, R., Lampert, C., Diamond, C., & Kaye, W. (2000). Controlled family study of anorexia nervosa and bulimia nervosa: Evidence of shared liability and transmission of partial phenotypes. *American Journal of Psychiatry, 157*, 393–401.—The largest family-genetic epidemiological study of eating disorders published to date. Findings suggest shared familial diathesis for anorexia nervosa, bulimia nervosa, and partial syndromes.

Wade, T. D., Bulik, C. M., Neale, M., & Kendler, K. S. (2000). Anorexia nervosa and major depression: Shared genetic and environmental risk factors. *American Journal of Psychiatry 157*, 469–471.—A study of the heritability of anorexia nervosa, using a broad definition of the disorder.

Woodside, D. B. (1993). Genetic contributions to eating disorders. In A. S. Kaplan & P. E. Garfinkel (Eds.), *Medical issues and eating disorders: The interface* (pp. 193–211). New York: Brunner/Mazel.—A review of methods in psychiatric genetics and their applications to research on eating disorders.

# 43

# Molecular Genetics of Eating Disorders

## DAVID A. COLLIER

As discussed in Chapter 42, the findings from twin studies suggest that about half the vulnerability to develop eating disorders is inherited. This points to the possibility of finding variation in genes that alters susceptibility to eating disorders—the subject of this chapter.

### CONCEPTUAL ISSUES

Unlike Mendelian genetic disorders such as Huntington's disease, which are caused by the effect of a single gene in each person, "complex" diseases are caused by the interaction of multiple genes with the environment. Thus, for example, a major unfavorable life event might have a much greater effect on somebody who carries a genetic vulnerability to depression than someone who does not. This genetic vulnerability is likely to take the form of many genes of small effect that might increase risk two- or three-fold. These genes will be neither necessary nor sufficient to cause disease (i.e., many, if not most, people who carry them will not become ill). An accumulation of these genes, together with adverse environmental factors, increases risk until the disease develops in those carrying the greatest genetic and environmental loading. This is known as the liability–threshold model.

 Although you cannot change your genes any more than you can reverse the event of childhood abuse, complex disease genetics is not deterministic genetics. Risk factors for complex genetic disorders cannot be reliably used to predict who will become ill. Instead, the usefulness of vulnerability genes is in the guidance they provide to the understanding of pathophysiology, which in turn must be helpful in designing new treatments. Finding genes does not mean that psychological treatments will be superseded or neglected; they are an important method of treatment and will remain so.

## METHODS AND FINDINGS

### Choosing the Phenotype

An important consideration in psychiatric genetics is the definition of the phenotype, the diagnostic criteria or traits used to classify participants in a family as affected or unaffected. This usually involves using a diagnosis such as anorexia nervosa, but narrower classifications such as the restricting type of anorexia nervosa have also been used. A narrower diagnosis may reduce heterogeneity, but it makes it harder to find multiply affected families, thereby reducing statistical power. Conversely, a broader diagnosis including all eating disorders makes it easier to find families with more than one person affected, but it probably introduces greater heterogeneity. An alternative approach is to use quantitative traits, which are measures continuously distributed in the population, such as body mass index. In eating disorders, this might involve using continuous scores from the Eating Disorder Inventory (such as Drive for Thinness) that appear to have a heritable component, or using scales measuring obsessional or perfectionist traits.

### Linkage Analysis

Linkage analysis involves a search of the human genome in a collection of families, with the aim of finding the rough location of susceptibility gene(s). No information on the type of gene that might be involved is required. There are two types of methods: parametric, in which the pattern of inheritance of the disease (i.e., dominant, recessive, etc.) must be specified, and nonparametric or "model-free" methods. Since a clear pattern of inheritance is not seen in psychiatric conditions such as eating disorders, nonparametric methods of linkage are usually used.

The ideal sample for linkage analysis is an extended family with many members affected, since this gives maximum statistical power. However, eating disorders do not tend to cluster densely in families, and single, large affected kindreds or large, extended families are very rare. Collecting such volunteer families is too difficult to be cost-effective and to accrue a sufficient sample size, so an alternative design using affected relative pairs has been proposed. An affected relative pair consists of a family with two affected members, for example, a sibling–sibling or an aunt–niece pair. These families are much easier to find therefore, much larger samples can be recruited.

With nonparametric linkage, the basic measure is simple: the degree of genetic identity for a given marker between the affected siblings. If a particular locus is involved in susceptibility to the disorder under study, then pairs of siblings with that disease should inherit the same copy of that locus more often than expected by chance. Since linkage is a statistical approach, a cutoff point must be specified, below which evidence is not considered significant. For single-gene disorders, this value is accepted by convention to be a "LOD score" of 3, equivalent to a $p$ value of .001. The stringency of this cutoff comes from the need to avoid false positive results that occur merely by chance. For complex disorders, the cutoff has been revised to 3.3, since the statistical methods used are somewhat different.

The results of a recent genome scan in affected relative pairs provide the first tentative evidence for a genetic susceptibility locus for anorexia nervosa. This study used 200 families with anorexia nervosa but found no evidence for linkage using a broad phenotype (i.e., both subtypes of anorexia nervosa—see Chapter 28). Using the narrower diagnostic category of restricting anorexia nervosa, a nonparametric LOD score found in one region of the genome. Genes that play a role in feeding behaviors and that map to this linkage region are now being analyzed for association with anorexia nervosa. The next stage in the process will be to screen for genetic variation in the gene, and determine if any of these polymorphisms are found to differ in frequency between participants with anorexia nervosa and control subjects without an eating disorder.

## Candidate Gene Analysis

The candidate gene approach involves the selection of a gene on the basis of its perceived relevance to the suspected pathophysiology of the disorder under study. For eating disorders, this includes genes involved in influencing feeding, mood, responses to stress, and personality traits. Where the pathophysiology of a disease is not well understood, finding a susceptibility gene using the candidate gene approach alone may involve as much luck as judgment.

Two sample designs may be considered in evaluating the role of a particular gene in a complex disorder: case-controls and family trios. Case-control analysis relies on the fact that a genetic variant of a gene (an allele) that causes a disease or trait will occur more often in people with that disease or trait than in people without it. Because this is not an all-or-nothing effect, and differences in allele frequency could occur by chance, statistical measures are required. Usually the chi-square test is used. Family trios consist of an affected child and both parents. Instead of using healthy volunteers as controls, the alleles that the parents do not pass on to their child are used as "controls" instead. Two tests are used: the haplotype-based haplotype relative risk and the transmission disequilibrium test, which also measures linkage as it considers heterozygous parents only. These two methods avoid the common problem of poor matching between cases and controls that can otherwise lead to false positive results. To attain sufficient statistical power, a panel of several dozen (if not hundreds of) cases or families is required.

Candidate gene studies in eating disorders have so far focused on genes encoding proteins implicated in the regulation of feeding and body composition, and genes involved in neurotransmitter pathways regulating behavior. The agouti-related melanocortin-4 receptor gene, which is involved in appetite regulation, has also been examined for association based on its role in regulating feeding behavior. Preliminary evidence suggests that a polymorphism in this gene is associated with anorexia nervosa.

Genes involved in serotonergic neurotransmission have also been examined because of the potency of serotonin as an appetite suppressant and its involvement in some of the behaviors associated with eating disorders such as obsessive and perfectionist behavior. One such gene encodes the serotonin neurotransmitter receptor type 2A or 5-HT2A. An association has been found with a polymorphism in the promoter region of the 5-HT2A gene (−1348G/A) and anorexia nervosa, in which the A allele of the polymophism appears to increase risk. This finding was subsequently replicated in a sample of anorexia nervosa patients and controls from Italy and the United States, but not in a sample from Germany or a second sample from the United Kingdom. Meta-analysis of both published and new data has been unable to clarify whether there is a significant association; this finding, therefore, remains controversial. One possibility is that this polymorphism is associated specifically with restricting anorexia nervosa.

## FURTHER READING

Collier, D. A., Sham, P. C., Arranz, M. J., Hu, X., & Treasure, J. (1999). Understanding the genetic predisposition to anorexia. *European Eating Disorder Review*, 7, 96–102.—This review describes some of the basic methodological approaches to the genetics of anorexia nervosa and presents a combined analysis of the association data with the 5-HT2A gene.

Kaye, W. H., Lilenfeld, L. R., Berrettini, W.H., Strober, M., Devlin, B., Klump, K. L., Goldman, D., Bulik, C. M., Halmi, K. A., Fichter, M. M., Kaplan, A., Woodside, D. B., Treasure, J., Plotnicov, K. H., Pollice, C., Rao, R., & McConaha, C. W. (2000). A search for susceptibility loci for anorexia nervosa: Methods and sample description. *Biological Psychiatry*, 47, 794–803.—This paper describes the overall strategy and methodology behind the systematic search of the human genome for anorexia nervosa genes.

Plomin, R., De Fries, J. C., McLearn, G. E., & Rutter, M. (1997). *Behavioral genetics*. New York: Freeman.—This excellent textbook describes the role of genes, environment, and their correlations and interactions in behavior and psychopathology.

Schalling, M., Johansen, J., Nordfors, L., & Lonnqvist, F. (1999). Genes involved in animal models of obesity and anorexia. *Journal of International Medicine*, 245, 613–619.—A good general review.

Sham, P. (1999). *Statistics in human genetics*. New York: Freeman.—This intermediate-level, general reference book explains the basic theory and methods used in human genetics.

Vink, T., Hinney, A., van Elburg, A. A., van Goozen, S. H., Sinke, R. J., Herpertz-Dahlmann, B. M., Hebebrand, J., Remschmidt, H., van Engeland, H., & Adan, R. A. (2001). Association between an agouti-related protein gene polymorphism and anorexia nervosa. *Molecular Psychiatry*, 6, 325–328.—This paper describes an association between the agouti-related protein (a peptide expressed in the hypothalamus that regulates feeding behavior) and anorexia nervosa.

Ziegler, A., Hebebrand, J., Gorg, T., Rosenkranz, K., Fichter, M., Herpertz-Dahlmann, B., Remschmidt, H., & Hinney, A. (1999). Further lack of association between the 5-HT2A gene promoter polymorphism and susceptibility to eating disorders and a meta-analysis pertaining to anorexia nervosa. *Molecular Psychiatry*, 4, 410–412.—This paper describes a combined analysis of published data and a set of new data from Germany to test for association between the 5-HT2A gene and anorexia nervosa.

# 44

# Risk Factors for Eating Disorders

## ULRIKE SCHMIDT

The causation of eating disorders is widely thought to be "multifactorial," a term so broad as to render it useless without further qualification. Myriad individual risk factors have been studied. As in other areas of research, there are definite fashions here. For example, during the 1960s and 1970s, an "anorexogenic family environment" was thought to be crucial for the development of anorexia nervosa, and during the 1980s and 1990s, childhood trauma, in particular, childhood sexual abuse, was promoted as causally important, mainly for bulimia nervosa. With the advent of new biotechnologies (molecular biology, brain scanning), we are seeing a revival of the interest in biological factors. Several important classes of risk factors are discussed in detail elsewhere in this book (e.g., genetic factors—see Chapters 42 and 43; sociocultural risk factors—see Chapters 45 and 47; personality factors—see Chapter 36; family factors—see Chapter 38). The focus of this chapter is threefold: on some of the methodological issues affecting this kind of research; on research that attempts to integrate our knowledge about the relative contribution of different risk factors; and on some of the newer lines of investigation in this area.

## METHODOLOGICAL ISSUES

In order to appreciate the methodological difficulties in studying risk factors, it is useful to remember the definition of a "risk factor"; a factor that is associated with a disorder and may support a causal connection. Evidence supporting a causal link between a risk factor and a disorder is provided by (1) the factor preceding the disorder being studied; (2) the repeated appearance of the same risk factor in multiple risk factor studies; (3) the risk factor being associated with one disorder only; and, most importantly, (4) the finding that an experimental intervention that eliminates the risk factor also eliminates the disorder. Many studies of eating disorders, especially those using cross-sectional designs, violate the first point regarding temporal precedence and, while purportedly being interested in identifying risk factors, do not attempt to identify what occurred first—the putative risk factor or the eating disorder. To disentangle this requires dating the onset of the risk factor and the careful definition and dating of the onset of the eating disorder (which is not as straightforward as it sounds). While it may be possible to determine the time point when someone developed a disorder of clinical severity, this may have been preceded by many months of subthreshold symptoms that can be more difficult to date precisely.

Two main types of study are used to investigate risk factors, the case-control study and the cohort study, both of which have important advantages and disadvantages. The main advantage of case-control studies is that they are valuable when the condition of interest is relatively rare, as is the case in anorexia nervosa. The disadvantages relate to the many potential biases in the comparison of cases and controls. Recall bias (generally due to underreporting of exposure in the control group) is a common problem, as is the inaccuracy of retrospective data, especially where detailed recall of relatively "soft" information is required. The use of semistructured interviews, which help patients to remember information in relation to autobiographical anchor points, and which use multiple probes to allow detailed description and encourage behavioral examples, can reduce these types of problems considerably. Important considerations also include how cases and controls are selected, for example, whether patients or community subjects are studied, and whether the two groups are matched on variables that might confuse the comparison.

The population-based case-control study of adolescent anorexia nervosa by Råstam, Gillberg, and colleagues and the Oxford risk factor studies by Fairburn and colleagues overcome many of these methodological difficulties. Both use semistructured interviews that build on and extend previous risk factor research. The particular strength of the Swedish study is that subjects were weighed and mothers were used as informants. The particular strength of the Oxford studies is that different eating disorders were compared with both healthy and psychiatric controls.

Prospective cohort studies allow careful control of the nature and quality of the data recorded. However, these kinds of studies have problems of their own. Given the relative rarity of eating disorders, they require extremely large numbers and may also need to be very long-term to detect associations between certain risk factors and onsets that may occur many years later. The interpretation of some cohort studies has been impaired by the use of only two measurement points and uncertain reliability in the measurement of both eating disorders and putative risk factors. Another major problem is loss to follow-up, especially if subjects are lost for some reason that is related to the outcomes being studied. Individuals with anorexia nervosa do actively avoid detection and have been found to be overrepresented among nonparticipants in population-based studies. Many of these limitations have been overcome in a prospective study of eating disorders in nearly 2,000 Australian secondary school students by Patton and colleagues. Other large, prospective studies designed to address these difficulties are ongoing.

## RISK FACTORS FOR DIFFERENT TYPES OF EATING DISORDERS

### Anorexia Nervosa

There is general consensus that a genetic vulnerability increases the risk for developing anorexia nervosa (see Chapters 42 and 43); however, it is not yet known what it is that might be inherited and how this interacts with environmental risk factors. A predisposition for leanness may be important (see Chapter 4). Another possibility, for which there is converging evidence, is that genetic risk is conveyed via personality traits of perfectionism, obsessionality, negative self-evaluation, and extreme compliance (see Chapter 36). Additionally, women with anorexia nervosa have high levels of exposure to a broad range of risk factors shared with other psychiatric disorders, including premorbid behavioral problems and psychiatric disorder, parental psychiatric disorder, and childhood adversity, including abuse and death among close relatives. Dieting seems to be relatively unimportant once the influence of other groups of risk factors has been taken into account.

A class of risk factors that so far has received relatively little attention is perinatal factors. A recent Swedish study found that girls born with a cephalhematoma and those born prematurely have an increased risk of developing anorexia nervosa. These associations seem to be specific. Speculatively, the authors suggest that subtle brain damage may result in early feeding difficulties, a factor that in other studies has been shown to predate the onset of anorexia nervosa. They also raise the possibility of a secondary interactional dysfunction between mother and child, for which there is support from work focused on the attachment patterns and early parenting of patients with anorexia nervosa.

## Bulimia Nervosa

Evidence from case-control and cohort studies converges in suggesting that bulimia nervosa arises as the result of exposure to (1) premorbid dieting and related risk factors (e.g., premorbid and parental obesity; critical comments by the family about weight, shape or eating) and (2) general risk factors for psychiatric disorders. Both classes of risk factors contribute independently to the risk. While childhood environmental risk factors also contribute, there is little evidence to suggest a specific link between childhood trauma and the later development of bulimia nervosa.

## Binge Eating Disorder

Risk factors for binge eating disorder have been less well studied than those for anorexia nervosa and bulimia nervosa. Adverse childhood experiences, vulnerability to obesity, and repeated exposure to negative comments about shape, weight, and eating have been implicated, but, compared with the wide range of risk factors found for bulimia nervosa, individuals with binge eating disorder seem to have lesser degrees of exposure.

## OUTLOOK FOR THE FUTURE

The challenge for the future is to improve our understanding of the interplay between, and relative significance of, different types of risk factors for different eating disorders. In particular, it will be crucial to bring together research on biological and environmental risk factors. Exploratory work along these lines has been done by the Maudsley group in examining genetic and environmental factors in sisters discordant for anorexia nervosa. A large European collaborative study now under way takes this line of research further. A better understanding of risk moderators, mediators, and mechanisms is also needed.

## FURTHER READING

Altman, D. G. (1991). *Practical statistics for medical research*. London: Chapman & Hall.— Chapter 5 provides an excellent introduction to the methodological difficulties inherent in the different types of risk factor design.

Baron, R. M., & Kenny, D. A. (1986). The moderator–mediator variable distinction in social psychological research: Conceptual, strategic and statistical considerations. *Journal of Personality and Social Psychology, 51*, 1173–1182.—A classic paper on the differences between moderators and mediators of risk factors.

Cnattingius, S., Hultman, C. M., Dahl, M., & Sparén, P. (1999). Very preterm birth, birth trauma, and the risk of anorexia nervosa among girls. *Archives of General Psychiatry, 56*, 634–638.— A study of perinatal risk factors.

Fairburn, C. G., Cooper, Z., Doll, H. A., & Welch, S. L. (1999). Risk factors for anorexia nervosa: Three integrated case-control comparisons. *Archives of General Psychiatry, 56*, 468–476.— One of three papers in the *Archives* describing findings from an integrated series of case-control studies of the development of anorexia nervosa, bulimia nervosa, and binge eating disorder, respectively.

Gillberg, C., & Råstam, M. (1998). The aetiology of anorexia nervosa. In H. W. Hoek, J. L. Treasure, & M. A. Katzman (Eds.), *Neurobiology in the treatment of eating disorders* (pp. 127–141). Chichester, UK, and New York: Wiley.—A succinct overview of the different classes of risk factors of anorexia nervosa.

Karwautz, A., Rabe-Hesketh, S., Hu, X., Zhao, J., Sham, P., Collier, D. A., & Treasure, J. L. (2001). Individual-specific risk factors for anorexia nervosa: A pilot study using a discordant sister-pair design. *Psychological Medicine, 31*, 317–329.—An exploratory risk factor study combining different lines of investigation.

Palmer, R. L. (1998). Aetiology of bulimia nervosa. In H. W. Hoek, J. L. Treasure, & M. A. Katzman (Eds.), *Neurobiology in the treatment of eating disorders* (pp. 143–159). Chichester, UK, and New York: Wiley.—An integration of our knowledge of different risk factors for bulimia nervosa.

Patton, G. C., Selzer, R., Coffey, C., Carlin, J. B., & Wolfe, R. (1999). Onset of adolescent eating disorders: Population based cohort study over 3 years. *British Medical Journal, 318*, 765–768.—A prospective study of the development of eating disorders.

Schmidt, U., Tiller, J., & Treasure, J. (1993). Setting the scene for eating disorders: Childhood care, classification and course of illness. *Psychological Medicine, 23*, 663–672.—This paper assesses childhood risk factors in a large patient sample of different types of eating disorders.

Ward, A., & Gowers, S. (in press). Attachment and childhood development. In J. Treasure, U. Schmidt, E. van Furth, & C. Dare (Eds.), *Handbook of eating disorders* (2nd ed.). Chichester, UK, and New York: Wiley.—A thoughtful review bringing together evidence on early interactional factors in anorexia nervosa.

# 45

# Gender, Ethnicity, and Eating Disorders

## RUTH H. STRIEGEL-MOORE
## LINDA SMOLAK

The pronounced gender differences in the distribution of anorexia nervosa and bulimia nervosa (see Chapter 33) have prompted the question of why eating disorders are so disproportionately more common among girls and women than among boys and men. The answer likely lies in gender differences in both biological and environmental factors. However, research on the contribution of biological factors is in its infancy. Evidence concerning genetic influences is inconclusive (see Chapters 42 and 43), and current pharmacological treatments have limited efficacy (see Chapters 58 and 64), raising the possibility that biological factors are not at the core of eating disorders. Little prospective research establishes that hormonal or neurotransmitter dysfunction predate eating disorders. One of the most promising findings, that dieting may trigger lowered 5-HT in women but not in men, underscores the interaction of a culturally induced behavior (dieting) and biological vulnerability.

Research on gender differences has focused largely on cultural factors. In this line of research, risk for the development of an eating disorder has been hypothesized to derive from women's subordinate position in society, female gender role socialization, and the contemporary female beauty ideal of extreme thinness. Few would dispute the validity of the cultural model's core assertions that, as a group compared to males, females are more likely to have less access to positions of power, earn less money, experience more sexual abuse and harassment, and be socialized toward adopting traditionally feminine behaviors of caring for and nurturing others and of pursuing physical attractiveness. There also is substantial empirical evidence linking some of these experiences, especially the internalization of the culturally defined thin ideal and exposure to sexual harassment and abuse, to risk for developing an eating disorder.

The emphasis on the role of cultural factors in the etiology of eating disorders is often justified further by the observation that eating disorders are significantly less common among females residing in non-Western, nonindustrialized nations (see Chapter 47) and, perhaps, certain ethnic minority groups within the United States. Indeed, some experts have conceptualized eating disorders as "culture-bound syndromes." In these accounts, eating disorders are described as predominantly a problem of white females in Western, industrialized societies. This cultural view of eating disorders does allow for the possibility that non-Western and nonwhite females may be at risk if they emigrate from unaffected cultures to Western societies, or if they emulate the social norms and behaviors of white individuals in Western societies.

There is substantial debate, however, regarding the nature and extent of the contribution of cultural factors to the etiology of eating disorders. Several methodological problems complicate efforts to evaluate their role.

## TERMS AND CONCEPTS

There is general confusion regarding terminology. The terms "race," "culture," and "ethnicity" are used inconsistently, interchangeably, or, at times, incorrectly, in this literature. "Race" is considered by many to be an outdated term, due to its history as a biological category: Rather than being based in biology, race is defined by cultural practices. "Ethnicity" is used to define populations by their ancestry, language, and customs, and does not necessarily imply specific physical characteristics such as skin color. Although the term "ethnicity" by itself does not imply minority status, typically, it is used to refer to a population group that is in the minority in terms of its size or its relative political dominance within a society. "Culture" is a broad term encompassing a multidimensional, complex construct that includes shared institutions, values, norms, and language. Members of a particular ethnic group may participate in and share values of a culture while simultaneously preserving and practicing values, norms, and languages of their ethnic group (e.g., individuals of African descent residing in the United States; individuals of Indian descent residing in Great Britain). Terms such as "gender" and "ethnicity" are summary terms (i.e., they capture a variety of factors under a general rubric). In practical use, they may be confounded with other variables such as differences in educational attainment, income, or other indices of socioeconomic status. Hence, studies purporting to examine gender or ethnic effects need to specify what about gender or ethnicity may be influential in the development of eating disorders.

In defining the precise influence of gender and ethnicity, researchers need to move beyond current conceptualizations of risk factors. The ethnicity literature, for example, has focused mainly on body ideal as a risk factor. There is little research on peer and media influences, levels of sexual abuse and sexual harassment, and the effects of ethnic discrimination.

## MEASUREMENT

Measurement problems abound in research on gender, ethnicity, and eating disorders. There are at least three common problems: (1) Operational definitions are inconsistent, as exemplified by measures of acculturation; (2) many instruments have only been validated in majority populations and in women; (3) current diagnostic categories may not adequately reflect the nature of eating disorders among men and ethnic minority women. For example, in some individuals, pathological behavior such as binge eating and steroid abuse might be a response to a desire to be bigger, yet there are few measures that acknowledge the possibility that people might want to be larger, much less that they might engage in problematic eating behaviors to achieve this goal.

## SAMPLES

The most rigorous epidemiological studies of anorexia nervosa and bulimia nervosa have been conducted either in countries with relatively homogeneous Western populations, or with samples selected to represent only one ethnic group (white European ancestry) and, frequently, only women. Hence, the distribution of these eating disorders among non-Western populations, ethnic minority populations residing in Western countries, and men is largely unknown. Arguments that females from ethnic minority groups are less likely to develop an eating disorder are generally based on the observation that clinical samples are typically composed of white females. The importance of studying representative samples rather than samples of convenience is underscored by a growing literature showing that members of ethnic minority groups with an eating disorder are significantly less likely to access or receive treatment.

It has been hypothesized that eating disorders among white women have increased during the last century (see Chapter 41), and this increase has been attributed to cultural changes. Empirical evidence only partially supports this claim: The increase in the number of cases of anorexia nervosa may be the result of better detection and increased use of medical services rather than any genuine increase in incidence. In contrast, the weight of evidence does support a real increase in the incidence of bulimia nervosa during the 1970s. It is plausible that the cultural factors that may underlie this increase (and are not specified in studies of changes in the incidence and prevalence of eating disorders) may raise the risk for eating disorders not only among majority populations but also ethnic minority groups. One might hypothesize, therefore, that the rates for eating disorders among ethnic minority groups might subsequently rise. Experts have suggested that ethnic minority groups lag behind majority groups in exposure to cultural risk factors but are "catching up" with the majority. Similarly, men exposed to media images of muscular bodies may develop body dysmorphic disorder (see Chapter 21), a condition that shares some features with anorexia nervosa.

## ASSOCIATION OR CAUSATION

Studies comparing ethnic minority groups to ethnic majority groups on characteristics that are thought to contribute to the risk for developing an eating disorder often reach the conclusion that their findings prove ethnic differences in risk exposure. However, even when differences in exposure are observed (e.g., as is typically the case for body image dissatisfaction when comparing black American and white American females), such differences do not permit the conclusion that the particular variable of interest operates in the same way in the two groups. Risk for eating disorders is multifactorial and may involve more than one pathway toward the development of an eating disorder.

## DIFFERENT TYPES OF EATING DISORDERS

Studies examining the role of culture and ethnicity in the etiology of eating disorders tend to collapse all types of eating disorder into one group. However, preliminary evidence suggests that the gender and ethnic distribution of eating disorders varies depending on the particular eating disorder under investigation. For example, binge eating disorder appears to be relatively more common among males and among members of ethnic minority groups than is anorexia nervosa or bulimia nervosa (see Chapter 31). Relatedly, the proportion of males relative to females, and of ethnic minority individuals relative to majority individuals, is less skewed in binge eating disorder than in anorexia nervosa or bulimia nervosa. This raises the possibility that the cultural (and biological) factors involved in binge eating disorder differ from those in anorexia nervosa or bulimia nervosa. Similarly, two lines of evidence suggest that culture may play a more prominent role in the etiology of bulimia nervosa than that of anorexia nervosa. First, unlike bulimia nervosa, it is not clear whether the incidence of anorexia nervosa has increased during the past century (see Chapter 41); and second, cross-cultural research suggests that in certain non-Western countries anorexia nervosa may be as common as in Western cultures (see Chapter 47).

## CONCLUSIONS

Overall, the research findings do suggest that gender and ethnicity are important in understanding the etiology and maintenance of eating disorders. However, this research is subject to notable shortcomings that preclude drawing strong conclusions. For future research to delineate the nature of putative etiological influences, investigators will need to define and operationalize terms appropriately, select measures that have psychometric validity with all included participants, and recruit representative epidemiological samples.

## FURTHER READING

Crago, M., Shisslak, C., & Estes, L. (1996). Eating disturbances among American minority groups. *International Journal of Eating Disorders, 19,* 239–248.—One of the first reviews of the prevalence of eating disorders among American ethnic groups and still one of the few to consider all major American ethnic groups.

Douchinis, J., Hayden, H., & Wilfley, D. (in press). Obesity, body image, and eating disorders in ethnically diverse children and adolescents. In J. K. Thompson & L. Smolak (Eds.), *Body image, eating disorders, and obesity in youth.* Washington, DC: American Psychological Association.—An exhaustive review of the occurrence of eating problems and eating disorders among girls from all major ethnic groups in the United States.

Fairburn, C. G., Welch, S. L., Norman, P. A., O'Connor, M. E., & Doll, H. A. (1996). Bias and bulimia nervosa: How typical are clinic cases? *American Journal of Psychiatry, 153,* 386–391.—An important epidemiological study that illustrates the biases involved in clinic-based sampling of eating disorder cases.

Goodwin, G. M., Fairburn, C. G., & Cowen, P. J. (1987). Dieting changes serotonergic function in women not men: Implications for the etiology of anorexia nervosa? *Psychological Medicine,*

*17*, 839–842.—A study revealing a biological difference that might contribute to the uneven gender distribution of eating disorders.

Hoek, H. W., van Harten, P. N., van Hoeken, D., & Susser, E. (1998). Lack of relation between culture and anorexia nervosa: Results of an incidence study on Curaçao. *New England Journal of Medicine, 338*, 1231–1232.—A study of eating disorders in Curaçao.

Rodin, J., Silberstein, L., & Striegel-Moore, R. H. (1985). Women and weight: A normative discontent. In T. B. Sonderegger (Ed.), *Nebraska Symposium on Motivation: Psychology and gender* (pp. 267–308). Lincoln: University of Nebraska Press.—This now classic paper introduced the first comprehensive analysis of gender as a risk factor for eating disorder.

Smolak, L., & Murnen, S. K. (2001). Gender and eating problems. In R.H. Striegel-Moore & L. Smolak (Eds.), *Eating disorders: Innovations in research and practice* (pp. 91–110). Washington, DC: American Psychological Association.—Provides a comprehensive review of the literature on gender and disordered eating.

Smolak, L., & Striegel-Moore, R. H. (2001). Challenging the myth of the Golden Girl: Ethnicity and eating disorders. In R. H. Striegel-Moore & L. Smolak (Eds.), *Eating disorders: Innovations in research and practice* (pp. 111–132). Washington, DC: American Psychological Association.—Offers a detailed review of studies examining the role of ethnicity as a risk or protective factor in the development of eating disorders.

Striegel-Moore, R. H. (1993). Etiology of binge eating: A developmental perspective. In C. G. Fairburn & G. T. Wilson (Eds.), *Binge eating: Nature, assessment, and treatment* (pp. 144–172). New York: Guilford Press.—Discusses in detail how gender-role socialization increases risk for the development of eating disorders with binge eating as the core clinical symptom.

Striegel-Moore, R. H., & Cachelin, F. M. (in press). Risk factors for eating disorders. *Journal of Counseling Psychology.*—A comprehensive review of risk factor studies, with a particular emphasis on ethnicity as a potential moderating factor.

# 46

# Sport, Occupation, and Eating Disorders

## SUSAN M. BYRNE

During the 1980s, a series of case studies, anecdotal reports, and press accounts began to emerge about eating disorders in individuals belonging to specific "high-risk" populations, such as athletes, dancers, fashion models, and those involved in the entertainment industry. An increasing amount of research has since begun to examine the extent and nature of eating disorders in such groups, although, so far, the research has almost exclusively focused on athletes and ballet dancers. This chapter begins by outlining some reasons why these groups are considered to be at particular risk for developing eating disorders, and then review existing studies of eating disorders in athletes and dancers, highlighting various methodological limitations of these studies. Finally, some guidelines for the prevention and management of eating disorders in high-risk groups are suggested, along with directions for future research.

## REASONS FOR THE INCREASED VULNERABILITY OF "HIGH-RISK" GROUPS

### Performance Enhancement and Aesthetic Appeal

The most prominent line of thinking stems from the proposed link between sociocultural pressure to conform to an unrealistically thin body ideal and the development of eating disorders (see Chapter 19). It is suggested that in addition to this pressure, which particularly impinges on females, athletes and dancers may come under specific pressure from within their highly competitive subcultures to manipulate their eating and weight in order to maximize their performance and/or improve their aesthetic appeal. This pressure is likely to be particularly intense for athletes competing in sports with strict weight restrictions (such as lightweight rowing or wrestling) or those that require a lean body shape or a low body weight for reasons of performance or appearance (including distance running, rhythmic and artistic gymnastics, and figure skating, as well as ballet).

## Personality Characteristics

Individuals in these high-risk groups have been observed in some studies to be perfectionist, competitive, and intensely concerned with achievement. This same constellation of personality traits has also been linked, independently, to individuals with eating disorders (see Chapter 36), so while these qualities might lead to excellence in athletic or artistic performance, they may also place an athlete or dancer at increased risk for developing an eating disorder. However, despite these shared characteristics, athletes with eating disorders appear to present a clinical profile that differs from that shown by other individuals with eating disorders, reporting higher levels of self-esteem, lower levels of body dissatisfaction, and fewer depressive symptoms than nonathletes with eating disorders. This difference may reflect the highly purposive motivation driving athletes' attempts to lose weight as opposed to the underlying psychopathology that is characteristic of other individuals with eating disorders.

## Age of Onset

The onset of eating disorders is typically during adolescence or early adulthood, a time of life when most elite athletic competition takes place, and when dancers, for example, are vying for positions in professional ballet schools and companies. The onset of puberty and the accompanying rapid changes in body shape may be of particular significance to female athletes and dancers, affecting not only their appearance but also their performance.

## RESEARCH METHODS AND FINDINGS

While the overall impression from existing studies is that athletes and dancers do show a relatively high prevalence of eating disorders, many studies have been limited both conceptually and methodologically. There have been three main problems. First, the majority of studies have been uncontrolled, which, coupled with their inconsistent findings, makes it difficult to draw firm conclusions. However, even studies comparing athletes to a control group of nonathletes have produced inconsistent results, with some studies documenting a greater range of disturbed eating behavior in athletes, but many reporting no differences, or even lower rates of eating problems. Second, sample sizes have often been too small to ensure adequate statistical power. Those studies with sufficiently large samples have often aggregated athletes from widely different sports, thereby possibly masking important differences. Many studies have increased the heterogeneity of their samples by recruiting athletes and dancers from a broad range of competitive levels rather than focusing on those who, competing at an elite level, are likely to be subject to especially intense pressure to conform to a particular body shape. Third, most studies have used self-report questionnaires rather than clinical interviews to make eating disorder diagnoses, a practice that is unsatisfactory in normal circumstances and especially problematic in this context.

Given these limitations, the considerable variation in estimates of the prevalence and symptoms of eating disorders in these groups is not surprising. The best information to date has come from a small group of studies comparing athletes participating in sports that emphasize leanness or impose weight restrictions (thin-build sports), athletes participating in sports that do not emphasize leanness (normal-build sports), and control groups of nonathletes. The two most methodologically sound studies, one from Norway and the other from Australia, used a two-stage design in which participants were first screened using a self-report questionnaire (the Eating Disorder Inventory) and then assessed by clinical interview in subgroups. In this way it was possible to estimate the prevalence of eating disorders in large samples of athletes and dancers. The Norwegian study identified eating disorders in 25% of female thin-build athletes, 12% of female normal-build athletes, and 5% of female nonathletes. The Australian study (by the author) concluded that it is only athletes competing in sports that emphasize thinness (including dancers) who appear to be at particularly high risk, with 15% of athletes in this group evidencing diagnosable eating disorders compared to 2% of normal-build athletes and 1% of nonathletes. This study had the added strength of having both male and female athletes in the sample. The results suggested that the increased risk associated with being an athlete competing in a thin-build sport was not exclusively associated with being female. Five percent of male athletes in this category had eating disorders. Little attention has otherwise been paid to the problem of eating disorders in male athletes, although some uncontrolled studies have reported a high rate of disturbed eating behavior among male athletes in sports such as rowing, wrestling, and bodybuilding.

## PREVENTION, TREATMENT, AND FUTURE RESEARCH

The relatively high rate of diagnosable eating disorders found in both male and female athletes and dancers engaged in "thin-build sports" has implications for the wide range of professionals concerned with these high-risk populations. Far-reaching prevention programs (see Chapter 67) need to educate not only these athletes but also their coaches, officials, and other responsible authorities. The emphasis should be on the deleterious effects an eating disorder is likely to have not only or overall health and well-being but also on athletic and artistic performance. In recent years, sporting organizations, particularly in the fields of gymnastics and athletics, have begun to recognize the need for eating disorder prevention programs (although less progress has been made in the traditional world of ballet, and in other fields such as modeling and the theater). However, there is still a need for evaluation of these programs, since their effectiveness has yet to be demonstrated. There is also a need to identify the conditions required to encourage athletes to be forthcoming about eating problems, and to develop sensitive screening procedures to ensure referral to the most appropriate source of help.

Additionally, research is needed to clarify the relationship between these pursuits and the development eating disorders. Specific recommendations include: conducting longitudinal studies of elite athletes and dancers; studying both male and female subjects; recruiting large, appropriately selected samples, with matched control groups; employing clinical interviews to assess eating disorder features and to make diagnoses; and developing improved measures of the perceived and actual intensity of pressures to be thin.

## FURTHER READING

Brownell, K. D., Rodin, J., & Wilmore, J. H. (Eds.). (1992). *Eating, body weight, and performance in athletes: Disorders of modern society.* Philadelphia: Lea & Febiger.—A comprehensive book that addresses many aspects of eating and weight issues for athletes.

Byrne, S. M., & McLean, N. (in press). Elite athletes: Effects of the pressure to be thin. *Journal of Science and Medicine in Sport, 4,* 145–160.—A recent, controlled Australian study of the prevalence of eating disorders in both male and female elite athletes.

Byrne, S. M., & McLean, N. (in press). Eating disorders in athletes: A review highlighting methodological issues of the literature. *Journal of Science and Medicine in Sport.*—A review of the research on eating disorders in athletes highlighting methodological issues.

O'Connor, P. J., & Smith, J. C. (1999). Physical activity and eating disorders. In J. M. Rippe (Ed.), *Lifestyle medicine* (pp. 1005–1015). Malden, MA: Blackwell Science.—An overview of the evidence linking eating disorders with involvement in physical activity and sport.

Powers, P. S., & Johnson, C. L. (1999). Small victories: Prevention of eating disorders among elite athletes. In N. Piran, M. P. Levine, & C. Steiner-Adair (Eds.), *Preventing eating disorders: A handbook of interventions and special challenges* (pp. 241–254). Philadelphia: Brunner/Mazel.—A discussion of the complicated issues involved in the prevention of eating disorders in athletes. This chapter includes examples of prevention programs offered by different sporting organizations in the United States.

Smolak, L., Murnen, S. K., & Ruble, A. (2000). Female athletes and eating problems: A meta-analysis. *International Journal of Eating Disorders, 27,* 371–380.—Reviews the research into eating problems in athletes and concludes that while participation in some sports may increase the risk for an eating disorder, participation in other sports may be protective.

Sundgot-Borgen, J. (1993). Prevalence of eating disorders in elite female athletes. *International Journal of Sport Nutrition, 3,* 29–40.—A methodologically sound Norwegian study of the prevalence of eating disorders in elite female athletes.

Sundgot-Borgen, J. (1994). Risk and trigger factors for the development of eating disorders in female elite athletes. *Medicine and Science in Sports and Exercise, 26,* 414–419.—Based on the same sample as the previous reference, this study attempted to identify some specific risk factors for eating disorders in female elite athletes.

Thompson, R. A., & Sherman, R. T. (1993). *Helping athletes with eating disorders.* Champaign, IL: Human Kinetics.—A practical guide to management strategies for athletes with eating problems.

Vincent, L. M. (1989). *Competing with the sylph: The quest for the perfect dance body.* Princeton, NJ: Princeton Book Company.—An insight into the pressure to achieve an ideal body shape in classical ballet, written by a former dancer who now works with dancers as a medical practitioner.

Wilmore, J. H. (1995). Disordered eating in the young athlete. In C. J. R. Blimkie & O. Bar-Or (Eds.), *New horizons in pediatric exercise science* (pp. 161–178). Champaign, IL: Human Kinetics.—An overview of the prevalence of eating disorders and other related problems in young athletes.

# 47

# Cross-Cultural Perspectives on Eating Disorders

## SING LEE
## MELANIE A. KATZMAN

A decade ago, eating disorders in the forms of anorexia nervosa and bulimia nervosa were predominantly confined to the developed West. However, anorexia nervosa and, more recently, bulimia nervosa are becoming common clinical problems among young females in high-income Asian societies such as Japan, Hong Kong, Singapore, Taiwan, and the Republic of Korea. They have also appeared in major cities in low-income Asian countries such as China, Malaysia, the Philippines, and Indonesia. They have even been identified in unexpected places such as India and Africa.

Drawing on clinical and research experience in Asian and, in particular, Chinese populations, this chapter addresses four main questions: (1) How common are eating disorders, and why are they emerging in Asian females? (2) Are eating disorders more likely to present atypically in Asian patients? (3) Are Western research instruments valid in Asian populations? (4) What are the implications of atypical eating disorders for the etiology, diagnosis, treatment, and prevention of eating disorders in general?

## THE EMERGENCE OF EATING DISORDERS

Accurate, two-stage community estimates of eating disorders are even rarer in Asian than Western populations, but rough estimates provide good reason for concern. Several community studies in Hong Kong have indicated that 3–10% of young females suffer from disordered eating. Rates of referrals to clinics suggest that eating disorders increased in prevalence in the 1990s and are affecting ever younger subjects. In several Asian countries, the mass media have repeatedly informed the public about the increased use of extreme weight-control behavior, dramatic cases of women who have died from untreated eating disorders, and celebrities who suffered from or recovered from anorexia nervosa.

For reasons that are far from clear, eating disorders in these societies seem to be unusually rare among men.

At an outpatient psychiatric clinic where the first author worked, the number of referrals of patients with eating disorders (primarily anorexia nervosa) increased from two per year in the early 1990s to at least one per week in mid-2000. In the 3 months that followed the opening of the Hong Kong Eating Disorders Center, over 200 Chinese women phoned in to seek help for eating problems, predominantly bulimia nervosa. This indicates that the latter is grossly undertreated in Asian societies.

Through the late 20th century the collective fear of fatness in Western cultures was the predominantly accepted sociocultural cause and discourse for disordered eating. (See Chapters 19 and 45 for further discussion of sociocultural influences.) However, cross-cultural investigations, especially when combined with feminist studies, are challenging this simplistic view. At the start of the 21st century, the rising identification of eating disorders in diverse places has extended not only the boundaries of imagination but disciplines as well. The future may see not only more sophisticated community prevalence studies, involving traditional and local healers as well as medical professionals, but also a parallel examination of shifting political and economic forces.

The experiences of Asian women who starve their already thin bodies has been a poignant example of how the experiences of women outside Western laboratories and languages may topple vaulted Western assumptions. Various speculations as to why eating disorders are emerging despite the fact that young Asian females are manifestly slim include the ubiquity of media forms that powerfully associate ultraslimness with such positive qualities as control, attractiveness, success, and efficiency. In this climate, no female is too thin. The other common belief is that globalized Western fast-food shops and eating styles have undermined appetite and weight control in women who are psychosocially vulnerable. Less obvious explanations are the rapid social transformation that has exaggerated both the conflicting opportunities and constraints pertaining to production and reproduction that take their toll on young females in patriarchal societies and the commodification of the female body.

## ATYPICAL EATING DISORDERS

While bulimia nervosa appears to "breed true" in Asian populations, the case of anorexia nervosa is more complex. DSM-IV criteria require that food refusal or emaciation in anorexia nervosa be solely attributed to an intense fear of fatness. (See Chapter 28 for discussion of the DSM-IV diagnostic criteria.) However, not all Asian anorexic patients exhibit fat concern, especially when they are evidently emaciated (and this is also true of some "atypical" Western patients). In the context of a retrospective study, Lee and colleagues in Hong Kong found that 41 (59%) of 70 Chinese anorexic patients, despite a compelling resemblance to their Western counterparts, attributed food refusal to stomach bloating, loss of appetite, no hunger, and other rationales not connected with fat concerns. A recent study by Nakamura and coworkers showed that atypical patients still commonly occur in Japan.

Three common explanations for the absence of fat phobia in these patients are "denial" of fat concerns, the disorder being a form of somatized depression, and the fact that these women were already premorbidly thin and so have never been sensitized to fatness.

A further explanation is that they come from subcultures in which fat phobia is not an effective idiom of distress: rather, rationales such as stomach bloating provide more irrefutable excuses for food refusal in their local worlds of interpersonal experience. This explanation is supported by ethnographic as well as prospective studies that have asked patients to identify reasons for their food refusal at different time points in their anorexic illness. These studies indicate that when the disorder is defined less restrictively, fat phobia is not an immutable core symptom of voluntary self-starvation. This is also supported by research in Georgia (of the former Soviet Union), which found that women who do not "own" the terms anorexia nervosa and bulimia nervosa still engage in the relevant behavior for what may be considered social control. Thus, patients with eating disorders do not live in a DSM diagnostic laboratory. As points of entry into the dynamic interpersonal processes of illness, patients' attributions for disordered eating connect with diverse illness narratives and rationales that are revealed only by experience-sensitive methods of research and "non-fat" focused clinicians.

Psychiatric researchers may be predisposed to exaggerate what is universal in mental disorders according to the DSM paradigm and to deemphasize what is culturally particular and often locally valid. In fact, the occurrence of atypical anorexia nervosa is congruous with historical, clinical, as well as community studies showing that attributions regarding weight and shape are not static but vary with chronicity of illness, age, degree of weight loss, and contextual factors. In a prospective study that involved a 15-year longitudinal design, Strober and coworkers compared the long-term outcome of typical and atypical anorexic inpatients. They defined atypical anorexia nervosa by the definite absence of fat phobia throughout subjects' inpatient stay. They found that atypical patients remained non-fat phobic, exhibited fewer bulimic symptoms, and had a more benign outcome than their fat-phobic counterparts. This is the first systematic study to conclude that anorexia nervosa without fat phobia is a valid nosological entity. (Atypical eating disorders are discussed in Chapter 30.)

## VALIDITY OF RESEARCH INSTRUMENTS

One factor that hampers community surveys in Asian and other non-Western populations is the lack of simple and valid research instruments. It should be noted that community epidemiological studies using familiar instruments such as the Eating Attitudes Test are fraught with methodological difficulties in Western populations. These surveys typically yield a very low prevalence of anorexia nervosa. One reason may be that disordered eating attitudes pertaining to fat rejection do not capture the experiential salience of eating disorders. For example, anorexic subjects may not necessarily endorse items on the Eating Attitudes Test such as "I am terrified of gaining weight" (No. 16) and "I am preoccupied with the desire to be thinner" (No. 32) when they are manifestly emaciated. As a result, some of them will be screened out as "noncases." (See Chapter 26 for further discussion of assessment instruments and their use.)

Even if Western instruments were accurately translated into the local language, whether they exhibit contextual validity in non-Western settings remains uncertain. Using the Chinese version of Eating Disorder Inventory (EDI-1), Lee and coworkers found that although the profile of fat-phobic patients was similar to that of Canadian patients with restrictive anorexia nervosa, that of non-fat-phobic patients was anomalous. The latter patients displayed significantly more "general psychopathology" than control subjects but exhibited even less "specific" or fat-phobic psychopathology as measured on the Drive for Thinness subscale. Likewise, non-fat-phobic anorexic patients scored atypically low on the Eating Attitudes Test.

A possible means of enhancing the sensitivity of existing instruments is to include items grounded in the local idioms used by self-starving subjects to explain their food denial. Research in mainstream psychiatric epidemiology has already shown that small but culturally relevant changes to the stem questions of research instruments originally based on the DSM system can result in significant changes in the rates of detection of nonpsychotic disorders. The obvious cultural basis of eating disorders notwithstanding, this approach has yet to be explored in this field.

## IMPLICATIONS

Cross-cultural and feminist studies can shed light on the etiology, diagnosis, treatment, and prevention of eating disorders in general. They suggest that the portrait of disordered eating as an appearance disorder incurred by young women lost in the world of calorie restricting is a belittling stereotype that not only camouflages women's real worries but also misses the universal power of food refusal as a means of proclaiming needs for self-control. It is worth noting that a connection between eating disorders and control was long underscored by Hilde Bruch. The notion was later contextualized by feminist researchers and incorporated into cognitive-behavioral therapies.

As regards diagnosis, if atypical eating disorders are common globally, the current classificatory systems cannot be considered adequate. We need to surrender essentializing diagnostic criteria that shun large portions of patients as dishonest deniers in favor of polythetic definitions that transcend local variations in the content of the anorexic illness.

In the psychological treatment of non-fat-phobic patients, since fatness does not define their interaction with clinicians, the treatment process may bring to light the interplay of economic, political, and social forces that influence women's self-image and psychological health in general. Such insights may prove useful for the primary prevention of eating disorders.

Predictably, the rising rate of eating disorders in non-Western societies poses a public health challenge. In nearly all of these societies, specialized treatment facilities and support groups are barely available. Patients frequently have to detour around various practitioners before they receive some sort of psychological treatment. Many more are not being treated. The outcome for these patients remains unknown, and the prevention of their distress is an intriguing social challenge.

## FURTHER READING

Bruch, H. (1973). *Eating disorders: Obesity, anorexia nervosa, and the person within.* New York: Basic Books.—A classic book that describes atypical anorexia nervosa.

Fallon, P., Katzman, M. A., & Wooley, S. C. (1994). *Feminist perspectives on eating disorders.* New York: Guilford Press.—Provides a comprehensive, gender-sensitive view of eating disorders.

Katzman, M., & Lee, S. (1997). Beyond body image: The integration of feminist and transcultural theories in the understanding of self-starvation. *International Journal of Eating Disorders, 22,* 385–394.—A rare paper that integrates cross-cultural and feminist perspectives, and concludes that fear of losing "control," not fatness, may underlie eating disorders.

Lee, S. (1995). Self-starvation in contexts: Towards the culturally sensitive understanding of anorexia nervosa. *Social Science and Medicine, 41,* 25–36.—Discusses from an ethnographic viewpoint how non-fat-phobic rationales serve as local idioms of distress for two atypical anorexic patients.

Lee, S., Ho, T. P., & Hsu, L. K. G. (1993). Fat phobic and non-fat phobic anorexia nervosa a comparative study of 70 Chinese patients in Hong Kong. *Psychological Medicine, 23,* 999–1017.—The largest systematic comparison of the clinical characteristics of Chinese typical and atypical anorexic patients in Hong Kong.

Lee, S., & Lee, A. M. (2000). Disordered eating in three communities of China: A comparative study of female high school students in Hong Kong, Shenzhen, and rural Hunan. *International Journal of Eating Disorders, 27,* 317–327.—A paper that demonstrates a consistent gradient of female fat concern across three Chinese communities that lie on a spectrum of societal modernization. Indicates that global change will make eating disorders a growing public health challenge to Asian countries.

Lee, S., Lee, A. M., & Leung, T. (1998). Cross-cultural validity of the eating disorder inventory: A study of Chinese patients with eating disorder in Hong Kong. *International Journal of Eating Disorders, 23,* 177–188.—Provides empirical evidence that a widely used Western research instrument lacks contextual validity in a non-Western population.

Nakamura, K., Yamamoto, M., Yamazaki, O., Kawashima, Y., Muto, K., Someya, T., Sakurai, K., & Nozoe, S. (2000). Prevalence of anorexia nervosa and bulimia nervosa in a geographically defined area in Japan. *International Journal of Eating Disorders, 28,* 173–180.—A recent hospital-based survey revealing that about one-third of Japanese patients with eating disorders belong to the "not otherwise specified" category. The rates of eating disorders are lower than in the West, but higher rates of anorexia nervosa than bulimia nervosa suggest that the sample is clinically biased.

Nasser, M., Katzman, M. A., & Gordon, R. (Eds.). (in press). *Eating disorders: Cultures in transition.* London: Routledge.—A unique volume that tracks, both cross-culturally and cross-disciplinarily, the psychological, economic, and political contributions to the identification and presentation of eating disorders around the world. Each chapter focuses on a different geographic region and is followed by two stimulating commentaries.

Strober, M., Freeman, R., & Morrell, W. (1999). Atypical anorexia nervosa: Separation from typical cases in course and outcome in a long-term prospective study. *International Journal of Eating Disorders, 25,* 135–142.—The first longitudinal empirical study in the West that validates atypical anorexia nervosa.

Tchanturia, K., Troop, N. A., & Katzman, M. A. (in press). Same pie, different portions: Shape and weight-based self-esteem and eating disorder symptoms in an Georgian sample. *European Journal of Eating Disorders.*—This article explores the unexpected presentation of eating disorders in Georgia (former Soviet Union) in the absence of a relevant vocabulary.

# Medical and Physical Aspects
of Eating Disorders

# 48

# Physiology of Anorexia Nervosa and Bulimia Nervosa

## KATHERINE A. HALMI

Most physiological abnormalities present in patients with anorexia nervosa and bulimia nervosa are secondary to an underweight state, dieting, or behavior directed toward losing weight, such as self-induced vomiting, laxative misuse, and excessive exercising. With nutritional rehabilitation and cessation of weight-losing behaviors, the physiological changes are reversed. Medical complications of anorexia nervosa and bulimia nervosa are described in Chapter 50.

## ENDOCRINE ABNORMALITIES

Endocrine changes in anorexia nervosa and bulimia nervosa involve the hypothalamic–pituitary–ovarian, adrenal, and thyroid axes, as well as growth hormone, insulin, neuropeptides, endogenous opioids, leptin, and neurotransmitters. (See Chapter 49 for a description of neurotransmitter abnormalities.)

Amenorrhea is an essential clinical feature in the diagnosis of anorexia nervosa. In underweight patients, basal levels of luteinizing hormone (LH), follicle-stimulating hormone (FSH), and estrogen are decreased. The 24-hour LH secretion pattern is abnormal and similar to that found in prepubertal females. With weight restoration, normal LH secretion occurs in most patients. The return of normal menstrual cycles lags behind, with resumption associated with psychological improvement and cessation of dietary restriction. Regular injections of gonadotropin-releasing hormone (GnRH) in underweight patients produce ovulation. These findings suggest that the pituitary cells producing LH and FSH are understimulated due to hyposecretion of GnRH in the hypothalamus. Dysfunction in the neurotransmitter systems that influence GnRH release is most likely present in anorexia nervosa.

Menstrual irregularities occur in many women with bulimia nervosa. Intermittent dieting, purging behaviors, and psychological stress factors could contribute to the neuroendocrine changes responsible for these menstrual abnormalities.

Mild hypercortisolism, with a blunting of diurnal rhythm, is commonly present in anorexia nervosa. Elevated levels of corticotropin-releasing hormone (CRH) are present but return to normal with weight restoration. Hypersecretion of endogenous CRH most likely produces the characteristic hypercortisolism, along with the increased half-life of cortisol found in starvation. Increased CRH, a potent anorectic hormone, may have a role in maintaining anorectic behaviors and encouraging relapse. Conflicting CRH and cortisol findings in bulimia nervosa patients are probably related to dieting behavior. The secretion of both GnRH and CRH is highly influenced by the neurotransmitters, norepinephrine, and serotonin, which help to regulate eating behavior and influence mood.

A blunted or delayed thyroid-stimulating hormone (TSH) response to thyrotropin-releasing hormone is present in anorexia nervosa. There is a reduced peripheral conversion of thyroxine ($T_4$) to triiodothyronine ($T_3$) and an increased conversion of $T_4$ to inactive reverse $T_3$. These changes are seen in other starvation states and probably represent an adaptive response to inadequate caloric intake. $T_4$ levels are in the low normal range, $T_3$ levels are depressed, and TSH levels are normal. Clinical evidence of hypothyroidism includes hypothermia, bradycardia, constipation, dry skin, and delayed relaxation of the tendon reflexes. All of these changes reverse with refeeding and weight gain. There are contradictory reports of thyroid functioning in bulimia nervosa. This may be due to the differences in the severity of these patients' dieting behavior.

Dopamine, norepinephrine, serotonin, growth hormone–releasing hormone and peripheral feedback mechanisms all influence the secretion of growth hormone from the pituitary gland. Patients with anorexia nervosa have dysregulation of growth hormone secretion. This likely is a response to the starvation state. However, an impaired growth hormone response to pharmacological challenge tests in both emaciated and weight-restored anorectic patients indicates a disturbance at the hypothalamic level. Basal prolactin levels are normal in anorexia nervosa but prolactin responses to challenge tests are impaired in weight-restored patients, suggesting a dysfunction at the postsynaptic dopaminergic receptor site. Growth hormone secretion studies in bulimia nervosa patients are contradictory and suggest that the occasional growth hormone aberrations could be a response to fasting. The most consistent finding is that growth hormone secretion seems to be abnormally sensitive to TSH.

Insulin and fasting blood sugar levels are decreased or in the low-normal range in anorexia nervosa. Glucose tolerance is also commonly impaired and likely reflects the starvation state.

Neuropeptides have a role in regulating satiety, appetite, mood and neuroendocrine functions and thus may contribute to the pathophysiology of eating disorders. Satiety may be produced by several gastrointestinal hormones such as cholecystokinin (CCK), glucagon, somatostatin, and bombesin. Studies in anorexia nervosa and bulimia nervosa patients indicate that these hormones are unlikely to make any meaningful contribution to the initiation or maintenance of the eating disorder.

Studies of the two central appetite stimulants, neuropeptide Y and peptide YY, have been conducted in only one center. The meaning of minor aberrations present in cerebrospinal fluid levels remains to be determined.

Patients with anorexia nervosa have an impaired ability to concentrate urine, which is related to the inconsistent secretion of vasopressin. Both vasopressin and oxytocin secretion return to normal with weight restoration.

Dopamine and opioids have a role in modulating eating behavior and pleasure–reward responses to food. The abnormal pleasure–reward response seen in both anorexia nervosa and bulimia nervosa patients could be related to an impairment in this system. Abnormalities of opioid activity seem to be state-related in that they reflect active bingeing, purging, or severe food restriction.

Initially, leptin was regarded as a signal to reduce feeding and hence reduce body weight. However, numerous studies show leptin levels in anorexia nervosa patients correlate positively with body mass index and amount of adipose tissue; that is, emaciated patients have extremely low levels of leptin that increase as the patients gain weight. These findings support the hypothesis that leptin is a signal of energy deficiency, and when leptin levels in the blood fall, energy intake is reduced. Thus, in starvation, falling leptin levels should promote increased food or energy intake, decreased energy expenditure, and the metabolism of calories into fat.

## ELECTROLYTE AND METABOLIC ABNORMALITIES

Electrolyte abnormalities are associated with poor fluid intake, vomiting, laxative abuse, and diuretic abuse in both anorexia nervosa and bulimia nervosa. For those who engage in purging behavior, a metabolic alkalosis may occur. This is a condition with low chloride and potassium levels (hypokalemia) in the blood and elevated bicarbonate levels. It produces physical symptoms of weakness, lethargy and, at times, cardiac arrhythmias (see below). Hypomagnesemia may be present and can interfere with the correction of hypokalemia. Hypophosphatemia may also occur in anorexia nervosa as a result of poor dietary intake. It can also be a dangerous complication of refeeding, since inorganic phosphate moves intracellularly as it is required for protein synthesis. This may result in a sudden drop in serum phosphatase levels, which can aggravate mild cardiac dysfunction.

Acutely ill patients with anorexia nervosa have a low total energy expenditure and resting metabolic rate. They also have proportionately less body fat and gain much of their weight initially as body fat (requiring more calories than are required to gain lean body mass). Newly weight-restored patients need more calories to maintain weight than normal controls: In contrast, patients with bulimia nervosa need fewer calories to maintain their weight. The reasons for this are unclear, but it is an unfortunate fact.

Elevated levels of beta-hydroxybutyric acid and free fatty acids may be found in starving anorectics. Hypercholesterolemia is more often present in children than in adults. It is unlikely to be dietary in origin, since patients with anorexia nervosa typically exclude saturated fat and cholesterol from their diet. Beta-carotene levels are often raised, the cause of which is uncertain, but this may reflect dietary intake of carotene. Vitamin deficiencies are uncommon. Studies of the zinc status of anorexia nervosa patients have yielded conflicting findings.

## CARDIAC AND CARDIOVASCULAR DISTURBANCES

Bradycardia and orthostatic hypotension are common findings in patients with anorexia nervosa, who frequently have a resting heart rate below 60 beats per minute and a diastolic blood pressure below 60. Dizziness and frank syncope are not unusual. Electrocardiographic (EKG) changes are common and usually reflect electrolyte disturbance.

These changes include low voltage, sinus bradycardia, and ST segment depression. At times, cardiac arrhythmias occur with hypokalemia in which case myocardial repolarization may be delayed, resulting in a prolonged QT interval. The QT interval reflects electrical signals from the start of ventricular depolarization to repolarization, the stage that prepares the ventricles for the next beat. The repolarization–depolarization process needs to happen more rapidly as the heart rate increases. The QTc, the corrected QT interval, adjusts for this. Patients with hypokalemia are vulnerable to have prolonged QTc, which may be associated with ventricular tachycardia (*torsade de pointes*) and sudden death. Adverse cardiac affects can occur when the $CYP_{450}$ $3A_4$ enzyme system is inhibited by certain medications, leading to elevated levels of medications that prolong the QT interval.

Patients who use ipecac to induce vomiting may develop a cardiomyopathy from ipecac intoxication. This is an irreversible condition of cardiac failure that usually results in death. Symptoms of pericardial pain, dyspnea, and generalized muscle weakness associated with hypotension, tachycardia, and EKG abnormalities should alert one to possible ipecac cardiac intoxication.

## GASTROINTESTINAL COMPLICATIONS

In anorexia nervosa, delayed gastric emptying is common and associated with feelings of fullness and bloating. Persistent laxative abuse may decrease the motility of the colon and result in true constipation. Patients who binge and purge are at risk for acute dilatation of the stomach or esophageal tears, which are usually accompanied by shock. There is some indirect evidence that the vagal afferent system in patients with bulimia nervosa is dysfunctional. These patients have been found to have an increased threshold for both pain and temperature stimuli. It is possible that dysfunctional vagal afferent input from the gastrointestinal tract to the brain concerning satiation may be a factor in their inability to stop eating.

## OTHER ABNORMALITIES

Elevation of serum enzymes may reflect fatty degeneration of the liver and is present in emaciated patients with anorexia nervosa and during their refeeding. Emaciation can also produce abnormalities in hematopoiesis, such as leukopenia and relative lymphocytosis (see Chapter 50). Impaired temperature regulation has also been observed in emaciated patients with an abnormal autonomic response to cold. They also have a sudden abnormal increase in core temperature in response to liquid feeding. Thus, the stability of their temperature regulation is impaired.

The EKG abnormalities found in some patients with anorexia nervosa and bulimia nervosa are probably related to fluid and electrolyte disturbance. Studies using computerized tomography and magnetic resonance imaging have revealed cerebral atrophy and ventricular dilatation. In most cases, this appears to be reversible. Functioning imaging methods have not revealed consistent findings, but more studies are needed.

Osteopenia and fractures are not uncommon in patients with chronic anorexia nervosa. The pathophysiology is not understood, but estrogen deficiency and excess cortisol secretion may be responsible. Current methods of treatment, such as estrogen replacement, have not proved effective.

## FURTHER READING

Eckert, E. D., Pomeroy, C., & Raymond, N. (1998). Leptin in anorexia nervosa. *Journal of Clinical Endocrinology and Metabolism*, *83*, 791–794.—A comprehensive study of leptin physiology in underweight and weight-restored anorexia nervosa patients.

Flier, J. S. (1998). What's in a name?: In search of leptin's physiologic role. *Journal of Clinical Endocrinology and Metabolism*, *83*, 1407–1413.—An excellent review of leptin studies in humans and a new hypothesis about its function.

Halmi, K. A. (1995). Basic biological overview of eating disorders. In F. E. Bloom & D. J. Kupfer (Eds.), *Psychopharmacology: The fourth generation of progress* (pp. 1609–1615).—New York: Raven Press.—A comprehensive review of the biological aspects of eating disorders.

Oborzanek, E., Lesem, M., & Goldstein, D. S. (1991). Reduced resting metabolic rate in patients with bulimia nervosa. *Archives of General Psychiatry*, *48*, 456–462.—A meticulous study of metabolic rate in patients with bulimia nervosa.

Reilly, J. G., Ayis, S. A., & Ferrier, I. N. (2000). QTc—interval abnormalities and psychotropic drug therapy in psychiatric patients. *Lancet*, *355*, 1048–1052.—A detailed explanation of QTc changes in drugs used for psychiatric patients.

Rock, C. L., & Curran-Celentano, J. (1994). Nutritional disorder of anorexia nervosa: A review. *International Journal of Eating Disorders*, *15*, 187–203.—A thorough review of nutrition problems in anorexia nervosa.

Salisbury, J., Levine, A. S., & Crow, S. J. (1995). Refeeding, metabolic rate, and weight gain in anorexia nervosa: A review. *International Journal of Eating Disorders*, *17*, 337–345.—A critical discussion of metabolic studies in anorexia nervosa.

Schweiger, U., Pirke, K. M., & Laessle, R. G. (1992). Gonadotropin secretion in bulimia nervosa. *Journal of Clinical Endocrinology and Metabolism*, *74*, 722–727.—A study of the hypothalamic–pituitary–ovarian axis in patients with bulimia nervosa.

Weiner, H. (1989). Psychoendocrinology of anorexia nervosa. *Psychiatric Clinics of North America*, *12*, 187–206.—A thorough review of the menstrual cycle physiology of anorexia nervosa patients.

# 49

# Central Nervous System Neurotransmitter Activity in Anorexia Nervosa and Bulimia Nervosa

## WALTER H. KAYE

It is common to consider eating disorders as being caused by cultural pressures for thinness, since dieting and the pursuit of thinness are common in industrialized countries. (See Chapters 19, 45, and 47 for discussions of sociocultural influences.) However, the disparity between the high prevalence of pressures for thinness and the low prevalence of eating disorders (see Chapter 41), combined with clear evidence of anorexia nervosa occurring at least several centuries ago (see Chapter 27), as well as the stereotypical presentation, predominance in females, premorbid anxiety, and developmentally specific age-of-onset distribution, underscore the possibility of contributing biological vulnerabilities. Other evidence of biologic risk factors includes indications that both anorexia nervosa and bulimia nervosa are familial and heritable disorders (see Chapter 42).

In the past few decades, a substantial number of neurotransmitters that contribute to the regulation of feeding behaviors have been identified. This in turn has raised the question of whether some disturbance of neurotransmitter function may contribute to the pathophysiology of anorexia nervosa and bulimia nervosa. However, it is difficult to answer this question with *in vivo* studies in humans because the central nervous system has been relatively inaccessible. In the living human brain, methods of characterizing neurotransmitter function have relied upon relatively indirect measures, such as levels of neurotransmitters in cerebrospinal fluid or endocrine responses to challenges of neurotransmitter function.

Another difficulty in the study of neurotransmitter activity in people with eating disorders is that disturbances of neuropeptide or monoamine activity could be secondary to dietary abnormalities or premorbid traits that contribute to a vulnerability to develop anorexia nervosa or bulimia nervosa. One way to tease apart cause and effect is to study people with anorexia nervosa or bulimia nervosa at various stages in their illness, that is, while they are symptomatic and after recovery. Neurotransmitter abnormalities that persist after recovery might indicate trait-related disturbances that may contribute to the etiology of anorexia nervosa or bulimia nervosa.

## NEUROPEPTIDES

There has been considerable interest in the neuropeptides reputed to have appetite stimulant or repressive properties. The most direct technology for assessment of these orexigenic and anorexigenic peptides *in vivo* in humans is measurements of concentrations in cerebrospinal fluid (CSF). While alterations in the concentrations of many neuropeptide systems have been found in ill patients with anorexia nervosa or bulimia nervosa, most disturbances normalize after recovery. However, neuropeptide disturbances may substantially contribute to symptoms in the ill state, and even to the high relapse rates in anorexia nervosa and bulimia nervosa. For example, people with anorexia nervosa who are underweight have increased plasma cortisol secretion that is thought to be a consequence of hypersecretion of endogenous corticotropin-releasing hormone (CRH). Both measures normalize after weight restoration, thus suggesting that activation of the hypothalamic–pituitary axis is precipitated by weight loss. Still, increased CRH activity is of great theoretical interest in anorexia nervosa, since intracerebroventricular CRH administration in experimental animals produces many of the physiological and behavioral changes associated with the disorder, including hypothalamic hypogonadism, decreased sexual activity, decreased feeding behavior, and hyperactivity.

Underweight patients with anorexia nervosa have increased CSF levels of neuropeptide Y, a potent appetite stimulant, which may be a compensatory physiological response to starvation but does not appear to counter the pursuit of thinness in anorexia nervosa. Animal studies suggest that elevated neuropeptide Y may contribute to altered gonadal hormone secretion, decreased sexual activity, high plasma CRH and cortisol, and hypotension in anorexia nervosa. A related, highly orexigenic peptide YY has been found to be increased only during recovery in bulimia nervosa. Activity of this system may contribute, at least in part, to urges to binge and purge, and thus contributing to relapse in bulimia nervosa.

Leptin, which is secreted predominantly by adipose tissue cells and is thought to contribute to the regulation of body fat, may decrease food intake and reduce body weight by reducing neuropeptide Y activity. Malnourished and underweight patients with anorexia nervosa have consistently been found to have significantly reduced plasma and CSF leptin concentrations compared to normal-weight controls. This strongly implies a normal physiological response to starvation. While leptin levels normalize after long-term recovery, one study found that CSF leptin concentrations reach normal values before full weight restoration, which might contribute to patients' difficulty in achieving and sustaining a normal weight.

Galanin is an orexigenic neuropeptide that may particularly stimulate fat intake. Interestingly, one study found normal CSF galanin in a group of largely weight-restored, but not menstrual-cycle-restored, patients with anorexia nervosa who showed large variations of this neuropeptide during recovery. Our group recently found a reduction of CSF galanin in women with long-term recovery from anorexia nervosa (with normal menses).

These data raise the question of whether alterations in brain galanin activity play a role in food restriction and fat avoidance in anorexia nervosa.

Oxytocin (OXT) and vasopressin (AVP), produced in the hypothalamic supraoptic and paraventricular nuclei, are released peripherally via pituitary projections to the neurohypophysis and are also centrally directed into the brain. In the periphery, AVP controls free-water clearance of the kidney, whereas OXT promotes uterine contraction and milk letdown. In the brain, these peptides are long-acting neuromodulators that exert complex behavioral effects. OXT administration to rats disrupts memory consolidation and retrieval, whereas AVP administration enhances memory function. In animal models, OXT has anxiolytic actions, whereas AVP has anxiogenic effects. Altered concentrations of OXT and AVP have been found in people with eating disorders. Our group studied people with eating disorders after recovery and found that persistently elevated levels of CSF AVP were related to having a lifetime history of major depression. In comparison, CSF OXT levels were normal in recovered subjects. The findings also suggested that elevated levels of CSF OXT after recovery from bulimia nervosa might be related to use of the birth control pill. Thus, the AVP findings may help in understanding why some people with eating disorders are more susceptible to major depression.

In summary, the correction of most of the neuropeptide disturbances after recovery from an eating disorder suggests that such disturbances are secondary to malnutrition or weight loss and not the cause. Still, an understanding of these neuropeptide disturbances may shed light on why many people with anorexia nervosa or bulimia nervosa cannot easily "reverse" their illness. In anorexia nervosa, malnutrition may contribute to the downward spiraling circle in which malnutrition sustains and perpetuates the desire for more weight loss and dieting. Symptoms such as increased satiety, as well as obsessions and dysphoric mood, may be exaggerated by these neuropeptide alterations and thus contribute to this downward spiral. Even after improved nutrition and weight gain, many people with anorexia nervosa have much difficulty normalizing their behavior. The persistence of some neuropeptide disturbances after long-term recovery provides several possible explanations for this phenomenon. First, these disturbances may be strongly entrenched and not easily corrected by improved nutrition or weight normalization. If correct, this would support the need to sustain therapy for months after weight normalization. Alternatively, the persistence of certain disturbances after long-term recovery raises the question of whether these are trait-related alterations that contribute to the pathogenesis of eating disorders or comorbid symptoms.

## MONOAMINES

There has been considerable interest in the role that serotonin may play in anorexia nervosa and bulimia nervosa, since this neuronal system contributes to the modulation of feeding, mood, and impulse control (both obsessional and impulse undercontrol). The most compelling evidence for a disturbance of monoamine activity is the positive response to antidepressant-type medications (see Chapter 58). In addition, when underweight, patients with anorexia nervosa have a significant reduction in basal concentrations of the serotonin metabolite 5-hydroxyindoleacetic acid (5-HIAA) in the CSF compared to healthy controls, as well as reduced [3H]-imipramine binding and blunted plasma prolactin response to drugs with serotonin activity. Together, these findings suggest reduced serotonergic activity. This might be a consequence of diet-related reductions of tryptophan, the amino acid precursor of serotonin. In contrast, CSF concentrations of 5-HIAA are elevated after long-term recovery from anorexia nervosa. Likewise, women who are ill with bulimia nervosa have evidenced altered response to serotonin challenges and low-to-normal CSF 5-HIAA levels that are inversely related to their frequency of binge eating and purging. After recovery, they show elevated concentrations of CSF 5-HIAA in response to serotonin-specific challenges.

It has been found that *low* levels of CSF 5-HIAA are associated with impulsive and nonpremeditated, aggressive behaviors that cut across traditional diagnostic boundaries. Thus, it is of interest that women who have recovered from anorexia nervosa or bulimia nervosa have elevated CSF 5-HIAA concentrations. Behaviors found after recovery from anorexia nervosa and bulimia nervosa, such as obsessionality with symmetry and exactness, and perfectionism, tend to be opposite in character to those displayed by people with low 5-HIAA levels. Together, these studies contribute to a growing literature that suggests that CSF 5-HIAA concentrations may correlate with a spectrum of behavior; that is, reduced CSF-5 HIAA levels appear to be related to behavioral undercontrol, whereas increased concentrations may be related to behavioral overcontrol.

## COMMON AND SPECIFIC VULNERABILITIES

The possibility of a common vulnerability for anorexia nervosa and bulimia nervosa may seem puzzling given well-recognized differences in behavior in these disorders. However, recent studies suggest that anorexia nervosa and bulimia nervosa have a shared etiological vulnerability; that is, there is a familial aggregation of a range of eating disorders in relatives of probands with either anorexia nervosa or bulimia nervosa, and these two disorders are highly comorbid in twin studies (see Chapter 42). Both disorders are characterized by high levels of harm avoidance, a personality trait hypothesized to be related to increased serotonin activity. Other features in common include a drive for thinness, perfectionism, and preoccupation with symmetry and exactness. (See Chapter 36 for discussion of the personality characteristics of people with eating disorders.) These data raise the possibility that a disturbance of serotonin activity may create a vulnerability for the expression of a cluster of symptoms that are common to both anorexia nervosa and bulimia nervosa.

Other factors that are *independent* of a vulnerability for the development of an eating disorder may contribute to the development of eating disorder subtypes. (See Chapters 28 and 30 for a description and discussion of the subclassification of eating disorders.) These other factors may be related to extremes of impulse control and mood stability. For example, only people who have recovered from restricting-type anorexia nervosa have been found to have reduced CSF concentrations of homovanillic acid, a major metabolite of dopamine. Dopamine neuronal function has been associated with motor activity, reward, and novelty seeking. These behaviors are altered in restricting-type anorexia nervosa compared to other eating disorder subtypes. A trait-related disturbance of dopamine metabolism may therefore contribute to a vulnerability to develop this subtype of eating disorder.

## FUTURE DEVELOPMENTS

New technologies in brain imaging offer the potential for increased understanding of previously inaccessible brain function and its dynamic relationship with human behaviors. For example, recent data from our group suggests that a disturbance of serotonin (5-HT) neuronal pathways persists in the orbital frontal cortex after recovery from an eating disorder. Both 5-HT activity and frontal lobe function have been associated with extremes of self-control such as obsessionality and impulsive, aggressive behaviors. We have postulated that people with eating disorders have an inherent disturbance of 5-HT circuits, including the orbital frontal cortex, which causes a vulnerability for imprecise and poorly modulated behavioral control. Advances in technology, using a range of brain imaging devices, offer the promise of the ability to identify regional localization of altered brain function and correlations with behavior and neurotransmitter functional activity.

Genomics is another promising technology. (See Chapter 43 for a discussion of the molecular genetics of eating disorders.) Complex traits that lead to the development of anorexia nervosa and bulimia nervosa do not have a simple, or Mendelian, mode of transmission. To date, conventional methods, such as linkage analysis, have failed to identify which critical regions of the genome are responsible for the inheritance of complex disease susceptibility. This is thought to be due to the oligogenic and oligoallelic nature of complex traits. The lack of power of linkage methods has led to the suggestion that association studies should be used. Such association methods provide evidence for connection between a specific allele at a locus (a candidate gene) and a phenotype. In fact, the findings from some, but not all, studies suggest that a polymorphism ($-1438$G/A) in the promoter region of the gene for the $5$-HT$_{2A}$ receptor may make a minor contribution to anorexia nervosa. There is the possibility that this polymorphism may be particularly associated with the restricting-type of anorexia nervosa and obsessive–compulsive disorder, but not bulimia nervosa. It is not known if this polymorphism has functional activity. The weakness of the candidate gene strategy has been the relative lack of both novel candidates and polymorphisms at those candidates. However, this problem will soon be solved as a result of the human genome sequencing efforts. When genome-wide single nucleotide polymorphism (SNP) maps and high-throughput scanning for SNPs in candidate genes become widely available, there will be a convergence of the association and candidate gene strategies, with the exciting possibility of eventually identifying genes that contribute to eating disorders.

## FURTHER READING

Brewerton, T. D., (1995). Toward a unified theory of serotonin dysregulation in eating and related disorders. *Psychoneuroendocrinology, 20,* 561–590.—Review and hypotheses about serotonin and eating disorders.

Collier, D. A., Arranz, M. J., Li, T., Mupita, D., Brown, N., & Treasure, J. (1997). Association between 5-HT2A gene promoter polymorphism and anorexia nervosa [Letter]. *Lancet, 3,* 350–412.—First of several reports on an altered frequency of a gene variant in anorexia nervosa.

Jimerson, D. C., Lesem, M. D., Kaye, W. H., Hegg, A. P., & Brewerton T. D. (1990). Eating disorders and depression: Is there a serotonin connection? *Biological Psychiatry, 28,* 443–454.—Review and hypotheses about serotonin and eating disorders.

Kaye, W., & Strober M. (1999). Neurobiology of eating disorders. In D. S. Charney, E. J. Nestler,

& B. S. Bunney (Eds.), *Neurobiology of mental illness* (pp. 891–906). New York: Oxford University Press.—Overview of neurobiology, including recent monoamine and neuropeptide alterations and their potential relationship to behavior.

Kaye, W. H., Greeno, C. G., Moss, H., Fernstrom, J., Fernstrom, M., Lilenfeld, L. R., Weltzin, T. E., & Mann, J. J. (1998). Alterations in serotonin activity and psychiatric symptomatology after recovery from bulimia nervosa. *Archives of General Psychiatry, 55,* 927–935.—Recent data supporting a persistent and possibly trait-related disturbance of serotonin.

Mantzoros, C., Flier, J. S., Lesem, M. D., Brewerton, T. D., & Jimerson, D. C. (1997). Cerebrospinal fluid leptin in anorexia nervosa: Correlation with nutritional status and potential role in resistance to weight gain. *Journal of Clinical Endocrinology and Metabolism, 82,* 1845–1851.—Intriguing report on the role of leptin in anorexia nervosa

Schwartz, M. W., Woods, S. C., Porte, D., Jr., Seeley, R. J., & Baskin, D. G. (2000). Central nervous system control of food intake. *Nature, 404,* 661–671.—Useful review.

Smith, K. A., Fairburn, C. G., & Cowen, P. J. (1999). Symptomatic relapse in bulimia nervosa following acute tryptophan depletion. *Archives of General Psychiatry, 56,* 171–176.—Recent data supporting a persistent and possibly trait-related disturbance of serotonin.

Srinivasagam, N. M., Kaye, W. H., Plotnicov, K. H., Greeno, C., Weltzin, T. E., & Rao, R. (1995). Persistent perfectionism, symmetry, and exactness after long-term recovery from anorexia nervosa. *American Journal of Psychiatry, 152,* 1630–1634.—Paper describing persistent symptoms after recovery from anorexia nervosa.

Treasure, J., & Campbell, I. (1994). The case for biology in the etiology of anorexia nervosa. *Psychological Medicine, 24,* 3–8.—Discussion of nature and nuture and eating disorders.

# 50

# Medical Complications of Anorexia Nervosa and Bulimia Nervosa

## CLAIRE POMEROY
## JAMES E. MITCHELL

Despite a growing literature outlining the medical complications of anorexia nervosa and bulimia nervosa, patients, families, and providers too often are so focused on the psychiatric aspects of the illness that they overlook the physical damage that these conditions can cause. In this chapter, the medical complications of eating disorders are reviewed. (Physiological abnormalities are described in Chapter 48.) It is important to emphasize that awareness of these potentially tragic consequences is the responsibility of all health professionals caring for these vulnerable patients, and that the management of these complications is an essential aspect of the overall management of eating disorders.

## RENAL AND ELECTROLYTE ABNORMALITIES

Decreased oral intake in restricting anorectic patients and purging behaviors in bulimic patients can result in severe disruptions of fluid homeostasis and potentially life-threatening electrolyte abnormalities. The most frequent serious electrolyte disturbance is hypokalemia, which usually occurs in patients with potassium loss due to self-induced vomiting or diuretic and laxative abuse. Simultaneous loss of fluid and stomach acid often results in an accompanying hypochloremic contraction alkalosis.

Hypokalemia may result in cardiac arrhythmias, one of the major causes of death in patients with eating disorders, and may also contribute to intestinal dysmotility and skeletal muscle myopathy. It is now recognized that chronic hypokalemia can cause nephropathy, with elevated serum creatinine levels, and eventually result in chronic renal failure severe enough to require dialysis.

A number of other electrolyte abnormalities occur less frequently. Hypomagnesemia is not uncommon in anorectic patients and may be associated with hypocalcemia or hypokalemia that will only resolve if magnesium is replaced concurrently. Hypophosphatemia can occur during refeeding and hyperphosphatemia may rarely complicate frequent vomiting.

Careful monitoring of serum potassium and other electrolytes is vital to the management of patients with eating disorders. Asymptomatic, mild hypokalemia can often be successfully treated with oral potassium supplementation. It is important to remember that metabolic contraction alkalosis will attenuate the efficacy of potassium replacement and must therefore be treated simultaneously, hopefully by cessation of purging behaviors. Intravenous replacement of potassium may be necessary in the patient with severe or symptomatic hypokalemia.

Persistent restricting and purging behaviors can result in a hypovolemic state, which stimulates the renin–angiotensin–aldosterone system as the body's homeostatic mechanisms attempt to conserve fluids. Patients who abuse diuretics or laxatives are particularly at risk of developing overstimulation of this hormonal axis. When patients attempt to curtail abuse of these substances, the persistent hyperaldosteronism may result in temporary reflex edema that can last for several weeks. If patients who attempt to discontinue laxatives develop constipation, they should be urged to avoid resuming use of stimulant laxatives and advised to use bulk-type laxatives, increase dietary roughage, and pursue regular exercise to maintain bowel function.

## CARDIOVASCULAR SYSTEM

Cardiovascular abnormalities occur frequently in patients with eating disorders, especially very low weight anorectic patients, and bulimic patients with electrolyte abnormalities. Restricted oral intake can cause low blood pressure and sinus bradycardia, reflecting a physiological adaptation to the hypometabolic state of starvation and not requiring specific therapy. Patients who restrict fluid intake or are dehydrated secondary to purging behaviors may develop hypovolemia and orthostatic hypotension. Symptoms of dizziness or fainting can be treated with fluid repletion.

Sudden death due to ventricular arrhythmias is a well-described consequence of eating disorders. Hypokalemia and other electrolyte abnormalities are major risk factors. Another cardiac complication is cardiomyopathy secondary to ipecac abuse. The drug accumulates in cardiac tissue and can cause prolonged and sometimes irreversible cardiac dysfunction. In anorectic patients, a refeeding cardiomyopathy may also result from overly aggressive, rapid refeeding.

Mitral valve prolapse has been described as a complication of anorexia nervosa, but the true prevalence remains controversial. Both mitral valve prolapse and anorexia nervosa are common in young women in the general population and the observed association may be coincidental. However, at least in some cases with extreme inanition, it appears that decreased left ventricular size accompanies the weight loss, resulting in a poor fit between the ventricle and the normal-size mitral valve, with consequent prolapse of the valve.

Electrocardiogram (EKG) abnormalities in patients with eating disorders have been reported with varying frequency. While sinus bradycardia and sinus arrhythmia are common in low-weight patients with anorexia nervosa, they do not appear to pose any increased risk. In contrast, serious arrhythmias can occur, usually in patients with disturbed electrolyte balance. Conduction defects, especially prolonged QT interval, are of major concern and warrant evaluation of electrolytes and consultation with an internist or cardiologist.

## GASTROINTESTINAL SYSTEM

The gastrointestinal (GI) complications of eating disorders can manifest in every portion of the GI tract. Swelling of the parotid or submandibular glands is often one of the few physical examination clues to the diagnosis of bulimia nervosa. Parotid hypertrophy may result in elevated serum amylase levels, and measurement of amylase isoenzymes can help differentiate this benign finding from pancreatitis.

Esophageal problems complicating eating disorders range from mild esophagitis to life-threatening esophageal rupture. Exposure to stomach acid secondary to self-induced vomiting can cause esophagitis, erosions, ulcerations, and eventually the development of esophageal strictures, or Barrett's esophagus. Recurrent retching can lead to Mallory–Weiss tears, which may result in significant GI blood loss. Esophageal rupture (Boerhove's syndrome) is an unusual but catastrophic complication that requires surgical intervention.

Acute gastric dilatation may occur in bulimic patients during binge eating and in anorectic patients during refeeding. Gastric dilatation can usually be treated medically with nasogastric suction, and fluid and electrolyte replacement. In rare cases, gastric rupture occurs and requires immediate surgical therapy. In anorexia nervosa, abdominal pain can also be due to the superior mesenteric artery syndrome. Acute pancreatitis can complicate refeeding in patients with anorexia nervosa and can occur during binge eating in bulimic patients.

Several studies have documented abnormal GI motility in many patients with eating disorders. Impaired gastric emptying may contribute to the symptoms of bloating and early satiety. Altered intestinal motility may manifest as prolonged whole-gut transit times and cause abdominal discomfort and ileus. Colonic dysmotility can play a pathogenic role in constipation, exacerbating the severity of symptoms due to dehydration and hypokalemia.

Laxative abuse is a major cause of GI complications in patients with eating disorders. Chronic use of stimulant laxatives results in loss of normal peristaltic function, often resulting in GI cramping and intermittent bouts of diarrhea and constipation. Evidence of GI bleeding, inflammation, and blackish discoloration known as melanosis coli can be seen on colonoscopic examination. Less frequently, anemia secondary to chronic GI blood loss and malabsorption, steatorrhea, or protein-losing gastroenteropathy can complicate prolonged abuse. Rarely, cathartic colon can eventually necessitate colonic resection.

## ENDOCRINE ABNORMALITIES

Extensive perturbations of the endocrine system characterize anorexia nervosa and, to a lesser extent, bulimia nervosa. Abnormalities may reflect dysfunction of the hypothalamic–pituitary (HP) axes, including the HP–gonadotropin (HPG), HP–adrenal (HPA), and HP–thyroid (HPT) axes.

## Hypothalamic–Pituitary–Gonadotropin Axis

Amenorrhea is a diagnostic criterion and hallmark feature of anorexia nervosa. It remains unclear if the absence of menses in these patients is merely a secondary effect of caloric restriction. Alternatively, amenorrhea and anorexia nervosa might both result from a common stressor or from a primary, possibly hypothalamic, abnormality. In the majority of cases, menses resume after normalization of body weight. However, menstruation ceases before any weight loss in some patients, and menstrual abnormalities sometimes persist after weight gain. Patients with anorexia nervosa have low levels of plasma estradiol, luteinizing hormone and follicle-stimulating hormone, such that the HPG axis function resembles that of premenarchal girls. In those with bulimia nervosa, HPG axis dysfunction is less frequent, and a pattern of irregular menses rather than frank amenorrhea is usually observed.

## Hypothalamic–Pituitary–Adrenal Axis

Sustained hypercortisolism is characteristic of anorexia nervosa and may result in nonsuppression of cortisol by dexamethasone. High cortisol levels have been attributed both to increased production and decreased clearance, but the exact stimulus for the HPA axis remains unknown. The HPA system has been less extensively studied in patients with bulimia nervosa. Many bulimic patients have normal cortisol levels, but some have abnormalities akin to those observed in anorexia nervosa. Abnormal dexamethasone suppression test results in patients with bulimia nervosa may be due to hypercortisolism but in other cases may merely reflect erratic absorption due to altered GI motility.

## Hypothalamic–Pituitary–Thyroid Axis

Thyroid function tests may be abnormal in patients with anorexia nervosa, but most frequently these abnormalities represent a physiological adaptation to starvation and not thyroid gland dysfunction. The most common finding in anorectics is normal thyroxine ($T_4$), decreased triiodothyronine ($T_3$), and normal thyroid-stimulating hormone. This "low $T_3$ syndrome" or "euthyroid sick syndrome" is observed in many chronic illnesses. It is important to note that the low $T_3$ syndrome does not require treatment with thyroid hormone replacement. Particular caution should be exercised because thyroid hormone abuse has been used as an illicit weight loss strategy. A subset of patients with bulimia nervosa may also have thyroid function tests consistent with a low $T_3$ syndrome, but most have normal values.

## Other Endocrine Abnormalities

Anorexia nervosa is associated with impaired or erratic release of vasopressin. As a result, patients may develop partial neurogenic diabetes insipidus, with symptoms of polyuria and polydipsia. In nearly all cases, no specific therapy is indicated. Asymptomatic hypoglycemia is quite frequent in patients with anorexia nervosa. Acute symptomatic hypoglycemia has been reported anecdotally. Elevated growth hormone levels probably reflect decreased production of somatomedin C and result in promotion of gluco-neogenesis and reduced peripheral use of glucose, representing a protective physiological adaptation to starvation.

# METABOLIC ABNORMALITIES

## Osteopenia

The increased availability of new diagnostic techniques such as bone densitometry has allowed identification of the high frequency of osteopenia in anorexia nervosa. Decreased bone density (osteopenia) may be as severe as that observed in women with post-menopausal osteoporosis and results in increased fracture risk. The extent of bone demineralization has generally been found to correlate with body mass index, nadir body weight, and duration of illness.

The pathogenesis of osteopenia in anorexia nervosa is complex, and further studies are needed to completely elucidate the etiology. Osteopenia appears to reflect a low turnover state associated with increased bone resorption without concomitant bone formation, a pattern that differs from that of postmenopausal women. The low estrogen levels are the most important cause of osteopenia in anorexia nervosa, but additional nutritional factors appear to play a role. Elevated cortisol or interleukin-6 levels may also contribute.

Treatment of osteoporosis in anorexia nervosa patients remains controversial. Many experts have utilized hormone replacement therapy, hypothesizing that correction of the estrogen deficiency would have beneficial effects comparable to those observed in postmenopausal women. Other experts are reluctant to subject young women to prolonged estrogen therapy and its potential complications, and prefer to emphasize treatment of the underlying eating disorder.

## Other Metabolic Abnormalities

In most, but not all, studies, hypercholesterolemia has been reported to be frequent in patients with anorexia nervosa. Elevated serum carotene levels are found in nearly 75% of anorectic patients and may be associated with frank carotenodermia. Deficiencies of zinc, other trace metals, and vitamins have been reported in a few patients.

# PREGNANCY AND REPRODUCTIVE FUNCTION

Unrecognized eating disorders have recently been implicated as a cause of infertility. Screening for eating disorders before embarking on expensive infertility workups is now recommended. A dietary review and careful historical evaluation to detect disordered eating should be part of the routine assessment of patients who experience difficulty conceiving.

Pregnancy can be challenging for patients suffering from an eating disorder. Higher rates of miscarriage, obstetric complications, and postpartum depression have been reported. Discomfort with body image may be exacerbated by the physiological changes that accompany pregnancy. The obstetrician must remain closely attuned to ensure that caloric intake remains adequate in patients with anorexia nervosa and that purging behaviors are curtailed to ensure adequate nutrition in bulimic patients. Women with bulimia nervosa appear to have a significantly greater incidence of hyperemesis gravidum. Babies born to mothers with eating disorders are at increased risk of low birth weight, low APGAR scores, and poor weight gain during infancy. (See Chapter 39 for discussion of the child rearing of patients with eating disorders.)

If feasible, it is reasonable to advise consideration of postponing pregnancy until the eating disorder is controlled. When a woman with a history of an eating disorder does become pregnant, ongoing collaboration among the eating disorder specialist, the obstetrician, and later the pediatrician is critical to maximizing the chances of a healthy baby.

## DERMATOLOGICAL ABNORMALITIES

Dermatological manifestations of starvation in anorexia nervosa include loss of scalp hair, dry skin, and brittle nails. Nearly one-third of patients with severe weight loss will develop fine, downy facial hair, termed "lanugo hair." In contrast to patients with other forms of starvation, anorectic patients may develop an orange discoloration of their skin due to hypercarotenemia.

Self-induced vomiting may be signaled by the physical examination finding of Russell's sign. In these patients, calluses, abrasions, or bruising of the dorsum of the hand or thumb are the classic clue to bulimia nervosa. Damage to the skin occurs when the teeth injure the fingers or thumb used to manually stimulate the gag reflex. Less commonly, conjunctival hemorrhages or facial petechiae or purpura can result from the increased thoracic pressure generated during purging.

Some laxatives and diuretics contain ingredients that may result in dermatological clues to abuse of these substances. For example, photosensitivity reactions to thiazide diuretics have been reported. Finally, self-induced excoriations or hair loss due to trichotillomania may be noted as manifestations of concomitant psychiatric conditions.

## DENTAL COMPLICATIONS

Dental damage is a major problem in patients with eating disorders who engage in recurrent self-induced vomiting. Erosion of the surface of the teeth, termed perimylolysis, occurs when gastric acid bathes the teeth and can result in extensive decalcification. Increased incidence of caries has also been reported in some but not all series. Frequent examinations performed by a dentist experienced with the complications of eating disorders are a vital part of complete health care delivery for these patients. Using bicarbonate rinses after vomiting may attenuate enamel erosion, but it is important to emphasize that prescription of this therapy should not be interpreted as acceptance of the purging behaviors. Bulimic patients should be advised to use fluoridated mouth rinses, and their dentists should provide topical fluoride treatments as part of routine dental care.

## NEUROLOGICAL SYSTEM

The availability of new brain scanning techniques has stimulated interest in defining potential central nervous system abnormalities in patients suffering from eating disorders. Patients with anorexia nervosa may have enlarged ventricles and external cerebrospinal fluid spaces, findings termed "pseudoatrophy." These abnormalities tend to normalize with weight gain and their pathogenic significance is unclear. However, some studies suggest persistent changes, raising the possibility of permanent damage. PET scans used to study brain function have shown alterations in glucose metabolism patterns in patients with anorexia nervosa.

## HEMATOLOGICAL AND IMMUNE SYSTEMS

Leukopenia, anemia, and thrombocytopenia have all been reported in patients with anorexia nervosa, and rare cases of bone marrow necrosis have occurred. Leukopenia usually reflects decreased neutrophil numbers accompanied by a relative lymphocytosis. The impact of leukopenia on infection risk remains controversial. While some studies have reported an increased risk of bacterial infections, other studies have reported a normal risk, possibly because bone marrow neutrophil reserves are normal. It does appear that during periods of starvation, patients are relatively protected from viral illness, or possibly just the symptomatic manifestations of infection.

A variety of perturbations of the immune system have been reported in patients with eating disorders. Although the available findings are not consistent, most studies report that patients with marked weight loss have impaired delayed-type hypersensitivity skin testing, abnormal neutrophil function, decreased complement levels, low immunoglobulin levels, and abnormal percentages of T-lymphocyte subsets. Emerging research suggests that cytokines, polypeptides which act as molecular messengers in the immune system, may be abnormal in patients with eating disorders.

## FURTHER READING

Abdel-Rahlman, E. M., & Moorthy, A. V. (1997). End-stage renal disease in patients with eating disorders. *Clinical Nephrology, 47*, 106–111.—Report of four cases of endstage renal disease in women with eating disorders, suggesting that chronic hypokalemia plays an important etiologic role in the renal failure.

Anderson, L., Shaw, J. M., & McCarger, L. (1997). Physiologic effects of bulimia nervosa on the gastrointestinal tract. *Canadain Journal of Gastroenterology, 11*, 451–459.—Overview of the gastrointestinal consequences of bulimia nervosa.

Becker, A. E., Grinspoon, S. K., Klibanski, A., & Herzog, D. B. (1999). Eating disorders. *New England Journal of Medicine, 340*, 1092–1098.—Overview of eating disorders, including discussion of the spectrum of medical complications.

Devuyst, O., Lambert, M., Rodhain, J., Lefebvre, C., & Coche, E. (1993). Hematologic changes and infectious complications in anorexia nervosa: A case study. *Quarterly Journal of Medicine, 86*, 791–799.—Summary of the position that anorexia nervosa is associated with increased risk of bacterial infections.

Franko, D. L., & Spurrell, E. B. (2000). Detection and management of eating disorders during pregnancy. *Obstetrics and Gynecology, 95*, 942–946.—Suggested guidelines for obstetricians to use as part of a team approach to management of the pregnant patient with an eating disorder.

Grinspoon, S., Miller, K., Coyle, C., Kremplin, J., Armstrong, C., Pitts, S., Herzog, D., & Klibanski, A. (1999). Severity of osteopenia in estrogen-deficient women with anorexia nervosa and hypothalamic amenorrhea. *Journal of Clinical Endocrinology and Metabolism, 84*, 2049–2055.—Comparison of women with anorexia nervosa and hypothalamic amenorrhea finds that osteopenia is more severe in anorexia nervosa, suggesting that, in addition to the estrogen deficiency, nutritional factors may be pathogenic in anorexia nervosa–associated bone disease.

Lennkh, C., deZwann, M., Bailer, U., Strnad, A., Nagy, C., el Giamal, N., Wiesnagrotski, S., Vitiska, E., Huber, J., & Kasper, S. (1999). Osteopenia in anorexia nervosa: Specific mechanisms of bone loss. *Journal of Psychiatric Research, 33*, 349–356.—Study of osteopenia in anorexia nervosa, confirming the positive correlation between duration of illness and minimal body weight, and suggesting that the mechanism of disease may be distinct from that of postmenopausal osteoporosis. Reviews controversies regarding therapy.

Milosevic, A. (1999). Eating disorders and the dentist. *British Dental Journal, 186*, 109–113.—An up-to-date discussion of the dental complications and management in patients with eating disorders.

Morgan, J. F. (1999). Eating disorders and reproduction. *Australia and New Zealand Journal of Obstetrics and Gynecology, 39*, 167–173.—A review of the impact of eating disorders on menstruation, ovarian function, fertility, sexuality, and pregnancy.

Turner, J., Batik, M., Palmer, L. J., Forbes, D., & McDermott, B. M. (2000). Detection and importance of laxative abuse in adolescents with anorexia nervosa. *Journal of the American Academy of Child and Adolescent Psychiatry, 39*, 378–385.—A recent report confirms and updates the high frequency and potential for medical complications of laxative abuse in patients with eating disorders.

# 51

# Eating Disorders in Diabetes Mellitus

## GARY M. RODIN

Type 1 diabetes mellitus is a common metabolic disorder in which there is impaired glucose utilization due to deficiency of insulin secretion by the pancreas. Its treatment involves multiple, daily insulin injections, regular monitoring of blood sugars, and restriction in the type and timing of food intake in order to normalize blood sugars. The latter diminishes short-term complications of diabetes, such as ketoacidosis, and long-term microvascular complications affecting the kidney, retina, heart, and peripheral blood vessels.

## EPIDEMIOLOGY

Eating disorders may occur in young women with type 1 diabetes on a coincidental basis, since both are relatively common conditions in this age group. Whether there is a more specific link between the two conditions is controversial, since some studies have reported negative findings, while others have found an increase in risk. Jones and colleagues recently conducted a large, case-controlled multisite study in which the prevalence of eating disorders in 356 girls age 12–19 years with type 1 diabetes was compared to that in 1,098 matched control subjects. Eating disorders that met DSM-IV diagnostic criteria for bulimia nervosa or eating disorders not otherwise specified ("atypical eating disorders"—see Chapter 30) were more than twice as common in subjects with diabetes as in controls (10% vs. 4%) and subthreshold states were also almost twice as common (14% vs. 8%).

## MEDICAL COMPLICATIONS

Eating disorders in which there is binge eating and insulin omission are associated with elevated blood sugars and more frequent episodes of ketoacidosis. In a 4-year follow-up study of 91 girls age 12–19 years, Rydall and colleagues demonstrated that disordered eating behavior was associated with a threefold increase in diabetic retinopathy at follow-up. Eating disorders were, in fact, more predictive of retinopathy than was the duration of diabetes, a well-established risk factor for microvascular complications. No specific association has been demonstrated between anorexia nervosa and type 1 diabetes, but hypoglycemia, growth retardation, and delayed secondary sexual characteristics may result when these conditions occur together.

## ETIOLOGICAL MODEL

We have postulated that the dietary restraint and higher body mass index (BMI) resulting from standard diabetes treatment may trigger dietary dysregulation, leading to a cycle of binge eating, purging by insulin omission, and further dietary restriction (see Figure 51.1).

Diabetes treatment is associated with increased BMI, particularly in adolescent girls. Increased BMI heightens body dissatisfaction and may lead to restrained eating, a risk factor for bulimia nervosa (see Chapters 17 and 44). Dietary restraint may also amplify dietary dysregulation, particularly in vulnerable individuals who are less aware of internal cues for hunger and satiety. Girls who develop diabetes at puberty, with its additional

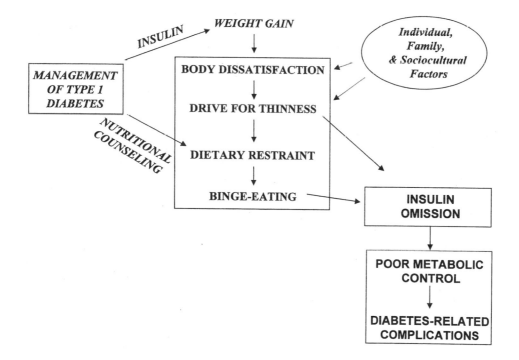

**FIGURE 51.1.** Model of the interactions between eating and weight psychopathology, diabetes management, and outcome in young women with type 1 diabetes. From Daneman, D., Olmsted, M., Rydall, A., Maharaj, S., & Rodin, G. (1998). Eating disorders in young women with type 1 diabetes mellitus: Prevalence, problems, and prevention. *Hormone Research, 50*(Suppl. 1), 79–86. Copyright 1998 by S. Karger AG, Basel. Reprinted by permission.

weight gain and bodily changes, may be most vulnerable to develop disturbed eating attitudes and behavior. Family relationships may contribute to diminished awareness of internal perceptions. Mother–daughter interactions of teenage girls with type 1 diabetes
and disordered eating attitudes and behavior are characterized by less affective engagement, less appropriate attunement, and less empathy.

Some evidence suggests that chronic medical illnesses other than diabetes are associated with an increased risk of disordered eating. However, this risk appears to be greatest
with medical illnesses such as diabetes or phenylketonuria, whose treatment imposes dietary restraint. Conditions such as cystic fibrosis, in which there may be food preoccupation without dietary restraint, have not been found to be associated with a higher rate of
eating disorders.

## MANAGEMENT

Eating disorders may present in a covert fashion in the diabetes clinic setting. Clinicians
should maintain a high index of suspicion in young women with diabetes who have unexplained, poor metabolic control, repeated episodes of ketoacidosis, or weight fluctuations. Inquiry about body dissatisfaction, dieting, binge eating, or purging by deliberate
insulin omission or other methods, using a brief self-report format can reliably identify
clinically significant eating disorders.

Modifications to the standard approach to diabetes management may prevent or alleviate development or progression of disordered eating attitudes and behavior in young
women. Emphasizing normalization of eating behavior and appropriate insulin administration rather than dietary restriction may diminish disordered eating. Education about
nutrition, blood sugar control, and the dangers of dietary restriction and insulin omission
may also be of value. Family counseling may help to support parents in providing practical and emotional support for children in their diabetes management, and in permitting
age-appropriate autonomy in these tasks.

Clinic-based group interventions for young women with eating disorders and diabetes are a practical and nonstigmatizing approach to prevention and early intervention.
Preliminary studies indicate that a six-session, clinic-based psychoeducational intervention for girls with type 1 diabetes and their parents leads to a reduction in disturbed eating attitudes and behavior for up to 6 months. Those with more severe eating disorders
may benefit from the usual range of interventions, including cognitive-behavioral therapy
(see Chapters 54 and 55), interpersonal psychotherapy (see Chapter 57) or dynamic therapy, and, in more severe cases, day hospital or inpatient treatment. Although the majority
of eating disorders associated with diabetes are mild and responsive to treatment, the
presence of diabetes inevitably complicates the treatment and outcome of those with
more severe eating disorders.

## SUMMARY

Eating disorders that meet DSM-IV criteria may be found in 10% of teenage girls with
type 1 diabetes, approximately twice the rate among their nondiabetic peers. The dietary
restriction and increased BMI associated with diabetes treatment are most likely responsi-

ble for the increased prevalence of eating disorders in this group. Deliberate insulin omission, the most common method of purging in these young women, contributes to the increased rate of hyperglycemia, ketoacidosis, and long-term diabetes-related medical complications.

Early identification of disordered eating attitudes and behavior in the diabetes clinic setting may help to prevent clinical eating disorders. Clinic-based group interventions may be effective for prevention or early intervention, although more severe eating disorders likely require specialized mental health referral. The major health risks resulting from eating disorders associated with type 1 diabetes make their early identification and treatment a matter of particular urgency.

## FURTHER READING

Affenito, S. G., Backstrand, J. R., Welch, G. W., Lammi-Keefe, C. J., Rodriguez, N. R., & Adams, C. H. (1997). Subclinical and clinical eating disorders in IDDM negatively affect metabolic control. *Diabetes Care, 20,* 182–184.—Study demonstrating the impact of eating disorders on blood sugar control in type 1 diabetes.

Diabetes Control and Complications Trial (DCCT)/Epidemiology of Diabetes Interventions and Complications (EDIC) Research Group. (2000). Retinopathy and nephropathy in patients with type 1 diabetes four years after a trial of intensive therapy. *New England Journal of Medicine, 342,* 381–389.—The most conclusive research demonstrating the link between metabolic control and medical complications.

Jones, J. M., Lawson, M. L., Daneman, D., Olmsted, M. P., & Rodin, G. (2000). Eating disorders in adolescent females with and without type 1 diabetes: Cross-sectional study. *British Medical Journal, 320,* 1563–1566.—Largest controlled study to date of the prevalence of eating disorders in female adolescents with type 1 diabetes.

Maharaj, S., Rodin, G., Connolly, J., Olmsted, M., & Daneman, D. (in press). Eating problems and the observed quality of mother–daughter interactions among girls with type 1 diabetes. *Journal of Consulting and Clinical Psychology.*—This paper reports the findings from the first systematic, controlled observational study of mother–daughter activation in young women with type 1 diabetes mellitus.

Neumark-Sztainer, D., Story, M., Resnick, M. D., Garwick, A., & Blum, R. W. (1995). Body dissatisfaction and unhealthy weight-control practices among adolescents with and without chronic illness: A population-based study. *Archives of Pediatrics and Adolescent Medicine, 149,* 1330–1335.—The largest population-based study of eating disorders and chronic illness.

Peveler, R. C., & Fairburn, C. G. (1992). The treatment of bulimia nervosa in patients with diabetes mellitus. *International Journal of Eating Disorders, 11,* 45–53.—A paper describing a cognitive-behavioral approach to the treatment of eating disorders associated with diabetes.

Peveler, R. C., Fairburn, C. G., Boller, I., & Dunger, D. (1992). Eating disorders in adolescents with IDDM: A controlled study. *Diabetes Care, 15,* 1356–1360.—An example of a study that did not confirm an increased prevalence of eating disorders associated with diabetes.

Pumariega, A. J., Pursell, J., Spock, A., & Jones, J. D. (1986). Eating disorders in adolescents with cystic fibrosis. *Journal of the American Academy of Child and Adolescent Psychiatry, 25,* 269–275.—A study of cystic fibrosis and eating disorders.

Rodin, G., & Daneman, D. (1992). Eating disorders in IDDM: A problematic association. *Diabetes Care, 15,* 1402–1412.—A comprehensive review of insulin-dependent diabetes mellitus and eating disorders, including the earlier studies.

Rydall, A. C., Rodin, G. M., Olmsted, M. P., Devenyi, R. G., & Daneman, D. (1997). Disordered eating behavior and microvascular complications in young women with insulin-dependent diabetes mellitus. *New England Journal of Medicine, 336,* 1849–1854.—A longtitudinal study showing the effect of both clinical and subclinical eating disorders on the development of diabetic retinopathy.

Steel, J. M., Young, R. J., Lloyd, G. G., & Clarke, B. F. (1987). Clinically apparent eating disorders in young diabetic women: Associations with painful neuropathy and other complications. *British Medical Journal, 294,* 859–862.—An early study showing the impact of eating disorders on the medical complications of diabetes.

# Treatment and Prevention of Eating Disorders

# 52

# Eating Disorder Services

## ALLAN S. KAPLAN

In devising comprehensive specialized programs in the new millennium to treat patients with eating disorders, it is important for health care administrators and providers to attend to the organization of services so that available resources are utilized in the most expedient and cost-effective manner. In particular, attention needs to be paid to the philosophical and conceptual characteristics of such programs, their clinical and educational components, their role in advocacy, and their administrative structure. This chapter addresses each of these characteristics in turn. More detailed consideration of many of these topics may be found in subsequent chapters in this book.

## CONCEPTUAL CHARACTERISTICS

The ideal comprehensive treatment program for eating disorders should have the following characteristics:

1. *The program should be multidisciplinary.* Because of the complex nature of eating disorders, a multidimensional–multidisciplinary treatment approach is required in order to provide competent care. Ideally, the members of the multidisciplinary team should be clinicians who have experience treating patients with severe and persistent mental illness. The team should include a psychiatrist trained in the assessment and treatment of patients with the full range of eating disorders (viz., anorexia nervosa, bulimia nervosa, and atypical eating disorders), including their medical management. The nonmedical clinicians should include psychologists trained in those evidence-based psychotherapies, both group and individual, known to be effective in the treatment of eating disorders; a nutritionist experienced in the nutritional care of these patients; a social worker experienced in working with the families of patients with eating disorders; an occupational therapist skilled in the psychosocial rehabilitation of patients with anorexia nervosa and bulimia

nervosa; and nursing staff familiar and comfortable in dealing with the medical and psychiatric needs of these patients.

2. *The program should follow up-to-date published treatment guidelines.* These should describe the mainstream, generally accepted approach to the treatment of these conditions. An example is the American Psychiatric Association's *Practice Guidelines for the Treatment of Patients with Eating Disorders*, published in January 2000. In addition, the program should provide care that is eclectic, encompassing a wide range of modalities: nutritional rehabilitation; medical stabilization; individual, group, and family psychotherapy; and pharmacotherapy. Such treatments should be focused on both the normalization of disturbed eating behaviors, including weight gain where appropriate, and the psychiatric care required to normalize disturbed attitudes and beliefs about weight and shape, and to treat comorbid conditions.

3. *The program should provide evidence-based care.* It is necessary, but not sufficient, that the program utilize interventions that have been described in the literature as effective for the treatment of patients with anorexia nervosa and bulimia nervosa. The program needs to clearly establish that its own delivery of such interventions is effective in alleviating core eating disorder symptoms. This requires a database that evaluates the pre- and posttreatment status of patients as part of a comprehensive and ongoing system of program evaluation.

4. *The program should provide care that is cost-effective.* This can be accomplished by providing a range of treatment intensities in a "stepped care" fashion, so that the least intensive, least costly interventions are given to the largest number of patients initially, with the more intensive, more costly treatments (i.e., inpatient and day treatments) being reserved for the sickest, most treatment-resistant patients who have not benefited from less intensive, less expensive outpatient treatments.

## CLINICAL COMPONENTS

The clinical components of a comprehensive "stepped care" treatment program should ideally include the following eight elements.

1. *Systematic and comprehensive initial evaluation.* A system of intake is needed that provides initial assessment of patients referred from the community. This initial assessment should be conducted by a psychiatrist trained in the psychiatric and medical care of patients with eating disorders. It should include a complete psychiatric history and mental status, as well as a medical evaluation, including appropriate laboratory investigations and recommendations for appropriate pharmacotherapy. (See Chapters 58 and 64 for discussions of the use of medication in the treatment of eating disorders.) Following such an evaluation, the patient should be referred to one of the clinical components of the program for treatment. (Chapter 53 discusses the conduct of the initial assessment appointment.)

2. *A brief psychoeducational program.* This is needed to provide patients with detailed information relevant to their understanding of the psychobiology of eating disorders. While most patients with eating disorders require specialist outpatient or in-hospital treatment, it has been demonstrated by Olmsted and colleagues that group psychoeducation on its own leads to a significant reduction in bulimic symptoms in a small minority

of patients with bulimia nervosa. In contrast, such an intervention is largely ineffective in inducing weight gain in patients with anorexia nervosa.

3. *Outpatient psychotherapy.* This should include cognitive-behavioral therapy (CBT) provided on an individual or group basis. It is generally agreed that CBT is the treatment of choice for bulimia nervosa, and it may also be effective for the treatment of anorexia nervosa, especially for relapse prevention once weight has been restored. Such treatment should follow the published guidelines of Fairburn and others for effective CBT in the treatment of anorexia nervosa and bulimia nervosa. Additional outpatient psychotherapy should include motivational enhancement therapy focused on increasing motivation to accept the changes necessary for recovery, as well as family or marital therapy. (Chapters 54 and 55 describe the cognitive-behavioral treatment of bulimia nervosa and anorexia nervosa, respectively, and Chapter 56 discusses family therapy.)

4. *Nutritional counseling.* This provides individualized meal planning focused on increasing caloric intake and expanding macronutrient selection. The goals of such nutritional rehabilitation should include reducing starvation-related symptoms, achieving adequate, medically safe weight gain, correcting nutritional deficiencies, and encouraging healthy exercising.

5. *An intensive day hospital treatment program.* Ideally, this should run for 5 days per week, 8 hours per day. It should provide structured, supervised meals, ongoing medical monitoring, pharmacotherapy when appropriate, and intensive group and individual therapy for seriously ill patients with bulimia nervosa, and seriously ill but medically stable patients with anorexia nervosa. The efficacy of this partial hospitalization approach for patients with eating disorders, especially bulimia nervosa, has been demonstrated by Kaplan and others. (See Chapter 59 for discussion of day patient treatment.)

6. *An inpatient program.* This should provide 24-hour in-hospital care for seriously ill, medically unstable patients with anorexia nervosa. The goal of such a program should be to stabilize patients medically and begin the process of nutritional and psychosocial rehabilitation, which can then continue in a partial hospitalization program. (See Chapter 60 for discussion of inpatient treatment.)

7. *An aftercare and chronic care program.* The aftercare program should focus on relapse prevention as well as vocational retraining and the provision of psychosocial support. Such support is also important for those treatment-resistant patients who continue to have significant symptoms despite having been involved in intensive treatment programs. (Chapter 62 discusses the management of intractable eating disorders.)

8. *Specialized interventions for subgroups of patients.* Certain patients have special clinical needs. Included in this group are patients with an eating disorder and comorbid physical illnesses such as diabetes mellitus (see Chapter 51); obese individuals who binge eat (see Chapters 63, 64, and 94); men with eating disorders (see Chapter 33); and chronically ill, treatment-resistant patients (see Chapter 62).

## EDUCATIONAL COMPONENTS

Educational components include the following:

1. *Public education.* A comprehensive eating disorder program should be responsive to its community and provide educational material as well as regular forums for public

education to its consumers. One way to accomplish this is to have within the program a telephone information and referral service (and possibly a web site) that provides the public with information about eating disorders and available treatment resources in the community, and makes available program staff who are willing to be present in schools, agencies, and at public forums.

2. *Professional education.* In addition to educating students of all disciplines who train within the clinical services, a professional education outreach program that focuses on educating and training local clinicians about eating disorders is an important component of a comprehensive eating disorder service. Such a "hands on" approach enables clinicians to develop key competencies in the treatment of patients with eating disorders, thereby allowing some patients to be treated in their local community without referral to a specialized treatment center, especially if clinicians feel supported by experts to whom they can turn for advice.

3. *Advocacy.* An increasingly important role for a program in eating disorders is to act as an advocate in lobbying government and third-party payers for adequate insurance coverage and the financial resources needed in order to be able to adequately treat patients with severe eating disorders. This role requires evidence-based data to demonstrate the importance, for example, of extended hospitalization for anorexia nervosa patients in order to achieve full weight restoration.

## ADMINISTRATIVE STRUCTURE

The administrative structure of a comprehensive eating disorder program should include a clearly designated head of the program who is responsible for program development, staff hiring and evaluation, budgetary management, and liaising with institutional officials. Budgetary control over the resources earmarked for eating disorder services is critical to maintaining the integrity of the program, including the quality and quantity of care offered.

## FURTHER READING

American Psychiatric Association. (2000). Practice guideline for the treatment of patients with eating disorders (Rev.). *American Journal of Psychiatry, 157*(Suppl. 1), 1–39.—A detailed description of all of the current recommended treatment approaches for eating disorders, with detailed references to support or refute each type of treatment.

Kaplan, A. S., & Garfinkel, P. E. (2001). General principles of outpatient treatment for anorexia nervosa and bulimia nervosa. In G. Gabbard (Ed.), *The treatment of psychiatric disorders* (3rd ed., pp. 2099–2117). Washington, DC: American Psychiatric Press.—This review provides a description of the general considerations relevant to the outpatient treatment of anorexia nervosa and bulimia nervosa, including the role of outpatient care in relation to more intensive interventions.

Kaplan, A. S., Olmsted, M. O., & Mollcken, L. (1997). Day treatment of eating disorders. In D. Jimerson & W. Kaye (Eds.), *Balliere's clinical psychiatry* (pp. 275–287). London: Balliere Tindall.—This review contains a detailed description of a comprehensive "stepped care" program for eating disorders and the role of a day hospital in such a program.

Kaplan, A. S., & Olmsted, M. O. (1997). Partial hospitalization. In D. M. Garner & P. E. Garfinkel

(Eds.), *Handbook of treatment for eating disorders* (pp. 354–360). New York: Guilford Press.—An up-to-date and comprehensive review of day treatment for eating disorders, including relevant outcome data.

Koran, L. M., Agras, W. S., Rossiter, E. M., Arnow, B., Schneider J. A., Telch, C. F., Raeburn, S., Bruce, B., Perl, M., & Kraemer, H. C. (1995). Comparing the cost effectiveness of psychiatric treatments: Bulimia nervosa. *Psychiatry Research*, *58*, 13–21.—This paper provides the only published, retailed cost-effectiveness analysis of various treatments for bulimia nervosa.

Olmsted, M. P., Davis, R., Rockert, W., Irvine, M. J., Eagle, M., & Garner, D. M. (1991). Efficacy of a brief group psychoeducational intervention for bulimia nervosa. *Behaviour Research and Therapy*, *29*, 71–83.—This is the only published study of the efficacy of pure group psychoeducation as a treatment for bulimia nervosa.

# 53

# Clinical Assessment of Patients with Eating Disorders

## ROBERT L. PALMER

The assessment of an adult presenting with a probable eating disorder involves the coming together of a clinician and a sufferer in pursuit of several ends. These include the clinician's attempts to make an adequate description and diagnosis of the clinical state of the patient, to achieve some understanding of the patient's experience, to decide what may be offered to the patient, and to start to establish a working relationship with the patient. Pursuit of the last end will inevitably involve a further process. The sufferer will be making a parallel assessment of the assessor. Does the clinician seem competent, understanding, and trustworthy? Or not? Each of these aspects of assessment is discussed separately, although in practice they all occur together. The style of the encounter will depend to an extent upon the setting and the background of those involved, but, ideally, it will take place within a conversation that feels authentic and fairly comfortable for both parties.

All patients also require some assessment of their physical state. (See Chapter 50 for a discussion of the medical complications of anorexia nervosa and bulimia nervosa.) It goes without saying that the assessment of an anorexia nervosa sufferer at very low weight or someone with exceptionally severe bulimia nervosa will require more attention to the physical than would be the case with less precarious disorders. Likewise, some such cases may demand more urgent intervention. However, this chapter concentrates upon the general issues involved in assessing a typical adult patient.

## ESTABLISHING A WORKING RELATIONSHIP

The patient will characteristically have mixed feelings. She—or sometimes he (see Chapter 33 for a discussion of eating disorders in men)—may want help but will often be wary about what it may involve. Typically, the anorexia nervosa sufferer will fear losing the tenuous sense of being in control that the disorder provides. The bulimia sufferer may fear exposing behavior of which she feels ashamed or from which she may sometimes derive guilty gratification. Opening up to a stranger about the private world of an eating disorder requires nerve.

The clinician needs to explore such mixed feelings. The sooner they are put into words the better. A simple question about what the sufferer feels about coming along may be sufficient to open up the issue. If the reluctant patient says that she would rather not be there, it may be a good idea to offer to end the consultation. Given the opportunity to opt out, almost all sufferers opt in. Time spent discussing mixed feelings is usually well spent. Furthermore, the issues that arise may begin to teach the clinician about the particular concerns of the sufferer.

It is worth bearing in mind that the clinical setting may well be unfamiliar to the patient. She may have erroneous or distorted ideas about what to expect. It is useful to spell out the purpose, nature, and content of the assessment. Getting implicit agreement about what will happen is important. The patient should retain a sense of autonomy, although with this comes responsibility. If the patient declines to cooperate with particular parts of the assessment, such as weighing or blood tests or certain topics of discussion, then she should not be bullied, although she does need to share responsibility for the assessment being less complete in these respects.

A useful first question is to ask what she, the patient, distinct from anyone else, is concerned about or might want in the way of help. It is a good idea to suggest that she state the obvious and not assume what the clinician knows.

## MAKING A DIAGNOSIS

Diagnosis is useful and using one of the available frameworks—DSM-IV or ICD-10—is a helpful discipline (see Chapters 28 and 30). However, merely slotting a patient's problem into a category is at best part of the job and many disorders fit only the ragbag category of "eating disorder not otherwise specified" (EDNOS; see Chapter 30 for a discussion of atypical eating disorders). Furthermore, many patients have diagnosable comorbid psychiatric disorders (see Chapters 34, 35, and 36); therefore, a general mental state examination should be part of routine assessment.

A presumptive diagnosis of anorexia nervosa may be easy. However, its confirmation or the diagnosis of other eating disorders requires *systematic inquiry about the sufferer's behavior and beliefs and their history*. It is a good idea to explore the timing of onset of any difficulties with weight or eating. For instance, a patient may understandably date the onset of her disorder to the time when she first binged and induced vomiting. However, a prior history of, say, childhood obesity and teenage slimming may be relevant. After taking a history, the clinician should have in mind or on paper a *lifetime weight graph* for the patient and the times of onset of notable behaviors. Asking about what weight the patient would ideally like to be may begin to open up wider issues.

Currently relevant behaviors include the patient's *recent pattern of eating*. The clinician needs to allow the patient to describe both what she intends to eat and what she actually eats. The pattern may be rigid or it may vary. If the diet seems surprisingly "normal," then detailed questions about quantity may be required. Patients do not commonly lie but they may mislead when describing behavior that for them is emotionally charged.

*Bingeing* may be objective, with consumption of unusually large quantities of food and a sense of loss of control, or subjective, when the latter occurs with average or meager intake. Questions should be asked about *abnormal weight-control behavior* such as self-induced vomiting, laxative use, excessive exercise, chewing and spitting, and the use of appetite suppressants. Is the patient drinking adequately or engaging in potentially dangerous behaviors such as washing out after vomiting?

Inquiry about behavior needs to be combined with *exploration of associated beliefs and attitudes*. Eating restraint is almost, but not quite, universal in people with eating disorders. What set it off, and what sustains it? Fear of fatness and an exaggerated view of the importance of body weight are cited in the diagnostic criteria, but often the motivation for eating restraint may be more complex and occasionally quite idiosyncratic. *Guilt and fears of loss of control* may be associated with eating, but so may feelings of forbidden pleasure or a blotting out of painful emotions. *Distortion of body image* should be discussed, but it is rarely straightforward. Such specific psychopathology may be measured with questionnaires and standard interviews (see Chapter 26) but these are neither essential in clinical practice nor should they be used as substitutes for the clinical interview.

The clinician making an assessment may not go into the richer details of the patient's beliefs. However, he or she should gain some understanding and, importantly, the patient should feel understood. The clinician should ask questions with confidence but allow the patient to talk. The patient should feel that the clinician is familiar with eating disorders in general but also able to hear about ways in which she may be different.

The psychopathology related to weight or eating may be thought of as entangling these matters with wider personal issues. Characteristically, these include low self-esteem and negative beliefs. The clinician needs to explore these wider issues and try to relate them to the patient's life. Sometimes the history will reveal patterns of behavior and relationships that suggest the diagnosis of a comorbid personality disorder (see Chapter 36).

## TELLING A STORY

Within the limits of the available time, the clinician needs to try to learn the outline narrative of the patient's life. Such history taking has little that is specific to people with eating disorders, although the clinician should inquire about a history of eating disorders, obesity, and weight-related concerns in the family. Otherwise, a good history should explore the patient's family relationships, upbringing, education, and sexual experiences, together with any abuse and adversity. Likewise, the clinician needs to create a picture of the patient's life now—her strengths and her vulnerabilities. All of this serves two functions. First, it enables the clinician to begin to develop a "story" about *why* the patient came to have an eating disorder and why she remains stuck within it. Second, it enables the clinician to use this story to understand what may be involved for the patient in changing. Of course, the clinician should treat the story as provisional. At best, it will be incomplete, and it may be wrong; however, it is usually better than nothing. Such "story-telling"—or empathetic understanding, to use a more fancy phrase—is the stuff of human interaction. Clinical assessment is the start of the human business of helping the patient to feel safe enough to change. This is linked with the clinician's expert judgment as to what way forward to recommend.

## INVOLVING OTHERS

The involvement of third parties—family or friends—in assessment is potentially helpful. It is usually best that the patient be present when others are seen and that this take place after she has had her say. Meeting with others can enrich the view of the clinician, make the patient feel cared about, and support the people that are involved in the patient's life. It may help a process of change. However, it can also complicate matters and should not be undertaken lightly or routinely. The adult patient needs to feel that she has a choice and that it is she who has the prime relationship with the clinician.

## OFFERING HELP

This fostering of autonomy should continue in the offer of help that is the culmination of clinical assessment. Together with general information and advice, the clinician should share his or her view of the particular patient's state and options. Except in extreme circumstances, when compulsion is being considered (see Chapter 61), these options will always include the possibility that the patient may decide to stay as she is. Discussing this option openly may be more helpful than to avoid mentioning it. By facing up to the difficulties of staying as she is, the patient may be better enabled to face the demands of changing. The clinician should help her to feel that change is possible. However, the clinician should not fudge the issues. Not all treatments are equally appealing, but neither are they equally efficacious. The patient is owed the clinician's informed advice. If she is to recover, the patient has hard choices to make and difficult experiences to go through. These choices are hers, and she should feel supported rather than taken over by the clinician. The encounter between clinician and patient at assessment sets the scene for change. Done well, it can itself be the start of therapy.

## FURTHER READING

Crowther, J. H., & Sherwood, N. E. (1997). Assessment. In D. M. Garner & P. E. Garfinkel (Eds.), *Handbook of the treatment of eating disorders* (2nd ed., pp. 34–49). New York: Guilford Press.—An account of assessment methods, including the assessment interview, assessment measures (see also Chapter 26), and self-monitoring.

Fairburn, C. G., & Cooper, Z. (1993). The Eating Disorder Examination (12th ed.). In C. G. Fairburn & G. T. Wilson (Eds.), *Binge eating: Nature, assessment, and treatment* (pp. 317–360). New York: Guilford Press.—The key reference for the most widely used research interview.

Nathan, J. S., & Allison D. B. (1998). Psychological and physical assessment of persons with eating disorders. In H. K. Hoek, J. L. Treasure, & M. A. Katzman (Eds.), *Neurobiology in the treatment of eating disorders* (pp. 47–96). Chichester, UK, and New York: Wiley.—An account of assessment methods, including measures of body composition (see also Chapter 22), energy balance (see also Chapters 23, 24, and 25), and specific and general psychopathology (see Chapter 26).

Palmer, R. L. (2000). *Helping people with eating disorders.* Chichester, UK: Wiley.—Chapter 6 gives an extended account of the author's views on assessment.

Wilson, G. T. (1993). Assessment of binge eating. In C. G. Fairburn & G. T. Wilson (Eds.), *Binge eating: Nature, assessment, and treatment* (pp. 227–249). New York: Guilford Press.—Reviews the various methods for assessing binge eating, including self-report questionnaires, clinical interviews, self-monitoring, and laboratory methods.

# 54

# Cognitive-Behavioral Therapy
# for Bulimia Nervosa

## CHRISTOPHER G. FAIRBURN

A specific form of cognitive-behavioral therapy (CBT) is the leading evidence-based treatment for bulimia nervosa and is widely accepted as the treatment of choice. In this chapter, the theory underpinning the treatment is first described. Then, the treatment is outlined and the data on its effectiveness are presented. Finally, future developments are discussed. (The cognitive-behavioral treatment of anorexia nervosa is discussed in Chapter 55.)

## THE COGNITIVE-BEHAVIORAL THEORY OF BULIMIA NERVOSA

A characteristic cognitive disturbance is a prominent feature of anorexia nervosa and bulimia nervosa, and it has long been regarded as their "core psychopathology." In both disorders, thinness and weight loss are sought, and there are strenuous attempts to avoid weight gain and any perceived "fatness." At the heart of this psychopathology is the tendency to judge self-worth largely, or even exclusively, in terms of eating, shape and weight, and their control. Rather than evaluating self-worth on the basis of perceived performance in a variety of domains (e.g., interpersonal relationships, work, parenting, sport, artistic ability, etc.), people with anorexia nervosa and bulimia nervosa evaluate themselves primarily in terms of their eating, shape, and weight.

To a varying degree, there may be other, more general, forms of cognitive disturbance, the most common of which is low self-esteem. Many of these patients have deep-seated and long-standing doubts about their self-worth. These doubts encourage self-evaluation in terms of controlling eating, shape, and weight, since dieting and weight loss are socially reinforced in women, and since appearance, and especially weight, seem more controllable than many other aspects of life. Extreme perfectionism is the other characteristic cognitive disturbance. Both low self-esteem and perfectionism tend to antedate the development of the eating disorder.

According to the cognitive-behavioral theory of the maintenance of bulimia nervosa, these patients' overevaluation of eating, shape, and weight, and their control, is the central cognitive disturbance and is of primary importance in maintaining the disorder (see Figure 54.1). Most of the other clinical features can be understood as being secondary to it. They include the extreme weight control behavior (viz., rigid dietary restraint, self-induced vomiting, misuse of laxatives and diuretics, and overexercising) and the preoccupation with thoughts about food, eating, shape, and weight.

The binge eating is the only feature that is not obviously a direct expression of the overevaluation of eating, shape, and weight. The cognitive-behavioral theory proposes that binge eating is largely the product of these patients' particular form of dietary restraint. Rather than having general guidelines about how they should eat, these patients adopt multiple extreme and highly specific dietary rules. These rules (which are one expression of their perfectionism) concern when they should eat, what they should eat, and

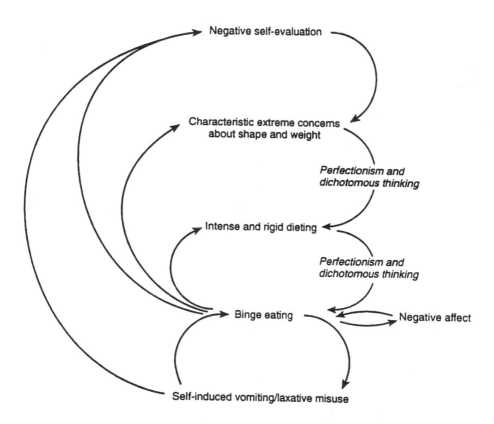

**FIGURE 54.1.** The cognitive-behavioral view of the maintenance of bulimia nervosa. From Fairburn, C. G. (1997). Eating disorders. In D. M. Clark & C. G. Fairburn (Eds.), *The science and practice of cognitive behaviour therapy* (pp. 209–241). Oxford, UK: Oxford University Press. Copyright 1997 by Oxford University Press. Reprinted by permission.

the overall amount of food that they should consume. Most patients attempt to follow many such rules, but in practice, this often proves impossible.

Accompanying the dietary rules is the tendency to react negatively to breaking them. Patients view even minor dietary slips as evidence of their lack of self-control and typically respond by temporarily abandoning their efforts to restrict their eating. This is a major trigger of binge eating. As a result, a highly distinctive pattern of eating develops, in which extreme dietary restraint is punctuated by repeated episodes of binge eating. The binge eating maintains the central cognitive disturbance by magnifying patients' concerns about their ability to control their eating, shape, and weight. In turn, this reinforces the dietary restraint and thereby increases the risk of further binge eating.

The binges do not occur at random; rather, they are particularly likely to happen at times of negative mood, with adverse moods in general tending to undermine patients' attempts to control their eating. Binge eating, however, also has the effect of temporarily neutralizing such mood states, with the result that, for some patients, it becomes a habitual means of mood modulation.

A further vicious circle links binge eating and the compensatory "purging" (viz., self-induced vomiting or misuse of laxatives or diuretics) seen among those with the purging form of bulimia nervosa. These patients (mistakenly) view purging as an effective means of minimizing the risk of weight gain following binge eating, with the result that a barrier against overeating is removed. And, as illustrated in Figure 54.1, repeated binge eating and purging tend to lower self-esteem, thereby further contributing to the perpetuation of the problem.

## Evidence for the Theory

A sizable body of research supports this cognitive-behavioral theory of the maintenance of bulimia nervosa. This includes descriptive and experimental studies of the clinical characteristics of these patients and research on dietary restraint and "counterregulation," a possible analogue of binge eating (see Chapters 15, 16, and 17). However, it is the research on the effects of treatment that provides the strongest support. Indirect support comes from the large body of evidence indicating that CBT has a substantial and lasting impact on bulimia nervosa (see below). More direct support comes from the finding that "dismantling" CBT by removing those procedures designed to produce cognitive change attenuates its effects and results in patients being markedly prone to relapse. The most direct support comes from the finding that, among patients who have recovered in behavioral terms, the severity of concerns about shape and weight at the end of treatment predicts the likelihood of subsequent relapse.

## Implications of the Theory

This cognitive-behavioral theory of the maintenance bulimia nervosa has important implications for treatment. Specifically, it suggests that the focus of treatment should not simply be binge eating—these patients' principal complaint. Rather, their dieting also needs to be tackled, as does their overevaluation of eating, shape, and weight, and their control.

## THE COGNITIVE-BEHAVIORAL TREATMENT

CBT for bulimia nervosa is outpatient-based and generally involves 15–20 one-on-one treatment sessions over 5 months. A therapist's manual is available. The treatment has three overlapping and evolving stages.

### Stage One

Stage One has three major aims. The first is to engage the patient by explaining and individualizing the rationale underpinning the treatment and, in particular, the need not only to tackle binge eating but also to address dietary restraint and the overevaluation of eating, shape, and weight. The second aim is to educate patients about the disorder and to correct any misconceptions about dieting and weight control. All relevant information is available in an accessible form in cognitive-behavioral self-help books. The third aim is to help patients start to regain control over eating. The most important strategy in this regard is establishing a pattern of regular eating, since this usually has the effect of displacing most episodes of binge eating.

### Stage Two

In this stage there is continuing emphasis on regular eating, but in addition, treatment broadens in scope to address dieting in general, together with the overevaluation of shape and weight, and its various behavioral expressions (e.g., the repeated checking of aspects of body shape). The therapist uses a combination of cognitive and behavioral procedures. With some patients, progress is limited by associated problems such as extreme perfectionism, low self-esteem, and poor impulse control. Outside events may also interfere with progress. In such cases, the scope of treatment may need to be broadened and extended in length.

### Stage Three

In the final stage, the aim is to ensure that progress is maintained in the future. There are two elements: First, patients must have realistic expectations, a common problem being that many hope never to binge again; and second, patients need to have a well-developed plan for dealing with any setbacks.

## THE RESEARCH ON COGNITIVE-BEHAVIORAL THERAPY

Given that bulimia nervosa has only recently been described, there has been a remarkable amount of research on its treatment. Over 50 randomized controlled trials have been completed and there have been over 20 studies of CBT. Although almost all of these studies have been "efficacy" rather than "effectiveness" trials, there are reasons to think that their findings are pertinent to routine patient care, not least because the patients have closely resembled those seen in ordinary clinical practice.

The main findings are as follows:

1. The dropout rate at most centers is about 15–20%. This is less than that with drug treatment.

2. CBT has a substantial effect on the frequency of binge eating and purging. Among treatment completers, there is, on average, about an 80% reduction in the frequency of binge eating, and a cessation rate of 40–50%.

3. The effects of CBT appear to be well maintained over the following 6 to 12 months. There are few data on the long-term effects of CBT. (The course and outcome of bulimia nervosa are discussed in Chapter 40.)

4. CBT has an impact on most aspects of the psychopathology of bulimia nervosa, including the binge eating, purging, dietary restraint, and overevaluation of shape and weight. In common with other treatments for bulimia nervosa, the level of depression decreases as the frequency of binge eating declines. Social functioning and self-esteem also improve.

5. CBT is more effective than delayed treatment, pharmacotherapy (see Chapter 58), and other psychological treatments (other than interpersonal psychotherapy, which is comparable in its effects but slower to act—see Chapter 57). Among the psychological treatments with which CBT has been compared are supportive psychotherapy, focal psychotherapy, supportive–expressive psychotherapy, interpersonal psychotherapy, hypnobehavioral treatment, stress management, nutritional counseling, behavioral versions of CBT, and various forms of exposure with response prevention.

6. The most powerful predictors of response to CBT are the frequency of binge eating and purging at the start of treatment (the higher the frequency, the worse the prognosis) and the extent of their reduction over the initial few weeks.

7. The mechanisms of action of CBT have yet to be identified. It seems that the cognitive elements of the treatment are required for progress to be maintained, since behavioral versions of the treatment are associated with a greater risk of relapse.

8. There is evidence that the combination of CBT and antidepressant medication may be somewhat more effective than CBT alone in reducing the anxiety and depressive symptoms associated with bulimia nervosa. Some nonresponders to CBT benefit from treatment with antidepressant drugs. (The drug treatment of bulimia nervosa is discussed in Chapter 58.)

9. Simpler forms of CBT show promise. These include brief versions of the treatment, designed for use in primary care, and cognitive-behavioral self-help in which patients follow a cognitive-behavioral self-help book either on their own or with limited supervision (see Chapter 65).

## FUTURE DEVELOPMENTS

There are two priorities. The first is the dissemination of CBT and the simpler versions of it, since many patients are not receiving optimal treatment. An evidence-based "stepped care" approach to management seems warranted. This involves patients receiving a simple treatment first and only having a more complex and specialized treatment if this proves insufficient. On the basis of the research evidence to date, the initial two steps should be cognitive-behavioral self-help (preferably supervised) and full CBT.

The second priority is improving the effectiveness of CBT, since less than half those who embark on CBT make a full and lasting response. There are a number of ways in which the existing form of CBT could be enhanced, but none has been put to the test. These include more direct measures for addressing the overevaluation of shape and weight, and its various behavioral expressions, and procedures for tackling low self-esteem, perfectionism, and difficulties tolerating and regulating adverse mood states.

## ACKNOWLEDGMENTS

I am grateful to the Wellcome Trust for their support (Grant No. 046386).

## FURTHER READING

Agras, W. S., Crow, S. J., Halmi, K. A., Mitchell, J. E., Wilson, G. T., & Kraemer, H. C. (2000). Outcome predictors for the cognitive behavioral treament of bulimia nervosa: Data from a multisite study. *American Journal of Psychiatry, 157,* 1302–1308.—Predictors of outcome from a large study of the efficacy of CBT.

Agras, W. S., Walsh, B. T., Fairburn, C. G., Wilson, G. T., & Kraemer, H. C. (2000). A multicenter comparison of cognitive-behavioral therapy and interpersonal psychotherapy for bulimia nervosa. *Archives of General Psychiatry, 57,* 459–466.—A large-scale replication of the original CBT-IPT (interpersonal psychotherapy) comparison of Fairburn and colleagues.

Fairburn, C. G. (1981). A cognitive behavioural approach to the management of bulimia. *Psychological Medicine, 11,* 707–711.—The original report on CBT for bulimia nervosa.

Fairburn, C. G. (1995). *Overcoming binge eating.* New York: Guilford Press.—A book for people with bulimia nervosa that includes a CBT self-help program.

Fairburn, C. G., Jones, R., Peveler, R. C., Hope, R. A., & O'Connor, M. (1993). Psychotherapy and bulimia nervosa: The longer-term effects of interpersonal psychotherapy, behaviour therapy and cognitive behaviour therapy. *Archives of General Psychiatry, 50,* 419–428.—A well-known study in which CBT was compared with a behavioral version of the treatment and IPT.

Fairburn, C. G., Marcus, M. D., & Wilson, G. T. (1993). Cognitive-behavioral therapy for binge eating and bulimia nervosa: A comprehensive treatment manual. In C. G. Fairburn & G. T. Wilson (Eds.), *Binge eating: Nature, assessment, and treatment* (pp. 361–404). New York: Guilford Press.—The CBT manual that has been used in most of the recent treatment studies.

Vitousek, K. M. (1996). The current status of cognitive-behavioral models of anorexia nervosa and bulimia nervosa. In P. Salkovskis (Ed.), *Frontiers of cognitive therapy* (pp. 383–418). New York: Guilford Press.—A review of cognitive-behavioral theories of anorexia nervosa and bulimia nervosa.

Wilson, G. T. (1999). Cognitive behavior therapy for eating disorders: Progress and problems. *Behaviour Research and Therapy, 37,* S79–S95.—A review of the current status of CBT across the eating disorders.

Wilson, G. T., & Fairburn, C. G. (1998). Treatments for eating disorders. In P. E. Nathan & J. M. Gorman (Eds.), *A guide to treatments that work* (pp. 501–530). New York: Oxford University Press.—A review of studies of the treatment of eating disorders (including bulimia nervosa).

Wilson, G. T., Fairburn, C. G., & Agras, W. S. (1996). Cognitive-behavioral therapy for bulimia nervosa. In D. M. Garner & P. E. Garfinkel (Eds.), *Handbook of treatment for eating disorders* (pp. 67–93). New York: Guilford Press.—A supplement to the Fairburn, Marcus, and Wilson (1993) CBT manual.

# 55

# Cognitive-Behavioral Therapy for Anorexia Nervosa

## KELLY BEMIS VITOUSEK

In the persistent absence of data, "best practice" standards for the treatment of anorexia nervosa continue to be defined by the "best guess" opinions of experts rather than the "best evidence" criteria of research. In this unsatisfactory context, cognitive-behavioral therapy (CBT) represents an educated guess. The approach is a strong candidate for inclusion in clinical trials and a defensible interim choice for clinicians, who clearly cannot defer treating anorexic patients until these trials are completed.

A CBT model for understanding and treating this disorder was first described by Garner and Bemis in 1982, and further elaborated in a series of papers that specified some components of the complex treatment package. Until the past few years, the treatment was virtually untested—a state of affairs that contrasts sharply with the extensive study of Fairburn's CBT for bulimia nervosa (see Chapter 54) but matches the general status of treatment research in anorexia nervosa. Recently, this area has been invigorated by proposals for shifts in emphasis in the basic CBT model, offered both by its originators and other CBT experts in the eating disorder field. Like the initial approach, however, these suggested revisions are based on clinical experience rather than accumulated evidence about the strengths or weaknesses of existing models. Since we know very little about how well the "traditional" CBT approach to anorexia nervosa works, how it might be improved remains a matter of conjecture.

## COGNITIVE-BEHAVIORAL THEORY

Cognitive models focus on the variables that initiate and maintain anorexic symptoms rather than on remote etiological factors. According to cognitive theories, the core disturbance is a characteristic set of beliefs associated with the desire to control eating and weight. A fundamental premise is that the worth of the self is represented in the size and

*conclusion*

shape of the body. This dominant idea influences individuals to engage in stereotypical eating and elimination behaviors, to be responsive to eccentric reinforcement contingencies, to process information in accordance with predictable cognitive biases, and, eventually, to be affected by the physiological and psychological sequelae of starvation—all of which strengthen the underlying premise.

Although some of the consequences that maintain anorexia are automatic and unmotivated, dietary restraint and weight loss also serve valued functions for these individuals. To a greater extent than other models, cognitive accounts stress the positively reinforced and "simplifying" functions of anorexia nervosa, noting that these explain its most unusual features better than the avoidance-based functions that are also present and influential. These distinctive features include a sense of "specialness," moral certitude, competitiveness, and positive identification with the disorder. Because these elements make a disproportionate contribution to the problems we face in treatment, CBT is organized around efforts to address them more directly and effectively.

Assessment research supports most of the predictions of cognitive theory that have been examined to date. Anorexic (and bulimic) individuals are distinguishable from normal women in the content, intensity, and absolutism of their beliefs about eating and weight, and display some of the expected differences in the processing of related information. Investigators have not yet assembled a compelling case for several of the most distinctive hypotheses of cognitive theory, however, and few efforts have been made to identify cognitive factors that distinguish anorexic from bulimic patients.

## COGNITIVE-BEHAVIORAL INTERVENTION

CBT for anorexia nervosa is based on the approach delineated by Beck for the treatment of depression and anxiety, with adaptations to address specific features of this disorder. These include (1) the ego-syntonic nature of symptoms; (2) the interaction between physical and psychological elements; (3) specific beliefs related to food and weight; and (4) pervasive deficits in self-concept. In theory and in practice, these issues are so interdependent that it seems artificial to assign them to different subheadings for discussion. The general sequence of CBT for anorexia nervosa tracks the order outlined here; however, all four issues are addressed throughout the course of therapy, and many techniques target multiple areas simultaneously.

### Format

This intervention should be delivered on an individual basis by a therapist who is well trained in the general CBT approach and familiar with the specialized problems of this population. One-to-one sessions are essential to address idiosyncratic beliefs, as well as to modulate the pace and emphases of treatment for these ambivalent patients. Individual therapy may be supplemented by family or group psychoeducational treatment. Meal planning is usually incorporated into regular sessions and conducted by the primary therapist, although additional nutritional counseling sessions are sometimes desirable, as long as the consulting dietitian subscribes to a compatible model.

The recommended duration of therapy is 1 to 2 years for patients who accomplish weight restoration on an outpatient basis, and approximately 1 year for those who enter therapy at a reasonable weight after hospital discharge. CBT favors treatment on an outpatient basis, when possible, to maximize personal responsibility for decision making and the transfer of gains to the natural environment. In some cases, brief inpatient or partial hospital care is essential. Guidelines are available for using CBT principles in these settings.

## Developing and Sustaining Motivation for Change

In descriptions of CBT for anorexia nervosa, considerable space is devoted to suggested strategies for engaging patients' interest in the prospect of change and then translating that interest into action. These include recommendations for how to understand the patient and her disorder (empathy and validation elements), how to talk with the patient (stylistic elements), and what to talk about (content themes). Four emphases seem strongly linked to the promotion of change in anorexia nervosa:

1. Thoughtful, nonconfrontational use of *psychoeducational* information to help the patient reassess the perceived risks and benefits of her symptoms and reconstrue their meaning.
2. Endorsement of the *experimental* approach, which casts each proposed step in therapy as an opportunity to gather information rather than an irrevocable commitment to change.
3. Emphasis on exploring the *functional* effects of patients' choices rather than challenging their rationality or validity. The functional emphasis is reiterated through simple question strategies (e.g., "From your perspective, how well has that been working out?") as well as systematic reviews of the advantages and disadvantages of alternative courses of action.
4. Exploration of *philosophical* issues that bear on patients' attachment to symptoms and fear of change. CBT advocates working through each patient's personal values to convince her that her anorexic way of life violates key principles that are even more fundamental to her sense of identity.

The ego-syntonic nature of symptoms seems to shape therapists with diverse orientations toward the collaborative, nonconfrontational stance and the Socratic questioning style favored by CBT. Recent enthusiasm for motivational interviewing in the eating disorder field has contributed to a wider dissemination of these shared principles. While motivational interviewing is often conceptualized as a discrete intervention (delivered in one to five sessions), CBT views the emphasis on motivation as an integral, ongoing part of all treatment efforts. Resistance to change is not an initial barrier that is cleared as soon as anorexic patients are persuaded to enter treatment and begin the "real work" of psychotherapy. In many ways, dealing with motivational issues *is* the "real work" of psychotherapy for this population and should be considered in designing all of its elements.

## Managing Eating and Weight

Efforts to improve nutritional and weight status are essential to the clinical agenda from the inception of treatment. The processes of dietary rehabilitation and weight restoration are not carried out in isolation from the rest of CBT but are closely integrated with the ongoing examination of patients' beliefs and values.

A goal weight range and targeted rate of gain are established on an individual basis, taking a variety of medical and psychological factors into account. The invariant principle is that because the starved organism is not only physically but cognitively and affectively impaired, there are sharp limits to the progress that can be achieved at low weight. Weight is assessed at each session by the therapist and shared with the patient, since changes in weight are vital to the interpretation of data by *both* parties in the collaboration.

Anorexic patients need considerable structure and support in planning their dietary intake. Initially, they are encouraged to eat in a "mechanical" fashion according to prescribed guidelines for the composition, quantity, and spacing of meals, rather than attempt to interpret the signals of hunger and satiety that have become confused by their belief systems and starved state. In outpatient treatment, meal planning begins gradually, working within the patient's own framework of food choices, while systematically introducing larger amounts and avoided food types.

*In vivo* therapy sessions are consistent with the CBT emphasis on experimentation and exposure, and are strongly recommended for work with anorexic patients. For example, eating sessions can be focused on the reintroduction of "forbidden foods" and exposure to avoided situations (such as fast-food restaurants), whereas body image sessions can be focused on trying on clothes or going to the gym. Patients are encouraged to experiment with new behaviors on their own; however, *in vivo* sessions are invaluable when patients are unwilling to consider changes or are too anxious to attempt the more difficult exercises that these sessions can accommodate.

Work on eating behavior and weight restoration invariably provides access to important cognitive material. When patients are asked to live differently, rather than simply encouraged to talk about their inability to do so, both patients and therapists get a much clearer view of the beliefs supporting anorexic symptoms. In turn, unless specific concerns about food and weight are addressed throughout this process, it is unreasonable to expect patients to continue experimenting with behavior change.

## Modifying Beliefs about Weight and Food

Across disorders, the essence of the CBT method is "collaborative empiricism." The therapist works with the patient to formulate her beliefs as testable hypotheses, to collect and analyze relevant data, and to draw (and then act upon) more accurate conclusions. Formal strategies for evaluating beliefs are imparted in therapy sessions and practiced through the completion of homework assignments. In this way, the patient is helped to map out her network of associations about weight and food, and to identify her expectations about what might occur if she violated self-imposed rules. Whenever possible, these predictions are translated into specific hypotheses, and the therapist and patient collaborate in designing experiments to check out their validity. Contrary to stereotype, skilled CBT therapists seldom resort to logical disputation. Instead, they draw on a blend of factual, functional, and values-related material in encouraging patients to reexamine the relationship between anorexic symptoms and their own goals and ideals.

## Modifying Views of the Self

During the course of therapy, attention gradually shifts from the focal symptoms of anorexia nervosa to the more general aspects of the self that may have predisposed the individual to develop her disorder. While none of these underlying disturbances is unique to anorexia nervosa, characteristic themes can be discerned, prominently featuring deficits in self-concept and concerns about achievement, control, maturity, and morality. It is not necessary to shift from a cognitive to a dynamic paradigm to address these issues, since CBT offers mode-consistent principles for work on this level. In the later stages of therapy, clients are encouraged to experiment with new strategies for achieving their goals, new sources of positive reinforcement, and new standards for gauging personal worth.

## EMPIRICAL EVIDENCE

During the first 7 years after the approach was proposed, only case studies and one small, controlled trial were reported. Very recently, three comparative studies have been completed and others are in progress, so that substantially more information is becoming available.

Two controlled trials have attempted to compare CBT to nutritional counseling. A study by Serfaty and colleagues broke down after 100% of the patients assigned to nutritional counseling dropped out and refused further contact; 92% of those allocated to CBT persisted to completion. The unpublished findings from a study by Pike and colleagues confirm this pattern. After inpatient weight restoration, adult patients were randomly assigned to a year of individual CBT or nutritional counseling and medical management. Fewer patients in the CBT condition terminated prematurely (27% vs. 53%) and more met criteria for "good" outcome at the end of treatment (44% vs. 6%).

Another controlled trial comparing CBT, fluoxetine, and combined treatment conditions for weight-restored anorexics is still in progress. Interim results reported by Halmi and colleagues suggest that CBT alone, or in combination with drugs, also confers some protection against premature termination compared to drugs alone. The high dropout rates already evident by midtreatment across *all* conditions in this study are troubling, however, and inconsistent with other investigations.

Collectively, these findings support the tentative conclusion that CBT does further at least two of the goals it was expressly designed to accomplish: higher rates of initial engagement and treatment persistence in these notoriously "resistant" patients. While it is tempting to attribute this effect to the strong emphasis CBT places on the development of motivation for change, such speculations are premature. Since these studies compared CBT to a nonpsychological intervention, they suggest only that *psychotherapy*—perhaps, but not necessarily, in the specific form of CBT—produces better outcomes than nutritional counseling and/or drug treatment alone. Ironically, the choice of weak comparison conditions has limited our ability to test the efficacy of CBT. Further investigation of its merits requires the identification of alternative treatments that are comparably effective in reducing attrition rates.

To date, only two investigations have examined the effects of CBT relative to other forms of psychotherapy. One early study suggested that CBT produced results equivalent to behavior therapy and unspecified treatment-as-usual, although there were some indications that CBT was better accepted by patients; however, extremely small sample size and serious design flaws prevent clear conclusions. In a recent unpublished study by Ball, CBT and family therapy yielded comparable improvements.

## FUTURE DIRECTIONS

At present, CBT is slightly *better established* than alternative forms of individual therapy for anorexia nervosa; however, it has yet to be demonstrated that CBT *works better*. In order to evaluate its relative efficacy, direct comparisons between CBT and other psychotherapies designed for this population are the obvious next step. Since the few data available already indicate that many anorexics fail to achieve full symptom remission with CBT (or any other tested modality), thoughtful modifications to the existing approach should also be tested.

## FURTHER READING

Bowers, W. A., Evans, K., & Andersen, A. E. (1997). Inpatient treatment of eating disorders: A cognitive therapy milieu. *Cognitive and Behavioral Practice, 4,* 291–323.—Descriptive article with suggestions for applying CBT principles during the inpatient phase.

Cooper, M. (1997). Cognitive theory in anorexia nervosa and bulimia nervosa: A review. *Behavioural and Cognitive Psychotherapy, 25,* 113–145.—Critical review of the evidence supporting specific hypotheses of cognitive theory.

Fairburn, C. G., Shafran, R., & Cooper, Z. (1999). A cognitive behavioural theory of anorexia nervosa. *Behaviour Research and Therapy, 37,* 1–13.—Proposal for shifts in emphasis in CBT theory and therapy, with closer focus on control over eating.

Garner, D. M., & Bemis, K. M. (1982). A cognitive-behavioral approach to the treatment of anorexia nervosa. *Cognitive Therapy and Research, 6,* 123–150.—The initial proposal of a cognitive-behavioral model for understanding and treating anorexia nervosa.

Garner, D. M., Vitousek, K. M., & Pike, K. M. (1997). Cognitive-behavioral therapy for anorexia nervosa. In D. M. Garner & P. E. Garfinkel (Eds.), *Handbook of treatment for eating disorders* (2nd ed., pp. 94–144). New York: Guilford Press.—A more detailed presentation of the therapeutic strategies outlined in Garner and Bemis (1982).

Serfaty, M. A., Turkington, D., Heap, M., Ledsham, L., & Jolley, E. (1999). Cognitive therapy versus dietary counseling in the outpatient treatment of anorexia nervosa: Effects of the treatment phase. *European Eating Disorders Review, 7,* 334–350.—Example of an attempt to complete a controlled trial comparing CBT to another modality; the study failed due to attrition from the nutritional counseling condition.

Treasure, J., & Ward, A. (1997). A practical guide to the use of motivational interviewing in anorexia nervosa. *European Eating Disorders Review, 5,* 102–114.—Application of Miller and Rollnick's (1991) motivational interviewing approach for alcoholic patients to the eating disorder field.

Vitousek, K. B., & Hollon, S. D. (1990). The investigation of schematic content and processing in the eating disorders. *Cognitive Therapy and Research, 14,* 191–214.—Theoretical discussion of biased information-processing and self-schemas in anorexia nervosa, outlining an agenda for research.

Vitousek, K., Watson, S., & Wilson, G. T. (1998). Enhancing motivation for change in treatment-resistant eating disorders. *Clinical Psychology Review, 18,* 391–420.—Discussion of motivational issues in anorexia nervosa and proposal of clinical strategies for increasing patients' involvement in treatment.

Wilson, G. T. (1999). Cognitive behavior therapy for eating disorders: Progress and problems. *Behaviour Research and Therapy, 37,* S79–S95.—Critical review of the current status of CBT across the eating disorders.

# 56

# Family Therapy and Eating Disorders

## CHRISTOPHER DARE
## IVAN EISLER

Clinicians have long believed that the family of the patient has an important role to play in a complete management plan for anorexia nervosa. During the early parts of the 20th century, psychological models of eating disorders were temporarily replaced by physical etiological models, but by the middle of the century, the tide had again changed and the patient's family experiences were seen as having a pivotal role. Hilde Bruch, in proposing the importance of formative experiences in early mother–infant interactions, provided a major impetus for a family-based theory for anorexia nervosa. She suggested that, as a child, the anorexic patient's needs received insufficient and inaccurate feedback from the mother. This led to poor development of the child's interoceptive awareness, a distorted perception of self, and a pervasive sense of ineffectiveness.

Although these specific, clinically derived, theoretical conceptualizations have not been backed up by systematic research, a growing number of studies in the past 40 years support the general notion that family factors contribute importantly to the development and maintenance of eating disorders.

Accumulating clinical observations have been supplemented in a significant way by ideas and practice early in the evolution of family therapy. A number of influential figures in the family therapy field gave their attention to the treatment of eating disorders. Selvini-Palazzoli advocated a move from an individual therapy approach to whole-family intervention for anorexia nervosa, and Salvador Minuchin produced systematic clinical data to show the effectiveness of family therapy. The high level of prestige given to the observations of these two innovators gave great impetus to the application of family therapy to anorexia nervosa. This appeared to offer strong support to a specific belief about the etiology of anorexia nervosa in particular, and of eating disorders in general, a belief not confined to the adherents of the "family therapy movement": The disorders were thought to originate in specific, pathogenic family processes. This was true despite the fact that Minuchin himself had drawn attention to a variety of factors other than the family processes that he had described as the etiological sources of anorexia nervosa.

Selvini Palazzoli had also indicated the wider processes of social change as influencing the historical development of an upsurge of cases of anorexia nervosa in northern Italy.

The theory of a singular cause leading to a single treatment method can have a strong appeal. The different clinical evocations of Minuchin and Selvini Palazzoli were augmented by additional comments by other influential family therapists. Cumulatively, family therapists and clinicians, convinced by these arguments, came to believe that anorexia nervosa was the exemplar of a disorder originating in known family disturbance that could be treated by forms of therapy targeting these apparently well-established causative factors. In fact, a careful examination of the research literature does not support the notion that there is a distinctive and consistent pattern of family structure and functioning in patients with eating disorders (see Chapter 38). The differences that have been reported between families of patients with eating disorders and control groups are probably best understood as being associated with more severe or more chronic illness rather than as consistent etiological factors. Somewhat paradoxically, while the accumulating empirical evidence is against a family etiological model, the evidence for the importance of involving the family in the treatment is increasingly strong.

## FAMILY THERAPY AND ADOLESCENT ANOREXIA NERVOSA

Over the years, clinical practice in departments of child and adolescent psychiatry has utilized family therapy techniques to work with both anorexic and bulimic patients below the age of adulthood. This is much less true of departments in adult mental health or internal medicine. Several follow-up studies have suggested the efficacy of family therapy, particularly in adolescent anorexic patients. The strongest evidence has come from a series of randomized controlled trials of family therapy conducted by the authors and their colleagues at the Maudsley Hospital in London. In the first study, 80 consecutive admissions to an inpatient refeeding program were randomly assigned on discharge from the hospital to a 1-year course of family therapy or a supportive individual treatment. Patients with an early onset (before the age of 19 years) and a short history (less than 3 years at presentation) had a significantly better outcome when treated with family therapy in comparison with the control treatment, both at the end of treatment and at 5-year follow-up. Family therapy was not, however, universally beneficial. The more chronic patients—patients with a late onset of illness and those with severe bulimia nervosa—did not gain specific benefit from family therapy in comparison with the control treatment.

The results of the study had some important practical and theoretical implications. Practically, it suggested that family therapy might be used for the initial treatment of adolescent anorexia nervosa, leaving admission and other interventions for those cases with life-threatening physical symptoms and those that fail to respond to outpatient treatment.

The implications of the efficacy of family therapy in adolescence led to a further controlled study comparing two forms of family therapy: the "conjoint family therapy" so far found to be effective, and "separated family therapy" in which the parents are seen as a couple but separately from their daughter. The aim of this study was to elucidate the mechanisms underlying an effective family intervention. Both the conjoint and separated forms of family therapy have similar aims and generally follow a similar course. From the start, there is a strong focus on helping parents manage the symptomatic behavior of their daughter or son. The therapist has to help them overcome their sense of helplessness and find a way of mobilizing the family's resources to help themselves. The therapist at the same time makes it clear that the family is not seen by the therapist as the source of the problem but rather as the best resource for effective treatment. Later in the treatment, as the patient regains weight, discussion of wider adolescent and family issues takes place. Similar topics come up for discussion in the conjoint family therapy and in the separated family therapy sessions. However, in the latter, the patient is not seen together with the parents but is seen alone for half the treatment session by the same therapist who is working with the parents. This counseling involves exploration of the patient's feelings and beliefs about her problems with food, body image, self-esteem, and relationships (especially those with her parents, as they change their attitude to her dieting, bulimic, or other eating behaviors).

A pilot study involving 18 patients and a larger study of 40 patients have shown that both treatments are effective in bringing about a return to normal weight without recourse to inpatient treatment. The larger study suggests that the specific eating disorder symptoms (low weight and bulimic symptoms) are most rapidly helped by the separated family therapy, whereas the psychological concomitants of anorexia nervosa—the depression, low self-esteem, sense of ineffectiveness, and interpersonal distrust—are more helped, at least at the end of treatment, by the conjoint family therapy.

This study also produced some evidence that challenges the view of the family as a pathogenic agent. The measure taken to evaluate family affective communication, expressed emotion (EE), turned out to be a strong predictor of the outcome of family intervention. As has been found in previous studies, families in which one or the other parent displayed an above average level of critical comments that was not lowered during the course of the treatment tended to have a poorer response to treatment. However, when the results were examined separately for "high EE" and "low EE" families, the surprising finding was that the separated family therapy was associated with greater improvement in high EE families than the conjoint family therapy.

Two other findings from the earlier pilot study suggest a possible explanation. A 2-year follow-up of the families in the pilot study revealed important differences in how the families experienced the therapy in the two treatment modalities. While parents as well as patients in both treatments had found the major thrust of the therapy (highlighting the serious, life-threatening nature of the illness and helping the parents to take charge) helpful, those in the conjoint family therapy condition were not only much more likely to report having open conflicts or struggles with the daughter but also more likely to feel blamed. This was particularly true in those families in which the initial levels of criticism as measured by the EE scales were relatively high. Moreover, a measure of family satisfaction suggested that those families most satisfied with family life (especially their sense of closeness) at the beginning of therapy were the most associated with a beneficial outcome for their child's eating disorder. The low levels of affective communication as measured by EE in these families can be seen, possibly, as an aspect of what Minuchin describes as showing conflict avoidance. The findings suggest that a form of family therapy that does *not* challenge the family's characteristic patterns is associated with as good an outcome for anorexic patients as a form that has access to and challenges those family qualities. Furthermore, in some families, separated family therapy may be, in fact, more effective. This challenges the notion that the efficacy of family therapy stems from its ability to alter characteristic patterns of family interaction and family organization.

Robin and his colleagues compared a behavioral systems family therapy and an ego-oriented individual therapy. The latter treatment offered weekly individual treatment for the patient and three weekly sessions to the parents. Thus, the comparison had similarities to that of the Maudsley comparison of conjoint and separated family therapy, and, indeed, the results of the studies largely support each other.

## FAMILY THERAPY AND ADULT ANOREXIA NERVOSA

Further treatment studies at the Maudsley Hospital continue to refine our knowledge of the potential benefits of family therapy and its mode of action in groups other than adolescents with anorexia nervosa. Two studies (one published and the other not) have focused on the question of the role of family therapy in adult and mostly chronic anorexia nervosa sufferers. The two studies are not decisive concerning the effectiveness of family therapy in these patients. In the published study of patients treated solely with outpatient therapy, the results were modest. Both 1 year of family therapy and an individual psychodynamic therapy appeared to lead to a better outcome than a low-contact, year-long treatment, with statistically significant differences tending to favor both the psychoanalytic treatment and family therapy. While these findings are of interest, they have to be viewed as tentative, since they are based only on posttreatment results and need to be confirmed in longer-term follow-up.

## FAMILY THERAPY AND BULIMIA NERVOSA

While the role of family therapy in the treatment of anorexia nervosa is now well established, its place in the treatment of bulimia nervosa is less clear. Two of the Maudsley studies discussed earlier included subgroups of severe, low-weight bulimia nervosa patients. In the first study, their outcome both in family therapy and individual supportive therapy was generally quite poor, while in the second study a comparable group of patients responded better to family therapy than to either individual psychodynamic psychotherapy or individual supportive therapy. A small, pilot study of family therapy in adolescents with bulimia nervosa conducted at the Maudsley Hospital showed a response to treatment similar to that found in adolescent patients with anorexia nervosa.

Fairburn's recent finding that an individual therapy focusing primarily on the patient's personal relationships (interpersonal psychotherapy, or IPT) is highly effective in bulimia nervosa—a finding that has been replicated (see Chapter 57)—indicates that it might be useful to explore family therapy more systematically in this group of patients.

## CONCLUSION

Family therapy is now established as an effective treatment for anorexia nervosa in adolescence. Its importance in the treatment of adult anorexia nervosa is unclear. Family therapy is currently being evaluated in the treatment of adolescent patients with bulimia nervosa. The family therapy approaches that have been used with adults (both in bulimia nervosa and anorexia nervosa) tend to be less symptom-oriented than their counterparts with adolescents, and the evidence for the effectiveness of any particular approach is at present weak. In clinical practice, family therapy is widespread and a variety of approaches are used. The systematic evaluation of family therapy is being extended to centers other than the Maudsely Hospital and to different therapeutic approaches and contexts. Replications and modifications of the research described in this chapter are a pressing need, especially in the absence of any other evidence-based treatments for anorexia nervosa.

## FURTHER READING

Bruch, H. (1973). *Eating disorders: Obesity, anorexia nervosa, and the person within*. New York: Basic Books.—An important book that has influenced much of the later thinking about families and eating disorder.

Dare, C., Eisler, I., Russell, G. F. M., Treasure, J., & Dodge, E. (2001). Psychological therapies for adult patients with anorexia nervosa: A randomised controlled trial of out-patient treatments. *British Journal of Psychiatry*, 178, 216–221.—This study, which found that specific treatments had a better 1-year outcome than a low contact "standard psychiatric" treatment, suggests that family therapy and psychoanalytic psychotherapy are similarly effective.

Eisler, I., Dare, C., Russell, G. F. M., Szmukler, G., Le Grange, D. & Dodge, E. (1997). Family and individual therapy in anorexia nervosa. *Archives of General psychiatry*, 54, 1025–1030.—A 5-year follow-up of the Russell and colleagues (1987) paper showing that posttreatment differences in treatment response are predictive of longer-term status.

Eisler, I., Dare, C., Hodes, M., Russell, G. F. M., Dodge, E., & Le Grange, D. (2000). Family therapy for adolescent anorexia nervosa: The results of a controlled comparison of two family interventions. *Journal of Child Psychology and Psychiatry*, 41 727–736.—Forty adolescent anorexic patients were randomized to either a conjoint family therapy or a separated family therapy. End-of-treatment results showed good outcomes for both treatments, but differences in details suggest that different mechanisms may be involved.

Le Grange, D., Eisler, I., Dare, C., & Hodes, M. (1992). Family criticism and self starvation: A study of expressed emotion. *Journal of Family Therapy*, 14, 177–192.—The crucial and deleterious effect of family criticism of the patient on the outcome of family therapy for anorexia nervosa challenges the clinical descriptions of the "psychosomatic family."

Lock, J., Le Grange, D., Agras, W. S., & Dare, C. (2001). *Treatment manual for anorexia nervosa: A family-based approach*. New York: Guilford Press.—A systematic account of a slightly out-of-date version of the "Maudsley method" of family therapy.

Minuchin, S., Rosman, B. L., & Baker, L. (1978). *Psychosomatic families: Anorexia nervosa in context*. Cambridge, MA: Harvard University Press.—This classic work describes the clinical picture of families of anorexic patients and suggests a treatment model for changing the family pattern.

Robin, A. L., Siegel, P. T., Koepke, T., Moye, A. W., & Tice, S. (1994). Family therapy versus individual therapy for adolescent females with anorexia nervosa. *Developmental and Behavioral Pediatrics*, 15, 111–116.—This study compares a behavioral family systems therapy with an ego-oriented individual therapy and broadly supports the Maudsley studies, but with intriguing differences in the detail.

Russell, G. F. M., Szmukler, G., Dare, C., & Eisler, I. (1987). An evaluation of family therapy in anorexia nervosa and bulimia nervosa. *Archives of General Psychiatry*, 44, 1047–1056.—The first published, controlled trial of family therapy for eating disorders.

Russell, G. F. M., Dare, C., Eisler, I., & Le Grange, D. (1992). Controlled trials of family treatments in anorexia nervosa. In K. A. Halmi (Ed.), *Psychobiology and treatment of anorexia nervosa and bulimia nervosa* (pp. 237–261). Washington, DC: American Psychiatric Press.—The chapter describes a series of controlled trials of family therapy from the Maudsley Hospital, including preliminary data from the two more recent studies.

Schwartz, R. C., Barrett, M. J., & Saba, G. (1985). Family therapy for bulimia. In D. M. Garner & P. E. Garfinkel (Eds.), *Handbook of psychotherapy for anorexia nervosa and bulimia* (pp. 280–310). New York: Guilford Press.—A useful account of family therapy in the treatment of bulimia nervosa in an important handbook.

Selvini Palazzoli, M. (1974). *Self-starvation: From the intrapsychic to the transpersonal approach to anorexia nervosa*. London: Human Context Books.—This book, which influenced the development of family therapy, showing its evolution from psychoanalytic psychotherapy, propounds a view of the family etiology of anorexia nervosa.

# 57

# Interpersonal Psychotherapy for Eating Disorders

## CHRISTOPHER G. FAIRBURN

Interpersonal psychotherapy (IPT) is a short-term psychological treatment designed to help people identify and address current interpersonal problems. Its use in the treatment of psychiatric disorders is based on the premise that enhanced interpersonal functioning will result in an improvement in psychiatric state. IPT was developed as a treatment for outpatients with clinical depression and this remains its primary indication. It has been evaluated as a treatment for various other psychiatric disorders and increasing evidence supports its wider use. One of its strongest additional indications is for the treatment of bulimia nervosa. Some evidence supports its use in the treatment of binge eating disorder, and it is being investigated as a possible treatment for anorexia nervosa.

This chapter starts with a brief description of IPT, followed by a review of the research on it effectiveness. Finally, I consider future developments in this application of IPT.

## THE TREATMENT

IPT is designed to be used on an outpatient basis and generally involves 12–20 one-on-one treatment sessions over 3 to 5 months. Variations on this format have been developed, ranging from brief forms of IPT for use in primary care to longer-term "maintenance" IPT for preventing recurrence in depression. IPT has also been adapted for use with adolescents and the elderly. From the outset, IPT has been a manual-based treatment. The original manual (written by Klerman, Weissman, and colleagues; published in 1984) provided a clear, nontechnical account of how to implement IPT. It has been superceded by an updated version (by Weissman and colleagues in 2000).

IPT is one of the best examples of a noninterpretive focal psychotherapy, its focus being on current interpersonal problems. The treatment has three phases. In the first phase (which may occupy up to four sessions), interpersonal "problem areas" are identified through a detailed assessment of the interpersonal context within which the psychiatric disorder has developed and subsequently persisted. A novel aspect of IPT for bulimia nervosa is that this assessment also includes an evaluation of possible interpersonal triggers of individual episodes of binge eating, for it has long been recognized that binges are commonly precipitated by interpersonal events. The first phase culminates in the therapist and patient agreeing on the problem areas that will become the focus of the remainder of treatment.

The problem areas identified in IPT are categorized into four broad groups; grief (referring to abnormal grief reactions); interpersonal role disputes; difficulty with "role transitions" (such as leaving home, starting work, getting married, becoming a parent); and interpersonal deficits (referring to a paucity of satisfying relationships). Most difficulties encountered fall comfortably into one or another of these categories, with many patients having difficulties in more than one of them. Particularly common among patients with eating disorders are interpersonal role disputes and role transitions.

The second phase of treatment is the heart of IPT and typically involves a series of 10 or so weekly sessions. The therapist helps the patient think further about the agreed problem areas, the aim being that the patient eventually identifies potential solutions and then tries to implement them. To this end, the therapist is active and encouraging but not directive—rather, the goal is that patients find their own solutions. IPT sessions have little structure to them and there are few specific techniques, although sessions may include the detailed analysis of specific interpersonal exchanges ("communication analysis"), informal problem solving ("decision analysis"), and some role playing. IPT does not involve formal cognitive restructuring, nor does it include self-monitoring or homework tasks. Thus, IPT is quite unlike cognitive-behavioral therapy (CBT).

In the final phase in treatment (which usually involves three or four sessions, often at 2-week intervals) IPT become more future-oriented. Progress in addressing the problem areas is reviewed, outstanding difficulties are discussed, and remaining work is identified. In addition, thought is given to possible future times of difficulty and ways of minimizing the risk of relapse.

In addition to the focus on resolving interpersonal problems, IPT for depression sometimes includes limited practical measures designed to reduce disabling symptoms. The form of IPT used in bulimia nervosa has not included such procedures, partly for research reasons (to keep IPT distinct from CBT) and partly because clinical experience suggests that emphasizing symptomatic control can distract patients and their therapists from focusing on interpersonal matters. I return to this point later.

## THE RESEARCH ON IPT

### Bulimia Nervosa

The leading treatment for bulimia nervosa is a specific form of CBT (see Chapter 54). It has proved superior to all forms of treatment studied other than IPT. Results from a trial by the author and his colleagues suggested that IPT was less effective than CBT in the short-term (at the end of treatment and over the subsequent 4 months) but that it subse-

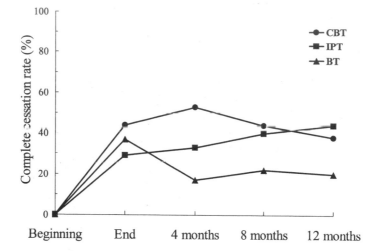

**FIGURE 57.1.** Complete cessation rates among patients with bulimia nervosa treated with interpersonal psychotherapy (IPT), behavior therapy (BT), or cognitive-behavioral therapy (CBT). Data from Fairburn, C. G., Jones, R., Peveler, R. C., Hope, R. A., & O'Connor, M. (1993). Psychotherapy and bulimia nervosa: The longer-term effects of interpersonal psychotherapy, behavior therapy and cognitive behavior therapy. *Archives of General Psychiatry, 50*, 419–428.

quently "caught up" and was thereafter as effective as CBT (see Figure 57.1). This finding has since been replicated in a large multisite study. The relative indications for IPT and CBT are not clear, however, since no treatment-specific predictors of outcome have been identified. Some unpublished evidence suggests that patients who do not benefit from CBT also do not benefit from IPT.

## Anorexia Nervosa

There are two reasons to think that IPT might also have a place in the treatment of anorexia nervosa: First, the psychopathology of anorexia nervosa is similar to that of bulimia nervosa; second, interpersonal factors have been implicated in the development and maintenance of the disorder. As yet, there are no data on this application of IPT, although it is currently being evaluated.

## Binge Eating Disorder

Little is known about the treatment of binge eating disorder (see Chapters 63 and 64). It appears to respond to a variety of treatments and the spontaneous remission rate also appears to be high. There has been one formal (unpublished) evaluation of true IPT (i.e., implemented according to the principles laid down in the IPT treatment manuals) and, interestingly, the treatment was administered in a group format. The comparison treatment was a group adaptation of CBT. Patients in both treatment conditions did well; indeed, their outcomes were virtually indistinguishable. This result is difficult to interpret, since it could represent a nonspecific response to psychotherapy and might therefore have been achieved with a much simpler intervention.

## FUTURE DEVELOPMENTS

The finding that IPT is a reasonably effective treatment for bulimia nervosa is interesting and raises many questions. For example, how does IPT achieve its effects? This is far from clear, although the mechanism is likely to differ from that of CBT in view of their distinctive time courses of action and their very different characteristics. If it were known how IPT operates, it might be possible to adapt the treatment to achieve its effects more efficiently. Alternatively, it might be possible to modify CBT so that it too addresses the mechanisms tackled by IPT. Conversely, it might be possible to potentiate IPT by incorporating symptom control measures of the type used in CBT, one possibility being to combine IPT with cognitive-behavioral self-help (see Chapter 65).

As noted earlier, the relative indications for CBT and IPT are unclear. All other things being equal, CBT is to be favored over IPT, since it achieves its effects more rapidly. On the other hand, IPT is probably easier for therapists to learn and is more widely applicable in its standard form. It may also be more acceptable to many therapists and patients. For these reasons, IPT may be more easier to disseminate than CBT.

The place of IPT in the treatment of anorexia nervosa and binge eating disorder is less clear. In anorexia nervosa, CBT must be the preferred option as matters stand (see Chapter 55), and simpler treatments may be as effective as IPT in binge eating disorder (see Chapters 63, 64, and 65).

## ACKNOWLEDGMENTS

I am grateful to the Wellcome Trust for their support (Grant No. 046386).

## FURTHER READING

Agras, W. S., Walsh, B.T., Fairburn, C. G., Wilson, G. T., & Kraemer, H. C. (2000). A multicenter comparison of cognitive-behavioral therapy and interpersonal psychotherapy for bulimia nervosa. *Archives of General Psychiatry, 57,* 459–466.—A large-scale replication of the original CBT–IPT comparison of Fairburn and colleagues.

Fairburn, C. G. (1997). Interpersonal psychotherapy for bulimia nervosa. In D. M. Garner & P. E. Garfinkel (Eds.), *Handbook of treatment for eating disorders* (pp. 278–294). New York: Guilford Press.—A description of the use of IPT in the treatment of bulimia nervosa.

Fairburn, C. G, Jones, R., Peveler, R. C., Hope, R. A., & O'Connor, M. (1993). Psychotherapy and bulimia nervosa: The longer-term effects of interpersonal psychotherapy, behavior therapy and cognitive behavior therapy. *Archives of General Psychiatry, 50,* 419–428.—A well-known study in which CBT was compared with a behavioral version of the treatment and interpersonal psychotherapy (IPT).

Klerman, G. L., Weissman, M. M., Rounsaville, B. J., & Chevron, E. S. (1984). *Interpersonal psychotherapy of depression.* New York: Basic Books.—The original IPT manual.

McIntosh, V. V., Bulik, C. M., McKenzie, J. M., Luty, S. E., & Jordan, J. (2000). Interpersonal psy-
    chotherapy for anorexia nervosa. *International Journal of Eating Disorders, 27,* 125–139.—A
    description of the use of IPT in the treatment of anorexia nervosa.
Weissman, M. M., Markowitz, J. C., & Klerman, G. L. (2000). *Comprehensive guide to interper-
    sonal psychotherapy.* New York: Basic Books.—The revised IPT manual.
Wilfley, D. E., MacKenzie, K. R., Welch, R. R., Ayres, V. E., & Weissman, M. M. (2000). *Interper-
    sonal psychotherapy for group.* New York: Basic Books.—A description of group IPT.

# 58

# Pharmacological Treatment of Anorexia Nervosa and Bulimia Nervosa

## B. TIMOTHY WALSH

There has been substantial research on the pharmacotherapy of eating disorders and medication is clearly of benefit for patients with bulimia nervosa. On the other hand, significant questions remain about when and for which patients with bulimia nervosa pharmacotherapy should be employed. Unfortunately, there is only meager evidence suggesting medication is useful in the treatment of anorexia nervosa. (The pharmacological treatment of binge eating disorder is discussed in Chapter 64.)

### ANOREXIA NERVOSA

As described in Chapter 29, individuals with anorexia nervosa exhibit a variety of psychological disturbances, some of which bear a strong resemblance to symptoms or conditions known to respond to pharmacotherapy. The occurrence of such disturbances, coupled with the often refractory nature of anorexia nervosa, has led to clinical trials of a variety of pharmacological agents. For example, the disturbance of thinking about shape and weight in anorexia nervosa at times becomes so severe as to suggest the presence of a delusion. It is not unreasonable to wonder whether antipsychotic medication might be of help in reducing patients' preoccupation with such thoughts. Similarly, depressed mood is commonly observed. Since many forms of depression respond well to treatment with medication, antidepressant medication would, on theoretical grounds, seem likely to be valuable.

In the decade after the introduction of the first antipsychotic medication, chlorpromazine, the potential utility of this class of medication for a number of psychiatric disorders, including anorexia nervosa, was enthusiastically touted. However, initial optimism about the benefits of chlorpromazine in anorexia nervosa was short-lived. The only two double-blind, placebo-controlled trials of antipsychotic medications, one of pimozide and the other of sulpiride, showed neither a statistically significant effect favoring weight gain nor any clear improvement in the core psychopathological features, including the distorted thinking about shape and weight. The lack of scientific evidence for benefit, coupled with an appreciation of the side effects of the typical antipsychotic agents, led to a loss of interest in the use of this class of medication for anorexia nervosa. In recent years, some interest has been reawakened by the introduction of newer "atypical" antipsychotic medications, such as olanzapine, which have fewer side effects and are associated with weight gain. Controlled trials are needed to ascertain the utility of such agents in the treatment of this disorder.

In the 1970s, attention focused on the presence of mood disturbance in anorexia nervosa. In part, this attention was prompted by the growing recognition of the utility of antidepressant medications for the treatment of mood disturbance. In addition, it was noted that some individuals who received tricyclic antidepressants for the treatment of depression described a marked increase in appetite and gained significant amounts of weight. Since patients with anorexia nervosa frequently exhibit depressed mood and would obviously benefit from gaining weight, the use of tricyclic antidepressants, particularly amitriptyline, was appealing. Open clinical trials of this medication were promising, but two double-blind, placebo-controlled trials produced minimal evidence of significant clinical utility. More recently, the selective serotonin reuptake inhibitor (SSRI) fluoxetine has also been found to provide no additional benefit compared to standard inpatient treatment for this eating disorder, either in increased weight gain or reduction of psychological symptoms.

The potential benefits of several other medications for underweight patients with anorexia nervosa have been examined under controlled conditions. Cyproheptadine, an antihistamine with antiserotonergic activity, was noted to be associated with weight gain, and was the subject of three trials in the 1970s and 1980s. Cyproheptadine, especially in relatively high doses of 32 mg/day, was of some small but statistically detectable benefit to hospitalized patients in promoting weight gain and relieving depression. In addition, unlike the other agents examined in controlled trials, cyproheptadine was relatively free of side effects in this medically ill population. Nonetheless, it is not commonly used.

Lithium was studied because of its mood-stabilizing effects and propensity to induce weight gain, but it was unimpressive. Cisapride, a gastric emptying agent recently withdrawn from the U.S. market because of cardiac effects, was examined and found to be of very limited benefit. Because of reports of possible zinc deficiency in patients with anorexia nervosa, several controlled trials of zinc supplementation have been conducted, yielding mixed results.

In recent years, several investigators have turned their attention from the acute "weight gain" phase of treatment of anorexia nervosa to the potential benefits of medication in helping to maintain recovery. Many patients who regain weight in a structured setting, such as an inpatient unit, relapse soon after the end of this phase of treatment. Based in part on the similarities between anorexia nervosa and obsessive–compulsive disorder, and on the utility of serotonergic agents in the treatment of obsessive–compulsive disorder, it was thought that the SSRI fluoxetine might be useful in preventing relapse in patients whose weight had been restored. The results of one controlled trial suggest that fluoxetine is of some benefit, and additional studies are currently under way.

In summary, despite the manifold biological and psychological disturbances of patients with anorexia nervosa, controlled medication trials have been few and no pharmacological agent has been demonstrated to have clinically significant utility. For this reason, the use of medication in anorexia nervosa is dictated not by the diagnosis of anorexia nervosa, but by other clinical features, and by the judgment of the responsible physician. One reasonable approach is not to initiate medication until any acute medical problems, such as disturbances of electrolytes or liver function, have been addressed and hopefully resolved, and the patient has gained a significant amount of weight. The presence of a moderate or more severe depression at that point might prompt consideration of treatment with antidepressants. Because their side effects are relatively few, and because of the suggestions of their utility in preventing relapse, SSRIs such as fluoxetine may be preferable to other classes of antidepressant medication. The use of antianxiety agents to relieve distress around meals has been suggested and may occasionally be helpful, but it is usually not of great value. Cyproheptadine appears benign, but its utility is unclear. The newer "atypical" antipsychotic agents, such as olanzapine, may be useful for difficult and refractory patients.

## BULIMIA NERVOSA

In contrast to the rather disappointing state of pharmacotherapy for anorexia nervosa, investigations of the benefit of medication for patients with bulimia nervosa have been clearly rewarding. The most convincing evidence of clinical utility is for antidepressant medications. Controlled trials of other agents including anticonvulsants, lithium, and the serotonin agonist fenfluramine have been either negative or equivocal, and these agents are only rarely used. An interesting recent study has suggested that the serotonin antagonist and antiemetic ondansetron may be helpful for refractory patients.

Investigations of antidepressant medication in the treatment of bulimia nervosa were prompted by the now widely accepted observation that there is an increased frequency of mood disturbance associated with this eating disorder. This observation led to a series of double-blind, placebo-controlled trials of antidepressant medication in bulimia nervosa. Most classes of antidepressant medication have been examined, including the tricyclic antidepressants, monoamine oxidase inhibitors, an SSRI, and atypical antidepressants such as bupropion and trazodone. In almost all the controlled trials, antidepressant medication has proven superior to placebo in terms of reduction of binge frequency. Generally, patients' mood disturbance and preoccupation with shape and weight also show greater improvement with medication than with placebo.

While the data from these studies represent a significant contribution to our knowledge of treatment strategies for bulimia nervosa, they have also raised a number of provocative and important questions. One major question that remains unresolved is why antidepressant medications are effective in the treatment of bulimia nervosa. Although the use of antidepressant medication was initially prompted by the presence of the depressed mood observed in many patients, it does not appear that the "antibulimic" efficacy of antidepressants is related to their effects on mood. In none of the controlled studies has the presence or degree of mood disturbance been found to be a significant predictor of response to antidepressant medication. In several studies, the response of patients with bulimia nervosa who were not depressed was compared to the response of similar patients who were depressed at the time of randomization. In general, the nondepressed patients obtained equivalent benefit to that obtained by the depressed patients. Thus, it does not appear that the pretreatment presence of depression is of any use in identifying those patients whose eating behavior is most likely to benefit from treatment with antidepressant medication.

Studies of the SSRI fluoxetine have provided another indication that the mechanism by which antidepressants lead to improvement in bulimia nervosa may differ from the mechanism responsible for relief of depression. In a clinical trial involving almost 400 patients, it was found that 60 mg of fluoxetine per day, but not 20 mg of fluoxetine per day, was clearly superior to placebo. Since fluoxetine at a dose of 20 mg per day is known to be effective in the treatment of depression, the observation that a higher dose is needed to treat bulimia nervosa suggests that the mechanism by which fluoxetine produces improvement is different from that by which it relieves depression.

The controlled trials of antidepressants for bulimia nervosa have also identified two significant clinical problems. First, in most studies, only a minority of patients achieve remission from binge eating and purging during medication treatment. Second, it is not clear that the improvement attained during medication treatment is sustained with continued medication, and even less clear that a time-limited course of medication will produce lasting improvement.

In addition, certain forms of psychotherapy, particularly cognitive-behavioral therapy (see Chapter 54), are clearly effective in the treatment of bulimia nervosa. The work conducted to date suggests that cognitive-behavioral therapy yields superior results when compared to a single course of a single antidepressant agent. The benefits of cognitive-behavioral therapy appear to be enhanced somewhat by the addition of medication. And there is also evidence that antidepressant medication can benefit patients whose response to psychological treatment is insufficient, or who relapse following the end of psychotherapy.

In presenting treatment options for a patient with bulimia nervosa, it may be helpful to summarize the current knowledge of the efficacy of both psychotherapy and pharmacotherapy. For patients who have not been previously treated and who are not seriously depressed, it is generally appropriate to recommend a trial of an evidence-based psychotherapy (especially cognitive-behavioral therapy) before initiating medication. Antidepressant medication should be considered particularly when the patient has failed or is failing to respond adequately to a course of good psychotherapy, or when the patient has a depressive syndrome sufficiently severe to merit treatment independent of its association with bulimia nervosa. While there is no evidence that any one antidepressant is superior in the treatment of bulimia nervosa, fluoxetine has two advantages: established efficacy when used at a dose of 60 mg/day and relative freedom from side effects. Additional studies are required to identify patient characteristics that identify persons most likely to benefit from treatment with antidepressant medication.

## FURTHER READING

American Psychiatric Association. (2000). Guideline for the treatment of patients with eating disorders (revision). *American Journal of Psychiatry, 157*(Suppl.), 1–39.—An authoritative review of the treatment of eating disorders, with suggestions regarding medication.

Attia, E., Haiman, C., Walsh, B. T., & Flater, S. R. (1998). Does fluoxetine augment the inpatient treatment of anorexia nervosa? *American Journal of Psychiatry, 155*, 548–551.—Evidence that fluoxetine does *not* provide additional benefits to patients receiving treatment on an inpatient unit.

Kaye, W. H., Nagata, T., Weltzin, T. E., Hsu, L. K. G., Sokol, M. S., McConaha, C., Plotnicov, K. H., Weise, J., & Deep, D. (2001). Double-blind placebo-controlled administration of fluoxetine in restricting and restricting-purging-type anorexia nervosa. *Biological Psychiatry, 49,* 644–652.—Evidence supporting the use of fluoxetine in the prevention of relapse in anorexia nervosa.

Mayer, L. E. S., & Walsh, B. T. (1998). Eating disorders. In B. T. Walsh (Ed.), *Child psychopharmacology* (pp. 149–174). Washington, DC: American Psychiatric Association Press.—A detailed review of the place of medication in the treatment of eating disorders, with comments regarding the use of medications in younger patients.

Walsh, B. T., Agras, W. S., Devlin, M. J., Fairburn, C. G., Wilson, G. T., Kahn, C., & Chally, M. K. (2000). Fluoxetine in bulimia nervosa following poor response to psychotherapy. *American Journal of Psychiatry, 157,* 1332–1334.—Evidence that fluoxetine may benefit patients who have not responded sufficiently to, or who have relapsed following, a course of psychotherapy.

Walsh, B. T., Wilson, G. T., Loeb, K. L., Devlin, M. J., Pike, K. M., Roose, S. P., Flciss, J., & Waternaux, C. (1997). Medication and psychotherapy in the treatment of bulimia nervosa. *American Journal of Psychiatry, 154,* 523–531.—Evidence that medication adds modestly to the benefits of psychological treatment.

# 59

# Day Hospital Treatment of Anorexia Nervosa and Bulimia Nervosa

## MARION P. OLMSTED

Day hospital treatment is intended to provide intensive multimodel treatment for moderately ill patients with anorexia nervosa and severely ill patients with bulimia nervosa. It is a cost-effective alternative to inpatient care and a forum for the provision of treatment that is more intensive and comprehensive than that typically available in an outpatient clinic. Day hospital treatment may also be used as a step-down intervention for patients with anorexia nervosa following complete hospitalization.

## STRUCTURE AND GOALS

Existing day hospital programs run 4, 5, or 7 days weekly. The weekly schedule includes supervised meals, a variety of therapy groups, and, in some programs, time for concurrent individual therapy. Family therapy, pharmacotherapy, and medical management are scheduled as needed. In addition to the schedule for patients, the program must include frequent and regular opportunities for staff to share information and make clinical decisions as a team.

Based on a biopsychosocial model of eating disorders, the treatment goals are to (1) normalize eating behaviors by following a balanced meal plan; (2) eliminate bingeing, purging (i.e., vomiting, laxative use, overexercising), and other unhealthy behaviors directed toward weight control; (3) facilitate weight gain for patients who are below a healthy weight range; and (4) address underlying issues. During program hours, patients are supported in their attempts to gain eating and symptom control, and over time, they learn to extend their new behaviors and strategies beyond the treatment setting. There is considerable variability across patients in the speed with which healthy behaviors are generalized. However, the guiding principle is that as treatment progresses, patients should try increasingly difficult eating tasks accompanied by decreasing support (i.e., graded task assignment). Underlying issues and stressors that maintain the eating disorder are identified and processed in group,

330

family, and individual therapy. The schedule for therapy groups should reflect the primary importance of body image concerns and the functional significance of the eating disorder (as a "solution" to life difficulties), as well as relationship issues of autonomy, intimacy and caring, past abuse, and ambivalence about recovery.

Under ideal circumstances, once patients stop bingeing and purging, and reach their target weight during day hospital treatment, they then have several more weeks to consolidate their new patterns and practice normalized eating. Follow-up treatment is essential. This supports the behavioral changes the patient has made and promotes ongoing work on body image and underlying issues.

## PATIENTS

Day hospital treatment is recommended for patients who have moderate to severe eating disorders and have not responded to less intensive outpatient interventions. In practice, this subgroup of patients has significant comorbidity related to depression, anxiety disorders, substance abuse, and personality disorders. Contraindications include acute medical problems, active substance abuse, and acute suicidal risk. For patients with anorexia nervosa, the American Psychiatric Association's Practice Guidelines note that the choice between inpatient hospitalization and day hospital treatment should be based primarily on medical status and degree of emaciation. Most patients with bulimia nervosa who have not responded to good, evidence-based outpatient treatment (viz., cognitive-behavioral therapy (see Chapter 54), interpersonal psychotherapy (see Chapter 57), or antidepressant medication (see Chapter 58) can be treated in a day hospital, but short, inpatient admissions prior to day hospital treatment may be helpful for patients with severe laxative abuse or poorly controlled type 1 diabetes mellitus. (See Chapter 51 for discussion of eating disorders and diabetes mellitus.)

Some day hospital programs are devoted exclusively to patients with anorexia nervosa, while others mix patients from the diagnostic subtypes (i.e., anorexia nervosa, bulimia nervosa, and atypical eating disorders, including binge eating disorder—see Chapters 28 and 30 for discussion of the classification of eating disorders). The composition of the patient group appears to relate to practical issues such as the mandate of the treatment facility rather than being evidence-based. In group therapy, cohesion is promoted by homogeneity in group members, but the similarity in therapeutic issues across diagnostic subtypes appears to be sufficient. It is preferable not to have one patient who is different from the others in the group (e.g., one patient with anorexia nervosa in a group otherwise composed of patients with bulimia nervosa), but for patients with less common characteristics (e.g., being male, having type 1 diabetes mellitus), this may be unavoidable. (See Chapter 33 for a discussion of eating disorders in men.) Women who are well above average weight constitute the subgroup of patients most likely to feel misunderstood and disliked by other group members.

## GROUP THERAPY FEATURES

A weekly schedule, a defined focus for group sessions, and an expectation that patients be punctual, present, and ready to work toward declared goals provide structure and safety for the group. The staff must take responsibility for adhering to the schedule and maintaining a therapeutic focus. These guidelines set a baseline for group homogeneity, for they require patients to be committed to the program and to clearly defined goals. In day hospital programs with an open group format, new patients join a preexisting group with members at various stages in their stay. A group culture has already been established, and most new members will quickly feel the pressure to join the group in working toward recovery. The empathetic realization that other group members may find it more difficult if one breaks group norms encourages a feeling of responsibility and commitment to the group. For some patients this operates at the level of reliable attendance or working with the group during program hours. For others, it may include taking food, body image, or interpersonal risks together. More senior group members may support newer patients by sharing strategies or offering to meet for a meal outside of program hours.

## PREPARATION FOR DAY HOSPITAL TREATMENT

Day hospital treatment can be stressful and demanding for patients. Before arranging an admission, clinicians need to inform patients about expectations regarding behavioral change, the interpersonal demands of participating in intensive group therapy, and the process of exploring underlying issues. Some patients will require a significant period of preparation after learning what day hospital treatment entails. This may involve a short, structured preparation phase of outpatient therapy or a longer period of contemplation or preparatory therapy.

While attending the day hospital, patients should be encouraged to view themselves as working toward recovery 24 hours per day, 7 days per week. This helps to emphasize the importance of practicing new behaviors outside program hours and limits expectations about meeting other life demands during this time.

Despite clinicians' best efforts to prepare patients, some patients will experience obstacles that make it difficult to engage with the treatment. Early in treatment, barriers may relate to patients' fear of change or weight gain, a lack of belief or hope that the treatment will work, or doubts that they can do what the treatment requires. Patients are encouraged to view change as an experiment and not a permanent commitment. However, if a patient has not made significant improvement by the fourth or fifth week of day hospital treatment, this should be discussed directly with him or her in the spirit of understanding what is happening and how to proceed. Some patients end up using a short first admission to increase their understanding of what recovery will demand of them, leaving the program with the knowledge that they are welcome to return for a future admission.

## UNDERLYING TREATMENT MECHANISMS

The multimodel nature of day hospital treatment makes it virtually impossible to identify the active ingredients. Common sense dictates that the components of the program should include treatments with empirically demonstrated effectiveness such as cognitive-behavioral therapy, interpersonal psychotherapy, family therapy, and specific pharmacotherapies (see Chapters 54, 55, 56, 57, and 58, respectively). In addition it may be speculated that day hospital treatment is more effective than the sum of its parts in two regards. First, it may be that different patients respond to different aspects of the treatment and that the matching of patients to their individual optimum treatment is circumvented by providing everyone with the whole package. Second, some components of treatment may have a synergistic effect on others. For example, the intimacy and group cohesion that can develop when patients spend 30–40 hours working together in groups each week appear to significantly augment the cognitive-behavioral structure of day hospital treatment. Similarly, patients who initially refuse to consider certain components of treatment (e.g., family therapy or pharmacotherapy) may become more willing after observing copatients' positive experiences with these treatments.

## EVIDENCE RELATED TO RESPONSE TO DAY HOSPITAL TREATMENT

Although there are only a few published reports documenting its effectiveness, day hospital treatment is viewed as an effective intervention for moderately to severely ill patients. Clearly, some patients with anorexia nervosa require inpatient hospitalization (see Chapter 60), but when clinically appropriate, day hospital treatment is a more cost-effective alternative. Dropout rates for day hospital treatment are not high, indicating that those patients who are willing to try this treatment find it acceptable. One 2-year follow-up study documented a relapse rate of 31% for bulimia nervosa patients following day hospital treatment; relapse was predicted by younger age, higher vomiting frequency, and higher bulimia scores on the Eating Attitudes Test (EAT-26; see Chapter 26) at admission to treatment.

Day hospital treatment "dose–response" has been examined for patients with bulimia nervosa. During the first week of treatment there was an 85% reduction in bingeing and vomiting, and this increased only slightly to a 95% reduction by the end of treatment. A large subgroup (41%) of patients who achieved symptom control during the first 4 weeks of treatment were considered to be "rapid responders." Rapid responders had an enduring response to treatment and a lower relapse rate at 2-year follow-up. This finding suggested that a lower dose of day hospital treatment might be adequate for some bulimia nervosa patients. However, when the 5-day program at Toronto General Hospital was reduced to 4 days per week, and the length of stay from 10 to 8 weeks on average, there was a significant reduction in the rates of abstinence from bingeing and vomiting. Interestingly, the 4-day program appeared to be just as effective as the 5-day program in terms of helping anorexia nervosa patients achieve weight restoration, their length of stay being kept constant at an average of 11 weeks. (In both the 4- and 5-day programs, 12 patients with various eating disorder diagnoses were treated at one time in an open group format.) Whether 7-day per week day hospital programs have superior effectiveness to 5-day programs has not been investigated. Similarly, the optimum length of stay has not been studied.

## FUTURE DIRECTIONS

The first specialized day hospital program for eating disorders, opened in Toronto in 1984, has had a number of years to refine its approach and study its effectiveness. In recent years, more day hospital programs have been developed, and this trend is likely to continue with the current emphasis on providing sound and cost-effective treatments. Inherent to the multimodal nature of day hospital treatment is the opportunity it provides for centers to create their own particular programs with distinct emphases and modes of operation. For example, programs may differ in their expectations regarding the speed with which patients should achieve symptom control or the degree to which symptomatic behavior is acceptable during program hours. It is to be hoped that, over the next few years, the newer day hospital programs will compile effectiveness data that allow for comparisons across centers and informed discussion regarding essential and active treatment ingredients.

## FURTHER READING

Gerlinghoff, H., Backmund, H., & Franzen, U. (1998). Evaluation of a day treatment programme for eating disorders. *European Eating Disorders Review*, 6, 96–106.—A description, and effectiveness data, for the day hospital at the Treatment Centre for Eating Disorders in Munich Germany.

Kaplan, A. S., & Olmsted, M.P. (1997). Partial hospitalization. In D. M. Garner & P. E. Garfinkel (Eds.), *Handbook of treatment for eating disorders* (2nd ed., pp. 354–360). New York: Guilford Press.—A description of the day hospital program at Toronto General Hospital, which includes the administration and financial structure and a section on the advantages and disadvantages of day hospital treatment.

Olmsted, M. P., Kaplan, A. S., & Rockert, W. (1994). Rate and prediction of relapse in bulimia nervosa. *American Journal of Psychiatry*, 151, 738–743.—A two-year retrospective follow-up study based on the Toronto General Hospital day hospital program.

Olmsted, M. P., Kaplan, A. S., Rockert, W., & Jacobsen, M. (1996). Rapid responders to treatment of bulimia nervosa. *International Journal of Eating Disorders*, 19, 279–285.—An empirical study of dose–response at the Toronto General Hospital day hospital program.

Olmsted, M. P., McFarlane, T., Molleken, L., & Kaplan, A. S. (2001). Day hospital treatment for eating disorders. In G. O. Gabbard (Ed.), *Treatments of psychiatric disorders* (3rd ed., pp. 2127–2137). Washington, DC: American Psychiatric Press.—A description of the current day hospital program at Toronto General Hospital and presentation of efficacy data for the 4-day versus 5-day program.

Piran, N., & Kaplan, A. S. (1990). *A day hospital group treatment program for anorexia nervosa and bulimia nervosa*. New York: Brunner/Mazel.—A detailed description of the original day hospital program at Toronto General Hospital.

Williamson, D. A., Duchmann, E. G., Barker, S. E., & Bruno, R. M. (1998). Anorexia nervosa. In J. Van Hasselt & M. Hersen (Eds.), *Handbook of psychological treatment protocols for children and adolescents* (pp. 423–465). London: Erlbaum.—A description of the day hospital program for anorexia nervosa at Our Lady of the Lake Eating Disorders Program in Baton Rouge, Louisiana.

# 60

# Inpatient Treatment and Medical Management of Anorexia Nervosa and Bulimia Nervosa

## D. BLAKE WOODSIDE

Rising costs and contractions of health care budgets and external limitations on insurability of severely mentally ill patients have focused attention on hospital based treatments for eating disorders in recent years. This interest has not been accompanied by an increase in research as to the effectiveness of various forms of inpatient treatment; as a result, there is little empirical evidence to guide clinicians. This chapter provides a brief overview of the nature of inpatient treatment and indications for the same. The typical medical complications encountered in such treatment are also discussed.

### INDICATIONS FOR INPATIENT TREATMENT

There is some consensus of expert opinion as to when patients should be hospitalized. These indications break down into two main groups: admission for medical management, where there is no expectation of ongoing change, and admissions for treatment, where change is expected to occur. Few patients with bulimia nervosa need to be hospitalized for either reason. Most patients are admitted are hospitalized for specific management of medical complications.

Patients with anorexia nervosa require hospitalization for both brief management and definitive treatment. Severity of weight loss is the usual criterion used as an indication for admission. Seventy-five percent of chart average is a figure often suggested as indicating a need for hospitalization. This translates to a body mass index (BMI; weight in kilograms divided by height in meters squared) of roughly 16.0 to 16.5. There are, however, no published studies examining the efficacy of attempting to treat patients under this weight in outpatient or partial hospitalization settings.

Other situations that suggest inpatient treatment rather than partial hospitalization or outpatient treatments include severe orthostatic hypotension, marked bradycardia (< 40 bpm), evidence of tachyarrhythmias, or hypokalemia (< 3.0 mmol/liter). Individuals with extreme levels of purging or exercise may also benefit from a more contained treatment setting. Finally, some individuals with comorbid medical conditions, such as diabetes mellitus, may require more intensive medical management and thus be suitable for inpatient admission.

There is considerable controversy as to the role of involuntary admission. Most clinicians agree that treatment is most likely to be successful when the patient is motivated to make changes and ready to engage in the treatment. Admissions for involuntary refeeding are most often viewed as an emergency measure that should not be confused with definitive treatment. (See Chapter 61 for a discussion of compulsory treatment.) There are no specific weight guidelines available for when to admit on an involuntary basis, or for how long to maintain a patient as involuntary. However, most patients with a BMI of 10 to 12 will become significantly medically unstable.

## NATURE OF INPATIENT TREATMENT

Inpatient treatment programs should have a mixture of elements, and there is some clinical consensus about what elements should be included. Required elements should include nutritional rehabilitation, medical rehabilitation, psychotherapeutic treatment, family treatment, and psychosocial rehabilitation. The precise mix of these different treatment modalities will vary depending on the age of the patient and his or her individual situation. Males are generally treated together with females, and there are no specific differences in the approach to treatment for men compared to women. (See Chapter 33 for discussion of eating disorders in men.)

Nutritional rehabilitation includes weight gain and the development of normal eating habits. A target of 1 to 2 kg/week weight gain is typical for inpatient settings, with a target BMI range of 18.5 to 20.0 usually being set. Providing patients with actual food is preferable to food supplements, although some patients will require very high caloric intake to gain weight and need to use supplements as part of their caloric intake. There is considerable debate as to what constitutes "normal" eating, with vegetarianism and red meat avoidance being the most typical issues raised. Approaches to this problem vary from totally permissive to rather restrictive. Nutritional rehabilitation should also include the provision of appropriate information about normal eating, and practice in shopping for and preparing food. Two studies suggest that individuals whose weight is not fully restored at the end of inpatient treatment have a poorer outcome than those whose weight is restored.

Most severely ill anorexic patients will benefit from a period of constrained activity, although forced bed rest is not usually required in voluntary programs. The extent to which such patients should be allowed to be physically active is unknown; however, physical activity should not interfere with weight gain, and patients should be provided with information about the physiology of weight restoration and the effects of exercise on this. As well, clinicians must pay attention to the underlying cognitions surrounding the drive to be active, helping patients to identify anorexia nervosa–related thoughts and develop strategies to resist acting on them.

Psychotherapeutic treatment may be provided on an individual or group basis. Specific foci will vary depending on the needs of the patient. While very starved patients can participate only to a limited extent psychotherapeutically, most can benefit from feeling supported. Attention to cognitive patterns typical of patients with anorexia nervosa and treatment focused on body image issues are common components of inpatient programs.

Traditional, more rigidly structured behavioral treatments are giving way to more "lenient" treatments focused on patients who are more ready to make changes, and these appear to have no worse success rates than more traditional, restrictive approaches. Even in strict behavioral settings, it is important to try to avoid having the treatment become a battleground between the patient and staff.

Family treatment is viewed by most clinicians as critical for younger patients and very valuable for older patients as well. There is some evidence to suggest that posthospitalization family treatment is preferable to individual treatment for weight-restored patients under the age of 18. Families should be involved from the beginning of inpatient treatment. A wider definition of "family" is often appropriate for older patients and may include friends, roommates, partners, spouses, and children. (See Chapter 56 for discussion of family therapy.)

Psychosocial rehabilitation is important for patients of all ages. For younger patients, this will focus mainly on schooling. For older patients, schooling or vocational rehabilitation is also important. Issues related to social relationships are almost always prominent among seriously ill anorexic patients, who may require long-term psychotherapeutic treatment after weight and eating have been normalized.

## MEDICAL MANAGEMENT OF INPATIENTS

To whatever extent possible, medical and psychological management should be provided in a coordinated fashion. All patients admitted to hospital will require some basic medical attention. At the very least, this should include a physical examination and measurement of blood count, electrolytes, kidney function, and possibly thyroid function. Care needs to taken to distinguish between starvation-related phenomena and other types of pathology. For example, it is typical for starved patients to have low thyroid indices: These patients do not require treatment with thyroid hormone! (See Chapter 50 for discussion of medical complications of anorexia nervosa and bulimia nervosa.)

Very underweight individuals (BMI < 12) may require close attention when being refed. Phosphate depletion is a common feature of malnutrition, and the carbohydrate load accompanying refeeding will drive phosphate intracellular, resulting in significant hypophosphatemia. Hypomagnesemia and hypocalcemia are often also seen. Abnormalities of sodium and chloride are occasionally seen in underweight patients, usually as a consequence of peripheral antidiuretic hormone resistance. Hypokalemia is not usually a problem in underweight patients who are not purging. An occasional patient will have a grand mal seizure early in the process of refeeding: A neurological consultation is required if this occurs.

Measurement of bone density may be indicated for chronically ill patients, primarily as an indicator of risk for pathological fractures. Unfortunately, no effective treatment has been developed for the osteopenia and osteoporosis of anorexia nervosa in underweight patients. Weight restoration may be accompanied by some increase in bone mass. The role of exogenous estrogens in weight-recovered patients is not known.

## MANAGING INVOLUNTARY PATIENTS

Some patients will require hospitalization against their will. (See Chapter 61 for a discussion of compulsory treatment.) This usually occurs when the patient is seriously ill but unwilling to agree to come into treatment or even to have attention paid to acute medical problems.

The conditions under which individuals may be admitted against their will vary across jurisdictions. Thus, specific indications for involuntary admission are variable, as are the duration of such admissions and the types of interventions that can be employed. However, risk of death due to very low weight, bradycardia, tachyarrhythmias, hypokalemia, cardiac chest pain and severe orthostasis are most often present in patients admitted against their will.

Generally, the least intrusive intervention should be provided. Thus, if the patient's weight is acceptable but her potassium is low, the appropriate intervention should be the administration of potassium rather than refeeding. The involuntary intervention should be as brief as needed to achieve the desired outcome. Thus, the goals of involuntary admission should be clear at the outset.

When patients need to be fed against their will, they should be informed as to the weight they must achieve to be discharged and offered a choice between eating food and being fed intrusively. If they will not agree to eat food, then nasogastric feeding is the preferred method. This requires consultation with a dietitian and a medical specialist, and entails careful medical monitoring. The medical problems most often encountered are hypophosphatemia and fluid overload. Parenteral feeding is much more complex and carries significant medical risk both for infection and fluid overload. This option should be reserved for the most desperate situations.

In any event, involuntary feeding should be performed in the most gentle and compassionate fashion possible under the circumstances, and for the briefest period of time required to meet the goals of the intervention. It should never be framed as a punishment.

## SPECIAL CIRCUMSTANCES

Patients with diabetes mellitus present a particular problem. Most who require hospitalization are markedly unstable, presenting with blood sugars as high as 60 mmol/L. Many such patients require close monitoring initially, and it is often difficult to transfer responsibility for glycemic control back to them. (See Chapter 51 for discussion of eating disorders in diabetes mellitus.)

Chronically ill patients are commonly encountered in hospital settings. For many such patients, formal attempts at treatment are not desired by the patient and are inappropriate. (See Chapter 62 for discussion of the management of intractable eating disorders.) Contracting with such patients about specific treatment or management goals is appropriate, and treatment should be delivered in a caring, nonjudgmental fashion. At times, the wishes of a chronically ill patient will conflict with those of his or her family. It is often beneficial to consult with a colleague about such a patient before a decision is made as to how to proceed.

## FUTURE DIRECTIONS

More research is needed to clarify what elements of inpatient treatment are required to provide a reasonable chance of recovery. At present, the role of involuntary treatment is poorly defined and would benefit from further examination. The role of the hospital in the treatment of chronically ill patients is also poorly understood.

## FURTHER READING

American Psychiatric Association. (2000). Practice guidelines for the treatment of patients with eating disorders (revision). *American Journal of Psychiatry, 157*(Suppl.), 1–39.—This document provides a consensus of clinical and research opinion as to the treatment of eating disorders, including inpatient treatment.

Baran, S. A., Weltzin, T. E., & Kaye, W. H. (1995). Low discharge weight and outcome in anorexia nervosa. *American Journal of Psychiatry, 152,* 1070–1072.—A study suggesting that lower discharge weight may predispose to relapse.

Kaplan, A. S., & Garfinkel, P. E. (Eds.). (1993). *Medical issues and eating disorders: The interface.* New York: Brunner/Mazel.—This book, which summarizes most of what is known about medical complications in eating disorders, is a valuable resource.

Russell, G. F., Szmukler, G. I., Dare, C., & Eisler, I. (1987). An evaluation of family therapy in anorexia nervosa and bulimia nervosa. *Archives of General Psychiatry, 54,* 1025–1030.—A study examining the benefits of family versus individual therapy for older and younger weight-restored patients.

Strober, M., Freeman, R., & Morrell, W. (1997). The long-term course of severe anorexia nervosa in adolescents: survival analysis of recovery, relapse, and outcome predictors over 10–15 years in a prospective study. *International Journal of Eating Disorders, 22,* 339–360.—A study that examines factors affecting recovery and harm reduction in adolescents with anorexia nervosa.

Touyz, S. W., Beumont, P. J., Glaun, D., Phillips, T., & Cowie, I. (1984). A comparison of lenient and strict operant conditioning programs in refeeding patients with anorexia nervosa. *British Journal of Psychiatry, 144,* 517–520.—An early descripion of more lenient approaches to inpatient treatment.

Yager, J., Gwirtsman, H. E., & Edelstein, C. K. (Eds.). (1992). *Special problems in managing eating disorders.* Washington, DC: American Psychiatric Press.—Contains chapters on specific approaches to difficult situations.

# 61

# Compulsory Treatment in the Management of Eating Disorders

## JANET TREASURE

The law in many countries recognizes that patients have the right to make their own treatment decisions as long as they posses the capacity to do so. Legal definitions of patient *capacity* require that the patient is able to do the following:

1. Take in and retain information material to the decision and understand the likely consequences of having, or not having, the treatment in question.
2. Believe the information. (Certain disorders and states, for example, intoxication, may interfere with belief in the information.)
3. Weigh the information as part of the process of arriving at a decision.

The clinical concept of *competence* may be wider than this, taking into account the consistency with which a decision is held.

## THE PHENOMENOLOGY OF ANOREXIA NERVOSA

Much of the focus of discussions of the psychopathology of anorexia nervosa is on the abnormal beliefs of these patients (see Chapter 29). In contemporary Western cultures, these beliefs center mainly on the conviction that there is a need to lose weight. As noted in Chapter 47, comparable beliefs in non-Western cultures often center on somatic symptoms (e.g., feeling bloated or full).

The abnormal beliefs of patients with anorexia nervosa are usually classed as overvalued ideas (see Chapter 29). However, the boundary between a delusion and an overvalued idea is blurred. The level of distress, preoccupation, and action associated with the beliefs of patients with anorexia nervosa are similar to those of patients with schizophrenia. The distinction between delusions and overvalued ideas is made in part by taking into account the evidence upon which the abnormal beliefs are based. For example, the beliefs of patients with schizophrenia may be built upon an abnormal perception, such as an auditory hallucination. The abnormal beliefs in anorexia nervosa may similarly be based upon a distorted perception (e.g., one of satiety) and on biases in data gathering and attribution. It could be argued that they, too, amount to delusions.

Whatever their phenomenological status, the beliefs of patients with anorexia nervosa interfere with criteria 2 and 3 of the previously cited legal definition of capacity. Thus, in many countries it is possible to use mental health law to impose treatment upon patients with anorexia nervosa if, for example, their health or safety is at risk.

## MODELS OF HEALTH BEHAVIOR CHANGE

The accepted role for ill individuals is to recognize their health problems and take action to remedy them. Patients with anorexia nervosa do not conform to this role. A classic feature of the illness is that people with anorexia nervosa do not perceive themselves as unwell. This stands in stark contrast to the overt signs of ill-health observed by others. There are many theoretical models in health psychology that explain an individual's drive for health. Many take a dimensional perspective on health-seeking behavior, placing the sick role at one extreme and self-destructive behavior at the other. Common to these models is the view that health-promoting or health-damaging behaviors are determined by the following:

1. Positive intention or predisposition.
2. Environmental barriers.
3. The requisite skills.
4. The belief that positive outcomes or reinforcement will follow.
5. Social pressures.
6. Health being consistent with self-image.
7. Psychological gains from ill-health.
8. Cues or enablers to act or engage in health-promoting behavior at the appropriate time and place.

If these features are examined with respect to anorexia nervosa, features 1, 4, 6, 7, and possibly 3, do not encourage health-seeking behavior. And when patients with anorexia nervosa were assessed at a specialized clinic using one of these models, Prochaska and DiClemente's transtheoretical model of change in which the health-seeking dimension is broken into stages, they were found to be in the "precontemplation" and "contemplation" stages rather than the "action" stage; that is, they were uncertain whether to classify themselves as unhealthy and needing treatment.

## AMBIVALENCE AND THE HEALTH DECISIONAL BALANCE

Patients with anorexia nervosa are ambivalent about their need to have treatment. Within the decisional balance, the positive aspects of anorexia nervosa outweigh the negative aspects. Anorexia nervosa, rather than health, fulfills criteria 4, 6, and 7 of the generic model. Anorexia nervosa is therefore ego-syntonic: It is seen positively; it fits with the person's self-image; and it provides positive reinforcement. A functional analysis of anorexia nervosa reveals many levels of reinforcement (see Chapter 55). Positive internal reinforcers include the sense of security, mastery, control, and achievement that the illness provides. Anorexia nervosa is also used to avoid negative reinforcers such as the necessity to achieve, to develop relationships, and to disengage from parents. Positive external reinforcers include care and concern from close others and even admiration and envy. Dysfunctional relationships and core values, and beliefs about the self, maintain many of these reinforcers. In contrast, the negative aspects of anorexia nervosa are discounted, reframed, or ignored. And aspects of treatment (e.g., weight gain) may produce adverse effects such as fluid retention, bloating, and a rebound of appetite and distress.

Thus, one of the main strategies in treatment is to accentuate the negative aspects of anorexia nervosa and reevaluate its positive, maintaining elements. This balance between the negative and positive aspects of change, which is underpinned by the severity of the phenomenology, contributes to insight and motivation to recover. (Chapter 55 also addresses motivation to change in anorexia nervosa.)

## ASSESSING THE DANGER

In some cases, the abnormal beliefs of people with anorexia nervosa are held with such tenacity, or the balance of maintaining factors is so tipped toward continuing anorexia nervosa, that the individual's health and safety are put at risk. Anorexia nervosa has the highest mortality of all psychiatric illnesses (see Chapter 50 for discussion of the medical complications of anorexia nervosa). It is therefore important to assess risk factors competently and be prepared to use the mental health law as necessary.

Risk assessment in anorexia nervosa is complex. Body mass index (BMI) is a key variable but there are no simple rules. For example, height, sex, developmental age, rate of weight loss, and other physiological variables, adjust the risk at any level of BMI. Careful, thorough monitoring by both the physician and caregivers is necessary.

## WHAT IS LAWFUL TREATMENT?

Many of the controversies surrounding compulsory treatment in anorexia nervosa relate to the type of treatment that may be given. Errors in logical reasoning contribute to the controversy and to confusion, as illustrated by the following common, invalid syllogism: *Patients with anorexia nervosa may be treated without their consent. Refeeding is part of the treatment of anorexia nervosa. Therefore, compulsory treatment for anorexia nervosa is force-feeding.*

Treatment for anorexia nervosa involves working with the cognitive, emotional, and behavioral factors that fix the patient into the ill role. Coercive behavioral regimes, in which the sole focus is on weight gain, are unacceptable because they are both ineffective and inhumane. In the hands of a skilled team, patients with anorexia nervosa rarely need instrumental feeding. Unfortunately, much of the controversy surrounding compulsion in the management of anorexia nervosa centers on the use of outdated and inappropriate treatments. Thus, although refeeding is accepted by law as a necessary part of treatment, it is also universally acknowledged by clinicians that it does not constitute sufficient treatment.

Another source of confusion, which arises from fuzzy thinking, is to liken a person with anorexia nervosa to an individual on a hunger strike. However, unlike a hunger striker, the individual with anorexia nervosa is not threatening to die to cause others to change their behavior. Therefore, laws about imposing nutrition on hunger strikers clearly do not apply.

## THE LAW AND THE THERAPEUTIC RELATIONSHIP

On the surface, there appears to be a basic contradiction between the collaborative, therapeutic relationship that is helpful in the management of anorexia nervosa (see Chapters 53 and 55) and the use of mental health legislation. However, this contradiction can be managed without confrontation. The therapist needs to be explicit about the boundaries of mental health law and ethical standards, and the need to work with the patient within these parameters. It is bad practice if the therapeutic relationship becomes a battle for power and control.

### FURTHER READING

Blake, W., Turnbull, S., & Treasure, J. L. (1997). Stages and processes of change in eating disorders: Implications for therapy. *Clinical Psychology and Psychotherapy*, 4, 186–191.—This paper describes the application of the transtheoretical model of Prochaska and DiClemente to patients with anorexia nervosa attending a specialized eating disorders clinic.

Dolan, B. (1998). Food refusal, forced feeding and the law of England and Wales. In W. Vandereycken & P. J. V. Beumont (Eds.), *Treating eating disorders: Ethical, legal, and personal issues* (pp. 151–178). London: Athlone Press.—A discussion of the legal status of compulsory treatment of anorexia nervosa in England and Wales.

Draper, H. (1998). Treating anorexics without consent: Some reservations. *Journal of Medical Ethics*, 24, 5–7.—This paper suggests that, for some people, living with anorexia nervosa and receiving therapy can become so burdensome that the prospect of death seems preferable.

Griffiths, R. A., Beumont, P. J. V., Russell, J., Touyz, S. W., & Moore, G. (1997). The use of guardianship legislation for anorexia nervosa: A report of 15 cases. *Australia and New Zealand Journal of Psychiatry*, 31, 525–531.—This paper discusses the use of Australian mental health legislation in the management of anorexia nervosa.

Griffiths, R., & Russell, J. (1998). Compulsory treatment of anorexia nervosa patients. In W. Vandereycken & P. J. V. Beumont (Eds.), *Treating eating disorders: Ethical, legal, and personal issues* (pp. 127–150). London: Athlone Press.—A discussion of the legal status of compulsory treatment of anorexia nervosa from an international perspective.

Ramsey, R., Ward, A., Treasure, J. L., & Russell, G. F. M. (1999). Compulsory treatment of anorexia nervosa. Short term benefits and long term mortality. *British Journal of Psychiatry*, 175, 147–153.—This paper discusses the use of mental health legislation in a specialized eating disorders clinic in the United Kingdom, comparing 81 cases treated compulsorily with 81 comparison cases from the same clinic.

Rathner, G. (1998). A plea against compulsory treatment of anorexia nervosa. In W. Vandereycken & P. J. V. Beumont (Eds.), *Treating eating disorders: Ethical, legal, and personal issues* (pp. 179–215). London: Athlone Press.—Argues against the compulsory treatment of anorexia nervosa.

Treasure, J. L., & Ramsey, R. (1997). Compulsory treatment of eating disorders. *Maudsley Discussion Paper No. 5.* Available at *www.iop.kcl.ac.uk/main.*—This booklet discusses controversies surrounding the use of mental health legislation in the United Kingdom.

# 62

# Management of Patients with Intractable Eating Disorders

## JOEL YAGER

Despite treatment advances, eating disorders of all types may prove refractory to treatment. Intractability may be associated with persistent physical, psychological, behavioral and social impairments, and contributing factors may include temperament, coping styles, comorbidity, and the quality of social support and treatment available. This chapter is concerned with the management of patients with such problems.

## ESTABLISHING A THERAPEUTIC CONTRACT

If patients do not agree with their treatment plan, little of substance is likely to be accomplished. To establish the rapport necessary for effective treatment alliance, clinicians must treat patients with respect and integrity, and convey by word and deed that the patient's well-being is their primary concern. Effective clinicians often convey affection for patients, proactively perform small acts of kindness, and show empathetic understanding for patients' feelings of despair, defiance, and mistrust. Clinicians lacking these qualities are often experienced as uncaring and coercive.

## MOTIVATIONAL ASSESSMENT

Patients with intractable problems vary in their motivation to change. Some maintain a sense of self-efficacy by convincing themselves that they *want* their symptoms. Others identify with aspects of their eating disorder psychopathology, particularly the pursuit of control over eating, shape, and weight. Some fear even contemplating the drastic changes required to overcome their disorder. Clinically, these patients appear unmotivated. Poor motivation may also result from the patient's judicious and experience-based appraisal of her past treatment failures and limitations. Intractable problems even occur in well-motivated patients who fully acknowledge their illnesses, exert good effort, and receive excellent treatment.

Treatment planning requires assessment of the patient's readiness for change. Using models developed in the substance abuse field, motivational stages may be classified as "precontemplation" (characterized by a preponderance of denial or minimization), "contemplation" (in which problems are acknowledged but no action plan is developed), "deliberation" (in which action plans are conceived), and "action" (in which effective activities are enacted). Whatever patients' initial motivational states, the clinician's role is to try to move them toward "action."

Strategies helpful in enhancing motivation include asking open-ended, evocative questions to elicit patients' inner experiences, expectations, wishes, and fears regarding change; listening reflectively; and affirming patients' perceptions and experiences.

## SETTING TREATMENT GOALS

Some interventions require considerable patient participation. Others require only acquiescence. For long-term, intractable problems, achieving consensus on clinical goals is sometimes problematic. When facing intractable problems, clinicians must guard against propensities for either undue therapeutic zeal or therapeutic pessimism. Clinicians should avoid setting unreachable goals. Unrealistic expectations may excessively pressurize patients, assure failure, and result in further shame, guilt, resentment, hopelessness, and, occasionally, suicide. In addition, they may lead clinicians to feel betrayed and resentful. On the other hand, setting therapeutic expectations too low may inadvertently promote chronicity. Steering between expecting too much and too little requires clinicians to constantly assess themselves and their patients.

## SPECIFIC CLINICAL STRATEGIES

• Realistically appraise all resources available for treatment over the long haul. These include access to the spectrum of medical services, social services, and support from families and other caregivers. Resources should not be squandered on treatments unlikely to have reasonable impact.

• Seek explanations for the success and failure of previous treatments from all those involved.

• Develop clear expectations for patients and caregivers, using behavioral contracts where appropriate.

• Establish specific parameters for weight and other key physical (e.g., serum potassium) and psychological variables (e.g., level of depression) beyond which the patient would require hospitalization.

• Communicate frequently with other providers to coordinate care and avoid splitting.

• Offer new forms of treatment if the patient (and, where relevant, his or her family) agrees that the potential advantages outweigh the foreseeable risks. Patients and their families should not be pushed to accept time-consuming (and perhaps expensive) psychotherapeutic, pharmacological, or psychosocial treatments unlikely either to effect sustained improvement or to significantly retard deterioration.

• If specific effective psychotherapies (e.g., cognitive-behavioral psychotherapy—see Chapters 54 and 55) have not been employed previously, weigh the potential benefits of a trial of such treatment.

• Consider new pharmacotherapies. (See Chapters 58 and 64 for discussion of the status of pharmacotherapy in the treatment of anorexia nervosa, bulimia nervosa, and binge eating disorder.) Medications worth considering include specific serotonin reuptake inhibitors (SSRIs) and other new classes of antidepressants. Some patients with intractable anorexia nervosa benefit from atypical neuroleptics, such as olanzapine and risperidone, used alone or to augment antidepressants. Similarly, thymoleptic anticonvulsants are increasingly tried when mood lability and impulsivity are persistent problems. Depending on comorbid conditions, naltrexone and antianxiety medications sometimes help. On the other hand, the potential value of medications should not be oversold. Using medications requires judgments of medical safety and efficacy based on scientific reports, consultation with psychopharmacological experts, informed consent, and close patient supervision.

• Assess patients' beliefs, concerns, expectations, and explanations regarding anticipated problems with proposed treatments. Assess the extent to which refusal of treatment reflects depressive or fearful distortions as opposed to judicious thinking.

• Avoid interventions that patients experience as dehumanizing, unless these interventions are essential for saving life. Treatments should never be inherently punitive.

• For patients whose symptoms are unlikely to change substantially, decide how to best provide humane, compassionate listening and support in a cost-effective manner.

• Offer food-refusing patients who risk death alternatives such as liquid diets, nasogastric tube feedings (including overnight gavage feedings and indwelling nasogastric tubes) or, very rarely, parenteral nutrition. Clinicians occasionally institute nasogastric feedings on a "good Samaritan" basis while seeking legal guardianship, but without patients' willing cooperation, such interventions are usually effective for only short periods of time.

• Electroconvulsive therapy is occasionally lifesaving.

• Leukotomy for unrelenting anorexia nervosa, followed by intensive psychotherapy, may be preferable to less impactful alternatives. Such considerations demand extensive consultations.

• Assess concerned families and provide them with education, counseling, and referrals.

• Direct patients and families to support and advocacy groups.

• Be particularly thoughtful when patients refuse treatment but families demand aggressive intervention. Some patients who are not in acute danger reject all treatments, appraising themselves as unlikely to change. Forcing treatment on chronic patients is rarely effective, but maintaining contact to keep the door open may help. These patients should be provided with food, clothing, and shelter, but no undue restrictions or impositions (except as necessary to sustain life). Families should be helped to accept such situations. Humane clinicians continue to treat these patients with compassionate listening, reinforced with motivational enhancement techniques. They provide ongoing education about available treatment options and offer assurances that they will help when patients request assistance.

• Request consultations frequently. Consultants can provide new perspectives, affirm treatment plans, and help clinicians deal with any negative reactions of their own.

• Unorthodox treatments require extensive prior consultation as well as signed consent and careful documentation.

• Use legal interventions judiciously to save life. (See Chapter 61 for discussion of compulsory treatment in the management of eating disorders.) Before undertaking legal interventions, all persons involved should realistically assess the probable, long-term consequences. The legal dilemmas of food-refusing patients parallel those of other chronically suicidal patients. Few facilities can hospitalize such patients indefinitely, and few patients or families can pay for prolonged confinement. Furthermore, sustained coercive confinement may prolong life but not necessarily improve its quality. Where available, ethics committee consultations may help. With patients who chronically engage in "subintentional" suicidal behaviors, it may help to get all caregivers together to review the case, to discuss possible clinical strategies, and to vent any negative attitudes toward the patient.

• Be realistic about suicide and the risk of death. Although compassionate clinicians cannot actively assist suicide, they understand that some patients are unable to struggle relentlessly. Clinicians and families, often unable to comprehend "rational" aspects of the desire to die, should be helped to accept the possibility of fatal outcomes. The events and issues surrounding death should be processed with survivors.

• Always hold out possibilities for improvement, even when cure is unlikely. For unclear reasons, some patients with chronic conditions experience spontaneous reductions in symptoms over time. Since our prognostic abilities are limited, steadfast pessimism is clinically unsound and humanistically untenable. Prognostications should always include the possibility of at least partial recovery. Telling patients about other patients whose "intractable" problems unexpectedly improved can be encouraging. Clinicians who lack examples should find other clinicians who know of such cases, and learn from them.

## FURTHER READING

Dresser, R. (1984). Legal and policy considerations in treatment of anorexia nervosa patients. *International Journal of Eating Disorders*, 3, 43–51.—A good review of the legal interventions to be considered with treatment-resistant patients in life-threatening situations.

Garner, D. M., & Garfinkel, P. E. (Eds.). (1997). *Handbook of treatment for eating disorders* (2nd ed.). New York: Guilford Press.—A gold mine of effective psychosocial interventions described in considerable detail.

Godil, A., & Chen, Y. K. (1998). Percutaneous endoscopic gastrostomy for nutrition support in pregnancy associated with hyperemesis gravidarum and anorexia nervosa. *Journal of Parenteral and Enteral Nutrition*, 22, 238–241.—An example of how use of aggressive interventions dealt successfully with two very difficult cases of anorexia nervosa.

Goldner, E. (1989). Treatment refusal in anorexia nervosa. *International Journal of Eating Disorders*, 8, 297–306.—A thoughtful review of why patients with anorexia nervosa refuse treatment.

Hamburg, P., Herzog, D. B., Brotman, A. W., & Stasior, J. K. (1989) The treatment resistant eating disordered patient. *Psychiatric Annals*, 19, 494–499.—Another good review that also synthesizes the combined experiences of several experienced clinicians.

Kaplan, A. S., & Garfinkel, P. E. (1999). Difficulties in treating patients with eating disorders: A review of patient and clinician variables. *Canadian Journal of Psychiatry, 44,* 665–670.—A review of patient and clinician-related factors contributing to perceptions of intractability and other difficulties in treatment.

LaVia, M. C., Gray, N., & Kaye, W. H. (2000). Case reports of olanzapine treatment of anorexia nervosa. *International Journal of Eating Disorders, 27,* 363–366.—This paper is representative of the current crop of new psychopharmacological strategies for use with intractable patients. Two patients with chronic anorexia nervosa who had failed multiple other treatments benefited from this medication. Larger studies are now under way.

Ludwig, A. M. (1971). *Treating the treatment failures: The challenge of chronic schizophrenia.* New York: Grune & Stratton.—A humbling account of how the best efforts of competent, hardworking, and well-intentioned clinicians dealing with intractable patients, in this case, patients with chronic schizophrenia, may often lead to frustrating failures and sometimes a few modest gains. For these cases at least, careful behavioral strategies occasionally effected at least modest improvement in some patients.

Miller, W. R., & Rollnick, S. (1991). *Motivational interviewing.* New York: Guilford Press.—Although this book addresses addictive behaviors, the strategies it offers may be usefully applied with patients who have eating disorders.

Morgan, J. F., & Crisp, A. H. (2000). Use of leucotomy for intractable anorexia nervosa: A long-term follow-up study. *International Journal of Eating Disorders, 27,* 249–258.—Three of four cases followed after 20 years appear to have been benefited, and, in spite of residual psychopathology, none regretted the operation or succumbed to the "avoidant position" of weight loss. The fourth patient committed suicide.

Vitousek, K., Watson, S., & Wilson, G. T. (1998). Enhancing motivation for change in treatment-resistant eating disorders. *Clinical Psychology Review, 18,* 391–420.—A review of motivational factors and strategies pertinent to patients with intractable eating disorders.

# 63

# Psychological Treatment of Binge Eating Disorder

## DENISE E. WILFLEY

Individuals with binge eating disorder (BED) typically present to treatment with the multiple problems of binge eating, varied eating disorder psychopathology (e.g., overeating in general and extreme concerns about eating, shape, and weight), psychiatric symptoms, and overweight (see Chapter 31). Accordingly, evaluation of treatments for BED need to take into consideration the impact of the intervention on these multiple problems in both the short and long term. Over the past decade, a number of controlled studies have been conducted on the treatment of BED. Promising, short-term findings have accrued for several conceptually and procedurally distinct psychological treatments, including specialist treatments, behavioral weight loss treatment, and self-help approaches. Positive, long-term outcomes have also been demonstrated for the two specialist treatments cognitive-behavioral therapy (CBT) and interpersonal psychotherapy (IPT). Nevertheless, central questions regarding the specificity of specialist treatment effects and whether BED patients require intervention beyond behavioral weight loss treatment remain unanswered.

## SPECIALIST TREATMENTS

To date, the two most intensively studied psychological treatments are CBT and IPT.

### Cognitive-Behavioral Therapy

CBT, the most frequently studied treatment for BED, uses similar cognitive and behavioral techniques as CBT for bulimia nervosa (see Chapter 54); however, modifications are necessary, because BED patients exhibit lower levels of dietary restraint, more chaotic eating patterns, and higher levels of overweight than bulimia nervosa patients. The adaptations include focusing on moderation of food intake such that it is neither over- nor underrestrictive (i.e., a healthy level of restraint is encouraged to aid in eliminating all forms of overeating); modification of harsh, stereotyped views of overweight; if applicable, promotion of the acceptance of a larger than average body size; and encouragement of weight-control behavior (e.g., increased physical activity, weekly weighing). Across a handful of studies, CBT has been shown to result in rates of binge-eating abstinence of approximately 50% at posttreatment compared to minimal change in assessment-only conditions. Moreover, findings from the author's recent study of CBT revealed long-term efficacy in binge-eating reduction and an abstinence rate of about 60% at 1-year follow-up. CBT also has a beneficial short- and long-term impact on decreasing dietary restraint, modifying distorted attitudes about body shape and weight, and decreasing psychiatric symptoms. Similar outcomes have been obtained in group and individual formats, and some data suggest that longer treatment programs (20 vs. 12 weeks) maximize the number of treatment responders.

## Interpersonal Psychotherapy

Two controlled studies have documented the effectiveness of IPT for BED. It helps patients identify and alter the interpersonal context in which the eating problem has developed and been maintained (see Chapter 57 for a description of IPT and its use in bulimia nervosa). Modifications of IPT for bulimia nervosa include adding strategies that encourage patients to examine the impact of their weight status on relationships and emphasis on addressing "interpersonal deficits," an interpersonal problem area that occurs more frequently in BED than bulimia nervosa. An initial study of CBT and IPT for BED revealed that both treatments were significantly more effective than a wait-list control group, but comparable to each other in reducing binge eating up to 1 year following treatment. In a second, unpublished study (by the author) with a substantially larger sample size, both CBT and IPT evidenced equivalent short- and long-term efficacy in reducing binge eating and associated specific and general psychopathology. Moreover, both treatments evidenced good maintenance of change on these outcomes, and 60% of the participants were abstinent from binge eating at 1-year follow-up (59% and 61% for CBT and IPT, respectively). The fact that CBT and IPT were remarkably similar in their effects raises the possibility that they operate through shared mechanisms. The one treatment-specific difference was a significantly greater reduction in dietary restraint among CBT patients at posttreatment and 4-month follow-up; however, by the 8- and 12-month follow-ups, IPT reached parity with CBT. Although these treatments resulted in a statistically significant decrease in weight over time, neither treatment produced a clinically significant reduction. This negative outcome for weight is consistent across the studies of CBT and IPT for BED; however, this study was the second to find that individuals who cease binge eating lose some weight, while those who remain even partially symptomatic tend to gain.

## BEHAVIORAL WEIGHT LOSS TREATMENT

Behavioral weight loss treatment (BWL) has also been evaluated as a treatment for BED, the goal being to reduce both binge eating and weight. In addition, BWL has several other potential advantages over the use of specialized psychological treatments. It can be used by a much wider range of health professionals, is less expensive, and it is therefore potentially more readily disseminated than specialized treatments. BWL interventions seek to modify weight via moderate caloric restriction, improved nutrition, and increased physical activity (see Chapter 94). BWL holds promise in the treatment of overweight individuals with BED; it appears to have the dual effect of decreasing binge eating and body weight, at least in the short-term. Of the two studies that have been completed with valid assessment of binge eating, both showed short-term reductions comparable in magnitude to those obtained with CBT and IPT. One of the studies also found that BWL evidenced significantly greater weight loss than CBT at posttreatment and equivalent reductions in specific eating disorder features. The long-term impact of BWL in BED is not known.

## SELF-HELP TREATMENT

Preliminary studies have begun to evaluate more cost-effective and disseminable methods of implementing CBT, particularly self-help treatment approaches (see Chapter 65). Two controlled studies offer evidence that both unguided (i.e., a book used independently by the individual) and guided (i.e., a book used in conjunction with guidance from a professional) self-help treatments produce significant reductions in both binge-eating frequency and associated psychopathology. Furthermore, one of the studies found that reductions in binge eating were well maintained over a 6-month follow-up for both guided and unguided self-help. Similar to specialized treatments, neither treatment produced weight loss. Findings from these studies suggest that brief, low-cost treatments can be effective for at least a subset of patients with BED. Future studies are required to establish the long-term efficacy of these treatments and to identify those patients for whom such brief, low-intensity interventions are indicated.

## CONCLUSIONS AND FUTURE DIRECTIONS

Compared to research on bulimia nervosa, the specificity and differential effectiveness of active treatments for BED remain largely unknown. Specialist psychological treatments have demonstrated short- and long-term reductions in binge eating and associated features, but not body weight. Preliminary but incomplete data suggest that BWL may be as effective as these specialist treatments. Since BWL in the treatment of obesity is associated with a high rate of relapse, its long-term effects need to be studied. Self-help approaches have demonstrated efficacy for BED in the short-term, and drug treatment can also be beneficial (see Chapter 64). Moreover, recent research on the use of dialectical behavior therapy adapted for BED supports its further investigation as a treatment for BED.

Studies are needed to clarify the most efficacious treatment for BED and to identify subtypes for whom specific treatments are indicated. Recently, a subtype of BED patients with high levels of negative affect has been reliably identified and shown to fare poorly in low-intensity treatments. Identifying different subsets of BED patients with distinct therapeutic needs will foster the development of more targeted and effective treatments.

## FURTHER READING

Agras, W. S., Telch, C. F., Arnow, B., Eldredge, K., & Marnell, M. (1997). One year follow-up of cognitive-behavioral therapy for obese individuals with binge eating disorder. *Journal of Consulting and Clinical Psychology, 65*, 343–347.—An important study of long-term treatment outcome, indicating that stopping binge eating appears critical to sustained weight loss in BED.

Carter, J. C., & Fairburn, C. G. (1998). Cognitive-behavioral self-help for binge eating disorder: A controlled effectiveness study. *Journal of Consulting and Clinical Psychology, 66*, 616–623.—The first controlled study to evaluate the effectiveness of two methods of administering a cognitive-behavioral self-help program for BED.

Loeb, K. L., Wilson, G. T., Gilbert, J. S., & Labouvie, E. (2000). Guided and unguided self-help for binge eating. *Behaviour Research and Therapy, 38*, 259–272.—A controlled study comparing the efficacy of therapist-guided and unguided use of a cognitive behavioral self-help program for binge eating.

Marcus, M. D. (1997). Adapting treatment for patients with binge-eating disorder. In D. M. Garner & P. E. Garfinkel (Eds.), *Handbook of treatment for eating disorders* (2nd ed., pp. 484–493). New York: Guilford Press.—A detailed description of cognitive-behavioral treatment modifications for BED.

Stice, E., Agras, W. S., Telch, C. F., Halmi, K. A., Mitchell, J. E., & Wilson, G. T. (2001). Subtyping binge eating-disordered women along dicting and negative affect dimensions. *International Journal of Eating Disorders, 30*, 11–27.—A cluster-analytic study that identified a "dietary-high negative affect" subtype characterized by more psychopathology.

Telch, C. F., Agras, W. S., & Linehan, M. M. (in press). Dialectical behavior therapy for binge eating disorder: A promising new treatment. *Journal of Consulting and Clinical Psychology.*—The first controlled study of dialectical behavior therapy for BED.

Wilfley, D. E., & Cohen, L. R. (1997). Psychological treatment of bulimia nervosa and binge eating disorder. *Psychopharmacology Bulletin, 33*, 437–454.—A comprehensive review of the research on the treatment of BED.

Wilfley, D. E., Frank, M. A., Welch, R., Spurrell, E. B., & Rounsaville, B. J. (1998). Adapting interpersonal psychotherapy to a group format (IPT-G) for binge eating disorder: Toward a model for adapting empirically supported-treatments. *Psychotherapy Research, 8*, 379–391.—A detailed description of IPT modifications for BED.

Wilfley, D. E., Friedman, M. A., Dounchis, J. Z., Stein, R. I., Welch, R. R., & Ball, S. A. (2000). Comorbid psychopathology in binge eating disorder: Relation to eating disorder severity at baseline and following treatment. *Journal of Consulting and Clinical Psychology, 68*, 641–649.—A study indicating that Cluster B personality disorders predict higher levels of binge eating at 1-year follow-up.

Wilson, G. T., & Fairburn, C. G. (1998). Treatments for eating disorders. In P. E. Nathan & J. M. Gorman (Eds.), *A guide to treatments that work* (pp. 501–530). New York: Oxford University Press.—A comprehensive review of the research on the treatment of BED.

Wilson, G. T., Vitousek, K. M., & Loeb, K. L. (2000). Stepped care treatment for eating disorders. *Journal of Consulting and Clinical Psychology, 68*, 564–572.—An up-to-date review of brief methods of treatment for BED.

# 64

# Pharmacological Treatment of Binge Eating Disorder

## MICHAEL J. DEVLIN

The state of the field in pharmacological management of patients with binge eating disorder (BED) is characterized more by questions than by answers. Studies of the risk factors for BED and of its phenomenology suggest that individuals who develop the disorder tend to be characterized by (1) a propensity toward obesity and dieting, and (2) a vulnerability to psychiatric disorders, particularly depression (see Chapter 31). In this regard, BED is similar to bulimia nervosa, except that patients who present for treatment for BED are usually overweight or obese, whereas bulimia nervosa treatment samples are typically of normal weight. In addition, the core behavioral feature of BED, binge eating, is similar to the binge eating seen in bulimia nervosa. It is therefore not surprising that clinical trials of medication for BED have been inspired by treatments of known (short-term) efficacy for bulimia nervosa or for obesity, namely, antidepressants and appetite suppressants, respectively.

In evaluating the outcome of medication trials for BED, it is important to keep in mind the target symptoms. Overweight or obese patients with BED (i.e., the subgroup recruited for the great majority of BED treatment trials) suffer from (1) a somatic disturbance of weight; (2) a behavioral disturbance of eating; (3) often a psychological disturbance of body weight/shape-related distress and, sometimes, depressive features. Any or all of these features are potential targets for treatment, and patients may selectively improve in one or more areas. It is also crucial to consider the long- as well as short-term outcome. Treatments that are helpful in the short term may fail to demonstrate any advantage when examined 1 to 5 years later and, arguably, may interfere with other forms of treatment. For patients who are doing well with short-term medication treatment, it is important to consider the effect of medication discontinuation or, alternatively, the pros and cons of chronic medication treatment.

Thus, the question in evaluating medication treatments for BED is not simply: Do medications work? Rather, one must ask: Are medications helpful in the short- and long-term? If so, what features of BED do they treat? Might they be a useful adjunct to psychological treatments? At what stage of treatment are they most useful? Are particular patients most likely to benefit from medication? Is there a downside to combining medication with other forms of treatment? And finally, if medication helps, does this benefit persist over time, and what happens after medication is discontinued?

## MEDICATION AS THE SOLE TREATMENT

Although the existence of a distinct syndrome of binge eating among obese persons has been recognized since the 1950s, the formulation of BED as an eating disorder in the early 1990s suggested new possibilities for pharmacological treatment. Specifically, the known short-term efficacy of antidepressants in the treatment of bulimia nervosa suggested that these medications might be helpful for patients with BED as well. Several clinical trials have demonstrated that treatment with antidepressant medications including tricyclic antidepressants and high-dose selective serotonin reuptake inhibitors (SSRIs), is associated with a short-term reduction in binge frequency of about 60–90%, substantially greater than the response to placebo. Weight loss is generally modest at best, although one recent trial using sertraline reported an estimated 12.3 pound weight loss in 6 weeks. Improvement in binge eating is variably associated with improvement in depressive symptoms and, as is the case for bulimia nervosa, does not appear to be mediated by improvement in these symptoms. Studies with follow-up information on patients following discontinuation of medication generally report substantial deterioration of beneficial effects.

An alternative pharmacological approach is the use of appetite suppressants (see Chapter 99 for discussion of their use in obesity). A study of dexfenfluramine for BED reported substantial short-term reduction in binge frequency that did not persist at 4-month postdiscontinuation follow-up and, surprisingly, was not accompanied by weight loss. Although fenfluramine and dexfenfluramine are no longer available, studies of sibutramine for patients with BED are under way.

Additional pharmacological approaches that have been the subject of small studies and case reports include the use of the opiate antagonist naltrexone and the anticonvulsant topiramate. Naltrexone (or, in one case report, naltrexone plus fluoxetine) appears to be associated with a reduction in the urge to binge-eat and in actual binge eating, but it is not clear that this exceeds the response to placebo. There is preliminary evidence that treatment with topiramate, an anticonvulsant and mood-stabilizer known to be associated with appetite suppression and weight loss, yields a short-term reduction in binge eating in patients with BED in the setting of a comorbid Axis I psychiatric disorder.

One notable feature of many clinical trials of medications for BED is the high short-term placebo response rate. In one study with a single-blind placebo lead-in, nearly half of the study subjects were withdrawn due to placebo response. This suggests a marked ability of many patients with BED to suppress binge eating in the short term, the importance of placebo-controlled trials, and the degree of caution needed in interpreting positive findings from noncontrolled studies and case reports.

## MEDICATION AS AN ADJUNCT TO PSYCHOSOCIAL TREATMENT

In theory, adding medication to psychological treatment for BED could have either positive or negative effects on outcome. (See Chapter 63 for discussion of psychological treatments for BED.) Medication may, for some patients, contribute to early improvement in binge eating and weight loss, and thereby enhance motivation to continue treatment. On the other hand, it is possible that concomitant medication treatment might mitigate the enhancement of self-efficacy that would otherwise accompany clinical improvement, or, by "artificially" suppressing binge eating, might interfere with the acquisition of psychological tools for managing binge eating. It has been suggested that in the treatment of obesity and bulimia nervosa, and presumably in the treatment of BED, medications act by enhancing dietary restraint. While this may conflict with psychotherapeutic treatments for bulimia nervosa that attempt to decrease dietary restraint, this would present less of a problem for patients being treated for BED.

There are few published studies of combined treatments for BED. In general, the short-term addition of tricyclic antidepressants to behavioral or cognitive-behavioral therapy appears not to markedly enhance binge reduction but may contribute to weight loss even 3 to 6 months after discontinuation of medication. Longer-term effects are unknown, although one open study using the combination of phentermine and fluoxetine as an adjunct to cognitive-behavioral therapy found ongoing improvement in binge eating but little evidence of long-term weight loss. One early study of fluoxetine as an adjunct to behavioral weight control treatment for obesity found that both binge eaters and non-binge eaters treated with fluoxetine for 1 year lost more weight than those treated with placebo, although this difference dissipated somewhat at 3- to 6-month follow-up off medication.

## CONCLUSION

As is the case for bulimia nervosa, medication treatment for BED, particularly with antidepressants, has demonstrable short-term benefits when compared to placebo. However, it is equally clear that relapse is common in the absence of other interventions. Lacking a sufficient database, treatment recommendations must be tentative and based on clinical common sense. Medication alone is probably not effective in the long term for most patients with BED, and it therefore makes sense to initiate treatment with behavioral weight loss treatment, cognitive-behavioral therapy, or interpersonal psychotherapy. (These treatments are considered in Chapter 63). One might consider adding medication for patients who do not achieve rapid binge reduction with these treatments, who relapse following treatment, or who have prominent depressive symptoms that require treatment in their own right. Further studies are needed to examine risks and benefits of longer-term medication treatment, the interactive effects of medication and psychosocial interventions on various outcome measures, and the possible existence of subgroups of patients who may be most likely to benefit from the addition of medication to the treatment regimen.

## FURTHER READING

Agras, W. S. (1997). Pharmacotherapy of bulimia nervosa and binge eating disorder: Long-term outcomes. *Psychopharmacology Bulletin, 33*, 433–436.—Discusses the problem of sequencing treatments to promote better long-term outcome.

Agras, W. S., Telch, C. F., Arnow, B., Eldredge, K., Wilfley, D. E., Raeburn, S. D., Henderson J., &

Marnell, M. (1994). Weight loss, cognitive-behavioral, and desipramine treatments in binge eating disorder: An additive design. *Behavior Therapy, 25,* 225–238.—Important study of combined psychotherapy and pharmacological treatment.

Craighead, L. W., & Agras, W. S. (1991). Mechanisms of action in cognitive-behavioral and pharmacological interventions for obesity and bulimia nervosa. *Journal of Consulting and Clinical Psychology, 59,* 115–125.—Discusses mechanisms of action and interactions of pharmacological and cognitive-behavioral treatments.

Devlin, M. J., Goldfein, J. A., Carino, J. S., & Wolk, S. L. (2000). Open treatment of overweight binge eaters with phentermine and fluoxetine as an adjunct to cognitive behavioral therapy. *International Journal of Eating Disorders, 28,* 325–332.—Open study that provides long-term follow-up data illustrating deterioration of benefits over time.

Hudson, J. I., McElroy, S. L., Raymond, N. C., Crow, S., Keck, P. E., Jr., Carter, W. P., Mitchell, J. E., Strakowski, S. M., Pope, J. G., Jr., Coleman, B. S., & Jonas, J. M. (1998). Fluvoxamine in the treatment of binge-eating disorder: A multicenter placebo-controlled, double-blind trial. *American Journal of Psychiatry, 155,* 1756–1762.—Large-scale study demonstrating short-term efficacy of an SSRI for reducing binge eating.

Stunkard, A., Berkowitz, R., Tanrikut, C., Reiss, E., & Young, L. (1996). d-Fenfluramine treatment of binge eating disorder. *American Journal of Psychiatry, 153,* 1455–1459.—Important trial with good description of practical issues, including recruitment of patients, their retention, and the high placebo response.

# 65

# Self-Help Books in the Treatment of Eating Disorders

## JACQUELINE C. CARTER

Although psychological treatments with proven efficacy for eating disorders exist, they are not widely available to those who need them. In an effort to facilitate the dissemination of evidence-based treatments, researchers have recently begun to study whether the active ingredients of established treatment protocols can be translated into self-help formats, so that they can be used by nonspecialist therapists or by sufferers to help themselves. Accumulating research evidence suggests that a significant proportion of those with eating disorders respond favorably to self-help interventions. Most of the research to date has focused on bulimia nervosa and binge eating disorder. Although self-help treatments for anorexia nervosa have not yet been studied, self-help is unlikely to be effective as a sole treatment for underweight individuals with eating disorders.

## MODES OF DELIVERY AND TARGET GROUPS

Self-help books may be used either by sufferers on their own ("pure" or "unguided" self-help) or in combination with guidance and support from a therapist who may, or may not, be a nonspecialist ("guided" self-help). Many self-help books are available for those with eating disorders. Since cognitive-behavioral therapy is the most extensively researched and well-validated treatment for eating disorders currently available (see Chapters 54 and 55), the focus of this chapter is on self-help books informed by cognitive-behavioral principles. Two such books have been published (see "Further Reading").

In the community, pure (unguided) self-help can provide an accessible form of information and advice for individuals with eating disorders who might not otherwise have access to expert help, or who may avoid seeking treatment due to factors such as shame or embarrassment. In primary care settings, guided self-help may be a useful initial intervention with those with bulimia nervosa or binge eating disorder, with the guidance being provided by a nurse or family doctor. Guided self-help usually involves about eight 30-minute sessions over 3 to 4 months. The therapist's role is to review progress, clarify material contained in the book, keep the patient on task, and provide support and encouragement. In specialized treatment settings, guided self-help may be a useful first step in a "stepped care" approach to treatment delivery, with only those who do not benefit going on to more intensive and costly treatments. Pure self-help may also have a role with patients who are on waiting lists for treatment. Another potential use of self-help is to facilitate, and perhaps abbreviate, therapist-administered cognitive-behavioral therapy. Self-help books provide a means of conveying much of the psychoeducational material that is a core element of cognitive-behavioral therapy (see Chapters 54 and 55). In addition, a cognitive-behavioral self-help book could be used as an adjunct to an entirely different form of treatment, such as interpersonal psychotherapy (see Chapter 57), thereby providing a means of directly addressing the eating disorder symptoms while concentrating on interpersonal issues during therapy sessions. Finally, self-help books focused on overcoming eating problems could be used with patients who are primarily being treated for another problem, such as an anxiety or mood disorder.

## RESEARCH ON EFFECTIVENESS

There have been seven studies of the effectiveness of written self-help material in the treatment of bulimic eating disorders (viz., bulimia nervosa or binge eating disorder). Four studies were conducted in specialized treatment centers. The first study found that 22% of bulimia nervosa patients referred to a tertiary care center were symptom-free over the previous week after receiving 8 weeks of unguided self-help. In the second study, two series of bulimia nervosa patients reported substantial reductions in the frequency of binge eating and vomiting following 8 sessions of cognitive-behavioral guided self-help. The third study, also of patients with bulimia nervosa, found that 8 biweekly sessions of guided self-help were as effective as 16 weekly sessions of individual cognitive-behavioral therapy. In this study, approximately two-thirds of patients in both conditions were free from binge eating and vomiting at follow-up. Both treatments also produced equivalent significant improvements in depression and self-esteem, providing evidence of the broader effects of cognitive behavioral self-help. In the fourth study, patients with bulimia nervosa received either fluoxetine or placebo, with or without an unpublished self-help manual, for 16 weeks. Patients who received fluoxetine in addition to the self-help manual reported the greatest decrease in binge eating and purging symptoms, although the difference between the drug-alone and drug plus self-help was not statistically significant.

There have also been three community-based studies. In the first (pilot) study, 9 women with binge eating disorder, recruited from the community, received eight telephone-based guided self-help sessions over 12 weeks. Of the 8 participants who completed the study, 5 reported a clinically significant reduction in binge eating. In addition, there was a significant reduction in general psychiatric symptoms. In the second study, a community-based sample of 72 women with binge eating disorder were randomly assigned to either pure (unguided) self-help, guided self-help, or a wait-list control condition for 12 weeks. Both forms of self-help produced a substantial and sustained reduction in the frequency of binge eating as well as improvements in general psychiatric symptoms, whereas there was little change in the wait-list condition. Overall, the results marginally favored guided self-help over pure self-help. In the third study, 40 women with binge-eating problems, recruited from the community, were randomly assigned to either guided or unguided cognitive-behavioral self-help. While participants in both conditions reported substantial improvements, guided self-help produced significantly greater reductions in the frequency of binge eating and its associated features.

In summary, these findings suggest that a substantial proportion of patients with bulimia nervosa or binge eating disorder benefit from self-help interventions, and that guided self-help produces somewhat better results than unguided self-help.

## STRENGTHS AND LIMITATIONS

Self-help is a potentially useful means of disseminating evidence-based treatment for eating disorders and may circumvent some obstacles to seeking help. Self-help is non-stigmatizing, and, if successful, may be experienced as empowering. Qualitative studies have found that self-help interventions decrease isolation and increase perceived support for sufferers, as well as helping them to overcome denial and shame. In addition, the use of self-help books, either independently or with guidance from a professional, might reduce the length and cost of treatment. The inclusion of self-help in stepped care treatment delivery programs might also reduce the number of people entering intensive and costly treatments. Finally, self-help books might play a useful role in helping to prepare and motivate patients for more intensive treatments.

On the other hand, not benefiting from a self-help program might have a negative impact on individuals' sense of self-efficacy and motivation for change. Not all self-help books are of equal merit, and there is currently no means of evaluating them—some may be disseminated without sufficient empirical study. Even with the best self-help books, only a subgroup of sufferers respond. The characteristics of those most and least likely to benefit have not yet been established, although there is some evidence that persons with the most severe symptoms and those with personality disorders do less well. It is important to ensure that the existence of self-help treatments does not delay those who require specialized treatment from receiving the help that they need.

## FUTURE DIRECTIONS

A priority for research is to identify the characteristics of persons who do and do not benefit from self-help books. In addition, it is important to study the impact of successful versus unsuccessful use of a self-help book on motivation for change, self-efficacy, and response to subsequent treatments. Finally, none of the studies to date have included attention-placebo control conditions. Studies are needed in which cognitive-behavioral self-help books focused specifically on the features of the eating disorder are compared with self-help programs designed to control for the "nonspecific" aspects of self-help, such as receiving a self-help book, being presented with a plausible rationale, and expecting to improve.

## FURTHER READING

Carter, J. C., & Fairburn, C. G. (1998). Treating binge eating problems in primary care. *Addictive Behaviors, 20,* 765–772.—A review of brief treatments for binge eating problems for use in primary care settings, including self-help.

Carter, J. C., & Fairburn, C. G. (1998). Cognitive-behavioral self-help for binge eating disorder: A controlled effectiveness study. *Journal of Consulting and Clinical Psychology, 66,* 616–623.— A community-based, controlled comparison of cognitive-behavioral self-help and guided self-help for binge eating disorder.

Cooper, P. J. (1993). *Binge eating and bulimia nervosa: A guide to recovery.* London: Robinson.— The first self-help version of cognitive-behavioral therapy for bulimia nervosa.

Cooper, P. J., Coker, S., & Fleming, C. (1996). An evaluation of the efficacy of supervised cognitive behavioral self-help for bulimia nervosa. *Journal of Psychosomatic Research, 40,* 281–287.— An open clinical trial of cognitive-behavioral guided self-help in a series of patients with bulimia nervosa referred to a specialized treatment clinic.

Fairburn, C. G. (1995). *Overcoming binge eating.* New York: Guilford Press.—A self-help manual based directly on the cognitive-behavioral approach to binge eating and bulimia nervosa.

Fairburn, C. G., & Carter, J. C. (1997). Self-help and guided self-help for binge eating problems. In D. M. Garner & P. E. Garfinkel (Eds.), *Handbook of treatment for eating disorders* (2nd ed., pp. 494–499). New York: Guilford Press.—A review of the use of self-help manuals in the treatment of eating disorders.

Loeb, K. L., Wilson, G. T., Gilbert, J. S., & Labouvie, E. (1999). Guided and unguided self-help for binge eating. *Behaviour Research and Therapy, 38,* 259–72.—A comparison of cognitive-behavioral self-help and guided self-help for women with binge eating disorder recruited from the community.

Mitchell, J. F., Fletcher, L., Hanson, K., Mussell, M. P., Seim, H., Al-Banna, M., Wilson, M., & Crosby, R. (2001). The relative efficacy of fluoxetine and manual-based self-help in the treatment of outpatients with bulimia nervosa. *Journal of Clinical Psychopharmacology, 21,* 298–304.—A randomized, placebo-controlled study examining the singular and combined effectiveness of fluoxetine and an unpublished self-help manual for bulimia nervosa.

Theils, C., Schmidt, U., Treasure, J., Garther, R., & Troop, N. (1998). Guided self-change for bulimia nervosa incorporating use of a self-care manual. *American Journal of Psychiatry, 155,* 947–953.—A comparison of guided self-help and individual cognitive-behavioral therapy for bulimia nervosa in a specialized treatment clinic.

Treasure, J., Schmidt, U., Troop, N., Tiller, J., Todd, G., Keilen, M., & Dodge, E. (1996). Sequential treatment for bulimia nervosa incorporating a self-care manual. *British Journal of Psychiatry, 168,* 94–98.—A controlled comparison of unguided self-help and individual cognitive-behavioral therapy for bulimia nervosa in a specialized treatment clinic.

Wells, A. M., Garvin, V., Dohm, F., & Striegel-Moore, R. (1997). Telephone-based guided self-help for binge eating disorder: A feasibility study. *International Journal of Eating Disorders, 21,* 341–346.—A community-based pilot study of telephone-administered guided self-help for binge eating disorder.

# 66

# Eating Disorders and the Internet

## ROZ SHAFRAN

This chapter aims to highlight the role that the internet can play in the lives of people with eating disorders and in the work of clinicians who treat them. The internet is a powerful tool, but there are many questions associated with its use. How accurate and useful is the information provided? Can people be treated effectively over the internet, and what are the implications of this? How can the internet best be used as an adjunct to face-to-face therapy? Does direct "on-line" counseling deter people in need from seeking more direct and evidence-based interventions? Do chat rooms perpetuate eating disorders? What ethical issues are raised by sufferers exchanging diet "tips," and should we try to guide our patients away from "pro-anorexia" web sites?

## INFORMATION

It is said that there are over 27,000 internet sites relating to eating disorders. Many provide information about the different types of eating disorder. The largest web site ("Something Fishy") contains over 400 pages, emphasizes recovery, and provides information on the physical and psychological consequences of having an eating disorder. Ensuring the accuracy of material on the internet is a perennial problem, although the information provided by governmental mental health web sites and specialized sites run by recognized eating disorder organizations is usually reliable. Such sites are also more commonly updated and may be more durable than sites that are primarily dependent upon the efforts of one person. Some web sites provide less than helpful information, such as those that deny the existence of adverse physical effects and sites that suggest that a body mass index (BMI) of 17 is entirely healthy.

Table 66.1 presents a small selection of some of the most prominent web sites related to eating disorders.

**TABLE 66.1. A Selection of Web Sites Related to Eating Disorders (as of July 2001)**

| Web site | Description |
|---|---|
| Academy for Eating Disorders *www.acadeatdis.org* | A multidisciplinary professional organization focused on eating disorders. It aims to bring together professionals working in the field. |
| American Anorexia and Bulimia Association *www.aabainc.org* | A nonprofit organization of concerned members of the public and health care industry dedicated to the prevention and treatment of eating disorders. Has outreach programs to provide education and advocacy in the community. |
| Anorexia Nervosa and Related Disorders, Inc. *www.anred.com* | A nonprofit organization that provides information about anorexia nervosa, bulimia nervosa, binge eating disorder, compulsive exercising, and "other less well-known food and weight disorders." Material includes details about recovery and prevention. |
| Eating Disorders Awareness and Prevention, Inc. *www.edap.org* | A nonprofit organization dedicated to increasing the awareness and prevention of eating disorders through education and community activism. |
| Mirror Mirror *www.mirror-mirror.org* | Linked to "Something Fishy," and provides similar services. Particularly easy to access information on physical signs and symptoms of eating disorders. |
| National Association of Anorexia Nervosa and Related Disorders (ANAD) *www.anad.org* | Aims to help people with eating disorders and their families by providing free "hotline" counseling, a network of support groups, referrals, a quarterly newsletter, and information packets. Other services are also provided. |
| National Eating Disorder Information Centre Canada *www.nedic.on.ca* | Information center focusing on eating disorders and health-related behavior of women. |
| Something Fishy *www.something-fishy.org* | The largest web site for eating disorders, with over 400 pages. Includes information, conference updates, chat rooms, a "treatment finder service," and help for family and friends. |

## RESEARCH

The internet facilitates access to many scientific journals. Several sites allow searches for evidence-based practice. Information about funding for medical research, including research on eating disorders, can also be found on-line. Participants for research projects can be recruited on-line and questionnaires can be transmitted and completed electronically, although it is difficult to gauge the nature of the sample being studied.

## TREATMENT

Many clinicians and organizations use the internet to advertise treatment programs much in the same way that they advertise using any other medium. Some provide a service to help find a local therapist for face-to-face therapy. General counseling sites offer treatment on-line for a fee, but there are also specific sites for the treatment of eating problems. One site offers guided self-help for binge eating based on Fairburn's cognitive-behavioral self-help book (*Overcoming Binge Eating*). The guidance takes the form of individual telephone calls and an on-line "private support group." (See Chapter 65 for a discussion of the use of self-help books in the treatment of eating disorders.) An on-line program for the treatment of body image concerns in female students has been evaluated in a controlled trial conducted in California, and was found to be helpful. In this program, the internet was used in conjunction with extensive weekly readings and assignments.

Therapists may use the internet in various ways. It can be used for simple administrative arrangements, such as organizing appointments. It can be used to maintain contact between appointments if treatment is disrupted for some reason, such as by a vacation. It can be used to supplement weekly appointments, for example, by asking patients to report on their progress every few days. Self-monitoring records can be transferred onto the internet and sent to the therapist. Internet communication can even be used instead of face-to-face treatment; indeed, it has been argued that some patients are more willing to disclose information via e-mail.

Because none of these therapeutic uses of the internet have been evaluated, therapists need to be aware of potential pitfalls. For example, providers of internet services may not be licensed to practice outside their geographical area, and they therefore may not be insured. They need to make sure that patients know that e-mail is an insecure medium, and they should obtain specific consent from the patient for its therapeutic use. There needs to be agreement regarding certain aspects of protocol—for example, whether e-mails are to be stored in the same way as written clinical records. It also needs to be established how frequently e-mails will be read and when patients can expect a reply. Patients also need guidance on aspects of clinical "netiquette," including the appropriate degree of formality, the range of content to be included in the messages, as well as their optimal length and frequency, and how the patient and therapist should refer to each other. In general, emoticons ("smileys"—codes such as :-) to convey affect) should be used sparingly and should not replace clarity in communication.

General internet-based sites that offer on-line counseling are potentially problematic, because it is possible that such "treatment" may delay the person from obtaining good, evidence-based care. Furthermore, there is no means of determining the validity of the therapist's qualifications or the quality of the intervention (although this can also apply to traditional forms of intervention, and it is possible to perform some credibility checks on-line).

## SOCIAL SUPPORT

Chat rooms provide accessible support at all hours. People can obtain comfort from knowing that they are not alone in their difficulties and be encouraged in their efforts to overcome them. As with any support group, there is the question as to whether such support can be counterproductive by giving patients the "identity" of someone with an eating disorder and reducing their motivation to change. Some web sites monitor their chat rooms and have rules to prevent the exchange of unhelpful information about weight and dieting. Unfortunately, there is an abundance of other web sites where such information can be obtained all too easily.

## PRO-ANOREXIA WEB SITES

These web sites unabashedly advocate having anorexia nervosa. They have "inspirational quotes," idealized body images, and dieting tips. Although such sites often carry warnings about their content and frequently require the user to register, clinicians should consider the possible negative impact of these sites on patients who are frequent users of the internet.

## SUMMARY AND FUTURE DIRECTIONS

The use of the internet to provide information and treatment about eating disorders is expanding rapidly. It has enormous potential but needs to be viewed with caution. Managed well, it can help patients obtain information about their disorder, identify a therapist, obtain solace, and it has the potential to enhance treatment. On the other hand, users may receive inaccurate information and be vulnerable to exploitation by bogus therapists. The self-regulation of those eating disorder practitioners who wish to advertise or provide therapeutic services over the internet would be of benefit.

## FURTHER READING

American Psychological Association. (1997). *Statement on services by telephone, teleconferencing and internet by the Ethics Committee of the American Psychological Association.*—A one-page general statement from the American Psychological Association's Ethics Committee addresses issues relating to the use of the internet within the broader code of conduct. *www.apa.org/ethics/stmnt01.html*

Fairburn, C. G. (1995). *Overcoming binge eating.* New York: Guilford Press.—Contains an evidence-based cognitive-behavioral self-help program. Its contents form the foundation for the 16-week program at *edrecovery.com*.

Pallen, M. (1995). Introducing the internet. *British Medical Journal, 311,* 1422–1424.—First of four articles to guide doctors in the use of the internet. Other articles can be found in the same volume on pages 1487 (use of email), 1552 (the World-Wide Web) and 1626 (describes logging in, fetching files, and reading news). A somewhat outdated but useful introduction.

Riley, S., & Veale, D. (1999). The internet and its relevance to cognitive behavioural psychotherapists. *Behavioural and Cognitive Psychotherapy, 27,* 37–46.—Straightforward, basic introduction to the internet, searching, chat rooms, and web sites. Considers issues relevant to cognitive-behavioral therapy over the internet.

Rothchild, E. (1997). E-mail therapy. *American Journal of Psychiatry, 154,* 1476–1477.—Letter highlighting the problems and pitfalls of using e-mail, including relationship, affective, ethical, and financial implications.

Schmidt, U. (1998). Food web: Eating disorders on the internet. *European Eating Disorders Review, 6,* 75–77.—An account of surfing the internet for eating disorder web sites.

Winzelberg, A. J., Eppstein, D., Eldedge, K. L., Wilfley, D., Dasmahapatra, R., Dev, P., & Taylor, C. B. (2000). Effectiveness of an internet-based program for reducing risk factors for eating disorders. *Journal of Consulting and Clinical Psychology, 68,* 346–350.—First controlled study to evaluate an internet-based health education program to improve body satisfaction and shape and weight concerns among college students.

Yager, J. (2001). E-mail as a therapeutic adjunct in the outpatient treatment of anorexia nervosa: Illustrative case material and discussion of the issues. *International Journal of Eating Disorders, 29,* 125–138.—Article illustrating the how therapy can be aided by the addition of e-mail.

# 67

# Prevention of Eating Disorders

## NIVA PIRAN

Prevention is a relatively new domain of research and discussion in the field of eating disorders. "Universal" or "primary prevention" refers to policies and programs that aim to lower the incidence of the disorder in a large population through reducing exposure to risk and enhancing exposure to protective or resilience factors. Both selective prevention, geared at groups at high risk of developing the disorder, and indicated prevention, geared at individuals already displaying low levels of symptoms, aim at reducing the rates of development of full-blown disorder through early identification and intervention (also termed "secondary prevention").

Most of the systematic study of the prevention of eating disorders has been conducted since 1990. Despite limited allocation of resources, the field has seen considerable growth in output, leading to the emergence of a cumulative body of knowledge that can help guide further developments. This chapter discusses the impact of risk factors research on eating disorder prevention, reviews results and trends in prevention outcome research, and examines current challenges in the field of prevention. (Chapter 112 addresses the prevention of obesity.)

## RISK FACTOR RESEARCH AND PREVENTION

Prevention work relies on the development of etiological models. The study of risk and protective factors, in turn, is guided by prevailing views about the target disorder. Until the past decade, most research and knowledge about eating disorders was derived from clinical samples reflecting a dichotomous, illness-based view of eating disorders. Accordingly, clinic-based risk factor research tended to emphasize disrupted familial and personality processes. However, as cross-sectional risk factor research, comparing eating disorder samples to controls, has progressed to prospective community-based designs aiming to identify risk factors that *predate* the development of eating disorders, most intraindividual and familial structural variables have been found to have little predictive value.

(See Chapters 38, 42, and 44 for discussion of familial and individual risk factors). The one factor that has consistently emerged from these studies as predicting the future development of eating disorders is weight concerns and the presence of eating disorder symptoms.

Most of the early prevention programs attempted to address a single social factor, namely, media-generated and culturally sanctioned pressures for thinness. This factor, derived through the use of correlational cross-sectional research designs rather than prospective designs, suggested an association between the rise in eating disorders and media-generated pressures for thinness. (See Chapter 19 for discussion of social and media influences on body image and dieting practices.) Following the social learning model, these prevention programs tended to emphasize healthy nutrition and healthy weight management, as well as ways to counter unrealistic pressures for thinness. While trying to address the social domain, these prevention programs were not yet informed by prospective risk factor research.

Several trends in eating disorder research have helped close the gap between prevention strategies and relevant research. First, the 1990s saw a rapid growth in community-based epidemiological studies of eating disorders, revealing a spectrum of disordered eating and weight preoccupation not easily classifiable into distinct clinical entities. In particular, a range of disordered eating patterns exist that, while not fulfilling clinical criteria, is associated with significant morbidity, highlighting the importance of preventing a larger spectrum of disorders rather than those subsumed under specified clinical diagnoses. Second, the study of social factors has expanded both in volume and nature. Social research moved beyond the unified media-generated pressures-for-thinness theory of eating disorders to reflect the multilayered and complex nature of social ecology. In terms of peer processes, cross-sectional empirical and qualitative research found an association between participants' own and peers' weight preoccupation, as well as between peer teasing about weight and disordered eating. Early co-occurrence of puberty and dating was found to be associated with disordered eating. Family-based studies also found a relationship between parental criticism and children's weight preoccupation. Exposure to the media was found in some studies to be associated with patterns of disordered eating. The third trend in risk factor research was to incorporate social factors into prospective research studies designed to predict the development of patterns of disordered eating. New prospective research has validated the predictive value of weight-related teasing as well as media exposure (in some studies) for the development of eating disorders. A fourth trend was to expand from the exclusive emphasis on weight-related variables to the study of other social variables, such as gender roles, the spectrum of violence in women's lives, and the influence of acculturation. However, the predictive power of these factors has not yet been explored in prospective designs. All these trends together reflect a greater attunement to social processes in the study of risk factors.

To conclude, with greater attunement to the contribution of social processes to the development of eating disorders, research is starting to yield information that can guide the construction of programs aimed at primary prevention. For example, prospective research suggests the importance of interventions with peers and parents that limit weight-related criticism and teasing, the potential relevance of media literacy skills, as well as the importance of intervening with higher-level structures and policies regarding media advertising. In terms of secondary prevention, prospective research has generated measures of early and lower-level weight concerns among children and adolescents that seem to predict the development of disordered eating patterns above and beyond the vulnerability factors of poor interoceptive awareness and negative affectivity. This will allow the identification of groups of individuals at risk for the purpose of secondary prevention.

## REVIEW OF THE OUTCOME OF EXISTING PROGRAMS

The number of studies examining the outcome of a variety of prevention programs has grown rapidly. To date, in the area of primary prevention, the findings of 17 outcome studies have been reported in which there has been a repeated measure experimental, or quasi-experimental, design comparing an intervention and control group, with at least 1-month follow-up. The programs themselves have included interventions as diverse as one lecture about the nature of eating disorders by partly recovered individuals through comprehensive and lengthy school programs that target schoolchildren as well as significant adults in the life of these children. The programs differ in their rationales, hypothesized active components, contents, length of interventions, age and gender composition of the participants, as well as in their emphases on individual, institutional, and societal levels of intervention. Most have not been anchored in risk and protective factors research.

Out of eight studies that measured knowledge acquisition related to topics such as diversity of natural weights or nutrition, seven reported significant differences between the experimental and control groups. Regarding attitudinal measures, such as body dissatisfaction, nine found a significant difference between the experimental and control groups on at least some of the measures during follow-up. In comparison, only seven (out of the 16 studies) found significant behavior changes, either at the completion of study or during follow-up, and in only two studies were these differences maintained throughout the period of follow-up.

Considering the pattern of results obtained in these 17 outcome studies, it appears that more favorable results were obtained as the 1990s progressed, probably related to somewhat changed prevention strategies over time. Knowledge acquisition, typically not correlated with attitudinal or behavioral change, was found in two studies to predict long-term attitudinal and behavioral change. Changes in attitudinal measures tended to show mixed and, at times, contradictory findings such as changes in body image but not drive for thinness measures, suggesting that key attitudinal dimensions and their relationship to behavioral change need to be explored separately. Regarding behavioral changes, four studies found long-term improvements in both the experimental and control groups. These studies recruited both their experimental and control groups from the same school setting and their interventions aimed at, among other things, creating new peer norms regarding weight-related prejudices and teasing. It is possible that these more systemic interventions may have resulted in a "spillover" effect that benefited the control group members. These results parallel the findings of one prevention study that focused almost exclusively on creating systemic changes in a school setting and found significant long-term improvements in individuals' eating patterns and negative body image.

Different research findings suggest that selected or targeted prevention (secondary prevention) is also a promising approach to the prevention of eating disorders. First, measures have been developed, in particular measures of early weight concerns, that successfully identify individuals at risk. Second, several studies that have implemented primary prevention programs have found that high-risk individuals respond particularly well to preventive interventions. Third, out of five controlled studies of selected prevention conducted to date, three obtained attitudinal change at follow-up, and two obtained behavior change. Two programs followed a psychoeducational and cognitive-behavioral approach, while the other used a dissonance-based program aimed at helping younger adolescents resist the slender ideal. It may be that the wealth of knowledge accumulated in clinical practice is more readily generalizable to secondary rather than to primary preventative programs.

## CONCLUSIONS AND CURRENT CHALLENGES

Within the relatively young field of prevention of eating disorders, unlike substance abuse or other prevention foci, no best practice models are yet available. While the field has seen considerable progress, many challenges remain. Current conceptual challenges in prevention interventions relate to the need for (1) enhanced reliance on risk and protective factor research in constructing prevention programs, and possibly the integration of risk factor and prevention research; (2) further expansion in the cross-sectional and prospective study of social etiological factors; (3) integration of knowledge derived from the broader field of primary and secondary prevention, particularly the emphasis on generic risk and protective factors (such as competence, self-esteem, life skills, and parental warmth), and on comprehensive programs; (4) incorporation of multilevel strategies and the assessment of consequent systemic changes at the policy, institutional, familial, and individual levels; and (5) examination of participatory context-specific models of health promotion strategies in schools, such as those developed by the World Health Organization. Methodological challenges relate to the need to (1) specify the goal, theoretical basis, rationale, and target population of each intervention strategy; (2) employ experimental designs with adequate sample sizes and follow-up periods that include more than one comparison group in more than one setting, and that allow for the examination of trends over time prior to the interventions being studied; (3) select outcome measures to match specific program goals, including the use of measures of systemic change and potential negative intervention effects; (4) specify implementation processes and requirements; (5) explore the pros and cons of alternative participatory approaches to health promotion interventions. As professionals systematically address these multiple challenges, the field continues to gain momentum and to work toward the development of best-practice models.

## FURTHER READING

Franko, D. L., & Orosan-Weine, P. (1998). The prevention of eating disorders: Empirical, methodological and conceptual considerations. *Clinical Psychology: Science and Practice, 5,* 459–477.—A thoughtful review of challenges in the prevention of eating disorders.

Gordon, R. A. (1999). *Eating disorders: Anatomy of a social epidemic* (2nd ed.). Malden, MA: Blackwell.—A valuable perspective on eating disorders as a social phenomenon.

Killen, J.D., Taylor, C. B., Hammer, L. D., Litt, I., Wilson, D. M., Rich, T., Hayward, C., Simmonds, B., Kraemer, H., & Varady, A. (1993). An attempt to modify unhealthful eating attitudes and weight regulation practices of young adolescent girls. *International Journal of*

*Eating Disorders, 13,* 369–384.—The first large-scale evaluation of the social learning approach to the prevention of eating disorders.

Levine, M. P., & Piran, N. (2001). The prevention of eating disorders: Towards a participatory ecology of knowledge, action, and advocacy. In R. Striegel-Moore & L. Smolak (Eds)., *Eating disorders: New directions for research and practice* (pp. 233–254). Washington, DC: American Psychological Association.–A comprehensive review and tabulated summary of outcome studies conducted to date in the prevention of eating disorders.

O'Dea, J. A., & Abraham, S. (2000) . Improving the body image, eating attitudes, and behaviors of young male and female adolescents: A new educational approach that focuses on self-esteem. *International Journal of Eating Disorders, 28,* 43–57.—An outcome evaluation of a prevention strategy that relied exclusively on general risk and resilience factors (such as self-esteem) rather than on risk factors specific to the development of eating disorders.

Piran, N. (1999). Eating disorders: A trial of prevention in a high risk school setting. *Journal of Primary Prevention, 20,* 75–90.—A study of a participatory approach to the prevention of eating disorders that relied on school-wide systemic changes.

Piran, N., Levine, M. P., & Steiner-Adair, C. (1999). *Preventing eating disorders: A handbook of interventions and special challenges.* Philadelphia: Brunner/Mazel.—A comprehensive volume that describes multiple approaches to the prevention of eating disorders.

Smolak, L. (1999). Suggestions for the content and structure of elementary school curricula for the primary prevention of eating disorders. In N. Piran, M. P. Levine, & C. Steiner-Adair (Eds.), *Preventing eating disorders: A handbook of interventions and special challenges* (pp. 85–104). Philadelphia: Brunner/Mazel.—A discussion of important considerations in developing prevention programs for children in elementary school.

Stice, F., Mazotti, L., Weibel, D., & Agras, W. S. (2000). Dissonance prevention program decreases thin-ideal internalization, body dissatisfaction, dieting, negative affect, and bulimic symptoms: A preliminary experiment. *International Journal of Eating Disorders, 27,* 206–217.—A successful secondary prevention study that obtained significant attitudinal and behavioral changes.

Thompson, K. J., Heinberg, L. J., Altabe, M., & Tantleff-Dunn, S. (1999). *Exacting beauty: Theory, assessment, and treatment of body image disturbance.* Washington, DC: American Psychological Association.—A comprehensive volume that reviews studies in the social domain of eating disorders.

# PART III

# OBESITY

# Clinical Characteristics
# of Obesity

# 68

# Definition and Classification of Obesity

## PER BJÖRNTORP

Obesity, now a worldwide epidemic, has recently been declared one of the major concerns for global health by the World Health Organization (WHO) (see Chapter 74). Obesity is associated with, or a precursor state to, numerous serious diseases, including type 2 diabetes mellitus, cardiovascular disease, stroke, and certain carcinomas (see Chapter 84). In order to identify the prevalence as well as diagnose the disease in clinical settings, it is necessary to define the condition by reliable measurements. Such measurements should not only include total body fat mass, but also distribution of body fat, because central localization of excess depot fat is associated with much higher risks for serious complications than more even, or peripheral, distribution of depot fat masses (see Chapter 11).

## MEASUREMENTS

Obesity is the condition with elevated fat masses in the body. A problem is how this should be defined. Depot fat is stored in essence only in adipose tissue as triglycerides. The function of adipose tissue is to supply the body with energy when needed. In the postprandial condition, fat is drawn from adipose tissue in the form of mobilized free fatty acids. This is then replenished by energy intake. In the absence of external sources of energy, adipose tissue is the major supplier of energy for bodily functions. A normal man or woman has about 10–15 kg of fat in adipose tissue, which is sufficient for survival during starvation for about a month. This is clearly an unnecessarily large reserve depot in current urbanized society, where food is immediately available when needed. One may then suggest that in terms of needs of reserve energy supply, the currently "normal" amount of fat in adipose tissue is not needed.

There is, however, another, more important aspect of this issue. When adipose tissue stores become enlarged, the risk for complicating diseases is elevated. There are good reasons for definition of obesity at a point where such risk is clearly apparent. This is, however, complicated, because there is no sharp delineation between health and disease at a certain body fat mass; in fact, the relationship between body fat mass and prevalence or incidence of various diseases is not even linear but often J- or U-shaped (see Chapter 76). There are several reasons for this. One is that smoking, which tends to decrease body fat, increases the risk for disease by other mechanisms. Another major cause for the relatively poor relationship between body fat and disease is the fact that the risk varies with the localization of excess fat. When distributed to central, abdominal, particularly intra-abdominal, visceral depots, the risk for disease increases sharply, under certain circumstances, even without a major increase in total body fat mass. It is therefore important to include measurements of the localization of excess body fat.

The gold standard for measuring total body fat mass are the imaging techniques, computerized tomography or magnetic resonance imaging (see Chapter 11). These methods also determine the localization of fat in the body. Such techniques are, however, not accessible everywhere, and are expensive in addition. Other methods include underwater weighing, determination of skinfold thickness, and anthropometric measurements. The latter are easily performed in both epidemiological and clinical settings.

Utilizing anthropometric measurements total body fat is estimated by the body mass index (BMI), which is calculated as body weight in kilograms divided by height, squared, in meters. This means that a person who has the height of 170 cm and a weight of 70 kg has a BMI of 22.9.

The WHO has recommended the following classification system based on the BMI:

Normal range:          18.5–24.9
Overweight:            ≥ 25.0–29.9
Obesity:               > 30

This means that the subject exemplified above would be obese at a body weight of about 87 kg. This seems to be a safe diagnosis, but the borderlines are obviously approximations and not necessarily valid for all ethnic groups.

Anthropometric measurements of body fat distribution include circumferences of the waist and hips as well as measurements of the abdominal sagittal diameter. The waist circumference is measured in the overnight fasting condition, in a normal respiratory position, horizontally, midway between the lower costal margin and the iliac crest. The hip circumference is measured horizontally over the widest parts of the gluteal region. The waist/hip circumference ratio (WHR) is then calculated. The abdominal sagittal diameter is measured, with the examined person in a supine position, as the distance between the examination table and the highest point of the abdomen.

When these simple measurements are compared with exactly determined fat mass by imaging techniques, it is clear that the sagittal diameter shows the strongest relationship to intraabdominal fat mass, while the circumference measurements are less precise. The problem is, however, that there are currently not sufficient data to evaluate the sagittal diameter as a risk factor for disease, and therefore no recommendations of borderlines can be given. There is, however, information on the associations between the circumference measurements and disease prevalence and incidence. The borderlines for the WHR of 1.0 in men and 0.85 in women have now been widely accepted for Caucasians. These borderlines are almost certainly different in other ethnic populations. For example, Pima Indians, Australian Aborigines, and some populations in the Pacific islands, who all suffer from a dramatic prevalence of obesity, also have a larger portion of excess fat in central depots.

The waist circumference alone is also useful, and the WHO has suggested the following borderlines for such measurements.

Risk for obesity-associated metabolic complications increased: Men ≥ 94 cm; women: ≥ 80 cm
Risk for obesity-associated metabolic complications substantially increased: Men: ≥ 102 cm; women: ≥ 88 cm

## CLASSIFICATION OF OBESITY

It is important to distinguish the subgroups of central, abdominal, or visceral obesity from peripheral, gluteofemoral obesity. Visceral obesity is associated with most of the established risk factors for cardiovascular disease, type 2 diabetes mellitus, and stroke. Prospective studies have shown that visceral obesity is an independent risk factor for these diseases. In addition, there is also a prospective association to mammary and endometrial carcinomas. In contrast, peripheral obesity is followed by less serious diseases such as varicose veins and joint–skeletal problems. The methods of circumference measurements seem most appropriate for this purpose both in epidemiological and clinical settings.

## PATHOGENIC FACTORS IN VISCERAL OBESITY

It then becomes important to examine what makes centralization of body fat such a powerful precursor to other diseases. A clue to detection of this association might be the similarities with Cushing's syndrome, which is characterized by a dramatic accumulation of body fat in central depots, as well as the same risk factors as those described in visceral obesity. The pathogenetic trigger in this syndrome is clearly an increased secretion of cortisol. The question then becomes, is central obesity a condition with elevated cortisol secretion?

Recent studies suggest that this probably is the case. Conventional clinical tools, utilized for the diagnosis of Cushing's syndrome, are not sensitive enough to be useful. If visceral obesity is caused by elevated cortisol secretion, it is a more subtle, milder abnormality, requiring more sensitive methods. Measuring the diurnal regulation of the hypothalamic–pituitary–adrenal (HPA) axis on an ordinary day in life can be accomplished by measuring cortisol in repeated saliva samples. With this method, it is possible to distinguish errors in HPA axis regulation, which are associated with centralization of body fat stores. Elevated cortisol secretion, with abnormal diurnal kinetics, is possible to identify in a majority of men with elevated sagittal diameter. This is seen more clearly after challenges of the HPA axis by perceived stress or food intake and is probably a causal association via known mechanisms. However, there is also a smaller group with low cortisol secretion, with a flat, rigid day curve, which shows strong associations to visceral obesity. Here, elevated cortisol could not be a causative factor. In this group, there are also diminished secretions of testosterone and growth hormone that might be responsible because these hormones antagonize the effects of cortisol on visceral fat accumulation. The decrease of testosterone and growth hormone might be a consequence of a perturbed HPA axis regulation.

In women, androgens, probably at least partly of adrenal origin, seem to be more important than cortisol. Elevated androgens might also be a consequence of an increased activity of the HPA axis. Women exposed to androgens accumulate visceral fat, although the detailed mechanisms are not clear.

It is thus apparent that visceral fat accumulation is a consequence of a neuroendocrine abnormality affecting several central endocrine axes. There is also evidence that the central regulation of the sympathetic nervous system is involved. Taken together, this is evidence for a central "arousal syndrome" affecting neuroendocrine and autonomic centers. Interestingly, the consequences of such an "arousal" in the periphery probably will be the generation of risk factors for disease via effects of the resulting endocrine and autonomic perturbations. The parallel between visceral fat accumulation and disease risk factors may therefore be due to a common trigger provided by the central arousal.

There are statistical associations of this syndrome with socioeconomic and psychosocial handicaps that, presumably via stress-reactions, lead to the "arousal syndrome." This is amplified by increased alcohol intake, smoking, and robust associations to depressive and anxiety reactions, which are factors known to activate central neuroendocrine and autonomic reactions. These might all be considered to be consequences of the current hectic, competitive lifestyle, which also contains excess availability of energy-rich food, and where muscular activity is seldom needed. These factors may together result in abdominal, visceral obesity.

## FUTURE RESEARCH DIRECTIONS

The difference between peripheral and visceral obesity is still not sufficiently appreciated in spite of conclusive documentation. This is of obvious importance for future obesity research. Epidemiological surveys would be more meaningful if obesity subgroups were separated. Furthermore, visceral obesity has most likely a different pathogenetic background than peripheral obesity, including such factors as those exemplified earlier. Since the obesity subgroups are associated with clearly different risks, they require different levels of ambition in the workup and treatment in clinical settings. In addition, the background factors and mechanisms for visceral obesity should attract further research efforts, because this condition is a precursor state to some of the most prevalent and serious diseases, leading to morbidity, mortality, and enormous economic costs.

## FURTHER READING

Björntorp, P. (1992). Visceral obesity: A civilization syndrome. *Obesity Research*, 1, 206–222.— Overview of epidemiological data and pathogenetic mechanisms.
Björntorp, P. (1996). The regulation of adipose tissue distribution in humans. *International Journal of Obesity*, 20, 291–302.—An overview of factors regulating distribution of body fat.

Björntorp, P. (1999). Neuroendocrine perturbations as a cause of insulin resistance. *Diabetes Metabolism Research and Reviews, 15,* 427–441.—An overview of factors regulating insulin resistance, with a focus on abdominal obesity.

Björntorp, P. (2001). Do stress reactions cause abdominal obesity and comorbidities? *Obesity Reviews, 2,* 73–76.—A review of the possibility that obesity, particularly the abdominal subtype, is caused by the neuroendocrine consequences of stress.

Björntorp, P., Holm, G., Rosmond, R., & Folkow, B. (2000). Hypertension and the metabolic syndrome: Closely related central origin? *Blood Pressure, 8,* 89–117.—Review of the evidence indicating common pathogenetic pathways for primary hypertension, abdominal obesity, and metabolic abnormalities.

Kirschbaum, C., & Hellhammer, D. (1994). Salivary cortisol in psychoneuroendocrine research: Recent developments and applications. *Psychoneuroendocrinology, 19,* 313–333.—A most useful methodological review.

Kissebah, A. H., & Krakower, G. R. ( 1994). Regional adiposity and morbidity. *Physiological Reviews, 74,* 761–811.—A comprehensive review of the associations between central obesity and disease.

McEwen, B. S. (1998). Protective and damaging effects of stress mediators. *New England Journal of Medicine, 338,* 171–179.—A review of stress mechanisms and consequences.

World Health Organization. (1998). *Obesity: Preventing and managing the global epidemic: Report of a WHO Consultation on Obesity* (WHO/NUT/NCD/98.1). Geneva: Author.—Provides a comprehensive overview of the global obesity problem.

# 69

# A Brief History of Obesity

## GEORGE A. BRAY

Past is prologue.

—WILLIAM SHAKESPEARE

The further backward you look, the further forward you can see.

—SIR WINSTON CHURCHILL

The real voyage of discovery consists not in seeking new landscapes but in having new eyes.

—MARCEL PROUST

In this chapter, I present highlights in the history of obesity. To do this, I first present a brief review of the major scientific advances with particular reference to obesity. Second, I indicate how these ideas have affected the understanding of obesity.

## KEY DEVELOPMENTS IN SCIENCE

### The Physical World

The beginning of modern science can be dated from 1450–1500 and the introduction of movable type printing by Gutenberg (Table 69.1). By 1500, printing presses were widely distributed and the classic writings were more available than ever before. Probably the major scientific development in the century following Gutenberg was the Copernican Treatise of 1543, arguing that the sun, not the earth, was the center of the universe. Late in the 16th century, Galileo took this argument to the point that the Catholic Church put him under house arrest for heresy. These early pioneers led the way to the Newtonian synthesis of the Laws of Motion in the 17th century. The Newtonian laws and the physics they spawned were followed by applications to biology and to human beings, and served us well until Einstein's Theory of Relativity. The so-called iatromechanical schools of medicine interpreted human physiology and disease in mechanical terms.

**TABLE 69.1. Major Events in the History of Science and Obesity since 1500 AD**

| | Physics | Chemistry | Biology | Obesity |
|---|---|---|---|---|
| 15th century | | Printing | | |
| 16th century | Copernicus (heliocentric theory)<br>Galileo | | Vesalius (anatomy) | |
| 17th century | Galileo (telescope) | Boyle (temperature and pressure) | Harvey (blood circulation)<br>Malpighi (pulmonary circulation)<br>Hooke (micrographia) | Santorio (metabolic balance) |
| 18th century | Walt (steam engine) | Hydrogen and oxygen discovered<br>Lavoisier (oxygen theory) | Morgagni (first pathology text)<br>Jenner (vaccination)<br>Lind (On Scurvy) | Lavoisier (respiratory exchange in humans)<br>Short (first monograph on corpulency) |
| 19th century | Photography<br>Electrical cell<br>Atomic theory<br>Electromagnetism<br>Internal combustion engine | Wohler (urea synthesized from inorganic molecules)<br>Mendeleev (periodic table of elements)<br>Bernard (liver glycogen)<br>Morphine, cocaine, quinine, amphetamine<br>Ions hypothesized | Laennec (stethoscope)<br>Helmholtz (ophthalmoscope)<br>Schwann (cell theory)<br>Morton (ether anesthesia)<br>Semmelweis (puerperal fever)<br>Lister (antiseptic surgery)<br>Darwin (Origin of the Species)<br>Mendelian genetics | Quetelet (BMI)<br>Helmholtz (conservation of energy)<br>Atwater (room calorimeter)<br>Wadd (On Corpulency)<br>Banting (first diet book)<br>Sleep apnea described<br>Fat cell identified |
| 20th century | Wright brothers' flight<br>Vacuum tube<br>Theory of relativity<br>$E = mc^2$ —atomic bomb<br>Quantum physics<br>Rockets<br>Transistor<br>Laser<br>CT scan | Sulfonamides<br>Nylon<br>DDT<br>Salvarsan<br>Vitamins | Secretin—first hormone<br>Reflex arc<br>Homeostasis<br>Inborn errors<br>Insulin<br>Penicillin<br>Conditioned reflexes<br>Polio vaccine<br>AIDS<br>Watson–Crick DNA hypothesis<br>Genetic engineering<br>Human genome<br>Operant behavior | Gastric contractions and hunger<br>Family study of obesity<br>Genetic obese animals<br>Amphetamine-treated obesity<br>CT/MRI scans for visceral fat<br>DXA and density for body fat<br>Doubly labeled water method<br>Leptin |

Newtonian physics reigned supreme through the 19th century. It was during the late 19th and early 20th centuries that quantum physics and the theory of relativity were promulgated. These two important theoretical advances were accompanied by many applications that have transformed the 20th century. The beginning of propelled flight in 1903 and rocket flight in 1927 led to jet airplanes that have shrunk the world. The transistor has replaced the vacuum tube and made possible the integrated circuits and today's computer revolution. Together with the laser, these technologies provided the base for replacing analogue devices, such as the phonograph and telephone, with digital information n laser and computer discs.

## The Chemical World

Some of the transformations in chemistry are shown in Table 69.1. The demonstration in 1815, that an organic molecule, urea, could be made from inorganic molecules, produced a revolution in thinking about chemistry and its interface with biology. Physiological chemistry, biological or biochemistry, and finally, molecular biology were outgrowths of this transformation.

Robert Boyle, in the 17th century, may be looked on as the father of chemistry. However, from the perspective of obesity and the study of energy balance, it is Lavoisier, at the end of the 18th century, who is the father of energy research. Although he discovered neither oxygen nor hydrogen, he had the genius to recognize the importance of oxidation. On this basis, he provided an entirely new classification of chemical elements in terms of oxidation and reduction.

Lavoisier was also the first to measure human oxygen consumption and the thermic effect of food. This set the stage for the law of conservation of energy, promulgated independently by Mayer and by Helmholtz in the middle of the 19th century. However, well before this, the idea of quantitative measurement had been introduced by Santorio Santorio with his human balance on which he ate food and drank beverages. Indeed, his use of the human balance to study metabolism may entitle him to being called the "Father of Obesity Research." The ultimate application of the law of conservation of energy to human beings came from the calorimeter built by Atwater and Rosa at the end of the 19th century.

The 19th century also saw the gradual isolation and then synthesis of many plant and animal products. Ether and chloroform were applied as anesthetics. Glycogen in liver was isolated by Bernard, opening the field of physiological chemistry. The 19th century and the first half of the 20th century might be called the Era of Chemistry. Chemistry was applied to therapeutics with Salvarsan's discovery to treat syphilis. Chemistry was applied to biology, with the development of contraceptives and pharmaceuticals. Chemistry was applied to everyday life, with the synthesis of nylon, polyethylene, and DDT.

## The Biological World

If the 17th century was the century of physics and the 19th century was the century of chemistry, the 20th century was the century of biology. Although anatomy was established as a discipline after 1543, and histology in the 17th century, it was the cell theory in the mid-19th century that provided the element to make biology a conceptual entity. Leeuwenhoek, Malpighi, and Hooke, working with simple microscopes in the 17th century, described many cellular events. However, it was Schwann and Schlieden who simultaneously recognized the unitary characteristics of cells as opposed to their diversity.

From this introduction of cellular biology, a cellular pathology followed shortly, just as organ and tissue pathology followed gross anatomy and tissue histology.

In addition to the cell theory, the 19th century provided two other stepping-stones to the 20th century. These were Darwin's *Origin of the Species* and Mendel's laws of inheritance, which were rediscovered by Bateson in 1895.

In the 20th century, the first hormone, secretin, was identified, and was followed in the rest of the century by a plethora of steroidal, thyroidal, and peptide hormones. The reflex arc and conditioned reflexes were discovered. Insulin was isolated, penicillin discovered, and inborn errors of metabolism identified. Surely, a key discovery in the 20th century was the double-helical structure, which was followed by cracking the genetic code and unraveling the entire genetic sequence of one human chromosome and that of several other organisms.

## KEY DEVELOPMENTS IN OBESITY

Table 69.1 provides an overview of the developments in obesity as a research problem. Obesity is a disease, and as with all disease concepts, it is a construct of the mind. I call it a disease because its etiology is a positive imbalance between the ingestion of food energy and the energy used by the body. This small daily surplus that in adults amounts to about a 10 kcal/day difference each year accounts for a weight gain of approximately 2.5 kg per decade, or 10 kg during adult life. This extra energy is stored as adipose cell triglyceride, producing hypertrophy of fat cells. Fat cell hypertrophy is the pathology of obesity. Big fat cells secrete more peptides and turn over more fatty acids. It is these increased peptides and free fatty acids that produce many of the clinical features of obesity such as diabetes, gallstones, atherosclerosis, and some forms of cancer. Other clinical problems, such as osteoarthritis, sleep apnea, and social stigmatization, arise from the consequences of an excessive physical mass of fat.

In one sense, Santorio Santorio, in the early 17th century, could be called the "Father of Obesity." What Santorio and William Harvey had both grasped by the end of the 16th century was the need for quantification of measurements and the indisputable value of experiment to separate truth from falsehood. Galileo in physics, and later, Boyle in chemistry, also grasped this fundamental premise of modern science. However, it took more than 1,500 years from the time of Hippocrates, Pythagoras, Aristotle, and Archimedes in Greece for this principle to be recognized as the hallmark of modern science. Why it took this long, and why it developed in Europe, not in China, Greece, Rome, the Middle East, or India, all with sophisticated cultures, is one of the fascinating questions in the history of science.

Lavoisier is the second pillar for the scientific basis of obesity. His measurement in the 18th century of human oxygen consumption and demonstration that metabolism is similar to combustion were fundamental contributions to energy balance. It was to take another century before application of these principles to human energy balance by Atwater showed that the Law of Conservation of Energy applied to human beings.

Even before Lavoisier, the first of a series of monographs about obesity began to appear. From the first small book by Short and a second by Flemyng, a long list in many languages has gradually accumulated. Banting's "Letter on Corpulence," written in a small edition in 1863, is probably the most famous. It is the first diet book written by a layman. It was translated into many languages and went through more than four editions. A recent Swedish translation is accompanied by pictures and the first edition has been republished in English.

In the 19th century, obesity received valuable intellectual input from several areas. Quetelet, an epidemiologist and mathematician in Belgium, published the concept of the body mass index (BMI) in 1835. It took nearly 150 years for this idea to be firmly embraced by the obesity research community. The clinical picture of sleep apnea was described, as were the first cases of hypothalamic obesity. Following the cell theory that became the basis of biology, the fat cell was identified and hypertrophy noted in obesity.

The 20th century has seen the application of basic sciences from other areas to improving the science of obesity. From physics, we have seen the use of hydrodensitometry, electrical conductivity, X-ray absorption, and magnetic resonance imaging to provide quantitative estimates of total body fat and regional fat distribution. Physical methods have also been used to measure the changes in isotopic enrichment of chemical compounds, with a special focus on the turnover of water as an indicator of energy expenditure. Chemical methods have been applied in the synthesis of new molecules to treat obesity. Peptide chemistry has unlocked the structure of many peptides.

The genome project and the impetus it has given to new techniques and new ideas has had a major impact on the study of obesity and will be a guiding force in the 21st century. The genes for all of the known Mendelian models of obesity have been cloned (see Chapters 4 and 5). Leptin and leptin receptor biology have opened up a wholly new study of the relation between fat tissue and the brain (see Chapter 6). The molecular and biological tools for overexpressing genes or targeting their destruction have led to numerous transgenic models that heighten our understanding of obesity. Coupled with the intense search for additional genetic targets for obesity, genetic approaches have been most productive.

The studies of diet have shown that no diet is ideal. Cannon showed that gastric contraction is a hunger signal modified by food in the stomach. Diets modifying every nutrient have been published for use by a gullible and optimistic public. If any of them had "cured" obesity, it is hard to see what the market would be for the next diet. The problem is the difficulty in curing obesity. The behavioral science of conditioned reflexes and operant behavior has been applied to the development of behavior therapy as a tool for treatment in all settings (see Chapter 94).

In contrast to these positive influences, the stigmatization of obesity is bad for the overweight individual, bad for the science of obesity, and bad for its practitioners (see Chapter 20). The idea that gluttony and sloth, two of the "deadly sins," are the cause of obesity is, sadly, a widely held view. This viewpoint hampers every aspect of the problem, producing real hurdles to research and treatment. The recent cloning of leptin has helped to remove some of the stigma, but a lot still remains as one of the challenges for the century ahead.

## FURTHER READING

Banting, W. (1863). *A letter on corpulence addressed to the public.* London: Harrison and Sons (Reprinted in *Obesity Research*, 1993, *1*, 153–163).—This is the original description of a metabolic respiration chamber for human beings. It was with this instrument that Atwater and Benedict carried out their classical studies on the first law of thermodynamics as it applies to human beings.

Bray, G. A. (1993). Commentary on classics in obesity: Science and politics of hunger. *Obesity Re-*

*search*, *1*, 489–493.—This paper comments upon a pivotal publication in history, which reveals that gastric contractions signal the recognition of hunger.

Bray, G. A. (1994). Commentary on classics in obesity: Lavoisier and scientific revolution: The oxygen theory displaces air, fire, earth, and water. *Obesity Research*, *2*, 183–188.—Lavoisier's commentary on development of the oxygen theory of metabolism. He understood that the burning of the candle is similar to the metabolism of a living organism.

Bray, G. A. (1994). Commentary on classics in obesity: Quetelet: Quantitiative medicine. *Obesity Research*, *2*, 68–71.—Quetelet was a 19th century mathematician, astronomer, epidemiologist who is recognized in medicine for his idea of the "normal man" and for the body mass index.

Bray, G. A. (1998). Historical framework for the development of ideas about obesity. In G. A. Bray, C. Bouchard, & W. P. T. James (Eds.), *Handbook of obesity* (pp. 1–29). New York: Marcel Dekker.—In-depth history of research and clinical approaches to obesity.

Flemyng, M. A. (1760). *Discourse on the nature, causes and cure of corpulency: Illustrated by a remarkable case, read before the Royal Society, November 1757 and now first published*. London: L. Davis & C. Reymers.—The monographs by Thomas Short and by Malcolm Flemyng were the first two English-language monographs to deal with obesity.

Quetelet, A. (1835). *Sur l'homme et le développement de ses facultés, ou essai de physique sociale*. Paris: Bachelier.—Quetelet was a 19th-century mathematician, astronomer, and epidemiologist recognized in medicine for his idea of the "normal man" and for the body mass index.

Santorio, S. (1720). *Medicina Statica. Being the Aphorisms of Sanctorius* (translated into English with large explanations). London: W. and J. Newton, A. Bell, W. Taylor and J. Osborne.—Santorio Santorio was professor of Medicine at Padua in the early 17th century. He developed a balance for weighing himself that he used daily to determine his changes in weight as he ate and performed other bodily functions. He might appropriately be called the "Father of Obesity Research."

Short, T. (1727). *Discourse concerning the causes and effects of corpulency together with the method for its prevention and cure*. London: J. Roberts.—(See Flemyng for commentary.)

# 70

# Obesity and Quality of Life

JACOB C. SEIDELL
MARJA A. R. TIJHUIS

## BACKGROUND

Health was defined by the World Health Organization (WHO) in 1947 as a state of complete physical, psychological, and social well-being. The concept of "quality of life" was developed to measure self-perceived health and can be interpreted as the individual's overall satisfaction with life. Fontaine and colleagues refer to health-related quality of life as the subjective evaluation by the patient of the effects of medical conditions on physical and mental functioning and well-being.

Many questionnaires have been developed to measure quality of life. The most frequently used are currently the Quality of Well-Being scale (QWB), consisting of 50 questions, the Nottingham Health Profile (NHP), consisting of 45 self-administered items, and the Medical Outcomes Study Short Form-36 Health Survey (SF-36). The latter, a well-validated, 36-item questionnaire, provides a comprehensive measure of physical, emotional, and social well-being. This chapter primarily reviews studies using the SF-36, so that results between different populations can be compared.

The SF-36 measures nine health concepts: physical functioning (10 items), role functioning limitations due to poor physical health (4 items), bodily pain (2 items), general health (5 items), vitality (4 items), social functioning (2 items), role functioning limitations due to poor emotional health (3 items), mental health (5 items) and health change in the past year (1 item). A score can be calculated for each concept, with a low score indicating poor health and a high score indicating good health. These scores can be standardized, so that they range from 0 to 100 and can be more readily compared across health concepts. Such a standardized score is calculated as follows:

$$\frac{\text{raw score} - \text{minimum score}}{\text{score range}}$$

## THE IMPACT OF OBESITY ON QUALITY OF LIFE

The impact of obesity on quality of life can be studied in a variety of ways:

1. Obesity and quality of life in the general population.
2. Prospective studies in the general population.
3. Cross-sectional studies in selected patient groups.
4. Effects of interventions on health-related quality of life.

### Cross-Sectional Studies in the General Population

Han and colleagues studied the SF-36 in detail in 1,885 men and 2,156 women ages 20–60 years in the Netherlands. The interpretation of the scores on the SF-36 is still relatively arbitrary and is often based on the distribution of scores in the general population. For example, in this Dutch study, a subject's particular health concept was classified as "poor" if his or her score was below 66.7% of the standardized score, and "good" if it was 66.7% or above. By these cutoff points, 10–15% of subjects were classified as having poor health for most health concepts. When body mass index (BMI) was classified in tertiles (cutoff points about 24.2 and 26.8 kg/m² in men and 22.7 and 25.6 kg/m² in women), the odds ratio for poor health was significantly higher in the upper tertile compared to the lower tertile in men for physical functioning, and in women for physical functioning, bodily pain, and general health. Within the concept of physical functioning, virtually all 10 items were significantly related to BMI. Within the concepts "mental health" and "general health," only some items were related to BMI. Table 70.1 shows the relative odds for poor physical function in obese compared to lean subjects. Impairment on most activities was about two to three times more common in obese compared to normal-weight women. The odds ratios for obese men were usually in the range of 1.5–2.0. Overweight in men was not clearly associated with impaired physical function, but in women, most activities were significantly associated with overweight.

A large population study from the United Kingdom also found that that obesity without other chronic conditions was associated particularly with the physical component of the SF-36 questionnaire and not with a constructed mental component. The presence of other chronic conditions in obese subjects further decreased physical functioning.

### Prospective Studies in the General Population

Several studies have assessed the role of weight and weight change as predictors of future quality of life. One study measured the BMI in 6,895 men and 3,413 women at four time points between the ages of 25 and 63 years. Only the physical functioning dimension of the SF-36 was used. BMI was a predictor of poor physical functioning in both men and women, although the relative risks were higher in women. Steady weight gain since age 25 was associated in women, but not in men, with poor physical functioning, independent of age, lifestyle factors, current BMI, and weight fluctuation. Weight fluctuation was also related in women to poor physical functioning, independent of current BMI and steady weight change.

Another study examined the effect of weight change on health-related quality of life over 4 years in over 40,000 U.S. female nurses. Weight gain was associated with de-

**TABLE 70.1. Odds Ratios for "Poor" Physical Functioning, Using the SF-36, by Categories of Body Mass Index**

| Items | Men | | Women | |
|---|---|---|---|---|
| | BMI 25–30 | BMI ≥ 30 | BMI 25–30 | BMI ≥ 30 |
| Vigorous activities | 1.1 | 1.8*** | 1.4** | 2.1*** |
| Moderate activities | 1.2 | 1.4 | 1.6*** | 1.5* |
| Lift/carry groceries | 1.1 | 1.4 | 1.4** | 1.6** |
| Walking several flights of stairs | 1.4* | 2.7*** | 1.6*** | 2.3*** |
| Walking one flight of stairs | 0.9 | 1.5 | 1.7** | 2.8*** |
| Bending, kneeling | 1.0 | 2.2*** | 1.7*** | 2.3*** |
| Walking more than 1 kilometer | 1.3 | 2.2*** | 1.4** | 2.0*** |
| Walking several blocks | 1.3 | 1.8** | 1.2 | 2.4*** |
| Bathing and dressing | 1.2 | 2.0 | 0.8 | 1.6 |
| Overall "poor" physical functioning | 1.4 | 2.6*** | 1.6** | 2.4*** |

*Note.* BMI of 20–25 kg/m$^2$ was used as the reference category in 5,887 men and 7,018 women from the Netherlands. Odds ratios were adjusted for age, smoking, education, alcohol consumption, physical activity, employment status, household composition, and parity in women. From Han, T. S., Tijhuis, M. A. R., Lean, M. E. J., & Seidell, J. C. (1998). Quality of life in relation to overweight and body fat distribution. *American Journal of Public Health, 88,* 1814–1820. Copyright 1998 by American Public Health Association. Reprinted by permission.

*$p$ < .05; **$p$ < .01; ***$p$ < .001.

creased physical functioning and vitality, and increased bodily pain regardless of baseline weight. Weight loss was associated with improved physical functioning and vitality, as well as decreased bodily pain. Again, weight change was more strongly associated with physical than mental health. The impact of weight change was just as strong in women 65 years and older as in women younger than 65. These two prospective studies suggest that minimal risk of poor physical functioning in women is obtained by maintaining a steady, moderate weight throughout adulthood. Weight gain should be avoided at all levels of BMI. Weight maintenance and, in cases of overweight, weight loss, are desirable and likely to be beneficial for physical function, vitality, and decreased bodily pain.

## Cross-Sectional Studies in Selected Patient Groups

Poor health-related quality of life has repeatedly been documented in obese patients participating in treatment programs. Specific, obesity-related quality-of-life questionnaires have been developed and validated for clinical purposes. One example is the Obesity-Related Well-Being questionnaire (ORWELL 97), developed by Mannucci and colleagues. It has two subscales, one related to physical symptoms and the other to psychological status and social adjustment. The SF-36 has been used in only a few studies.

Obese patients who sought treatment for obesity in an outpatient weight management program for their obesity in Baltimore had poorer quality of life (more impairment on bodily pain, general health, and vitality dimensions) when compared to obese patients who were not trying to lose weight. These differences persisted after adjustment for the degree of obesity, sociodemographic variables, and comorbidities. Eating behavior has not often been studied in relation to quality of life in obese patients. In a recent Italian study of 183 subjects who were seeking treatment at a university-based weight management center, a binge-eating pattern was identified in over 50% of the subjects. Binge eating appeared to be related to the mental domains of the SF-36 independent of the degree of obesity.

## Effects of Weight Loss on Health-Related Quality of Life

The SF-36 has been used to evaluate improved health-related quality of life resulting from treatment-induced weight loss (see Chapter 90). Many studies have been performed in morbidly obese patients undergoing surgical treatment of obesity (see Chapters 101 and 102). Quality of life at baseline in these patients is very poor and the dramatic weight losses induced by surgery lead to greatly improved quality of life. The postoperative quality of life tends to decrease with time. Fewer studies have evaluated quality of life following moderate weight loss in less severely obese subjects. One study of 38 slightly to moderately overweight persons undergoing a lifestyle modification treatment (average of 9 kg weight loss over 13 weeks) found increased scores on the physical functioning, role–physical, general health, vitality, and mental health domains of the SF-36. In a similar study, 80 women who participated in a lifestyle-based weight loss intervention were studied. Moderate weight loss (6 kg on average) resulted in improved physical function, vitality, and mental health. These findings illustrate that moderate weight loss achieved by lifestyle intervention may yield significant improvement in quality of life.

## SUMMARY AND DISCUSSION

Obesity (BMI of 30 or higher) in the general population is clearly associated with impaired physical functioning in both men and women. Mental and social functioning is generally not impaired (see Chapter 71). Moderate overweight (BMI between 25 and 30) is not accompanied by reduced quality of life. It seems that optimal quality of life can be achieved by maintaining a moderate weight throughout adulthood. In patients seeking expert treatment for obesity, health-related quality of life can be dramatically impaired depending on comorbidities, degree of obesity, and disturbances in eating behavior (e.g., binge eating). Weight loss tends to lead to improvement in all dimensions of quality of life (physical, psychological, and social), although some of these improvements may be attenuated with time even when weight loss is maintained (see Chapter 90).

## FURTHER READING

Doll, H. A., Petersen, S. E. K., & Stewart-Brown, S. L. (2000). Obesity and physical and emotional well-being: Associations between body mass index, chronic illness, and the physical and mental components of the SF-36 questionnaire. *Obesity Research, 8,* 160–170.—A cross-sectional study on BMI and the summary scores of the SF-36.

Fine, J. T., Colditz, G. A., Coakley, E. H., Moseley, G., Manson, J. E., Willett, W. C., & Kawachi, I. (1999). A prospective study of weight change and health-related quality of life in women. *Journal of the American Medical Association, 282,* 2136–2142.—A prospective study on weight change and the dimensions of the SF-36.

Fontaine, K. R., Barofsky, I., Andersen, R. E., Bartlett, S. J., Wiersema, L., Cheskin, L. J., & Franckowiak, S. C. (1999). Impact of weight loss on health-related quality of life. *Quality of*

*Life Research*, *8*, 275–277.—A physical activity intervention study on weight reduction and the dimensions of the SF-36.

Fontaine, K. R., Bartlett, S. J., & Barofsky, I. (2000). Health related quality of life among obese persons seeking and not currently seeking treatment. *International Journal of Eating Disorders*, *27*, 101–105.—A cross-sectional study on seeking treatment for obesity and the dimensions of the SF-36.

Han, T. S., Tijhuis, M. A. R., Lean, M. E. J., & Seidell, J. C. (1998). Quality of life in relation to overweight and body fat distribution. *American Journal of Public Health*, *88*, 1814–1820.—A cross-sectional study on BMI and the dimensions of the SF-36.

Lean, M. E. J, Han, T. S., & Seidell, J. C. (1999). Impairment of health and quality of life using new U.S. federal guidelines for the identification of obesity. *Archives of Internal Medicine*, *159*, 837–843.—A cross-sectional study on obesity and items of the physical functioning dimension of the SF-36 (Table 70.1).

Mannucci, E., Ricca, V., Barciulli, E., Di Bernardo, M., Travaglini, R., Cabras, P. L., & Rotella, C. M. (1999). Quality of life and overweight: The Obesity-Related Well-Being (ORWELL 97) questionnaire. *Addictive Behavior*, *24*, 345–357.—A description of an obesity-related quality-of-life questionnaire.

Marchesini G., Solaroli E., Baraldi, L., Natale, S., Migliorini, S., Visani, F., Forlani, G., & Melchionda, N. (2000). Health-related quality of life in obesity: The role of eating behaviors. *Diabetes Nutrition and Metabolism*, *13*, 156–164.—A cross-sectional study on binge eating in obesity and the dimensions of the SF-36.

Stafford, M., Hemingway, H., & Marmot, M. (1998). Current obesity, steady weight change and weight fluctuation as predictors of physical functioning in middle aged office workers: The Whitehall II Study. *International Journal of Obesity*, *22*, 23–31.—A prospective study on BMI and the physical functioning dimension of the SF-36.

Van Gemert, W. G., Adang, E. M., Greve, J. W., & Soeters, P. B. (1998). Quality of life assessment of morbidly obese patients: Effect of weight-reducing surgery. *American Journal of Clinical Nutrition*, *67*, 197–201.—An intervention study on weight-reducing surgery and the NHP.

# 71

# Psychological Consequences
of Obesity

## MICHAEL A. FRIEDMAN
## KELLY D. BROWNELL

In contrast to the concerted effort to document the physical consequences of obesity, there is much less knowledge about the psychological consequences of excess weight. Furthermore, an interesting paradox exists. Clinical impressions suggest that obesity is often associated with intense suffering, including shame, guilt, and poor body image. However, most studies comparing obese and nonobese groups on psychological variables have not found consistent differences, leading many researchers to conclude that obesity is not associated with general psychological problems (see Chapter 70). The absence of group differences in studies comparing obese and nonobese persons has led to the assumption that the obese population is homogeneous with respect to psychological functioning. It is clear, however, that the obese population is heterogeneous with respect to etiology, effects of excess weight on medical variables, and response to various treatments. An approach accounting for this heterogeneity is necessary to understand the psychological consequences of obesity.

## A GENERATIONAL APPROACH

Friedman and Brownell have proposed a generational approach, suggesting that the results of comparative studies of obese and nonobese groups are an expected, if not inevitable, outcome of the approach used. Most studies use small samples, do not represent the general obese population, and typically employ a single measure of only one aspect of psychopathology. These studies are helpful as a first generation of research in the area but may not prove a lack of psychological suffering among obese individuals. Rather, inconsistent findings reflect an inconsistent phenomenon (i.e., the effects of being obese vary across individuals). Obesity may create serious psychosocial problems in some individuals, mild problems in others, and perhaps no distress in others. For this reason, we have proposed that the field needs to move to a second generation of research that examines the effects of being obese and whether the psychological correlates of obesity vary across individuals, and if so, identify factors responsible for the variation. Ultimately, a third generation of research will take the associations found between specific risk factors and psychological characteristics among obese individuals and attempt to establish causal links. We can use reactions to social stigma as an example of how these research generations might apply (see Figure 71.1).

## OBESITY AND PSYCHOLOGICAL SUFFERING

Thirty years of research shows clearly that the stigma of obesity is widespread. Obese people are less liked and viewed less favorably than persons of normal weight. Compared

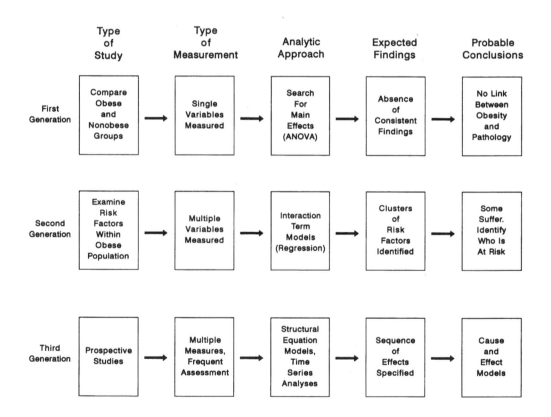

**FIGURE 71.1.** Diagram showing three generations of research methods and outcomes aimed at establishing links between obesity and psychological functioning. Nearly all existing research has been from the first generation, with some newer studies falling into the second generation. Third-generation studies will be needed to examine clearly the key associations. From Friedman, M. A., & Brownell, K. D. (1995). Psychological correlates of obesity: Moving to the next research generation. *Psychological Bulletin, 117,* 195–212. Copyright 1995 by American Psychological Association. Reprinted by permission.

to normal-weight individuals, obese individuals have been described as "lazy," "stupid," "cheats," and "ugly," among other characteristics. Furthermore, these negative attitudes often translate into prejudice and discrimination against obese individuals (see Chapter 20). Discrimination has been reported in employment, housing, and college admissions. In addition, individuals who were overweight as adolescents are less likely to be married, and have lower household incomes and higher rates of household poverty in future years than individuals who were normal-weight adolescents. By living in a culture that condemns their physical appearance and, perhaps more importantly, blames them for their condition, it is logical to assume that obese persons would suffer emotionally from the bias, negative attitudes, and discrimination.

## THE FIRST GENERATION OF STUDIES

The first generation of research sought to identify personality and psychopathology variables related to the etiology of obesity rather than the effects of being obese on the individual. The results of these studies, which examined constructs such as depression, anxiety, negative body image, and self-esteem, point to clear heterogeneity, both in etiology and consequences of obesity. The methodology used in these comparison studies of obese to nonobese individuals in homogeneous populations utilizing narrow measures was to some extent appropriate for determining if psychological functioning played a causal role in the onset of obesity. However, in light of the heterogeneity of etiological factors in the obese population, the predictable result was that some studies showed differences and others did not. The conclusion that there were no systematic psychological effects of obesity was perhaps inevitable, but it is contrary to our interpretation—that there are important but inconsistent effects. We feel that a second generation of studies is necessary to determine who suffers negative psychological consequences.

## THE SECOND GENERATION OF STUDIES: A RISK-FACTOR APPROACH TO DETERMINE WHO SUFFERS

We propose that a theoretical approach examining the psychological consequences of obesity *within* the obese population is necessary. The model identifies factors likely to place an overweight individual at risk for psychological problems. Instead of studying whether obese and nonobese people differ, the search would be for risk factors that explain why some obese individuals suffer negative psychological consequences and others do not. Although the field has not labeled them as such, results of some recent studies can be discussed within the second-generation framework.

### Binge Eating

An important development in the obesity field is the recognition that a distinct subset of the obese population is composed of binge eaters (see Chapters 18, 31, 63, and 73). Binge eating refers to eating large amounts of food in a short time, while feeling that the eating is out of control. This is qualitatively different from overeating, in that the amount eaten, frequency of episodes, compulsive nature of the eating, and psychological aftermath are striking. Binge eaters show a higher prevalence of psychopathology, particularly affective disorders, compared to obese non-binge-eaters. For example, Marcus and colleagues found that 60% of binge eaters met criteria for at least one psychiatric disorder versus 28% of non-binge-eaters. Similar results have been found in other studies. Obese binge eaters also tend to display more psychopathology than normal-weight binge eaters, indicating an important interaction of weight with binge eating. Binge eating can be considered a risk factor for psychological problems among obese individuals.

## Weight Cycling

Although there is a large literature on the metabolic effects and, to a lesser extent, the health effects of repeated cycles of weight loss and regain, much less is known about the effects of weight cycling on behavior and psychological factors. Furthermore, the data are decidedly mixed. One possible reason is that while more objective measures of weight loss and regain do not appear to be related to negative psychological consequences, an individual's perception of him- or herself as a weight cycler, or someone who has difficulty maintaining weight loss, does appear to be related to lower self-esteem, and poorer body and life satisfaction. While the mechanism by which weight cycling influences psychological functioning is unclear, it is possible that weight cycling perpetuates unhealthy eating behavior such as binge eating.

## Potential Demographic Risk Factors

There are three demographic variables that may represent risk factors for psychological suffering among the obese population: being female, being adolescent, and being severely overweight. For example, it is well known that obesity carries greater stigma in females than in males, and evidence suggests that there is a powerful fear of obesity among both obese and nonobese high school girls. Similarly, adolescence and early adulthood may represent a period of time when the stigma, and therefore psychological consequences, may be most intense. For example, a small number of studies have shown evidence of poorer self-concept in obese adolescents and college-age women than in normal-weight peers. Finally, when considering that obesity may be more noticeable in severely obese individuals, it is likely that both the associated stigma and psychological suffering may be greater for these individuals. At present, these demographic variables must be considered potential risk factors, as more research is needed.

## THE THIRD GENERATION OF RESEARCH

Second-generation studies have identified binge eating and weight cycling as likely behavioral risk factors for increased psychopathology among obese individuals and may represent a behavioral syndrome that is associated with increased psychopathology. These factors need to be studied in concert, utilizing a second-generation approach to determine whether they are truly associated with suffering in the obese population, and whether they interact or occur in sequence. The third generation should build on the second by establishing causal links between risk factors and psychopathology. Because the third generation must await the results of the second, and because the second generation is in its early stages, it is only possible to speculate about what the third generation will bring.

## CONCLUSIONS

Because so many individuals are obese, the potential for psychological problems is substantial. Existing studies have been useful in demonstrating an absence of clear and consistent differences between obese and nonobese populations in general. Hence, it is safe to say that not all obese people suffer psychological distress from their condition. We believe attention should turn from *whether* obese persons suffer psychological distress to *who* will suffer and in what ways. This philosophy suggests a risk-factor approach that will identify individuals in whom psychological problems may occur, conditions likely to promote suffering, and their interaction. Elucidating the psychological consequences of obesity may be important in establishing the pathogenesis and treatment of obesity, and in understanding the lives of obese individuals.

## FURTHER READING

Brownell, K. D., & Wadden, T. A. (1992). Etiology and treatment of obesity: Understanding a serious, prevalent, and refractory disorder. *Journal of Consulting and Clinical Psychology, 60,* 505–517.—Classic description of the heterogeneity of the obese population and the implications for treatment.

Friedman, M. A., & Brownell, K. D. (1995). Psychological correlates of obesity: Moving to the next research generation. *Psychological Bulletin, 117,* 195–212.—Original article that describes the generational approach to understanding psychological correlates of obesity.

Friedman, M. A., Schwartz, M. B., & Brownell, K. D. (1998). Differential relation of psychological functioning with the history and experience of weight cycling. *Journal of Consulting and Clinical Psychology, 66,* 646–650.—First study identifying that the experience of being a weight cycler is more highly associated with psychological problems than recalled history of cycling.

Gortmaker, A., Must, A., Perrin, J. M., Sobol, A. M., & Dietz, W. H. (1993). Social and economic consequences of overweight in adolescence and young adulthood. *New England Journal of Medicine, 329,* 1008–1012.—Important study documenting the widespread negative effects of obesity among children and adolescents.

Kiernan, M., Rodin, J., Brownell, K. D., Wilmore, J. H., & Crandall, C. (1992). Relationship of level of exercise, age and weight-cycling history to eating and weight disturbances in male and female runners. *Health Psychology, 11,* 418–421.—One of the original articles documenting the negative psychological consequences of weight cycling.

Klesges, R. C., Haddock, C. K., Stein, R. J., Klesges, L. M., Eck, L. H., & Hanson, C. L. (1992). Relationship between psychosocial functioning and body fat in preschool children: A longitudinal investigation. *Journal of Consulting and Clinical Psychology, 60,* 793–796.—Important study in which body fat was not related to self-concept in children.

Kolotkin, R. L., Revis, E. S., Kirkley, B. G., & Janick, L. (1987). Binge eating in obesity: Associated MMPI characteristics. *Journal of Consulting and Clinical Psychology, 55,* 872–876.—One of the first studies documenting the relation between binge eating and psychopathology among treatment-seeking obese individuals.

Marcus, M. D., Wing, R. R., & Hopkins, J. (1988). Obese binge eaters: Affect, cognitions and response to behavioral weight control. *Journal of Consulting and Clinical Psychology, 56,* 433–439.—One of the first studies to identify "obese binge eaters" as having more psychopathology than non-binge-eating obese persons.

Wadden, T. A., & Stunkard, A. J. (1985). Social and psychological consequences of obesity. *Annals of Internal Medicine, 103,* 1062–1067.—Important, early field-documentation of the pain and suffering potentially associated with obesity.

# 72

# Obesity and Body Image

## JAMES C. ROSEN

Obesity is viewed as physically unattractive and the result of personal misbehavior; hence, many overweight persons develop a negative body image. Distressing body image experiences are associated with psychological and eating disorder symptoms, and can influence the outcome of weight control programs (see Chapter 108). Although concern about physical appearance is a main reason that people seek weight reduction, specific intervention to improve body image has been neglected in the treatment of obesity.

## BODY IMAGE EXPERIENCES IN OBESITY

Studies of nonclinical samples indicate that obese persons do not have more severe mental health symptoms or maladaptive personality traits than nonobese persons (see Chapter 71). The only consistent obese–nonobese difference on psychological measures is body image. Obese persons are more prone to distort their body size, more dissatisfied and preoccupied with physical appearance, and more avoidant of social situations. Thus, all three components of body image are affected: perception, cognition–affect, and behavior.

### Types of Appearance Complaints

The most common aspects of physical appearance that are dissatisfying to obese *and* nonobese persons, especially women, are the waist or abdomen, whole body, thighs, lower body, and buttocks. Close to one-third of obese persons report concern with issues other than size of large body regions, including facial features, facial or head hair, skin blemishes, teeth, and breast size or shape. Morbidly obese persons in particular complain of other appearance problems, such as excessive facial hair or skin discoloration; these often are related to their extreme weight. Frame size and hip circumference in women are better predictors of body dissatisfaction than body fat and degree of overweight. Therefore, weight reduction by itself may be ineffective in reducing body dissatisfaction.

## Relation between Body Image, Weight, and Clinical Status

Treatment seeking does not necessarily predict a more negative body image. Obese persons in random, community samples report about the same body dissatisfaction as do people in behavioral, lifestyle, weight control programs, perhaps because most community subjects also are trying to lose weight. Two clinical populations with more negative body image are persons with binge-eating disorder and those who have had gastric bypass surgery. Body dissatisfaction increases with body mass index (BMI), and the severity in obesity surgery patients is comparable to that of people who seek treatment for diagnosable body image disorders. Extreme social isolation due to social phobia is not uncommon in morbidly obese patients.

## Definition of Body Image Disorder in Obesity

The boundary between normal and abnormal concerns about appearance is difficult to specify, and many people, including many mental health professionals, think dissatisfaction with body image in obese persons is reasonable; obese people do not just imagine their physical defect or social prejudice. This attitude represents a misunderstanding about the nature of body image disorder and is another form of negative bias toward obesity (i.e., obese people deserve to feel the way they do) (see Chapter 20). Obese people may not simply imagine being obese, as might a normal-weight person with bulimia. However, body size distortion is not a necessary feature of body image disorder. Obese persons with body image disorder experience upsetting preoccupation with their appearance, unrealistically believe their appearance proves something negative about their personal worth, avoid too many social situations because of their weight, and are overly concerned about hiding or disguising their body.

Although body image disorder occurs in obesity, lack of a standard definition is a major research and clinical problem. A diagnosis of body dysmorphic disorder is inappropriate, because it is reserved for essentially normal-looking people who imagine themselves to have physical defects (see Chapter 21). An alternative is to use a cutoff score on a standard measure of body image distress; however, for obese subjects, norms are not available for many popular body image measures. Another method is to use a diagnostic measure for body dysmorphic disorder, minus the criterion for "normal" appearance. This results in about 10% of obese weight control patients meeting the criteria for body image disorder. Moreover, about one-fourth of these patients show daily affective distress about their physical appearance and significant behavioral avoidance. Total body image symptoms correlate significantly with mental health symptoms and negative self-esteem.

## DEVELOPMENT OF NEGATIVE BODY IMAGE

Being overweight by early adolescence sets the stage for negative body image and predicts body dissatisfaction in adulthood. Presumably, obese adolescents become more self-conscious than normal about their physical appearance because of the negative stereotypes about obesity and the barrage of images of thin women and muscular men in the media (see Chapter 19). All obese persons are exposed to prejudice about obesity, but not all develop truly negative body images. Why do some obese persons become confident about their appearance and others become fearful and ashamed? Little research is available on the development of negative body image in obesity. Having good experiences in sports and family or friends who give positive self-esteem messages, such as "Accept yourself for who you are," are associated with positive body image and might be considered protective factors, whereas being teased or pressured by parents to lose weight is associated with negative body image.

Stigmatizing experiences for obese persons are not just occasional events (see Chapter 20) and include nasty comments from children, people's negative assumptions (e.g., obese people must have emotional problems), physical barriers, being stared at, inappropriate comments from doctors, and derogatory remarks from family or strangers. The frequency of stigmatizing situations is associated with negative body image, mental health symptoms, and BMI. Maladaptive coping responses to stigmatization predict more negative body image, whereas adaptive coping responses such as positive self-talk, seeing the situation as the other person's problem, refusing to hide the body, and self-love–self-acceptance strategies predict better adjustment.

## BODY IMAGE AND WEIGHT CONTROL

Despite the important health benefits of weight loss, obese persons usually enroll in weight control programs with the desire to improve their self-esteem and body image. Starting an exercise program and picking a specific weight loss goal also are more influenced by appearance concerns than by health problems or a doctor's recommendation.

Obese people can overcome their distressing preoccupation with physical appearance and social avoidance using proven cognitive-behavioral techniques, without trying to lose weight (see Chapter 108). This body image therapy, or learning to accept one's self, does not cause people to gain weight. But clearly, most people see weight loss as the way to eliminate negative body image. Is this effective? Some persons who successfully lose weight still feel overly fat, and some former morbidly obese persons still have social phobia after gastric bypass surgery. Body image symptoms can become deeply ingrained habits. Extra behavioral procedures are needed to eliminate them. However, on average, obesity surgery results in dramatic improvement in body image. Even a 5–10% weight loss in a behavioral, lifestyle weight control program leads to clinically significant reductions in negative body image (see Chapter 90). The graduates of such programs might still be obese and dissatisfied with their weight, but they experience more body image improvement than they predicted at the beginning of treatment, and in fact, are close to the normal range on standard measures.

The relapse problem in obesity treatment extends to body image. Even a small weight regain predicts a slip in body image, a consequence that people rate as more distressing than losing physical health benefits. Instruction in body image management during weight control reduces the effect of weight regain on body satisfaction. Also, it appears that body dissatisfaction at the end of weight control treatment predicts weight regain. Although addressing body image concerns during treatment might help with weight loss maintenance, more research into the reciprocal effects of weight loss and body image change is needed. Generally speaking, weight control appears to be good body image therapy.

## FURTHER READING

Foster, G. D., Wadden, T. A., Vogt, R. A., & Brewer, G. (1997). What is a reasonable weight loss? Patients' expectations and evaluations of obesity treatment outcomes. *Journal of Consulting and Clinical Psychology, 65,* 79–85.—An examination of the relation between body image improvement and expectations for losing weight.

Myers, A., & Rosen, J. C. (1999). Obesity stigmatization and coping: Relation to mental health symptoms, body image, and self-esteem. *International Journal of Obesity, 23,* 221–230.—Includes an empirically derived list of common stigmatizing situations and coping techniques.

Ramirez, E. M., & Rosen, J. C. (in press). A comparison of weight control and weight control plus body image therapy for obese men and women. *Journal of Consulting and Clinical Psychology.*—A clinical trial that details the degree of clinical improvement in body image.

Rosen, J. C. (1997). Cognitive-behavioral body image therapy. In D. M. Garner & P. E. Garfinkel (Eds.), *Handbook of treatment for eating disorders* (2nd ed., pp. 188–201). New York: Guilford Press.—A clinical guideline to identifying and modifying the symptoms of severely negative body image.

Rosen, J. C., & Reiter, J. (1996). Development of the Body Dysmorphic Disorder Examination. *Behaviour Research and Therapy, 34,* 755–766.—A clinically significant body image measure that is neither gender-biased nor limited strictly to weight concerns.

Sarwer, D. B., Wadden, T. A., & Foster, G. D. (1998). Assessment of body image dissatisfaction in obese women: Specificity, severity, and clinical significance. *Journal of Consulting and Clinical Psychology, 66,* 651–654.—An examination of types of appearance complaints in obesity and the rate of clinically severe body image disorder.

# 73

# Binge Eating in Obese Persons

## SUSAN Z. YANOVSKI

Binge eating is a common and serious problem in individuals with obesity. Depending on how it is defined, more than one-third of obese individuals undergoing weight loss treatment report difficulties with binge eating, although far fewer meet criteria for binge eating disorder (BED) when assessed by a clinical interview (see Chapters 18 and 31).

## DEFINING BINGE EATING

Binge eating, according to the fourth edition of the *Diagnostic and Statistical Manual of Mental Disorders*, is characterized by eating, in a discrete period of time, an amount that is larger than most others would consume in similar circumstances, and is accompanied by a sense of loss of control over what or how much one is eating. Both of these criteria (objectively large amount of food and loss of control) are necessary for an episode to be considered an objective binge. Many people report loss of control alone (without consuming a large amount of food), objective overeating without loss of control, or both loss of control and overeating, and it is common for individuals to report all three types of episodes at different times. When binge eating is frequent (i.e., more than twice weekly) and accompanied by behavioral indicators of loss of control and distress, BED may be diagnosed.

Occasional binge eating is commonly reported by overweight as well as non-overweight persons. It is not known whether subthreshold binge eating carries the same prognostic significance as that of binge eating disorder. Some studies suggest similar psychopathology and distress.

## NATURE OF BINGE EATING IN OBESITY

Binge eating in obese persons who do not purge or engage in other inappropriate compensatory behaviors appears to differ somewhat from the binge eating seen in those with bulimia nervosa. Binge episodes tend to be of smaller size and caloric content. In addition, because binges are not terminated by vomiting, discrete binge episodes may be difficult to identify. Some obese binge eaters describe "grazing," in which they see themselves as out of control most or all of an entire day. Studies analyzing recorded food intake find that obese binge eaters report binge episodes that vary greatly in caloric content, ranging from fewer than 50 to several thousand kilocalories. This suggests that both objective and subjective binge episodes are common.

## Laboratory Studies

Laboratory studies of eating behavior in obese individuals with BED shed light on how they differ from individuals with bulimia nervosa or obese non-binge-eaters. Studies using a standardized buffet meal of usual dinner and snack foods have found that obese binge eaters consume more than weight-matched non-binge-eaters when asked to "let yourself go." Of interest, however, those with BED also consumed more than obese non-binge-eaters when asked to eat normally, without identifying the large amount as a binge. This suggests that the presence of a large amount of palatable food may act to disinhibit food intake, regardless of instruction. This contrasts with subjects with bulimia nervosa who, when presented with a similar array, either restrict and eat very little or binge eat. There is little evidence for "carbohydrate craving" during binge episodes, with most studies suggesting similar macronutrient composition to usual meal foods, or an increase in percent fat and decrease in percent protein during the episodes. Women, in particular, tend to binge on combination foods containing large amounts of both sugar and fat.

## CAUSES OF BINGE EATING IN OBESITY

Binge eating is frequently presumed to be the consequence of dieting and restriction of food intake. In this model, prolonged dietary restriction interferes with food regulation and satiety, leading to compensatory binge episodes (see Chapters 15, 16, and 17). In bulimia nervosa, dieting almost invariably precedes the onset of binge eating. Among obese binge eaters, however, the relationship between dieting and binge eating is much less clear. About half of obese individuals with BED report dieting before the onset of binge eating, with the remainder reporting binge eating either prior to or at about the same time as the first diet.

It is possible that binge eating contributes to the development or worsening of obesity. Some studies, although not all, suggest that presence of frequent binge eating is associated with more severe obesity. Binge eating is also associated with a history of weight cycling, although causality cannot be determined. Numerous studies have found an association between binge eating and psychiatric disorders, particularly affective disorders such as depression (see Chapters 31 and 71). Personality disorders involving impulse control, as well as substance abuse disorders, have also been reported to be more common in this population. It is still unclear whether the binge eating precedes development of depression or is a consequence, but binge eating may be an attempt at affect regulation for some individuals.

While the relationship between dietary restraint and binge eating in obesity is not strong, a consistent association has been found between disinhibition and obesity. Disinhibition, defined as loss of control over eating in response to affective, cognitive, or pharmacological stimuli (such as alcohol), is strongly linked to binge eating and appears to improve with successful treatment (see Chapter 16). In contrast, cognitive restraint often stays the same or increases as binge-eating severity declines.

## WEIGHT LOSS TREATMENT AND BINGE EATING

Because many individuals who report frequent binge-eating episodes are obese, the response of binge eaters to weight loss treatment is important (see Chapter 63). Concerns center on two areas: (1) Does weight loss treatment worsen binge eating? (2) Is weight loss treatment less effective in binge eaters?

### Does Weight Loss Treatment Worsen Binge Eating?

Despite concerns that caloric restriction will worsen binge eating in those predisposed to the problem, there is little evidence from controlled studies that dietary restriction combined with behavioral weight loss treatments worsens binge eating. Studies using moderate (e.g., 1,200–1,500 kcal/day) as well as more severe (< 800 kcal/day) energy restriction have consistently shown that binge eating, on average, improves during weight loss treatment in those who report preexisting binge-eating difficulties—at least during the phase of active weight loss. Binge eaters are equally likely as non-binge-eaters to adhere to a diet but may have larger or more severe lapses, particularly as flexibility and choices increase, for example, during refeeding after a very-low-calorie diet. One study showed a temporary increase in "binge episodes" among non-binge-eaters exposed to a very-low-calorie diet; however, this was primarily limited to the period of dieting, and decreased within 3 months after termination of treatment. The responsiveness of binge eaters to weight loss treatment may be secondary to the support and structure provided by such programs. The long-term effects of standard weight loss treatments on binge eating have not been determined, and further studies are needed.

The impact of weight loss medications on binge eating has also not been clarified (see Chapter 64). One small study using dexfenfluramine in obese binge eaters found a significant decrease in binge eating with active drug relative to placebo; interestingly, the dexfenfluramine did not lead to weight loss in this group. Studies are currently ongoing to determine the effects of weight loss medications on both binge eating and weight loss in this population. The use of other medications, such as antidepressants, on binge eating is discussed in Chapter 64.

### Is Weight Loss Treatment Less Effective in Binge Eaters?

Although binge eating appears to decrease among those in weight loss programs, short- and long-term weight losses are more mixed. Most studies show similar decreases in body weight in response to weight loss treatment for binge eaters or non-binge-eaters, and some have even found greater weight losses among binge eaters. Several studies, however, suggest that obese binge eaters may be more likely to drop out of treatment prematurely, or to regain lost weight more quickly. In addition, the relationship between binge eating and weight loss may be mediated by other factors. A recent study found that although overweight binge eaters had a greater tendency to drop out of treatment and to have slightly lower weight losses at 18 months, the impact of binge status on weight loss or regain appeared to be mediated by degree of psychological dysphoria. It is likely that further research will clarify whether obese binge eaters need different weight loss treatment than non-binge eaters, and whether combining treatment targeting the disordered eating as well as weight loss will provide better and more lasting results (see Chapters 63 and 64).

Surgical weight loss treatment for obese patients with binge eating disorder has also yielded mixed results, with some studies reporting less weight loss in those with severe binge eating. Type of surgical procedure may have an impact on treatment outcome (see Chapters 101 and 102). For example, it has been reported that gastric restrictive procedures may be problematic for binge eaters, who can "out-eat" their procedure with frequent small amounts of energy-dense foods. Procedures such as gastric bypass, which would lead to increased symptoms of excess sweet consumption, may be more appropriate in this population, although controlled studies have not been reported.

## BINGE EATING AND THE PREVENTION OF OBESITY

Binge eating is a likely contributor to excess energy intake for many obese persons, leading to increasing weight gain and worsening comorbid conditions. Better understanding of factors underlying binge eating in obese individuals should lead to improved treatments that will decrease binge eating and enhance efforts at sustained weight loss. Perhaps more importantly, early identification and treatment of those at risk for binge eating have the potential to help prevent excessive weight gain from ever occurring, which may play one role in the primary prevention of obesity.

## FURTHER READING

Abbott, D. W., de Zwaan, M., Mussell, M. P., Raymond, N. C., Seim, H. C., Crow, S. J., Crosby, R. D., & Mitchell, J. E. (1998). Onset of binge eating and dieting in overweight women: Implications for etiology, associated features and treatment. *Journal of Psychosomatic Research, 44,* 367–374.—This study investigated differences between obese women who report binge eating prior to dieting and those who dieted first, and discusses the implication of different patterns on causes and severity of binge eating.

Gladis, M. M., Wadden, T. A., Vogt, R. A., Foster, G. D., Kuehnel, R. H., & Bartlett, S. J. (1998). Behavioral treatment of obese binge eaters: Do they need different care? *Journal of Psychosomatic Research, 44,* 375–384.—This paper presents data from one study and reviews the literature on binge eating and weight loss, concluding that binge eaters respond as well as non-binge-eaters to standard weight loss treatments.

Hsu, L. K., Benotti, P. N., Dwyer, J., Roberts, S. B., Saltzman, E., Shikora, S., Rolls, B. J., & Rand, C. W. (1998). Nonsurgical factors that influence the outcome of bariatric surgery: A review. *Psychosomatic Medicine, 60,* 338–346.—A review and discussion on how nonsurgical factors, including binge-eating behavior, may affect long-term outcome of bariatric surgery.

Mitchell, J. E., Crow, S., Peterson, C. B., Wonderlich, S., & Crosby, R. D. (1998). Feeding laboratory studies in patients with eating disorders: A review. *International Journal of Eating Disorders, 24,* 115–124.—Reviews laboratory studies of eating behaviors in a laboratory setting, including studies of BED.

National Task Force on the Prevention and Treatment of Obesity. (2000). Dieting and the development of eating disorders in overweight and obese adults. *Archives of Internal Medicine, 160,* 2581–2589.—Reviews the literature regarding the relationship between dieting and eating disorders, including psychological effects, impact of weight cycling, and obesity prevention.

Sherwood, N. E., Jeffery, R. W., & Wing, R. R. (1999). Binge status as a predictor of weight loss treatment outcome. *International Journal of Obesity and Related Metabolic Disorders, 23,* 485–493.—Presents data on the relationship between binge eating and weight loss in a large cohort of obese subjects undergoing treatment.

Spitzer, R. L., Devlin, M., Walsh, B. T., Hasin, D., Wing, R., Marcus, M., Stunkard, A., Wadden, T., Yanovski, S., Agras, S., Mitchell, J., & Nonas, C. (1992). Binge eating disorder: A multisite field trial of the diagnostic criteria. *International Journal of Eating Disorders, 11,* 191–203.—The original field study leading to the characterization of BED.

Stunkard, A. J., & Messick, S. (1985). The three-factor eating questionnaire to measure dietary restraint, disinhibition and hunger. *Journal of Psychosomatic Research, 29,* 71–83.—A description of the questionnaire used to assess three factors believed to be important in categorizing eating behaviors: restraint, disinhibition, and hunger.

Yanovski, S. Z. (1999). Diagnosis and prevalence of eating disorders in obesity. In G. Ailhaud & B. Guy-Grand (Eds.), *Progress in obesity research* (Vol. 8, pp. 229–236). London: John Libby.—A review of current knowledge about the prevalence of binge eating and other eating disorders among obese persons.

# Epidemiology, Etiology, and Course of Obesity

# 74

# A World View of the
# Obesity Problem

## W. PHILIP T. JAMES

A global perspective on obesity is now possible because all countries and the World Health Organization (WHO) have come to accept a general classification of normal weight, with different degrees of underweight, overweight, and obesity based on the body mass index (BMI) (see Chapter 68). The range of normal body weight is currently accepted internationally as a BMI of 18.5 to 24.9, the lower limit being determined on the basis of our classification of different degrees of underweight in adults, specifying increasing limitations in work capacity below a BMI of 18.5. The BMI of 25.0 was a compromise between the then-standard in North America based on U.S. analyses and an Asian concern that comorbidities emerged at lower BMIs. For reference purposes, BMIs of 25.0 and 30.0 will now allow estimates of regional and global overweight and obesity rates, respectively. Currently, WHO estimates that there are about 180 million obese adults, and the probability is that there are in addition at least twice as many adults who are overweight, with a BMI of 25.0 to 29.9.

Four issues of classification are important. First is the increasing recognition that waist circumference may be a particularly useful additional criterion for specifying comorbidity risks (see Chapters 68, 84, and 86). This is particularly important in the developing world where early poor growth *in utero* and postnatally could explain the increased propensity to abdominal obesity at modest increases in adult weight. Second, Latin American investigators highlight the spuriously enhanced BMIs of adults of short stature because they have short legs, having been "stunted" throughout childhood. By simply measuring sitting heights, however, it is possible to derive simple corrections for this feature. Short people (e.g., those living in Central America and Asia) need to accumulate substantially less total energy before their weight exceeds a BMI of 25.0, even with adjustments for sitting height. The smaller gain in energy is, however, sufficient to trigger similar comorbidities (e.g., with serum lipid changes, glucose intolerance, and hypertension) to those seen in taller Caucasians.

Third, many Asian experts consider lower cutoff points for both BMI and waist

411

circumference appropriate for their populations, since glucose intolerance, hypertension, and diabetes emerge as florid clinical problems and prevalent public health issues at BMIs above 23.0, with few of the population having a BMI of 30.0 or more. On this basis, a recent proposal suggests that BMIs of 23.0 should be considered as the upper limit of normal, with obesity as such specified as a problem at BMIs of ≥ 25.0. Similarly, preliminary sex-specific waist circumferences are suggested with lower limits than those applied by WHO on the basis of analyses of Caucasians. Coherent comparative analyses of the relationship of comorbidities to BMI and waist circumference are under way in different societies, with evidence from both the United States and Northern Europe of optimum BMIs of about 20.0, with clear evidence of comorbidities emerging within the specified normal range. Attributable risk analyses relating weight gain to comorbidities are awaited, but in China, the Caribbean, and affluent societies, BMI is of major importance in explaining both diabetes and hypertension. About two-thirds of the global burden of diabetes has been attributed to excess weight gain by WHO when the upper normal limit of BMI is set at 25.0. New evidence suggests that fetal and early childhood limitations on growth enhance the susceptibility to later comorbidities, especially if growth rates in later childhood accelerate markedly. Thus, Asian propensities toward hypertension and diabetes at modest weight gain may reflect early fetal and childhood programming mediated by nutrition and other factors. This is now of major public health concern.

The BMI index is a crude but valuable measure for comparative purposes; differences between groups may well prove to be of environmental origin, such as in the field of child growth, where postwar inappropriate assumptions were made about intrinsic ethnic differences. Currently, detailed studies of different ethnic groups reveal that at equivalent BMIs, adult Indians have substantially less lean tissue than Caucasians, with adults of Chinese origin having intermediate proportions of lean body mass per unit weight. Pacific Islanders have higher lean-to-fat ratios than Caucasians. Recognized individual differences in the control of lean–fat ratios have not been identified as genetically controlled in different ethnic groups.

Finally, throughout the world, there is concern about childhood obesity, with the International Obesity Task Force now having suggested preliminary reference BMIs on an age- and sex-specific basis for designating overweight and obese children (see Chapter 85). This proposal is based on taking nationally representative data from the United States (NHANES I survey), United Kingdom, the Netherlands, Hong Kong, Singapore, and Brazil and specifying cutoff points that are the average percentiles corresponding to those that, when girls and boys mature at the age of 18, equate to BMIs of 25.0 and 30.0. By choosing these values, it is now possible to gain some perspective on children's adiposity while recognizing that for individual clinical care, the cutoff points are far less useful because they lack the appropriate selectivity and specificity.

## THE GLOBAL PREVALENCE OF OBESITY

Recent analyses reveal the marked disparities in obesity rates among different countries within a region as well as substantial differences in obesity rates even in the developing world. Thus, in sub-Saharan Africa, the overall obesity rates are low, but in South Africa, the obesity rates in black women, even in rural areas, often exceed 30%. In Europe, obesity rates vary markedly from country to country, with Central and Eastern European countries having particularly high obesity rates (i.e., again exceeding 30%). Adults in some European Union countries (e.g., the Netherlands), have modest obesity rates for reasons that as yet have not been clearly documented. However, crude analyses based on questionnaires of physical activity levels suggest that those European Union countries in which adults are most sedentary have the highest obesity prevalence rates.

Traditionally, excess body weight was a sign of affluence but now, in both the developed and many developing countries (e.g., in Latin America), overweight and obesity are particularly marked in the lower socioeconomic classes. There is also an inverse linear relationship between the educational level of both men and women and their degree of excess weight gain, but it is difficult to distinguish between educational level and socioeconomic status. Obesity is now, therefore, seen as being closely linked to poverty and social exclusion in many countries.

The prevalence rates of obesity in adults are rising rapidly in most parts of the world, with increases, for example, in the United Kingdom, of 3–5% more adults being so classified in national surveys repeated every 5 years. The increments in BMI, again, vary with striking increases in comorbidity rates in Asian countries (e.g., China) as average BMIs rise by 0.3 to 0.5 units every 2–3 years. Thus, the problems associated with weight gain are assuming ever-greater public health importance.

Throughout the world, women in general have a higher prevalence rate of obesity than men, but more men are in the overweight category. Although there are a number of potential environmental explanations for this gender difference, the most likely explanation is the innate increase in the proportion of body fat that develops as girls go through pubertal changes. Detailed analyses of the propensity for lean-tissue gain as weight increases then show that to counter a sustained positive energy balance of an average 100 kcal per day involves women gaining much more weight and body fat. Only when their accumulation of excess lean tissue is sufficient for the basal energy requirement to rise, so that this, plus the cost of physical activity from the excess weight equates to the 100 kcal. excess intake, will body weight stabilize. Men, however, by having a higher lean-tissue mass (including muscle) and a greater capacity to accumulate the excess energy as lean tissue, will counter the 100 kcal excess at much more modest weight increases. So this probably explains the almost uniform finding of greater obesity rates in women and that, in Third World countries, middle-age women are the first to become obese as environmental circumstances change.

## THE ENVIRONMENTAL BASIS FOR WEIGHT GAIN INTERNATIONALLY

The WHO analysis of the basis for weight gain highlighted the importance of environmental factors when explaining population weight gains (see Chapter 78). As yet, there are no objective studies that demonstrate ethnic or genetic sensitivities relating to the "thrifty genotype" hypothesis. The age-related increase in overweight and obesity observed in most societies is most readily explained by the almost universally observed reduction in physical activity—dietary patterns are not coherently different on an age basis in the countries displaying age-related weight increases. Physical activity levels may not be as high as expected in rural communities in the developing world, but with the transfer to urban environments, there is usually a further reduction in physical activity and marked changes in diet. Ecological studies, some prospective analyses, and a range of physiological investigations with covertly manipulated diets show that an increasing energy-dense diet is particularly conducive to a positive energy balance and weight gain. Dietary density is a feature of modern Western diets, and dietary fat and the use of processed and refined carbohydrates increase dietary density. Dietary fat, however, usually contributes more to energy density, and dietary fat rather than sugar intake has been related to within-country and cross-country increases in weight. Few studies, however, have looked at the combination of fat and sugar in food items to assess the propensity to overeat these particular foods, which are recognized to be particularly attractive and energy-dense.

There appears to be an interaction between increases in dietary fat and increasingly sedentary behavior in explaining weight gain. Passive overconsumption of higher-fat diets readily occurs, whereas total food intakes should be low in individuals who are sedentary. Attempts to distinguish between dietary density and sedentary behavior as the factors inducing weight gain are made difficult because the usual food frequency surveys for assessing dietary fat are known to be very inaccurate, whereas crude indices of sedentary behavior (e.g., hours watching television or car ownership) are readily measured. Studies in developing countries show that once dietary fat increases to 20%, middle-age women display increasing rates of overweight and obesity even in societies where their physical activity would be considered appreciable in a Western context. The prevalence rate of overweight increases progressively in men as dietary fat rises above 15%; with fat intakes of 30% or more, a fall in physical activity below a level equivalent to about 90–120 minutes of active walking daily, that is, a physical activity level (PAL—expressed as total energy expenditure divided by estimated basal metabolic rates) of 1.80, then weight gain is much more likely. Equivalent levels of activity seem to be required for women in Western societies to prevent weight regain after slimming. The United Nations specified levels for moderate activity are PAL values of 1.76 in men and 1.68 in women. Levels above these seem to be required to minimize the risk of obesity in men and the likelihood of weight regain in formerly obese women in societies where Westernized diets with a high fat content are usual.

The nutrition transition affecting all societies in the world involves a technological revolution not only in work and leisure patterns but also in all aspects of the food chain. Traditionally, 80% of populations lived in a rural environment and had to work on the land to ensure a sufficiency of food. Moderately developed countries still have about 30% of their population engaged in farmwork. In affluent societies, however, this figure has fallen to about 5% and people rely on mechanized, intensive agriculture to produce food, at least 75% of which is processed and packaged. This processing usually involves a manipulation of the nutrient content and an alteration in the structure of foods to prolong their shelf life and make them both attractive and readily consumable, with a high dietary density. In addition, the demands for physical activity at work have been minimized by mechanization and the technological revolution, and housework and cooking have been reduced to a minimum by domestic appliances and the availability of ready-made meals and eating out. With many societies, such as the United States, planned and built primarily for ease of access and travel by motor car, the opportunity to walk or cycle as a routine daily activity is minimized or made virtually impossible.

## STRATEGIES FOR PREVENTING OVERWEIGHT AND OBESITY

So far, obesity experts have concentrated on a health educational approach for individual patients. This classic medical strategy neglects the all-pervasive inducements to overeat and societal constraints on physical activity (see Chapters 111 and 112). These are usually amplified by huge industrial interests (e.g., the food and drink industry). At-risk individuals therefore have to counter an "obesigenic" or "toxic" environment (see Chapter 78). Similar individualized approaches to therapy and prevention have been tried to ameliorate or prevent diabetes, hypertension, and other cardiovascular diseases. These approaches are of only modest benefit, with the affluent, better-educated, and intelligent members of society being more able to initiate long-term change.

Dramatic changes have, however, been achieved in combating chronic diseases in Scandinavia. Governments and professional groups have cooperated to change policies on diet and physical activity. Nutritional standards were set for schools and public catering outlets. Restaurants and catering services improved the nutritional quality of their meals and included vegetables and salads within the price of meals. Over a 20-year period, this strategy led to more than a 75% reduction in premature death rates from both heart disease and strokes in some parts of Scandinavia. Norway is unusual: It has transformed the population's approach to routine leisure activity, which in its egalitarian society is then not confined to the rich and well-educated. National strategies are also being developed to combat childhood obesity (e.g., in Singapore and Taiwan) and traffic control measures have been taken in some cities that spontaneously lead to children playing routinely in the street. The pedestrianization of city centers and the provision of walkways and cycle paths enhance routine physical activity and limit the need to undertake specific leisure-time activities that often require special facilities and commitment. These public health strategies have yet to be combined with novel approaches to industrial collaboration for public health benefit. The dilemma of prevention is the need to develop coherent national strategies when academics increasingly demand, from a pharmaceutical perspective, controlled trials to demonstrate efficacy before action is initiated. This would require decades of coherent national experiments at a time of an escalating obesity epidemic.

## FURTHER READING

Bray, G. A., & Popkin, B. M. (1998). Dietary fat intake does affect obesity rate. *American Journal of Clinical Nutrition, 68*, 1157–1173.—A coherent overview of the international data linking dietary fat with the prevalence of overweight.

James, W. P. T., & Reeds, P. J. (1997). Nutrient partitioning. In G. A. Bray, C. Bouchard, & W. P. T. James (Eds.), *Handbook on obesity* (pp. 555–571). New York: Marcel Dekker.—A review of the biological basis for differences in the deposition of lean and fat on weight gain, with evidence for the greater propensity for fat gain in women.

Martorell, R., Khan, L. K., Hughes, M. L., & Grummer-Strawn, L. M. (2000). Obesity in women from developing countries. *European Journal of Clinical Nutrition, 54*, 247–252.—The first analysis of Third World obesity rates, based on an evaluation of major international mother and child studies.

Peña, M., & Bacallao, J. (Eds.). (2000). *Obesity and poverty* (Pan American Health Organization, Scientific Publication No. 576; pp. 41–49). Washington, DC: Author.—Presents a coherent analysis of a wide spectrum of data on obesity in Latin America and the propensity toward obesity in the lower socioeconomic groups.

World Health Organization. (1998). *Obesity: Preventing and managing the global epidemic: Report of a WHO Consultation on Obesity* (WHO/NUT/NCD/97.2). Geneva: Author.—The first global report on all aspects of obesity.

World Health Organization. (1999). *Nutrition for health and development: Progress and prospects on the eve of the 21st century* (WHO/NHD/99.9). Geneva: Author.—This new analysis includes a summary of the huge burden of adult chronic diseases affecting, particularly, the developing world. It also provides the only available WHO analysis of obesity rates based upon governmental reports to WHO.

Yajnik, C. (2000). Interactions of perturbations in intrauterine growth and growth during childhood on the risk of adult-onset disease. *Proceedings of the Nutrition Society, 59,* 1–9.—This review covers most of Yajnik's emerging data on the interactions between poor fetal and child growth rates, and the susceptibility to glucose intolerance and higher blood pressure in fast-growing preadolescents.

# 75

## Prevalence and Demographics of Obesity

### RODOLFO VALDEZ
### DAVID F. WILLIAMSON

## MEASUREMENT OF OBESITY IN EPIDEMIOLOGY

Weight gain in most adults is due to body-fat accumulation. Obesity results when such accumulation becomes excessive and threatens health. Current methods for measuring excess body fat are impractical for large-scale use; therefore, epidemiologists must rely on simple body measurements to detect excess weight in individuals and populations (see Chapter 11). Some weight-by-height indices correlate well with body fat. Epidemiologists routinely use these indices in populations to estimate body weights with the lowest morbidity or mortality and to determine the health risks assumed by individuals who exceed those weights (see Chapter 76). There have been two major approaches to identifying healthy body weights.

First, the Metropolitan Life Insurance Company pioneered this effort with its widely used weight-by-height tables. The 1959 Metropolitan tables were based on data pooled from 26 insurance companies in the United States and Canada. These tables list ranges of body weights for specific heights, with the lowest mortality, extracted from 4.9 million insurance policies issued between 1935 and 1953. The ranges of the height-specific weights are listed by sex and three body frames (small, medium, large) for subjects between 25 and 59 years of age. Cases of heart disease, cancer, or diabetes were excluded. The most recent Metropolitan tables were issued in 1983, using a similar approach (25 companies, 4.2 million insurance policies issued between 1950 and 1971). At comparable heights, the weights with the lowest mortality in the 1983 tables were higher than those in the 1959 tables. The labels "ideal" or "desirable" introduced with these tables for recommended body weights remain popular in the obesity literature (see Chapters 76 and 91). However, despite their continued use and the richness of the data supporting them, the Metropolitan tables lack universal applicability. These tables are based on data from the insured, likely healthier, and mostly white segment of the North American population of several decades ago.

The second approach uses the body mass index (BMI). It is currently the index of choice for epidemiologists to detect overweight and obesity (see Chapter 68). BMI is defined as weight in kilograms divided by height in meters squared. The formula was developed about 130 years ago by Quetelet to compare weight in adults independently of height. In the last three decades, however, BMI has also become an index of adult body composition by virtue of its low correlation with height and its strong, although far from perfect, association with total body fat.

BMI has been tested in populations around the world and in nearly all of them is positively associated with morbidity and mortality. Echoing the Metropolitan tables, there are also ranges of BMI where morbidity and mortality reach minimum values. The recommended body weights from the Metropolitan tables overlap to some extent with the recommended weights found with BMI, though the latter have more appeal for epidemiologists.

## CURRENT GUIDELINES

As a tool to assess overweight in adults, BMI has quickly gained widespread acceptance in the scientific community. The U.S. National Institutes of Health (NIH) and the World Health Organization (WHO) have issued separate but consistent evidence-based guidelines for the identification and management of obesity. Both guidelines divide the BMI distribution into four major categories (units in kilograms divided by height in meters squared): underweight (BMI < 18.5), normal (18.5 ≤ BMI < 25), overweight (25 ≤ BMI < 30) and obese (BMI ≥ 30). Within the obese category are several subcategories, as the health risks sharply increase with BMI after the obesity threshold. Stimulated by this effort, Asian Pacific epidemiologists have been working on their own guidelines and have recently proposed lower BMI thresholds for overweight (BMI ≥ 23) and obesity (BMI ≥ 25) for their populations.

## PREVALENCE AND DEMOGRAPHICS
## OF OBESITY IN THE UNITED STATES

The rates of obesity in a population are affected by a host of demographic and behavioral factors such as age, sex, physical activity, diet, and socioeconomic status. Moreover, since racial and ethnic origins are important categories of vital statistics in the United States, they are included in the list of major factors associated with obesity in this country as well (see Chapter 79). Table 75.1 lists some important factors related to the prevalence of obesity in the United States.

This list has two caveats: First, these factors relate to groups and not necessarily to individuals; second, outside of the United States, factors such as ethnicity and socioeconomic status may have a different and even the opposite effect on the prevalence of obesity (see Chapter 74). Nevertheless, it is always important to know the social and demographic factors shaping the distribution of obesity in a particular population. The close

**TABLE 75.1. Demographic and Behavioral Factors Related to Obesity in the United States**

| Factor | Prevalence of obesity is increased if subjects are . . . |
|---|---|
| Age | Older |
| Sex | Female |
| Race or ethnicity | Of racial and ethnic minorities |
| Socioeconomic status | Of low socioeconomic status |
| Family history | Children of obese parents |
| Marital status | Married |
| Parity | Multiparous women |
| Smoking | Ex-smokers |
| Diet and physical activity | Chronically exceeding energy intake over energy expenditure |

association between obesity and several chronic diseases may help predict the distributions of these diseases as well.

A cross-sectional example of the interplay between demographic factors and the prevalence of obesity is presented in Table 75.2. The example is from the United States, where these associations have been studied extensively, but it could apply to other indus-

**TABLE 75.2. Distribution of Four BMI Categories and Their Associated Risk Factors in Three Racial/Ethnic Groups of the U.S. Population Ages ≥ 20 Years**

| | BMI category (kg/m$^2$) | | | |
|---|---|---|---|---|
| | < 18.5 Underweight | 18.5–24.9 Normal | 25.0–29.9 Overweight | ≥ 30.0 Obese |
| *Non-Hispanic white* | | | | |
| Sample size | 156 | 2,676 | 2,269 | 1,382 |
| Population represented | 2,771,093 | 49,937,568 | 37,438,793 | 24,109,659 |
| % women | 77.8 | 58.1 | 39.8 | 55.2 |
| Median age | 36.0 | 37.6 | 44.8 | 46.4 |
| Prevalence (%) | 2.4 | 43.7 | 32.8 | 21.1 |
| Mean BMI difference (women–men) | −0.1 | −0.9 | 0.0 | 1.4 |
| *Non-Hispanic black* | | | | |
| Sample size | 95 | 1,533 | 1,391 | 1,327 |
| Population represented | 352,745 | 6,020,743 | 5,427,631 | 4,906,705 |
| % women | 68.3 | 49.5 | 51.0 | 68.8 |
| Median age | 33.9 | 33.4 | 38.7 | 40.1 |
| Prevalence (%) | 2.1 | 36.0 | 32.5 | 29.4 |
| Mean BMI difference (women–men) | −0.5 | −0.1 | 0.2 | 1.8 |
| *Mexican American* | | | | |
| Sample size | 59 | 1,400 | 1,638 | 1,165 |
| Population represented | 104,287 | 2,706,269 | 3,036,958 | 2,121,462 |
| % women | 63.0 | 45.8 | 41.4 | 60.2 |
| Median age | 27.3 | 29.4 | 34.8 | 39.2 |
| Prevalence (%) | 1.3 | 34.0 | 38.1 | 26.6 |
| Mean BMI difference (women–men) | −0.3 | −0.4 | 0.1 | 1.4 |

*Note.* Data from NHANES III: 1988–1994.

trialized countries. Table 75.2 reveals that one in five non-Hispanic whites and about one in three non-Hispanic blacks or Mexican Americans are obese; that women are over-represented at both ends of the BMI distribution and they are heavier than men at the up-per end of this distribution; and that among minorities, half of the obese people are under 40 years of age.

## PREVALENCE OF OBESITY AROUND THE WORLD

Detailed international comparisons of the prevalence of obesity are difficult (see Chapter 74). Until recently, there was no consensus definition of obesity, and the demography of the populations vary widely from country to country. The substantial range of such variation is portrayed in Table 75.3, which presents recent prevalence data from selected countries.

## FUTURE DEVELOPMENTS

The recent NIH and WHO obesity guidelines represent a major step toward standardiz-ing the field of obesity epidemiology. The next step should be to consolidate standards for BMI-based definitions of overweight and obesity around the world. Then, these BMI standards should be complemented with simple, standard criteria for identifying abdomi-nal obesity. The ultimate goal would be to create a global typology of obesity in which all risk factors associated with it were identified and catalogued in a practical manner. Such typology should be implemented by all clinical practitioners and public health workers who deal with obesity and its related chronic health conditions.

**TABLE 75.3. Prevalence of Obesity in Selected Countries**

| Country | Age range (years) | Prevalence of obesity (BMI ≥ 30 kg/m$^2$) | |
|---|---|---|---|
| | | Men (%) | Women (%) |
| Australia | 25–64 | 12 | 13 |
| Brazil | 25–64 | 6 | 13 |
| Canada | 18–74 | 15 | 15 |
| China | 20–45 | 0.4 | 0.9 |
| England | 16–64 | 15 | 17 |
| Finland | 25–65 | 14 | 11 |
| Japan | ≥ 20 | 2 | 3 |
| Kuwait | ≥ 18 | 32 | 44 |
| Mauritius | 25–74 | 5 | 15 |
| Netherlands | 20–59 | 8 | 8 |
| New Zealand | 18–64 | 10 | 13 |
| Samoa, rural | 25–69 | 42 | 59 |
| Samoa, urban | 25–69 | 58 | 77 |
| Saudi Arabia | ≥ 15 | 16 | 24 |
| Sweden | 16–84 | 5 | 9 |
| United States | 20–74 | 20 | 25 |

*Note.* Data from World Health Organization. (1998). *Obesity: Preventing and managing the global epidemic: Report of a WHO Consultation on Obesity.*

## FURTHER READING

International Diabetes Institute. (2001). *The Asia-Pacific perspective: Redefining obesity and its treatment*. Melbourne, Australia. Available online at *http://www.idi.org.au/obesity_report.htm*.—Good document on the epidemiology of obesity internationally.

Keys, A., Fidanza, F., Karvonen, M. J., Kimura, N., & Taylor, H. L.(1972). Indices of relative weight and obesity. *Journal of Chronic Disease, 25*, 329–343.—Original and very detailed paper in which BMI was first proposed as an index of body composition.

Metropolitan Life Insurance Company. (1983). 1983 Metropolitan height and weight tables. *Statistical Bulletin, 64*, 2–9.—A very succinct account of the rationale and data behind the most popular weight-by-height tables.

National Heart, Lung, and Blood Institute, and the National Institutes of Health. (1998). Clinical guidelines on the identification, evaluation, and treatment of overweight and obesity in adults: the Evidence Report. *Obesity Research, 6*(Suppl. 2), 51S–209S. (Also available at http://www.nhlbi.nih.gov/guidelines/obesity/)—Report on the epidemiology, assessment, and treatment of obesity.

World Health Organization. (1998). *Obesity: Preventing and managing the global epidemic: Report of a WHO Consultation on Obesity* (WHO/NUT/NCD/97.2). Geneva: Author. (Also available at *http://www.who.int/home/info.html*)—The first document on the global problem of obesity.

# 76

# Epidemiology of Health Risks Associated with Obesity

JOANN E. MANSON
PATRICK J. SKERRETT
WALTER C. WILLETT

## HEALTH RISKS AND EXCESS WEIGHT

The relationship of body weight and total mortality, as well as the risk of developing several chronic diseases, have been examined in numerous epidemiological studies that provide insight into biological relationships and are used to develop ranges of desirable weights. Defining these ranges and applying them to individuals are controversial topics (see Chapters 75 and 91). In this chapter, we examine methodological issues, review known associations, and attempt to synthesize available data regarding desirable weights.

### Measures of Body Weight in Epidemiological Studies

Measuring body fat, which is diffuse and inaccessible, is possible but difficult (see Chapter 11). While fairly precise estimates can be made using hydrodensitometry, dual-energy X-ray absorptiometry, and computed tomography (CT) or magnetic resonance imaging (MRI), these measures are time-consuming and expensive. Because many thousands of subjects are needed for epidemiological studies relating adiposity to health outcomes, simpler, more widely available measures that combine weight and height are generally employed. Most frequently used is the Quetelet index, more commonly known today as the body mass index (BMI = weight in kilograms divided by the square of height in meters). To make them more understandable, BMIs are often converted to weight-for-height tables, or nomograms. BMIs are generally reliable because measures of weight and height tend to be quite accurate, even when self-reported. While the BMI has been criticized because it does not distinguish fat mass from lean mass, this simple measure is highly correlated with fat mass in young and middle-age adults ($r$ = approximately 0.9 for both men and women) and strongly predicts important health outcomes (see Chapter 11). Among older individuals, however, changes in weight often reflect losses in lean body mass resulting from inactivity or chronic disease, thus complicating the interpretation of data based on weight and height (see Chapter 81).

Measurements of the distribution of body fat, particularly waist and hip circumferences or the ratio of the two, have also received attention as possible predictors of serious disease based on evidence that intraabdominal fat is more metabolically active than fat in the hips, thighs, or buttocks (see Chapters 68, 84, and 86). Furthermore, the increased sensitivity of abdominal fat cells to lipolytic stimuli and their direct delivery of free fatty acids and glycerol to the liver via the portal circulation may induce insulin resistance. In an aging population, abdominal circumferences may be a better indicator of overall adiposity than indices based only on weight and height, due to the gradual replacement of lean tissue with adipose tissue with increasing age. However, BMI is not only strongly correlated with abdominal adiposity and waist-to-hip circumference ratio, it is also the most modifiable of these parameters.

Change in weight is another potentially useful predictor of disease risk (see Chapter 72). Because differences in weight are observed within the same individual, they tend to be uncorrelated with frame size, which is difficult to characterize, and more closely reflect changes in adiposity.

## Methodological Issues

Studies of weight and risk are conceptually quite simple: Measure the weight and height of all the individuals in a large population and then follow these individuals to determine who dies or develops specific diseases. Rates of death or disease can be calculated for various levels of body weight (adjusted for height, age, and gender) to determine a dose–response relationship. The nadir of this relationship defines the range of optimal weights. In practice, though, several problems can potentially distort true causal relationships between weight and health outcomes.

One critical issue is that other variables may be related to both weight and health and may thus distort the causal relationship. Smoking is a prime example: Smokers tend to be lean but have greatly increased risk of death, making lean individuals appear to have an elevated rate of mortality. Alcoholism and depression can have the same effect but are harder to characterize. While these effects can be partially controlled by statistical methods, the best estimates are likely to come from studies of persons who have never smoked and nonalcoholics.

Another problem is that statistical methods are sometimes used to control for the metabolic consequences of obesity such as hypertension, hyperlipidemia, and hyperglycemia or diabetes. This approach results in "overcontrol," which statistically removes the biological consequences of obesity that mediate its effects on disease incidence (see Chapter 70).

The assessment of the relationship between body weight and total mortality is even more problematic. While total mortality is attractive as the primary outcome, or "bottom line," in determining optimal weights, studies are prone to produce misleading conclusions. In addition to the methodological problems noted earlier, many individuals lose weight before death, so low weight may be the consequence, rather than the cause, of the underlying disease. Investigators have eliminated from analyses subjects who have known conditions, such as cancer, that might cause both weight loss and premature death, and have eliminated the first years of follow-up. However, some unrecognized conditions, such as preclinical cancers, depression, alcoholism, or early pulmonary or cardiac failure, may cause weight loss that begins many years before death. In addition, studies of total mortality are inherently insensitive because obesity, like almost any other single factor, is not likely to influence all specific causes of death. Thus, even important health effects will be diluted by unrelated causes of death, making them more difficult to detect except in extremely large investigations. Finally, mortality is a small part of the substantial burden of disease wrought by conditions such as angina pectoris, degenerative arthritis, diabetes, hypertension, and nonfatal cardiovascular disease, and does not contribute to biological understanding (see Chapters 82 and 84). Ultimately, we want to relate epidemiology to pathophysiology and basic biology. This requires information about the types of disease and metabolic perturbations caused by excess adiposity.

## Body Weight and Mortality

Each year, at least 280,000 deaths among U.S. adults are attributable to obesity. The issue of whether the relationship between body weight and mortality is linear, J-shaped, or U-shaped has been controversial, but this argument is not fundamentally fruitful. Overwhelming evidence exists that substantial adiposity increases morbidity and mortality and that extremely low body weight is deleterious. A more useful focus is to define the range of weights associated with optimal health.

Until recently, no study had fully addressed these methodological problems. For example, data used to compile the Metropolitan Life Insurance Company tables of desirable weights historically did not include information on cigarette smoking, thus biasing these tables toward higher recommended weight levels. This bias is more serious in recent data, since the full effect of smoking on health is not experienced until after many decades of smoking. Such an effect might account for the higher weights for height included in the 1983 revision of the Metropolitan Life tables than those used in the 1959 tables.

In an early study that tried to account for confounders, a large American Cancer Society cohort included nearly 1 million adults. Although the analysis did not account for early deaths due to preclinical disease, it did provide information separately for smokers and nonsmokers. Among nonsmokers, mortality was minimal, at or somewhat below the cohort's average relative weight. Excess mortality among the leanest individuals was mainly due to cancers of the lung, bladder, and pancreas, strongly implicating smoking. A reanalysis of these 12-year follow-up data using BMI instead of relative weights, and excluding smokers and those with a history of cancer or cardiovascular disease at baseline, as well as a new analysis of a second cohort of more than 1 million adults with 14 years of follow-up, showed a clearer pattern of increasing mortality with increasing weight. Among healthy people who had never smoked, optimal mortality was found at a BMI of 23.5–24.9 for men and 22.0–23.4 for women. These data confirm similar observations from a 27-year follow-up of more than 19,000 middle-age men in the Harvard Alumni Study and 40,000 middle-age men in the Health Professionals Follow-up Study followed for 10 years, as well as a 16-year follow-up of 115,000 middle-age women in the Nurses' Health Study. In the aggregate, these data support current U.S. guidelines setting the range for healthy weight at BMIs between 18.5 and 25.0.

Although some researchers have argued that the optimal weight increases with age, this observation is probably an artifact of the increasing prevalence of weight loss secondary to chronic disease among older individuals, the cumulative effects of cigarette smoking, the reduced reliability of BMI as a measure of adiposity with advancing age, and the enormous burden of comorbidity among older individuals. Studies from Framingham, a population of Seventh-Day Adventists, and the American Cancer Society cohorts indicate that although the strength of the association between body weight and mortality decreases with age, being overweight remains predictive of excess mortality (see Chapter 81). At least up to age 75, a BMI under 25 is associated with reduced total mortality.

## Excess Body Weight and Morbidity

A large body of evidence indicates that higher levels of body weight and fat are associated with increased risks of developing numerous adverse health outcomes (see Chapters 84 and 86). The incidence of coronary disease, the most common cause of death in the United States, is strongly related to excess weight in both men and women. The relationship appears to be linear, and even individuals of average weight (i.e., a BMI of 24 to 26) at midlife are at increased risk compared with leaner individuals. Excess body weight is also associated with the risk of ischemic, but not hemorrhagic stroke, although not as strongly as for coronary disease. Not surprisingly, excess weight is strongly associated with the major metabolic risk factors for coronary disease. It accounts for a high proportion of cases of hypertension and hyperglycemia, and is also associated with increases in low-density lipoprotein (LDL) cholesterol and triglyceride levels, and decreases in high-density lipoprotein (HDL) cholesterol levels (a constellation of metabolic aberrations attributable to insulin resistance that is known as "Syndrome X"; see Chapter 86). Consistent with the excess risk of coronary heart disease even among individuals with average weights, the Framingham Heart Study demonstrated that many individuals with BMIs between 23 and 25 had abnormalities in serum lipids, glucose tolerance, and blood pressure compared to those with BMIs less than 23, and almost all individuals with BMIs above 25 had such abnormalities. In support of a causal association between obesity and these metabolic abnormalities, even modest degrees of weight loss are associated with favorable alterations in blood pressure, lipid profile, insulin sensitivity, and glucose tolerance (see Chapter 88). The American Heart Association recently highlighted the association between weight and heart disease by adding obesity to its list of major risk factors for coronary heart disease.

Type 2 diabetes mellitus is extremely sensitive to excess weight, with a more than 50-fold gradient in risk seen from the leanest to the heaviest men and women in some cohorts. Even modest gains in weight (approximately 5 kg) between age 18 and midlife are associated with a severalfold increase in risk compared with maintaining a stable weight. Weight gains of more than 10 kg have been linked to elevated incidence rates of hypertension and coronary heart disease.

Incidence rates of endometrial and gallbladder cancer are several times higher among obese than among lean persons; however, these are relatively uncommon causes of cancer death. The incidence of the more common cancers, including those of the lung and prostate, are, at most, weakly associated with body weight. Weight is somewhat more strongly related to risk of colon, esophageal, renal, and postmenopausal breast cancer.

The increased mortality from breast cancer among obese women is due in part to the later detection of tumors in these women and to a worse prognosis independent of stage. Breast cancer during the premenopausal years is one of the few diseases that is inversely associated with body weight, possibly because of the increased occurrence of anovulatory menstrual cycles at higher weights. Even among premenopausal women, however, there is no reduction in breast cancer mortality with higher weight.

Incidence rates of osteoarthritis of the knees and hips are strongly associated with body weight. Fractures of the hip, in contrast, are only about one-fourth as common in obese women as in lean women. This may be due to the padding that extra weight provides during falls or the higher bone mass related to increased mechanical stress and/or higher endogenous estrogen levels. This apparent benefit from obesity, which is experienced primarily at the end of life, does not, however, outweigh the deleterious effects of overweight, because cardiovascular disease and diabetes are far more important causes of illness and disability; even the orthopedic complications of overweight counterbalance the reduced mortality due to hip fractures.

Increasing body weight significantly raises the risk of developing gallstones or requiring cholecystectomy. Data from the Third National Health and Nutrition Examination Survey show that the prevalence of gallbladder disease among women in the highest BMI quartile is nearly triple that of women in the lowest, and more than twice as high as that among men. Other health outcomes associated with overweight and obesity include deep venous thromboembolism, pulmonary dysfunction, sleep apnea, and a variety of reproductive problems in women, including menstrual irregularities, primary infertility, and gestational diabetes. Conditions that have also been associated with obesity, but for which the evidence is not yet as compelling, include asthma, gastroesophageal reflux disorder, and impaired wound healing.

Another measure of the cumulative burden of weight-related disorders is quality of life (see Chapter 70). In analyses from the Nurses' Health Study, both higher BMI and substantial weight gain during adulthood were strongly associated with reduced daily physical functioning and vitality, a greater burden of physical pain, and diminished feelings of well-being. The average decline in physical function experienced by a woman under age 65 years who gained 9 kg or more over a 4-year period was approximately three times the magnitude of that associated with cigarette smoking over the same period.

## CONCLUSIONS

For most adults, optimal health will be experienced if a healthy body weight is maintained throughout life by means of regular physical activity and, if needed, modest dietary restraint. In general, this corresponds to a BMI between 18.5 and 25.0, though the upper limit of the range may be lower for conditions such as hypertension and type 2 diabetes. This range of "healthy" BMIs is most appropriately used as a guide for persons who wish to prevent obesity-related morbidity and mortality during adulthood but may represent an unrealistic goal for persons who are already substantially outside this range (see Chapter 98). Treatment of overweight and the benefits of even modest reductions in weight are discussed elsewhere in this book (see Chapters 70 and 71). Individuals and health care providers should regard even modest weight gain (on the order of more than

5 kg) after age 21 as an important signal indicating the need for adjustments in activity and eating patterns to prevent further weight gain. The absence of weight gain, however, does not indicate that fat mass has not increased, particularly among men older than 50. After this age, muscle mass tends to be replaced by fat, much of it within the abdomen—a shift that maintains the BMI while significantly altering the risk for subsequent disease. Regular physical activity can minimize the loss of lean body mass and the redistribution of adipose mass.

## FURTHER READING

Allison, D. B., Fontaine, K. R., Manson, J. E., Stevens, J., & VanItallie, T. B. (1999). Annual deaths attributable to obesity in the United States. *Journal of the American Medical Association, 282,* 1530–1538.—Estimates annual rates of obesity-related deaths using relative hazard ratios from six large prospective cohort studies.

Baik, I., Ascherio, A., Rimm, E. B., Giovannucci, E., Spiegelman, D., Stampfer, M. J., & Willett, W. C. (2000). Adiposity and mortality in men. *American Journal of Epidemiology, 152,* 264–271.—A prospective cohort study of BMI, fat distribution, and mortality among male health professionals.

Calle, E. E., Thun, M. J., Petrelli, J. M., Rodriguez, C., & Heath, C. W., Jr. (1999). Body-mass index and mortality in a prospective cohort of U.S. adults. *New England Journal of Medicine, 341,* 1097–1105.—A detailed analysis of mortality in the second large American Cancer Society cohort, including separate analyses by smoking status and history of disease, and by age, race, and cause of death among healthy never smokers.

Garrison, R. J., & Kannel, W. B. (1993). A new approach for estimating healthy body weights. *International Journal of Obesity and Related Metabolic Disorders, 17,* 417–423.—A detailed study of the metabolic effects of overweight and obesity in the Framingham population.

Lee, I. M., Manson, J. E., Hennekens, C. H., & Paffenbarger, R. S., Jr. (1993). Body weight and mortality: A 27-year follow-up of middle-aged men. *Journal of the American Medical Association, 270,* 2823–2828.—A large-scale follow-up of body weight and all-cause mortality in men that includes a separate analysis of never smokers, excludes the first several years of follow-up, and provides long duration follow-up.

Lew, E. A., & Garfinkel, L. (1979). Variations in mortality by weight among 750,000 men and women. *Journal of Chronic Disease, 32,* 563–576.—The first American Cancer Society study of body weight and mortality, including analyses relating to nonsmokers.

Lindsted, K., Tonstad, S., & Kuzma, J. W. (1991). Body mass index and patterns of mortality among Seventh-Day Adventist men. *International Journal of Obesity, 15,* 397–406.—A study of body weight and mortality that largely accounts for methodologic biases because the population contains few smokers and follow-up was carried out for more than two decades.

Manson, J. E., Stampfer, M. J., Hennekens, C. H., & Willett, W. C. (1987). Body weight and longevity. A reassessment. *Journal of the American Medical Association, 257,* 353–358.—A critical review of studies of weight and total mortality.

Manson, J. E., Willett, W. C., Stampfer, M. J., Colditz, G. A., Hunter, D. J., Hankinson, S. E., Hennekens, C. H., & Speizer, F. E. (1995). Body weight and mortality among women. *New England Journal of Medicine, 333,* 677–685.—A large-scale epidemiological study of BMI and mortality among middle-age women in the Nurses' Health Study that accounts for several methodological biases.

National Task Force on the Prevention and Treatment of Obesity. (2000). Overweight, obesity, and health risk. *Archives of Internal Medicine, 160,* 898–904.—A detailed overview of the health risks associated with excess weight.

Stevens, J., Cai, J., Pamuk, E. R., Williamson, D. F., Thun, M. J., & Wood, J. L. (1998). The effect of age on the association between body-mass index and mortality. *New England Journal of Medicine, 338,* 1–7.—A reanalysis of data from the first American Cancer Society cohort that included men and women who had never smoked, had no history of cardiovascular disease or cancer at baseline, and no history of unexplained weight loss.

Willett, W. C., Dietz, W. H., & Colditz, G. A. (1999). Guidelines for healthy weight. *New England Journal of Medicine, 341,* 427–434.—A review of the problems associated with defining "healthy weights" and their clinical application.

# 77

## Epidemiology and Causes of Obesity in Children

### DENISE E. WILFLEY
### BRIAN E. SAELENS

Obesity in childhood is related to both negative psychosocial consequences and higher rates of obesity-related morbidities in adulthood (see Chapter 85). It frequently persists into adulthood, especially with increasing child age. This chapter examines the epidemiology of childhood obesity as well as commonly proposed etiological factors among children without specific known conditions (e.g., Prader–Willi).

### EPIDEMIOLOGY

The prevalence of childhood obesity is increasing worldwide (see Chapter 74). Although recent proposals have been advanced, there is no universally accepted definition of childhood obesity. This limits comparative evaluations of prevalence. A method of defining overweight in adults is based on data relating morbidity and mortality to various levels of weight (see Chapter 76). Defining childhood overweight in this manner is problematic because of sparse prospective data to support a classification system. Epidemiological studies have had to rely on statistical definitions of overweight based on selected percentiles for a given reference group (e.g., age and gender).

For population-based assessments, measurements must reflect excess body fat and still be simple to use, standardized, and able to demonstrate comparability across time. Body mass index (BMI) is a weight-for-height index that correlates with adiposity in children and is calculated easily. Commonly used BMI-for-age cut points include ≥ 95th percentile to identify children who are overweight and ≥ 85th and < 95th percentile to identify children at risk for becoming overweight. In children, BMI needs to be assessed using age-specific reference curves, because it changes dramatically with age, compared to adults, where BMI increases slowly with age and age-independent cutoff points can be used to grade weight status.

Regardless of the method used to classify obesity, studies examining obesity during childhood have reported high prevalence rates, with a dramatic increase in the past two decades. The most recent representative data in the United States shows that 11% of children ages 6–17 years have BMI at or above the 95%. This is a twofold increase since the mid-1970s. A similar trend was observed for U.S. preschool girls; the frequency of overweight in girls ages 4 to 5 years increased from 5.8% to 10.8%. The most pronounced increases in overweight are among the heaviest children, creating a grave medical situation.

## CAUSES OF CHILDHOOD OBESITY

Increased prevalence of childhood obesity has sparked interest in its cause. Numerous causal factors have been proposed and examined. Although far from determining the exact causes of this growing epidemic, many researchers have speculated that environmental change associated with affluence in developed countries (e.g., energy-saving devices, greater access to food) has contributed to pervasive positive energy balance (see Chapters 74 and 78). This exploration of environmental factors has been accompanied by the investigation of genetic and other biological factors that may promote obesity in childhood (see Chapters 3, 4, and 5).

### Prenatal and Familial Factors

Prenatal factors may affect children's weight in early childhood. Extreme caloric deprivation during critical periods in pregnancy is positively related to children being at a higher weight. Higher birth weight has also been linked to greater likelihood of being obese early in childhood. Children born to mothers with insulin-dependent diabetes are at greater risk for being overweight, even after controlling for maternal weight. Gestational diabetes, independent of insulin-dependent diabetes, may result in higher child birth weight but may not necessarily increase the likelihood of later obesity in childhood.

Familial impact on children's weight includes both genetic and shared lifestyle influences. Whereas twin, family, and adoption studies suggest a strong genetic contribution for childhood obesity, specific known genotypes for obesity account for few cases of childhood obesity. Similarly, few familial environment factors have been confirmed as causal. Cross-sectional and longitudinal evidence finds that parental obesity is positively linked with child weight status and is among the strongest obesity predictors known for very young children. A general familial environment marked by lower socioeconomic status promotes greater childhood adiposity, especially among girls. A longitudinal study documented that children reared in a family environment marked by neglectfulness had a substantially higher risk of being overweight young adults, with this association remaining even after controlling for socioeconomic factors (e.g., parent education).

Other individual familial factors have been less thoroughly examined and appear to have less influence upon child weight. For instance, parents' eating behavior, especially disinhibited eating, may contribute to higher child adiposity, but this finding requires further longitudinal examination. Cross-sectional research also suggests that high levels of parental control over children's eating is paradoxically related to higher weight among children, although parents' reports of control over children's eating does not differ between obese and nonobese siblings within the same family. Parents may be exerting more control after obesity has developed in their child.

## Energy Intake

Breast feeding has been proposed as protective against the future development of childhood obesity. Studies that examine early childhood weight and have the largest samples are most likely to support this claim. Not all studies have documented this finding and some suggest that this association is confounded by social class. There is no consistent evidence that obese children have higher caloric intake than lean children, although caloric reduction appears to be a necessary component of weight loss in childhood. No consistent evidence links specific macro- or micronutrient consumption with weight status. The use of more valid and prospective dietary assessment could help clarify this relationship.

## Energy Expenditure

Resting energy expenditure adjusted for absolute fat-free mass does not appear to differentiate obese and nonobese youth or predict weight gain in childhood. Many studies have found higher risk of childhood obesity associated with sedentary activity (e.g., television watching). Other research suggests that higher physical activity is related to lower weight in childhood and then into adulthood. Parental levels of physical activity appear to be positively associated with children's physical activity and therefore energy balance. As with dietary factors, the use of more accurate measures of physical activity (e.g., accelerometers) and measurement throughout childhood will better elucidate the magnitude and causal direction of the relation between children's physical activity and weight (see Chapter 25).

## SUMMARY

Childhood obesity continues to increase in prevalence. Unfortunately, many of the determinants of child weight status that have been examined are likely markers of other underlying mechanisms, prompting more questions than answers. For instance, the relation between children's weight status and socioeconomic status provides little information about the way in which lower socioeconomic status leads to positive energy balance. There are some reliable predictors of childhood obesity, though, including parent weight status, maternal diabetes, and socioeconomic status. More comprehensive models that evaluate environmental and biological influences, while accounting for these known predictors, will provide more complete answers regarding the causes of childhood obesity.

## FURTHER READING

Cole, T. J., Bellizzi, M. C., Flegal, K. M., & Dietz, W. H. (2000). Establishing a standard definition for child overweight and obesity worldwide: International survey. *British Medical Journal, 320*, 1240–1243.—This paper advances a new definition of overweight and obesity in childhood, based on pooled international data for BMI and linked to the widely used BMI cutoff points of 25 and 30 for adult overweight and obesity.

Kuczmarski, R. J., Ogden, C. L., Grummer-Strawn, L. M., Flegal, K. M., Guo, S. S., Wei, R., Mei, Z., Curtin, L. R., Roche, A. F., & Johnson, C. L. (2000). *CDC growth charts: United States. Advance data from vital health statistics; 314.* Hyattsville, MD: National Center for Health Statistics. (Available at http://www.cdc.gov/growthcharts)—This publication presents the U.S. growth charts using more representative data sets and more advanced statistical methods than were previously used.

Ogden, C. L., Troiano, R. P., Briefel, R. R., Kuczmarski, R. J., Flegal, K. M., & Johnson, C. L. (1997). Prevalence of overweight among preschool children in the United States, 1971 through 1994. *Pediatrics, 99,* 1–7.—This article presents cross-sectional estimates of overweight prevalence for preschool children between the ages of 2 months and 6 years in the United States.

Parsons, T. J., Power, C., Logan, S., & Summerbell, C. D. (1999). Childhood predictors of adult obesity: A systematic review. *International Journal of Obesity, 23,* S1–S107.—This comprehensive, qualitative review examines etiological factors in childhood that relate to adult obesity, while also reviewing the empirical literature on the predictors of obesity within childhood.

Troiano, R. P., & Flegal, K. M. (1998). Overweight children and adolescents: description, epidemiology, and demographics. *Pediatrics, 101,* 497–504.—Using preliminary data from the Centers for Disease Control's National Center for Health Statistics revised growth charts, this article provides epidemiological data on the prevalence of obese and overweight children and adolescents in the United States.

Troiano, R. P., & Flegal, K. M. (1999). Overweight prevalence among youth in the United States: Why so many different numbers? *International Journal of Obesity, 23,* 22–27.—This paper provides a comprehensive and thoughtful review of the challenging issues involved in defining, measuring, and establishing prevalence rates of childhood obesity.

Weinsier, R. L., Hunter, G. R., Heini, A. F., Goran, M. I., & Sell, S. M. (1998). The etiology of obesity: Relative contributions of metabolic factors, diet, and physical activity. *American Journal of Medicine, 105,* 145–150.—This article provides an overview of the metabolic and energy-balance behavioral factors that have been examined in relation to weight.

Whitaker, R. C., & Dietz, W. H. (1998). Role of the prenatal environment in the development of obesity. *Journal of Pediatrics, 132,* 768–776.—This review details prenatal influences on obesity development and considers mechanisms for such influences.

# 78

# The Environment and Obesity

## KELLY D. BROWNELL

In this chapter, I take a strident stand, namely, that the epidemic of obesity seen in the United States, and increasingly so in other countries, is caused by the environment. Genetic and psychosocial factors may determine who in a given population is susceptible to a damaging environment (see Chapters 3, 4, and 5), but the number of people affected, and hence the public health burden, is dictated by the environment. In the absence of a "toxic" food and physical activity environment, there would be virtually no obesity.

This position differs from the default explanation that obesity is caused by a combination of genetic and environmental variables. This is true when one focuses on why an *individual* is obese, based on the medical model in which causes are sought for individual cases, and treatment rather than prevention is the aim (see Chapter 111 for a comparison of medical and public health models). Adopting a public health model to ask why a *nation* is obese leads squarely to the environment as the cause.

The past 20 years have seen an explosion of research on the biology of obesity and, in recent years, on genetics. This research is important, to be certain, in the hope that we learn more about individual susceptibility and develop better methods for treatment. Yet excitement about genetics threatens to obscure the obvious: that genetic susceptibly, no matter how strong, will rarely create obesity in the absence of a bad environment.

Searching for obesity genes in the hope of establishing cause may be akin to pursuit of a gene explaining lung cancer in smokers. True, the discovery might identify those most at risk and perhaps lead to ways to counteract the disastrous effects of tobacco, but the cause of the cancer is environmental. Removal of the toxin would eliminate most of the disease.

Individuals in the United States and in many other countries are exposed to an environment in which energy-dense foods are widely available, inexpensive, and promoted heavily, while at the same time energy-saving devices and other changes in lifestyle increase sedentary behavior (see Chapters 74 and 83). The only hope for changing the prevalence of obesity is to address these environmental causes (see Chapters 111 and 112).

## EVIDENCE OF ENVIRONMENTAL INFLUENCES

Studies using a variety of methods have shown repeatedly that body weights change as the food and activity environment changes. Laboratory animals maintaining normal weight on unlimited access to healthy food will gain vast amounts when energy-dense foods are added to the available choices. In humans, studies tracking obesity in countries show increased obesity in case after case as the cultures become more modernized. Much as America is now an obese country, we face having an obese world.

Another method is to examine the prevalence of obesity in people who move from a less to a more obese country. Japanese individuals who move to Hawaii have increased obesity compared to people in Japan, but lower prevalence than Japanese people moving to the mainland United States. A stronger methodology yet is to compare individuals who move to a new country and their biological relatives who remain in the native country. This controls at least in part for genetics. Such studies show increased obesity in those moving to more modernized countries.

A dramatic example of this is the Pima Indians. Part of this tribe has migrated to Arizona, while many have remained behind in the native country, Mexico. Ravussin and colleagues have documented the striking differences between those in Mexico and their biological relatives in the United States (Figure 78.1). The percentage of calories from fat, near the desirable level in Mexico, is much higher for the Pimas in Arizona, and the prevalence of obesity and diabetes are among the highest in the world.

Based on research using this array of methods, it is clear that genetics may permit obesity to occur but a "toxic" environment causes it to occur. These influences have been recognized in authoritative reports of the Institute of Medicine (IOM) and the World Health Organization (WHO). For instance, the IOM report, *Weighing the Options*, concludes:

> Although it is clear that genetics has a modest influence on obesity on a population basis, by far the largest amount of variance in body weight is due to environmental influences . . . there has been no real change in the gene pool during this period of increasing obesity. The root of the problem, therefore, must lie in the powerful social and cultural forces that promote an energy-rich diet and a sedentary lifestyle. (pp. 53, 152)

## THE TOXIC ENVIRONMENT

### The Toxic Food Environment

It is difficult to imagine an environment that places people at greater risk for obesity than that seen in the United States. Sadly, the factors that make it so damaging appear to be growing worse. Food in this environment is available, inexpensive, and promoted in unprecedented ways. Several everyday examples underscore the situation.

The yearly marketing budget of McDonald's is $1.1 billion, and of Coca-Cola, $866 million, and these are just two companies. The budget of the National Cancer Institute to promote healthy eating is $1 million. Advertising for healthy foods versus that for fast foods, soft drinks, and so on, is a drop against a tidal wave. It is not a fair contest, and the outcome, a world with diets growing rapidly worse, cannot be considered surprising.

The number of fast-food restaurants has increased exponentially in the past 20 years.

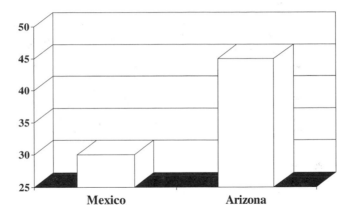

**% Calories from Fat**

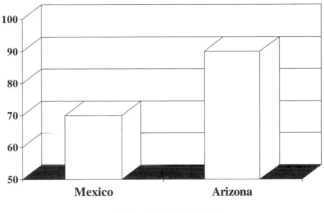

**Mean Weight (kg)**

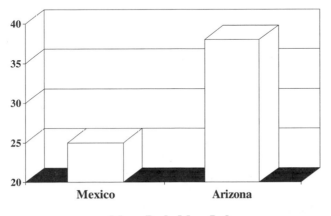

**Mean Body Mass Index**

**FIGURE 78.1.** Data abstracted from Ravussin and colleagues (1994) comparing diet, weight, and body mass index in Pima Indian women living in Arizona compared to biological relatives remaining in Mexico. Providing partial control for genetics, this study shows a strong environmental contribution to obesity.

Marketing advances such as drive-in windows, 24-hour service, and increasing portion sizes make it easier to obtain energy-dense foods. An example is the packaging of meals (e.g., what McDonald's calls "Super Value Meals"). These provide as a main feature a large hamburger or equivalent and large servings of french fries and soft drinks. One can also "supersize" the meal and have the largest size french fries and drinks, typically bringing the total to 900 calories or more before one eats the main item, the large hamburger. The power of this concept, and of this one fast-food chain, is clear when one considers that "supersize" is recognized as a verb. It may not be surprising, therefore, that one-fourth of all vegetables eaten in the United States come in the form of french fries.

The systematic increase in portion sizes is another example. Soft drinks in the 1950s were served in 8-ounce bottles. These yielded to 12-ounce cans, 16-ounce plastic bottles, and now 20-ounce plastic bottles. The 7-Eleven chain has the Big Gulp (32 ounces) and the Double Big Gulp (64 ounces). Combined with double quarter-pound hamburgers, much larger candy bars, chips, and other snack foods served in bags labeled "Big Grab," and the popularity of buffet restaurants, one sees the pervasive nature of large portion sizes.

Most disturbing is what occurs with children. The average child in the United States watches 10,000 televison advertisements for food each year, 95% of which are for foods in one of four categories: sugared cereals, candy, fast foods, and soft drinks. Even the most intrepid parents cannot compete with this. And no matter what occurs at home, children must go to school.

More than 5,000 schools in the United States have fast-food outlets in the cafeterias. These schools, and almost all others, also serve their own versions of fast foods. Rarely is the food service considered part of the child's education.

There are increasing numbers of school systems signing contracts with soft drink companies. A case example was reported from a school district in Colorado Springs, Colorado. In 1998, the school district signed a multiyear deal worth millions of dollars with the Coca-Cola company. In exchange for these large payments, the school district agreed that only Coke products would be available, and that in one of the first 3 years of the contract, at least 70,000 cases of Coke products would be sold. In the year prior to the contract being signed, the district sold 21,000 cases of these products.

In response to fear that the district was not selling enough Coke products to meet the contract demands, a school district official sent a letter to all principals encouraging them to take steps to increase sales. The letter asked that soft drink machines be moved "to where they are accessible to the students all day" and claimed that "research shows that vendor purchases are closely linked to availability. Location, location, location is the key." Teachers were encouraged to allow Coke products in the classrooms and told that "if soda products are not allowed in classes, consider allowing juices, teas, and waters" (quotes from the *Denver Post*, November 22, 1998).

If ones's aim were to make as many American children obese as possible, 10,000 captivating television ads, selling toys with fast foods, allowing fast-food franchises into school cafeterias, and having the schools collude in sales of soft drinks, a top grade would be warranted. We must ask what we are doing to our children.

## The Toxic Physical Activity Environment

Declining physical activity is also a major contributor to increasing obesity (see Chapters 74, 83, and 93). There is ample evidence of a major decline in activity from the early and even the mid-1900s. With energy-saving devices such as the automobile, elevators and escalators, computers, and the like, few people receive more than minimal activity at work or in day-to-day living. The Surgeon General's Report on Activity and Health found that more than 60% of American adults do not obtain regular physical activity and that 25% obtain no activity at all. More than half of young Americans (ages 12–21) are not regularly vigorously active. Participation in physical education classes in schools dropped from 42% to 25% just in the period from 1991 to 1995. The picture is not promising.

The computer, television, and video games have made sedentary behavior very appealing and engaging, especially for children. The number of hours children watch television or use the computer has risen steadily as the number of programs increases, the programming becomes more creative, and the internet provides instant access to friends and information of all sorts. In some cases, the sedentary lifestyle becomes institutionalized. Only 1 among the 50 U.S. states mandates physical activity in the schools at the state level.

Poor diet and physical inactivity probably act in synergistic ways. Poor diet makes it more difficult and less enjoyable for an individual to become physically active. Some data using both humans and animals suggest that physical activity is associated with better appetite control and healthier diet composition.

## Lack of Research on the Environment

With the environment being such an important contributor, it is surprising and discouraging that so little research on the topic has been done. In some cases, there is a literature but it is neither widely known nor assembled into authoritative reviews. The effects of food advertising aimed at children would fall into this category. Some issues of obvious importance have been addressed in only the most cursory fashion. The impact of school lunch programs and availability of fast foods and soft drinks in schools are examples. Money spent on biological research dwarfs that spent on documentation of environmental influences and understanding the mechanisms by which they influence behavior. The opposite may have been a more wise choice.

## SUMMARY

With pressures both to eat a poor diet and to be physically inactive, and their interaction, the environment exerts a powerful and unrelenting pressure on nation after nation to be heavier. The United States may be in the lead, but many other countries are showing alarming trends. Biology cannot explain the epidemic, and looking to biology for the solution (as would be inferred from funding priorities), is missing what is clear. The cause lies in the environment and so must the solutions.

## FURTHER READING

Brownell, K. D. (1994). Get slim with higher taxes [Editorial]. *The New York Times*, December 15, A-29.—One of the early calls for considering public policy as a means for reversing the rising prevalence of obesity, based on the assumption that the environment is the cause and that medical and personal responsibility models are ineffective.

French, S. A., Story, M., & Jeffery, R. W. (2001). Environmental influences on eating and physical activity. *Annual Review of Public Health*, 22, 63–89.—Excellent review dealing with environmental contributors to obesity, focusing on both diet and physical activity.

Horgen, K. B., & Brownell, K. D. (1998). Policy change as a means for reducing the prevalence and impact of alcoholism, smoking, and obesity. In W. R. Miller & N. Heather (Eds.), *Treating addictive behaviors* (2nd ed., pp. 105–118). New York: Plenum Press.—Overview of the effects of legislation and regulation that target diet, smoking, and alcohol consumption.

Horgen, K. B., Choate, M., & Brownell, K. D. (2001). Food advertising: Targeting children in a toxic environment. In D. G. Singer & J. L. Singer (Eds.), *Handbook of children and the media* (pp. 447–462). Thousand Oaks, CA: Sage.—Comprehensive review of the extent of food advertising aimed at children and research showing its impact on individuals and the culture at large.

Institute of Medicine. (1995). *Weighing the options: Criteria for evaluating weight management programs*. Washington, DC: National Academy Press.—Report from an expert panel dealing with causes of obesity, treatment, and prevention.

Nestle, M. (2000). Soft drink "pouring rights": Marketing empty calories. *Public Health Reports*, 115, 308–319.—Paper showing trends in soft drink consumption, with a critical view of marketing aimed at children and practices in the schools.

Ravussin, E., Valencia, M. E., Esparza, J., Bennett, P. H., & Schulz, L. O. (1994). Effects of a traditional lifestyle on obesity in Pima Indians. *Diabetes Care*, 17, 1067–1074.—Study showing dramatic differences in body weight in Pima Indians living in Arizona compared to relatives living in Mexico.

U.S. Department of Health and Human Services. (1996). *Physical activity and health: A report of the Surgeon General*. Atlanta, GA: U.S. Department of Health and Human Services, Centers for Disease Control and Prevention, National Center for Chronic Disease Prevention and Health Promotion.—Authoritative report on levels, determinants, and health effects of physical activity, and intervention and policy recommendations for increasing activity in the population.

Wadden, T. A., Brownell, K. D., & Foster, G. D. (in press). Obesity: confronting a global epidemic. *Journal of Consulting and Clinical Psychology*.—Paper that discusses etiology, treatment, and prevention of obesity, and covers approaches based in both medical and public health models.

World Health Organization. (1998). *Obesity: Preventing and managing the global epidemic: Report of a WHO Consultation on Obesity* (WHO/NUT/NCD/97.2). Geneva: Author.—The first global view, backed by substantial international data, on the obesity epidemic across the world.

# 79

# Obesity in Minority Populations

## SHIRIKI K. KUMANYIKA

There is particular concern about obesity in both children and adults in minority populations. This will intensify as the proportion of minorities in the U.S. population increases.

### MINORITY POPULATIONS

Three "racial" classifications (black or African American, Asian or Pacific Islander American, American Indian or Alaska Native) and one ethnic classification (Hispanic or Latino) are used to describe U.S. minority populations. These ethnic groups vary among themselves, and in relation to the nonminority (white) population, in the percentage who are immigrants, duration of residence within the United States, fertility rates, family structures, living arrangements, poverty, wealth, educational attainment, occupation, and residence distribution across U.S. regions and in inner-city, suburban, and rural areas. In spite of this diversity, when compared to non-Hispanic whites, minorities are more socially disadvantaged and have worse health profiles. This is least applicable to Asian Americans. Aggregate data for Asian Americans mask the presence of a bipolar distribution of socioeconomic status, with substantial proportions of both advantaged and disadvantaged individuals.

### PREVALENCE AND HEALTH IMPLICATIONS

Table 79.1 shows obesity prevalence estimates for adults in several minority populations—taken, of necessity, from various sources and with some differences in age groupings, cutoffs, and time lines. In spite of the recognized ethnic differences in percentage body fat and regional distribution of body fat at any given body mass index (BMI) level, a single set of cutoffs (e.g., BMI $\geq 25$ kg/m$^2$ for overweight and $\geq 30$ kg/m$^2$ for obesity) is considered advantageous when comparing across populations. However, the standard

**TABLE 79.1. Prevalence of Overweight or Obesity Ethnicity in U.S. Adults**

| Ethnic group and data source | Age range | Measured or self-reported data | Definition | Percent | |
|---|---|---|---|---|---|
| | | | | Males | Females |
| Non-Hispanic white, NHANES III[a] | ≥ 20 years | Measured | BMI ≥ 30 | 19.9 | 22.7 |
| Non-Hispanic black, NHANES III[a] | ≥ 20 years | Measured | BMI ≥ 30 | 20.7 | 36.7 |
| Mexican American, NHANES III[a] | ≥ 20 years | Measured | BMI ≥ 30 | 20.6 | 33.3 |
| Puerto Rican, HHANES[b] | 20–74 years | Measured | BMI ≥ 27.8* or 27.3** | 25.2 | 37.3 |
| Cuban American, HHANES[b] | 20–74 years | Measured | BMI ≥ 27.8 or 27.3 | 29.4 | 34.1 |
| American Indians, 1994–1996[c] | 18 years | Self-reported | BMI ≥ 27.8 or 27.3 | | |
|   Oklahoma | | | | 37.8 | 35.7 |
|   New Mexico and Arizona | | | | 32.9 | 34.4 |
|   Washington State and Oregon | | | | 33.3 | 43.2 |
|   North and South Dakota | | | | 46.0 | 47.3 |
| Alaska Natives 1996[c] | ≥ 18 years | Self-reported | BMI ≥ 27.8 or 27.3 | 40.8 | 38.9 |
| Native Hawaiians in Molokai[d] | 20–64 years | Measured | BMI ≥ 27.8 or 27.3 | 66 | 63 |
| Asian Americans[e] | 18–59 years | Self-reported | BMI ≥ 25 | | |
|   Entire sample | | | | 57 | 38 |
|   Chinese | | | | | 9 |
|   Japanese | | | | 17 | |
|   Vietnamese | | | | 42 | 9 |
|   Asian Indian | | | | | 25 |
| Samoans[f] | | | | | |
|   Manu'a, American Samoa | 20–74 years | Measured | BMI ≥ 27.8 or 27.3 | 56 | 77 |
|   Tuitila, American Samoa | | | | 62 | 79 |
|   Oahu, Hawaii | | | | 75 | 80 |

*Males; **females.

[a]1988–1994 National Health and Nutrition Examination Survey; see *Obesity Research* (1998), 6(Suppl. 2), 70.

[b]1982–1984 Hispanic Health and Nutrition Examination Survey; see *Obesity Research* (1998), 6(Suppl. 2), 142S.

[c]Behavioral Risk Factor Surveillance System; see Will, J. C., Denny, C., Serdula, M., & Muneta, B. (1999). *American Journal of Public Health*, 89, 395–398.

[d]See Kumanyika, S. (1994). *Obesity Research*, 2, 166–182.

[e]1992–95 National Health Interview Survey; see Lauderdale, D. S., & Rathouz, P. J. (2000). *International Journal of Obesity*, 24, 1188–1194.

[f]See McGarvey, S. T. (1991). *American Journal of Clinical Nutrition*, 53, 1586S–1594S.

cutoffs may substantially underestimate risks in populations of Asian descent. To account for obesity-related risks associated with abdominal fat in Asian populations with relatively low average BMI levels, cutoffs of BMI ≥ 23 kg/m² for overweight and ≥ 25 kg/m² for obesity have been suggested. This does not apply to Pacific Islanders or Native Hawaiians, who have high BMI levels.

As shown in Table 79.1, obesity is notably more prevalent among adults in one or both sexes in most minority populations compared to non-Hispanic whites (see Chapter 75). A parallel situation is evident with children in minority populations (not shown). Even when defined as BMI ≥ 25, obesity is least common in certain Asian American subgroups. To the extent that the data cover different time periods, the older estimates are probably underestimates. Recent data from the Centers for Disease Control Behavioral Risk Factor Surveillance System indicate increased obesity in U.S. whites, blacks, and particularly Hispanics (not disaggregated by subgroup) between 1991 and 1998. Obesity varies with socioeconomic status (see Chapter 75). However, the disproportionate prevalence of obesity in U.S. ethnic minority populations is only partly explained by socioeconomic variables.

Obesity is strongly linked to morbidity in minority populations. Cardiovascular diseases, cancer, and diabetes—all linked to obesity—are among the major causes of death in all U.S. ethnic groups. This is particularly evident for type 2 diabetes, which is more prevalent in all minority populations compared to whites. Data linking obesity, either generalized or in the abdominal region, to hypertension, dyslipidemias, subclinical atherosclerosis, coronary heart disease, left ventricular hypertrophy, sleep apnea, and musculoskeletal problems have been reported for one or more minority populations. Although the size of the associations may vary, the health consequences of obesity generally apply across ethnic groups. Where studied, an association between obesity and mortality in minority populations is not observed consistently. In addition to the limited data on this issue, such comparisons are complicated by ethnic differences in the timing and mix of death from various causes and the prevalence of critical, chronic disease risk factors other than obesity. In addition, the *relative* risks associated with obesity tend to decrease as the prevalence of obesity increases.

## ETIOLOGY, PREVENTION, AND TREATMENT

Whether the excess of obesity in minority populations can be explained on the basis of known or suspected obesity determinants is unclear. Depending on the scientific perspective, racial differences may imply primarily genetic or primarily environmental causation. The latter is more strongly supported in that U.S. racial and ethnic classifications do not define biologically homogeneous groups. Rather, these classifications differentiate population groups with common geographic and cultural origins in a very broad sense (e.g., all people with origins anywhere in Asia are in one category). The most viable hypothesis is that genes predisposing to greater efficiency in energy utilization conferred a survival advantage on certain populations during exposure to food shortages (see Chapters 3, 4, 78, and 83). Such genes—when identified—will presumably have higher frequency in minority populations. Although the concept that predisposing genes are involved is widely accepted, the polygenic nature of most obesity, as well as the high proportion of genes that are common to all racial and ethnic groups, argue against primarily genetic explanations. In addition, the predominance of environmental factors in obesity expression is supported by cross-cultural comparisons. Obesity is absent or less prevalent among populations that are genetically similar to U.S. minority populations but who have less Westernized lifestyles. In Asian American and Hispanic immigrants, obesity prevalence increases with successive generations of residence within the United States.

The frequent, although not universal, finding of lower resting energy expenditure (REE) in some minority populations, particularly African Americans, has been interpreted by some as evidence of a genetic predisposition to become or remain obese. However, it is unclear whether REE of African Americans is inappropriately low for metabolic size. The meaning of ethnic differences in the REE continues to be actively explored and debated. Other biological influences could occur during gestation (e.g., affecting infants born to obese mothers). This possibility has not been studied systematically. Given the higher fertility rates in minority compared to white women, excess weight gain or weight retention in association with childbearing may predispose to obesity. This can be demonstrated in African American women.

Environmental factors that potentially cause and perpetuate obesity in minority populations are relatively easy to identify, although these factors have not yet been synthesized into a definitive epidemiological picture. African Americans, Hispanic Americans, and American Indians are more likely than whites to live in communities where residents are ethnic minorities. Many of these communities are in socially disadvantaged urban or rural areas. In such environments, the available food and options for physical activity tend to be biased toward overconsumption of calories and fat, and underconsumption of dietary fiber, as well as underexpenditure of energy through physical activity. Specific environmental risk factors include lack of supermarkets in some neighborhoods combined with a high density of fast-food outlets, lack of neighborhood fitness and recreation facilities, and high neighborhood crime rates that discourage outdoor activities. Work environments (e.g., cafeteria or vended food and lack of fitness facilities) may provide limited food and physical activity options. Both discretionary income and discretionary time may be limited for individuals who have low incomes, high housing costs, more than one job, and child care or family responsibilities—further limiting lifestyle options.

Individual attitudes and preferences in minority communities may also be influenced by cultural norms that favor consumption of fried or other high-fat foods and sweetened beverages, or discourage physical activity or exercise. Stress among the socially disadvantaged may predispose to overeating. Excess caloric consumption in minority compared to white populations has been difficult to document, however, and may not be the relevant variable. Excess caloric consumption in relation to physical activity (i.e., chronic positive energy balance) is strongly implied by findings on physical activity levels in minority populations. There is convincing evidence that energy output is lower among minority populations than among whites, at least for African Americans, Hispanic Americans, and American Indians. How to increase physical activity in minority populations is an important public health issue.

Several studies in minority populations indicate cultural attitudes toward obesity or large body size that are less negative than those observed in whites. Such attitudes may be enhanced by a normative presence of obesity and a lack of awareness that obesity is linked to health. Furthermore, observation of thinness in association with wasting illnesses (e.g., tuberculosis or HIV/AIDS) or poverty-related food insufficiency may perpetuate the association of good health with a relatively large body size. Thinness, especially extreme thinness, is a far from universal criterion of female attractiveness. Taken together, these influences potentially reduce both the perceived importance of avoiding obesity and the social support for attempted weight control in minority compared to white populations. Motivations to control weight are lower, on average, in African American women, but this may not be the case for Hispanic and American Indian women. Relatively little attention has been given to weight control motivations of men in minority populations.

Conventional obesity treatment approaches appear to have lower efficacy among African Americans than among whites; no data on this question are available for other minority populations (see Chapter 105). This finding may reflect both client variables (biological factors, contextual and behavioral issues related to adherence) and treatment variables (theoretical frameworks or implementation approaches that fail to address cultural factors adequately).

## CONCLUSION

Identifying the obesity determinants that distinguish minority populations, qualitatively or quantitatively, from U.S. whites, and the factors within each population that promote and inhibit obesity, is of high priority. Prevention and treatment of obesity in minority populations are among the most challenging and significant domains for future obesity research.

## FURTHER READING

Deurenberg, P., Yap, M., & van Staveren, W. A. (1998). Body mass index and percent body fat: A meta-analysis among different ethnic groups. *International Journal of Obesity, 22,* 1164–1171.—Describes the relative over- or underestimation of percent body fat in various ethnic groups and discusses the implications of these differences for how obesity is defined in a public health setting.

Gannon, B., DiPietro, L., & Poehlman, E. T. (2000). Do African Americans have lower energy expenditure than Caucasians? *International Journal of Obesity, 24,* 4–13.—Careful examination of studies comparing components of energy expenditure—a possible determinant of obesity levels—in African American and white children and adults.

King, A. C., Castro, C., Eyler, A. A., Wilcox, S., Sallis, J., & Brownson, R. C. (2000). Personal and environmental factors associated with physical activity among different racial–ethnic groups of U.S. middle-aged and older-aged women. *Health Psychology, 19,* 354–364.—Results of a population-based survey of determinants of physical activity levels, with comparisons among black, Hispanic, and American Indian women.

Kumanyika, S. K. (1994). Obesity in minority populations: An epidemiologic assessment. *Obesity Research, 2,* 166–182.—Review of evidence on population-level disparities in obesity in U.S. racial and ethnic groups, and related implications for prevention and treatment.

Kumanyika, S. K., & Krebs-Smith, S. M. (2000). Preventive nutrition issues in ethnic and socioeconomic groups in the United States. In A. Bendich & R. J. Deckelbaum (Eds.), *Primary and secondary preventive nutrition* (pp. 325–356). Totowa, NJ: Humana Press.—Review of available data on nutrient- and food-intake patterns, and related health implications among U.S. minority groups.

Kumanyika, S. K., & Morssink, C. B. (1997). Cultural appropriateness of weight management programs. In S. Dalton (Ed.), *Overweight and weight management: The health professional's guide to understanding and practice* (pp. 69–106). Gaithersburg, MD: Aspen.—Detailed consideration of how cultural factors potentially influence the outcomes of weight management programs, with guidelines for improving cultural appropriateness.

Mokdad, A. H., Serdula, M. K., Dietz, W. H., Bowman, B. A., Marks, J. S., & Koplan, J. P. (1999). The spread of the obesity epidemic in the United States, 1991–1998. *Journal of the American Medical Association, 282,* 1519–1522.—Reports the continued increase in obesity prevalence in the United States among white, black, and Hispanic American respondents in the Behavioral Risk Factor Surveillance System.

National Heart, Lung, and Blood Institute Obesity Education Initiative. (1998). Clinical guidelines on the identification, evaluation, and treatment of overweight and obesity in adults. *Obesity Research*, 6(Suppl. 2), 51S–209S.—Comprehensive review that includes considerations of obesity prevalence, health implications, and treatment issues in minority populations in text, sidebars, and appendices.

Pollard, K., & O'Hare, W. (1999). America's racial and ethnic minorities. *Population Bulletin*, 54, 1–34.—Explains how race and ethnicity are defined in the United States and provides extensive descriptive information on the sociodemographics of U.S. minority populations.

Story, M., Evans, M., Fabsitz, R. R., Clay, T. E., Rock, B. H., & Broussard, B. (1999). The epidemic of obesity in American Indian communities and the need for childhood obesity-prevention programs. *American Journal of Clinical Nutrition*, 69(Suppl.), 747S–754S.—Reviews obesity as a health problem among American Indians and makes a case for the development of culturally appropriate prevention programs.

# 80

# Pregnancy and Weight Gain

## STEPHAN RÖSSNER

### BACKGROUND

A typical weight development pattern during pregnancy and after delivery is shown in Figure 80.1. The average reported lasting weight increase with pregnancies ranges from 0.4 to 3.8 kg compared with prepregnancy weights. However, several methodological complications must be considered when these data are evaluated.

- Women generally do not have recorded weight data available from the time of conception, so the initial body weight is difficult to obtain in a reliable manner.
- Weight increase during pregnancy consists of several components. For technical and ethical reasons, it is not possible to analyze all of these compartments in larger studies.
- Postpregnancy body weight is difficult to define. Many women may change their weight during a considerable period of time after delivery. The weight measurement taken soon after delivery may not be representative of the entire weight development associated with the pregnancy. If weight after delivery is recorded at a late stage, numerous other life changes, including a new pregnancy, may have taken place.

Body weight increases with age, whether women have children or not (see Chapter 75). The increase with age is more pronounced in women than in men. A further steep increase can be observed during onset of menopause. Basal metabolic rate normally decreases by about 1% per year. For an individual who maintains an identical lifestyle with regard to eating habits and exercise, this implies a weight increase of about 3–4 kg per 10 years.

### PREGNANCY AND LACTATION

On theoretical grounds, it can be assumed that the energy requirement for an entire pregnancy is about 80,000 calories, or about 300 calories per day, to cover the needs for fetal

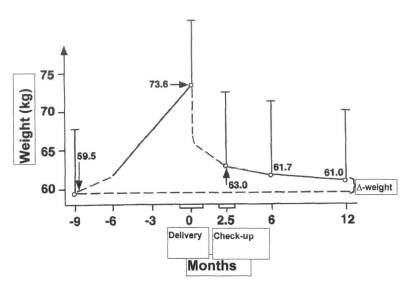

**FIGURE 80.1.** Weight development from conception (reported), during pregnancy (recorded), and until 1 year after delivery (recorded). Data from Öhlin, A., & Rössner, S. (1996). Factors related to body weight changes during and after pregnancy: The Stockholm Pregnancy and Weight Development Study. *Obesity Research*, *4*, 271–276.

growth and adipose tissue storage. Lactation has been assumed to facilitate weight loss, particularly if the period of lactation exceeds 2 months. Lactation has been calculated to increase the energy requirements by about 500 calories per day, which takes into account that production of milk is a process that requires energy.

The characteristics of adipose tissue change dramatically during pregnancy. Adipose tissue lipolysis in the femoral region is limited during pregnancy but can be easily stimulated hormonally during lactation. This seems to be a functional adaptation of the adipose tissue to the needs of the mother and the child.

The relationships between lactation, energy needs, and energy balance are not fully clarified. In some studies, no difference in energy intake was found between lactating and nonlactating women. Other studies suggest that lactation plays a minor roll in weight reduction after delivery. From a theoretical point of view, weight changes after delivery could also depend on changes in basal metabolic rate. The three mechanisms that may explain the lack of weight loss after delivery are (1) reduced basal metabolism, (2) impaired thermogenesis, and (3) reduced physical activity. These mechanisms could possibly account for reduction in energy requirements of up to about 240 calories per day. Thus, it is conceivable that the energy need for lactation can be provided from different sources, such as a combination of an increased energy intake, utilization of adipose tissue in storage, and a metabolic adaptation.

## PREGNANCY WEIGHT GAIN: STILL CONTROVERSIAL

During the past 50 years, recommendations for healthy weight change during pregnancy have been controversial. The initial concern mainly focused on safety for mother and infant, but the emerging obesity epidemic made it more important to scrutinize the extent to which an extensive and physiologically unnecessary weight gain during pregnancy could trigger overweight and obesity in the mother.

In countries with low socioeconomic status or with ethnic subgroups containing such individuals, it is clear that a low weight gain during pregnancy is an indicator of poverty, malnourishment, and future risk for high infant mortality, disability, and even mental retardation.

In the United States, in 1990, the Institute of Medicine (IOM) issued recommendations that were more liberal than before, causing considerable discussion. Some experts claimed that these IOM recommendations would not improve perinatal outcome and would have negative consequences for both infant and mother. It was suggested that the liberal weight increases advocated by the IOM would produce overgrown newborns, result in an increased frequency of cesarean sections, and eventually trigger obesity in the mothers.

Abrams and colleagues, in a recent review of all studies that examined fetal and maternal outcome, concluded that there is a steady increase in birth weight as the mean pregnancy weight gain increases, and that incidence of high birth weight (> 4,500 g) does not dramatically increase until pregnancy weight gains exceed 16 kg (the upper IOM limit). There is an impressive body of evidence indicating that weight gains within IOM recommendations are indeed associated with better pregnancy outcome, and little evidence that such pregnancy weight gains cause substantial postpartum weight retention. These conclusions are based on observational and not experimental studies. Maternal weight gain alone may not be a very helpful predictor of poor pregnancy outcome. A good pregnancy outcome can clearly be associated with a wide variety of weight development patterns throughout pregnancy. Furthermore, these studies are based only on data from an U.S. population.

## PREGNANCY TRIGGERING OBESITY

Many women seeking professional help for their weight report their pregnancies as major events in their weight development. Data from our own unit indicate that 73% of these obese women reported their pregnancies as major triggering events in their weight history. It has been recommended that women with a prepregnancy BMI > 27 kg/m² and those with a high weight gain during the first trimester should be more actively informed about the negative consequences of gaining too much weight (heavier infants, increased likelihood of cesarean sections, prolonged labor).

## SMOKING AND PREGNANCY WEIGHT DEVELOPMENT

Giving up smoking is one of the healthiest things a pregnant mother can do for herself and her child, even though several studies indicate that the weight increase in pregnancy is higher in women who give up smoking when they learn they are pregnant. It appears that the effects of smoking during pregnancy have effects on weight development of the child; children of smoking mothers not only weigh less at birth but also show feeding pattern differences. Smoking mothers tend to breast-feed their children for a shorter time. The reason is not clear, but physiological, physical, and social–environmental factors probably contribute. Smokers who have more difficulty maintaining milk supply may compensate by providing more solid food to their infant, thus increasing its weight. Nicotine withdrawal in the newborn as an effect of such reduced milk supply may induce a withdrawal syndrome and consequently more hunger for the child.

## PREGNANCY, WEIGHT DEVELOPMENT, AND PHYSICAL ACTIVITY

Research on physical activity to control adipose tissue development during pregnancy has received little attention. Studies mainly deal with the effects of exercise on the maternal cardiorespiratory system, the effects of exercise-induced trauma on mother and fetus, the effects of exercise on maternal heat production and fetal consequences, and the response of the fetus and the uterus to exercise.

Observational studies of exercise and pregnancy outcome rarely mention maternal weight development as an outcome. Most report effects on pregnancy complications, risk of prematurity, labor time and complications, and birth weight.

A 1998 review in *American Family Physician* is interesting in terms of what it does not tell about exercise during pregnancy as a method to improve weight control. The review concludes that there is sufficient evidence to justify specific exercise recommendations. Weight control is only mentioned to say that routine monitoring of maternal weight should occur, which probably does not surprise physicians or pregnant women. Nor is it surprising to note that boxing and wrestling are not recommended during pregnancy, whereas walking, stationary cycling, low-impact aerobics, and swimming are encouraged activities. The latter activities obviously agree with recommended programs to control inappropriate gain of adipose tissue.

## FURTHER READING

Abrams, B., Altman, S. L., & Pickett, K. E. (2000). Pregnancy weight gain: Still controversial. *American Journal of Clinical Nutrition, 71*(Suppl.), 1233S–1241S.—Extensive IOM analysis of the dietary recommendations in the United States during pregnancy and their implications.

Institute of Medicine. (1990). *Nutrition during pregnancy.* Washington, DC: National Academy Press.—IOM panel recommendations on both nutrition and weight gain during pregnancy.

Öhlin, A., & Rössner, S. (1996). Factors related to body weight changes during and after pregnancy: The Stockholm Pregnancy and Weight Development Study. *Obesity Research, 4,* 271–276.—A study of behavioral factors predicting weight development during and after pregnancy and during lactation.

Rebuffé-Scrive, M., Enk, L., Crona, P., Lonnroth, P., Abrahamsson, L., Smith, U., & Björntorp, P. (1985). Fat cell metabolism in different regions in women: Effects of menstrual cycle, pregnancy and lactation. *Journal of Clinical Investigation, 75,* 1973–1976.—Classic paper describing the changes in adipocyte lipolytic function during pregnancy and lactation.

Strychar, I. M., Chabot, C., Champagne, F., Ghadirian, P., Leduc, L., Lemonnier M.-C., & Raynauld, P. (2000). Psychosocial and lifestyle factors associated with insufficient and excessive maternal weight gain during pregnancy. *Journal of the American Dietetic Association, 100,* 353–356.—Recent update on behavioural aspects of weight development during pregnancy.

Wang, T. W., & Apgar, B. S. (1998). Exercise during pregnancy. *American Family Physician, 57,* 1846–1852.—Summary of exercise recommendations during early and late pregnancy.

# 81

# Age and Obesity

## REUBIN ANDRES

## BODY WEIGHT AND MORTALITY IN OLDER MEN AND WOMEN

In 1998, the World Health Organization (WHO) and the National Heart, Lung, and Blood Institute (NHLBI) issued comprehensive reports setting guidelines for the classification of overweight and obesity. These reports confirmed the well-known fact that weight increases with age (see Chapter 75). The key questions are then whether this is healthy, and how ideal weights should be determined for people at different ages.

The WHO and NHLBI reports agreed in recommending the use of body mass index (BMI) in contrast to weight-for-height tables, and in setting cut points at 25 and 30 kg/m² to define the separation of normal from overweight, and overweight from obesity (see Chapter 68). They also agreed in recommending the same cut points for adults of all ages.

These recent proposals have largely replaced the use of the tables issued periodically for the past 60 years by the Metropolitan Life Insurance Company, most recently in 1983. Those tables, which provided separate ranges of weights for men and women according to their heights and "body frame," for adults ranging in age from 25 to 59 years, provided no recommendations for those over age 60. A reanalysis of the insurance data upon which those tables are based showed that the relation of BMI to all-cause mortality was decidedly U-shaped (a quadratic function) in men and women for the decades of life ranging from 20–29 to 60–69 years. Furthermore, minimal mortality (the nadirs of the U-shaped curves) increased progressively, from about 20–27 kg/m² over the 40-year age span. Thus, the question of the need for age-specific weight tables was raised and became a topic of controversy that has continued for the past 15 years.

The literature is now vast: The NHLBI Evidence Report cites 768 references, and the WHO Consultation on Obesity cites over 600. In the present chapter, I have limited my analyses to reports of all-cause mortality in older men and women, published since the reviews noted earlier, that is, during the years 1997–2000.

Obesity is associated with a remarkably broad spectrum of health problems, including cause-specific mortality and morbidity, and disability (see Chapters 76 and 84). Yet, as noted in the NHLBI Evidence Report, the definitions of overweight and obesity were based on mortality per se and, over the years, all-cause mortality has been the "end point" considered most consistently.

Reports of the analysis of data relating body weight to mortality have been seriously criticized, as codified by Manson and her colleagues (see Chapter 76). Examples of major technical and analytical problems include the issue of adjustment or stratification for cigarette smoking and consideration of the impact of illness (overt or undetected) on body weight and mortality. These caveats have in turn received serious criticism from others. As a consequence, most results of the recent studies have been reported in exceedingly complex ways. Not only have men and women been reported separately, but also there have been variable groupings by age, differing BMI levels, smoking status, various times of follow-up, all-cause and cause-specific mortality, and an array of covariates. Furthermore, a wide variety of populations have been studied. What follows, then, may be an illustration of H. L. Mencken's aphorism that for every complex question, there is always a simple answer and it is always wrong. With that warning, the following reports demonstrate (1) that controversy persists; and (2) that a wide variety of studies in older men and women frequently show minimal mortality to occur at BMIs higher than the currently defined normal zone of 18.5 to 24.9 kg/m$^2$.

## SUMMARY OF RECENT STUDIES IN OLDER MEN AND WOMEN

There were 15 publications in the 1997–2000 time period reporting on the relation of BMI to all-cause mortality in populations of men and women whose mean ages were 60 years or higher. Of these reports, 13 presented data analyses that permitted identification of a BMI zone associated with minimal mortality. These are summarized in Table 81.1. In two studies, the BMI–mortality association is monotonically negative, that is, mortality decreases as BMI increases. For those reports, odds ratios, or hazard ratios, were computed. A 1998 report of elderly Chinese residents in Hong Kong, a random sampling of the "Old Age and Disability Allowance Schemes," presented an analysis of men and women 70 years of age and older. Mortality declined by 12% for each unit of BMI, that is, for each kg/m$^2$. A 1999 report of a random sample of men and women ages 65–84 years, the Italian Longitudinal Study of Aging, showed hazard ratios of less than one; that is, mortality decreased with increasing BMI. In the 75 to 84-year-old age decade, the results were statistically significant, with mortality declines of 6% in men and 3% in women for each kg/m$^2$ of BMI.

## IMPLICATIONS OF RECENT STUDIES IN OLDER INDIVIDUALS

The 15 recent reports demonstrate why controversy persists over the need for age-specific BMI recommendations. The two Cancer Prevention Studies presented data in several age groupings, and the two Seventh-Day Adventist Studies presented data in three follow-up periods. Several of the multiple groups of men and women derived from those two sets of studies show that minimal mortality occurred in the lower half of the normal BMI range (i.e., 18.5–21.7 kg/m$^2$). But, as the table demonstrates, these are exceptional results. All remaining studies report that the BMI range associated with minimal mortality is either

**TABLE 81.1. Publications (1997–2000) Relating Body Mass Index to All-Cause Mortality in Older Men and Women (in Order of Increasing BMI)**

| Study | Year | Sex | Age range (years) | BMI range (kg/m² at minimal mortality) |
|---|---|---|---|---|
| 1. Seventh-Day Adventist Study | 1997 | F | 55–74 | up to 21.3 |
| 2. Seventh-Day Adventist Study | 1998 | M | 55–74 | 14.3–22.5 |
| 3. Cancer Prevention Study I | 1998 | M/F | 65–74 | 19.0–21.9 |
| 4. Cancer Prevention Study II | 1999 | M | 65–74 | 19.5–21.9 |
| 5. Cancer Prevention Study II | 1999 | F | 65–74 | 22.0–23.4 |
| 6. Cancer Prevention Study I | 1998 | M | 75–84 | 22.0–24.9 |
| 7. Seventh-Day Adventist Study | 1997 | F | 55–74 | 23.0–24.8 |
| 8. Health Professionals Follow-Up | 2000 | M | 65–75 | 23.0–25.0 |
| 9. Cancer Prevention Study II | 1999 | M/F | 75+ | 23.5–24.9 |
| 10. Honolulu Heart Program | 1999 | M | 71–93 | 24.2–25.9 |
| 11. Gothenburg, Sweden | 2000 | M | 60 | 24.6–26.2 |
| 12. Cancer Prevention Study I | 1998 | M | 85+ | 25.0–26.9 |
|  |  | F | 75–84 | 25.0–26.9 |
|  |  | F | 85+ | 25.0–26.9 |
| 13. Buffalo Blood Pressure Study | 1997 | M | 65–96 | 25.2–27.4 |
| 14. Honolulu Heart Program | 1999 | M | 71–93 | 26.0–39.3 |
| 15. Iowa Women's Health Study | 2000 | F | 55–69 | 27.1–30.1 |
| 16. Longitudinal Study of Aging | 1997 | M/F | 70+ | 27.5–30.1 |
| 17. Seventh-Day Adventist Study | 1998 | M | 55–74 | 27.5–43.9 |
| 18. National Health Interview Survey | 1997 | F | 65+ | 29.3+ |
| 19. Cardiovascular Health Study | 1998 | M | 65–100 | 30.0–32.4 |
| 20. Panel Study of Income Dynamics | 1998 | F | 50–99 | 34.0 |

*Note.* BMI ranges for minimal mortality in the two Seventh-Day Adventist studies were presented for three follow-up periods for men and women: 15- to 26-year follow-up, female (1); 9- to 14-year and 15- to 26-year follow-up, male (2); 1- to 8-year and 9- to 14-year follow-up, female (7); and 1- to 8-year follow-up, male (17). BMI ranges for the Honolulu Heart Program study were presented for never-smokers (10) and for former + current smokers (14). BMI ranges for the two American Cancer Society studies were presented for three older age groups (Study 1) and for two older age groups (Study II), as indicated in the table.

the upper half of the normal range (21.8–24.9 kg/m²) or in the BMI zone defined as "overweight" (i.e., 25.0–29.9 kg/m²), or even the zone of obesity (i.e., above 30.0 kg/m²). To these tabulated results can be added the reports from Hong Kong and Italy noted earlier.

Obviously the data from diverse studies with such widely differing results should not simply be averaged out. There are so many putative flaws in such studies, considered by some to be "fatal," that it is not possible to define a narrow, best BMI zone for older men and women, especially since only all-cause mortality has been included in this brief summary. Still, a conservative message can be offered: Caution should be exercised in insisting upon the standards recommended for men and women in the later years of life by the WHO and NHLBI reports. It is obviously prudent to recommend avoidance of obesity at younger ages, but once old age has been achieved, it may not be advisable to recommend that the otherwise healthy person undertake vigorous efforts to achieve the BMI zone designated as "normal." Strawbridge and his colleagues recently updated data from the Alameda County Study and concluded from their results that the NHLBI and WHO guidelines stigmatize too many people as overweight and ignore the serious health risks associated with low weight and efforts to maintain an unrealistically lean body mass (see Chapters 15, 17, and 20). The advisability of weight loss at older age, discussed in the NHLBI report, is a topic that will require further consideration in the future.

## FURTHER READING

Allison, D. B., Faith, M. S., Heo, M., Townsend-Butterwork, D., & Williamson, D. F. (1999). Meta-analysis of the effect of excluding early deaths on the estimated relationship between body mass index and mortality. *Obesity Research, 7*, 342–354.—A test of the hypothesis that deaths occurring in the early follow-up period distort the BMI–mortality relationship.

Andres, R., Elahi, D., Tobin, J. D., Muller, D. C., & Brant, L. (1985). Impact of age on weight goals. *Annals of Internal Medicine, 103*, 1030–1033.—This study reanalyzed the insurance data, noted the U-shaped relationship between BMI and mortality, and demonstrated a progressive increase with age in the BMI associated with lowest mortality in men and women.

The BMI in Diverse Populations Collaborative Group. (1999). Effect of smoking on the body mass index–mortality relation: Empirical evidence from 15 studies. *American Journal of Epidemiology, 150*, 1297–1308.—A test of the hypothesis that studies not including data on cigarette smoking are fatally flawed.

Manson, J. E., Stampfer, M. J., Hennekens, C. H., & Willett, W. C. (1987). Body weight and longevity: A reassessment. *Journal of the American Medical Association, 257*, 353–358.—A codification of purported technical analytical problems in relating BMI to mortality.

Metropolitan Life Insurance Company. (1983). 1983 Metropolitan Height and Weight Tables. *Statistical Bulletin of the Metropolitan Life Insurance Company, 64* (January–June), 2.—The dominant reference base for judging body weight until superceded by NHLBI and WHO reports.

NHLBI Obesity Education Initiative Expert Panel. (1998). Clinical guidelines on the identification, evaluation, and treatment of overweight and obesity in adults. *Obesity Research, 6*, 51S–209S.—A comprehensive consensus report with extensive bibliographical support.

Strawbridge, W. J., Wallhagen, M. I., & Shema, S. J. (2000). New NHLBI clinical guidelines for obesity and overweight: Will they promote health? *American Journal of Public Health, 90*, 340–343.—A critique of the recent NHLBI and WHO recommendations based upon a literature review and data from the Alameda County Study.

World Health Organization. (1998). *Obesity: Preventing and managing the global epidemic: Report of a WHO Consultation on Obesity* (WHO/NUT/NCD/97.2). Geneva: Author.—A remarkable compendium of this complex field; includes extensive bibliographic information up to the time of publication.

# 82

# The Health Economics of Obesity and Weight Loss

Obesity[1] in the United States is a major public health problem with substantial economic consequences. Despite the known health risks, managed care organizations, health insurance plans, employers, and the government (i.e., Medicaid) do not consistently provide services to treat this growing epidemic (see Chapter 20). It is imperative that leaders who study and treat obesity be well versed in the economic consequences of obesity and weight loss, so that they can approach and educate health care decision makers regarding health care coverage of this chronic disease.

## DEFINITION OF TERMS

Economic costs represent the overall economic burden caused by disease, whether on the nation or on a payer of health care (i.e., managed care organization, employer). They are categorized classically into two components: direct medical costs, and indirect morbidity and mortality costs. Direct medical costs are the cost of preventive, diagnostic, and treatment services related to the disease (e.g., hospital care, physician services, medications). Indirect costs are the value of lost output due to cessation or reduction of productivity caused by morbidity and mortality. Morbidity costs are wages lost by people who are unable to work because of illness and disability. Mortality costs are the value of future earnings lost by people who die prematurely. This chapter focuses on direct and indirect morbidity costs; indirect mortality costs of obesity are incomplete estimates but will be available from large, long-term clinical trials, such as the Study of Health Outcomes of Weight Loss (SHOW) trial.

---

[1]Throughout this chapter, overweight is defined as a body mass index (BMI) $\geq 25$ kg/m$^2$, moderate overweight as a BMI $\geq 27.8$ kg/m$^2$ (men) and 27.3 kg/m$^2$ (women), and obesity as a BMI $\geq 30$ kg/m$^2$.

453

## DIRECT MEDICAL COSTS ASSOCIATED WITH OBESITY

### National Perspective

Approximately 22% of the U.S. population is obese (see Chapter 75). This has had a substantial impact on health care utilization and costs. The direct health care cost attributable to obesity in 1995 was estimated to be $51.6 billion, approximately 5.7% of the total U.S. health expenditure for that year. Compared to other chronic diseases, the economic impact of obesity is approximately the same as diabetes, 1.25 times greater than coronary heart disease, and 2.7 times greater than hypertension. It is estimated that approximately $16.1 billion will be spent in the United States during the next 25 years, just for the treatment of non-cancer-related illnesses associated with overweight in women ages 40–44. Mild obesity is projected (by modeling) to increase the expected lifetime medical care costs of specific conditions related to obesity (hypercholesterolemia, hypertension, type 2 diabetes, coronary heart disease, and stroke) by approximately 20%, while moderate obesity will increase them by about 50%, and severe obesity will nearly double the cost. The lifetime medical care costs of obesity are similar in magnitude to those of smoking. Because obesity is associated with increased mortality, direct health care cost estimates may be as much as 25% lower than projected.

The National Health Interview Survey (NHIS) was used to track the number of physician visits related to obesity. In 1988, 42.9 million physician visits were attributable to obesity; by 1994, the number of visits increased by 88% to 81.2 million visits per year. The sharp rise in visits was due to increases in both the prevalence of obesity and the average number of visits per year by obese patients.

### Payer's Perspective: Managed Care Organizations and Employers

Although cost-of-illness studies from a societal perspective are important to health care policymakers, managed care organizations are concerned with models and research using populations that are "managed" and hence reflect their membership. In the Northern California Kaiser Permanente population, the percentage of patients with one or more comorbid conditions increased as body mass index (BMI) increased. Relative to members with BMIs between 20.0–24.9 kg/m$^2$, mean annual costs were 25% greater among people with BMIs between 30–35 kg/m$^2$ and 44% greater among people with BMIs > 35 kg/m$^2$ (Figure 82.1). The magnitude of the increased inpatient and outpatient utilization among the Northern California Kaiser Permanente members was similar to that reported among the Northwest Kaiser Permanente members, showing that obesity does impact health care utilization and costs even among "managed" patients.

Among the HealthPartners population in Minnesota, investigators reported that for every 1-unit increase in BMI, there was a 1.9% increase in median costs. While this does not translate into large cost increases at the individual level ($11.26 per BMI unit increase per year), the costs can become considerable at the population level. One model projected that in a managed care organization with 1 million members, health care costs attributable to obesity would be approximately $345.9 million annually.

Studies have also evaluated health care claims and costs in an employer setting. Employees who were obese had 21.4% more health care expenditures than lean employees. This magnitude was comparable to or greater than other risk factors such as smoking, high blood pressure, poor exercise habits, high cholesterol levels, and high alcohol intake.

## Body Mass Index (kg/m$^2$)

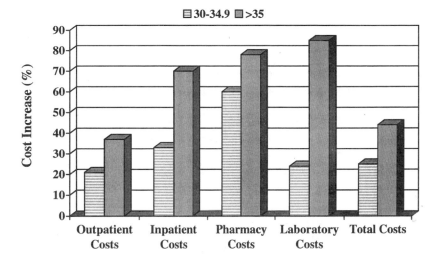

**FIGURE 82.1.** Increased health care costs in obese patients (BMI = 30–35 kg/m$^2$ and > 35 kg/m$^2$) relative to costs in lean patients (BMI = 20–25 kg/m$^2$). All participants are members of a managed care setting (the Northern California Kaiser Permanente Health Care System). Data from Quesenberry, C. P., Jr., Caan, B., & Jacobson, A. (1998). Obesity, health services use, and health care costs among members of a health maintenance organization. *Archives of Internal Medicine, 158,* 466–472.

One study (*n* = 843) reported that moderately overweight employees had on average $2,326 more health care costs over a 3-year period than did employees with lower BMIs. Health care costs doubled among obese employees who were older than 45. Age, however, has not been consistently found to increase health care costs among the obese population.

Overall, obesity is associated with greater health care utilization and cost, particularly pharmaceutical and laboratory costs. In most studies, there is no difference in utilization and costs among obese people by age. Obese women tend to utilize health services more than men, but, in general, this is true regardless of body weight. The dominant diagnoses relative to direct health care costs among the obese population are coronary heart disease, type 2 diabetes, hypertension, and osteoarthritis, suggesting that these comorbidities should be preferentially targeted when treating obesity.

## DIRECT MEDICAL COSTS ASSOCIATED WITH WEIGHT LOSS

All studies evaluating the economic impact of weight loss have focused on pharmaceutical cost savings after weight loss treatment and utilized small samples and less than 1-year follow-up. In one such report, pharmaceutical expenses for hypertensive and diabetic medications decreased 50% in 1 year among obese patients who lost 8% of their body weight. Other reports show that a modest weight loss (5–10%) results in net cost savings for the pharmaceutical use in the treatment of diabetes, hypertension, and hyperlipdemia, after accounting for costs of medications for treating obesity (see Chapters 87 and 88). Whether patients lose weight through pharmaceuticals or surgery, the cost savings are similar.

The impact of a sustained modest weight loss on lifetime health and health care costs was recently modeled. Depending on age, gender, and initial BMI, a 10% weight loss was projected to reduce patients' expected number of years with hypertension, type 2 diabetes, and coronary heart disease. Modest weight loss was also projected to affect hypercholesterolemia and stroke, but to a lesser degree. A sustained 10% reduction in body weight would decrease expected lifetime medical care costs of these diseases and conditions by $2,300 to $5,300 for men and $2,200 to $5,200 for women (Figure 82.2).

## INDIRECT MORBIDITY COSTS ASSOCIATED WITH OBESITY

### Productivity

Employers are the major payers and decision makers for health care coverage. They are concerned with both direct health care costs to their company and indirect morbidity

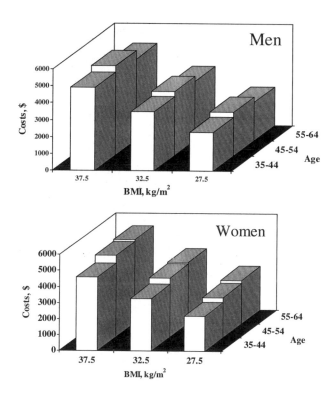

**FIGURE 82.2.** Savings in expected lifetime medical care costs (in 1996 U.S. dollars) of specific obesity-related diseases (coronary heart disease, stroke, hypertension, type 2 diabetes, hypercholesterolemia) with a sustained 10% weight loss by gender, age, and initial body mass index (BMI, kg/m²). Data from Oster, G., Thompson, D., Edelsberg, J., Bird, A. P., & Colditz, G. A. (1999). Lifetime health and economic benefits of weight loss among obese persons. *American Journal of Public Health, 89,* 1536–1542.

costs (short- and long-term disability, and restriction in activity). Obesity has a profound impact on indirect morbidity costs (measured by days missed at work due to illness; see Figure 82.3).

Approximately 27% of the U.S. labor force has a BMI $\geq 29$ kg/m². Obesity was estimated to cost U.S. businesses $12.7 billion in 1996, including $2.6 billion as a result of mild obesity and $10.1 billion due to moderate-to-severe obesity. Sixty-one percent of these costs were from health insurance expenditures, 19% from paid sick leave, 14% for life insurance expenditures, and 6% for disability insurance costs.

In 1994 alone, there were 39.2 million excess workdays lost among obese persons. The cost of the lost productivity amounted to $3.93 billion (in 1995 U.S. dollars). There was a 51% increase nationally in the number of missed work days between 1988 and 1994, due to increases in the prevalence of obesity and number of sick days per obese employee. The degree of obesity appears to affect the amount of lost productivity. Men and women with healthy body weights (BMI = 20.0–24.9 kg/m²) missed, on average, 4.5 and 5.0 days of work per year, respectively (based on the 1994 NHIS). Overweight men and women missed, on average, 4.0 and 7.4 days of work per year, respectively, and obese men and women missed an average of 5.7 and 7.9 days per year, respectively. In one company's estimation, employees who were moderately overweight had twice as many sick days (on average, 8.45 days/year) as employees with a healthy body weight (on average, 3.73 days/year). The cost of sick leave to employers was $863 per overweight employee during a 3-year period, which increased to $1,400 among older (> 45 years), overweight employees.

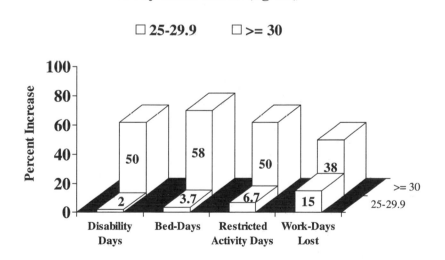

**FIGURE 82.3.** Percent increase in indirect morbidity outcomes in overweight (BMI = 25–29.9 kg/m²) and obese (≥ 30 kg/m²) people as compared to lean people (BMI = 20–25 kg/m²). Data from the National Health Interview Survey as reported in Wolf, A. M., & Colditz, G. A. (1998). Current estimates of the economic cost of obesity in the United States. *Obesity Research, 6,* 97–106; and Thompson, D., Edelsberg, J., Kinsey, K. L., & Oster, G. (1998). Estimated economic costs of obesity to U.S. business. *American Journal of Health Promotion, 13,* 120–127.

The association between obesity and absenteeism is supported in other studies as well. Among 10,825 employed adults, obese employees were more than twice as likely to experience high-level absenteeism (seven or more absences due to illness during the previous 6 months) and 1.49 times more likely to have moderate absenteeism (three to six absences due to illness during the previous 6 months) than lean employees. One study indicated that obesity increased the risk of some common diseases that in turn affected absenteeism. For instance, mental disorders were higher among obese than lean women (1.1 vs. 0.8 per 100), and musculoskeletal disorders and heart disease were higher among obese men (musculoskeletal disorders, 3.2 vs. 2.0 per 100; heart disease, 1.1 vs. 0.7 per 100). Finaly, obesity affected productivity. Similar to persons with other chronic disease risk factors (e.g., hypertension and hypercholesterolemia) and worse than those with other lifestyle risk factors (e.g., smoking and physical inactivity), moderately overweight employees with "at-risk BMIs" had lower productivity standards.

## Restricted Activity and Disability

Obesity can limit one's activity level and increase long-term disability (see Chapter 70). In 1994, there were 239 million excess restricted activity days and 89.5 million excess bed days among obese persons in the United States. This reflects a 36% increase in restricted activity and a 28% increase in the number of bed days among obese persons between 1988 and 1994. Most of the increase over time appears to reflect the rise in the prevalence of obesity.

There is also an association between the rate of disability and the degree of obesity. In 1994, 5.9% of men and 4.7% of women with a healthy body weight were unable to work. This compares to 5.6% of men and 7.9% of women unable to work in the overweight population, and 9.6% and 12.6%, respectively, in the obese population.

There is strong evidence that obesity affects productivity and potentially all indirect morbidity costs. Women appear to be driving the association between obesity and productivity. To date, there are no studies that evaluate whether weight loss influences productivity or other indirect morbidity outcomes.

## CONCLUSION

Obesity increases morbidity costs substantially, both directly and indirectly. The economic impact of obesity is comparable to that of smoking. There appears to be a dose–response relationship between economic costs and the degree of overweight/obesity, but further research is needed to confirm this finding. Economic costs are significantly elevated at BMIs greater than 30 kg/m$^2$. There is a suggestion of increased economic costs attributable to obesity over time but, again, more studies are needed to confirm this finding. Age and gender may have a differential impact on certain economic outcomes. While substantial data support the association between economic costs and obesity, relatively little data address the economic impact of weight loss. Much research in this area is needed.

# FURTHER READING

Burton, W. N., Chen, C.Y., Schultz, A. B., & Edington, D. W. (1998). The economic costs associated with body mass index in a workplace. *Journal of Occupational and Environmental Medicine, 40,* 786–792.—Provides useful information on the impact of obesity on health care claims, and short- and long-term disability from an employer's perspective.

Burton, W. N., Conti, D. J., Chen, C. Y., Schultz, A. B., & Edington, D. W. (1999). The role of health risk factors and disease on worker productivity. *Journal of Occupational and Environmental Medicine, 41,* 863–877.—Evaluates the impact of obesity on workers' productiveness and compares this to other health risk factors (i.e., smoking, hypertension).

Gold, M. R., Siegel, J. E., Russell, L. B., & Weinstein, M. C. (Eds.). (1996). *Cost effectiveness in health and medicine.* New York: Oxford University Press.—The gold standard text for understanding and completing cost-effectiveness studies.

Oster, G., Thompson, D., Edelsberg, J., Bird, A. P., & Colditz, G. A. (1999). Lifetime health and economic benefits of weight loss among obese persons. *American Journal of Public Health, 89,* 1536–1542.—Presents a model that examines the impact of a sustained, modest weight loss (10%) on health (i.e., type 2 diabetes) and health care costs over an obese person's lifetime.

Pronk, N. P., Goodman, M. J., O'Connor, P. J., & Martinson, B. C. (1999). Relationship between modifiable health risks and short-term health care charges. *Journal of the American Medical Association, 282,* 2235–2239.—Examines the financial impact of obesity and other health risks (i.e., smoking, physical inactivity) on short-term health costs within a managed care organization.

Quesenberry, C. P., Caan, B., & Jacobson, A. (1998). Obesity, health services use and health care costs among members of a health maintenance organization. *Archives of Internal Medicine, 158,* 466–472.—A very good cross-sectional examination of health care utilization and costs associated with BMI at different grades (i.e., overweight, obesity, grade I and grades II–III) in a managed care organization.

Thompson, D., Edelberg, J., Colditz, G. A., Bird, A. P., & Oster, G. (1999) Lifetime health and economic consequences of obesity. *Archives of Internal Medicine, 159,* 2177–2183.—This paper presents a model that examines the impact of obesity on health (i.e. years with type 2 diabetes) and health care costs over an obese person's lifetime.

Thompson, D., Edelberg, J., Kinsey, K. L., & Oster, G. (1998). Estimated economic costs of obesity to U.S. business. *American Journal of Health Promotion, 13,* 120–127.—This paper evaluates the cost of obesity to U.S. businesses at a national level.

Wolf, A. M., & Colditz, G. A. (1996). Social and economic impact of body weight in the United States. *American Journal of Clinical Nutrition, 63*(Suppl. 1), 466S–469S.—This paper examines the impact upon the nation of weight (overweight and obesity) and weight gain.

Wolf, A. M., & Colditz, G. A. (1998). Current estimates of the economic cost of obesity in the United States. *Obesity Research, 6,* 97–106.—Estimates the financial impact of obesity at a national level.

# 83

# An Overview of the Etiology of Obesity

## JAMES O. HILL

The current global epidemic of obesity is fueled by an environment that "overpowers" the body's energy balance regulatory system. The impressive stability of body weight seen in most individuals over time implies that the body does have a system to regulate energy balance. But the worldwide increase in body weights suggests that the capacity of this system to maintain energy balance at a "healthy" body weight in response to environmental challenges is limited. The current environment is exerting constant, unidirectional effects on energy balance that exceed the adaptive capacity of the system (see Chapters 74 and 78). Under these conditions, an increase in body weight and body fat mass is necessary for the achievement of energy balance.

## THE NATURE OF THE ENERGY BALANCE REGULATORY SYSTEM

We do not fully understand the physiological mechanisms in the body by which energy intake and energy expenditure are linked, but the existence of such a system is suggested by results of under- and overfeeding studies. In response to underfeeding, decreased resting energy expenditure tends to limit negative energy balance and minimize changes in body weight. Similarly, with overfeeding, resting energy expenditure increases in a fashion that opposes positive energy balance and weight gain. The adaptive response appears to be somewhat stronger to oppose weight loss than to oppose weight gain (see Chapter 8). Furthermore, body weights of these subjects return to baseline levels relatively quickly after the under- or overfeeding stops, suggesting an ability to restore the "usual" state of energy balance after the challenge to the system is withdrawn.

While there are clearly adaptive responses to under- and overfeeding, this physiological system has a limited capacity to maintain energy balance in the face of environmental challenges (e.g., under- or overfeeding). If such challenges are sufficiently large, energy balance is not maintained and body weight changes. If the challenges are constantly present, the system does not have an opportunity to return to the original state of energy balance regulation.

Within many environments, this physiological system serves to maintain energy balance and leads to a stable, nonobese body weight. For mankind's early history, this system allowed most people to maintain a nonobese body weight with little conscious effort. These environments consisted of day-to-day variations in energy intake and physical activity but were likely relatively small and consisted of bidirectional influences (i.e., promoting both positive and negative energy balance). While there may have been periods of more substantial under- or overeating and/or periods when physical activity varied significantly above or below usual levels, these were temporary, allowing the system to recover its usual state of energy balance when the challenge was withdrawn. Under such conditions, body weight stability could be maintained almost solely by physiological mechanisms.

## THE MODERN ENVIRONMENT AND ENERGY BALANCE REGULATION

The environment in which we live has changed substantially over the past few decades, and in the current environment, few people can maintain a nonobese body weight by relying exclusively on their physiological regulation of energy balance. This is because this environment is exerting exactly the types of pressures on energy balance—large, constant, and unidirectional—that overwhelm physiological regulation of energy balance (see Chapter 78).

Brownell (Chapter 78) has described these environmental pressures within the environment in the United States, and James (Chapter 74) has shown that the U.S. environment is being exported around the world. While the magnitude of changes in the environment have not been documented quantitatively, it seems likely that, over the past few decades, they have served to greatly reduce physical activity, and to increase energy intake.

Changes in society that have greatly reduced the need to be physically active in daily life have likely reduced the total energy expenditure of the population. In response to declining energy expenditure, obesity can only be avoided by comparable reductions in food intake. This does not seem to have occurred, and in fact, changes in the environment over the past few years have probably served to increase energy intake. Brownell (Chapter 78) has described many of these changes, including easy availability of inexpensive, high-energy foods, increased portion sizes, and increases in food advertising. The impact of the environment has been unidirectional, with few, if any, changes in the environment that promote decreased energy intake.

Furthermore, the pressures exerted by the environment on physical activity and energy intake are constant, forcing changes in the way in which energy balance is regulated. For example, cohort studies show that the average adult in the United States shows gradual weight gain during the adult years. Under these constant environmental conditions, the "desirable" state of energy balance cannot be maintained and weight gain occurs.

It is clear that, for most people, the current environment does not allow maintenance of a nonobese body weight without conscious effort. We can no longer rely solely on our physiology to keep us lean. However, the strength of current environmental influences on energy balance may even be greater. As our environment evolved from a low- to high-obesity-conducive environment, many people could likely maintain a nonobese body weight only with substantial cognitive effort (i.e., watching food intake, making conscious efforts to be physically active). The high prevalence of obesity despite the recognition of the cognitive need to manage energy balance suggests that, for more and more people, this environment may be overwhelming even cognitive efforts to maintain body weight at nonobese levels. In thinking about "curing" the environment, it may be unrealistic to attempt to return to totally physiological energy balance regulation and more realistic to seek an environment in which the majority of individuals can, with conscious efforts, maintain energy balance at a healthy body weight. Along with changing the environment, we must also look toward teaching the cognitive skills needed to achieve energy balance.

## OBESITY AS A NATURAL RESPONSE
## TO AN OBESITY-CONDUCIVE ENVIRONMENT

In one sense, the gradual increase seen in body weights of many populations can best be considered "normal" rather than "abnormal" physiology. The body seems to strive to reach a steady state of energy balance regulation in which energy intake equals energy expenditure. In response to environmental pressure toward constant positive energy balance, body weight and body fat increase. This in turn serves to restore energy balance. Becoming obese is one way to achieve energy balance in an environment that decreases physical activity and increases energy intake. If energy balance regulation within the obesity-conducive environment is not achieved behaviorally (e.g., by opposing environmental pressure to eat less or becoming less physically active), it must be achieved metabolically. The increase in body mass that occurs as a consequence of positive energy balance produced by environmental pressures on energy intake and physical activity leads to an increase in energy expenditure and fat oxidation. Both resting metabolic rate and the energy cost of physical activity increase with increasing body mass. As body mass increases, energy expenditure increases and lessens positive energy balance. A new steady state of energy balance is reached once the increase in energy expenditure is sufficient to match energy intake.

The increase in body fat mass also leads to an increase in fat oxidation. Flatt has described how reaching a steady state of energy balance requires achieving a balance between fat intake and fat oxidation. Positive fat balance exists during periods of positive energy balance, so that bringing the system back into steady state requires increasing fat oxidation. An increase in fat oxidation appears to accompany increases in body fat mass through mechanisms not yet fully understood.

It is likely that the increase in body weight and body fat mass may also increase signals to reduce food intake. Leptin, for example, which may be one such signal originating in adipose tissue (see Chapter 6), increases with increases in body fat mass and may signal the brain to reduce food intake. We do not currently understand the extent to which reducing food as a result of signals such as leptin helps to reachieve energy balance after a period of positive energy balance. This is an obvious area in need of further research.

The net result is that becoming obese is one way for the body to reach a steady state of energy and nutrient balance in an obesity-conducive environment.

## THE ROLE OF GENETICS

While the current obesity epidemic is driven largely by the environment, genetics certainly plays an important role in determining whether and to what extent any individual responds to the environment (see Chapters 3, 4, and 5). A great example of gene–environment interaction relative to body weight is provided by the Pima Indians. Pimas living on reservations are one of the fattest populations on record and have been considered to be genetically susceptible to obesity. However, Pimas living as subsistence farmers in remote parts of Mexico are not obese. In every environment, there are the rare genotypes that regulate some people's body weight differently from the majority of the population. For example, obesity is present to some extent even in environments characterized by low-fat, low-energy-dense diets and high levels of physical activity. Similarly, there are likely people in the most obesity-conducive environments that remain lean because of genetic factors.

Whether or not someone within a given environment actually becomes obese is determined not only by the nature of the environment but also by the degree of susceptibility to obesity. We do not fully understand what determines susceptibility to obesity, but one part of this could be the ability of the functional phenotype to adapt to influences on the metabolic and behavioral phenotypes. A high susceptibility to obesity would be associated with a low adaptive ability of the functional phenotype, and low susceptibility would be associated with a high adaptive ability of the functional phenotype. Genes are likely to be involved in determining the adaptive capacity of the functional phenotype.

## SUMMARY

Understanding the physiological regulation of energy balance is important and will explain why some individuals are obese within a given environment while others are lean. This information will help us devise treatment–prevention strategies targeted at those who are predisposed to obesity. To understand the etiology of the obesity epidemic we must understand and modify environmental pressures on energy balance that require the majority of people to become obese in order to achieve energy balance. The success in managing the global epidemic of obesity may lie more in modifying our environment than in modifying human physiology.

Finally, targeting the environment obviates the need to know prospectively who might become obese and who will not. Eventually, we may be able to screen individuals for susceptibility and to target other approaches. But until then, we seem destined to wait to react until individuals are obese. Targeting the environment may be the only way to stop the obesity epidemic before it gets worse (see Chapters 111 and 112).

## FURTHER READING

Flatt, J. P. (1988). Importance of nutrient balance in body weight regulation. *Diabetes–Metabolism Reviews*, 6, 571–581.—This paper describes how achieving fat balance is the key to achieving energy balance.

Hill, J. O., & Peters, J. C. (1998). Environmental contributions to the obesity epidemic. *Science*, 280, 1371–1374.—This paper describes how factors in the environment promote obesity.

Horton, T. J., Drougas, H., Brachey, A., Reed, G. W., Peters, J. C., & Hill, J. O. (1995). Fat and carbohydrate overfeeding in humans: Different effects on energy storage. *American Journal of Clinical Nutrition, 62,* 19–29.—This study of subjects overfed for 14 days on a high-fat diet and 14 days on a high-carbohydrate diet shows the differences in how excess energy is stored depending on whether the energy source is fat or carbohydrate.

Kriketos, A. D., Sharp, T. A., Seagle, H. M., Grunwald, G., & Hill, J. O. (2000). Effects of aerobic physical fitness on fat oxidation and body fatness. *Medicine and Science in Sports and Exercise, 32,* 805–811.—This study deals with the relationship among fat oxidation, body fat, and exercise.

National Institutes of Health. (1998). Clinical guidelines on the identification, evaluation, and treatment of overweight and obesity in adults—the Evidence Report. *Obesity Research, 6*(Suppl. 2), 51S–210S.—Guidelines for clinicians involved in managing obese patients.

Ravusssin, E., Lillioja, S., Anderson, T. E., Christin, L., & Bogardus, C. (1986). Determinants of 24-hour energy expenditure in man: Methods and results using a respiratory chamber. *Journal of Clinical Investigation, 78,* 1568–1578.—This comprehensive paper describes the components of energy expenditure and shows how each is related to body composition.

Ravussin, E., Valencia, M. E., Esparza, J., Bennett, P. H., & Schulz, L. O. (1994). Effects of a traditional lifestyle on obesity in Pima Indians. *Diabetes Care, 17,* 1067–1074.—In this paper, the authors' reports that Pima Indians living on reservations in Arizona are very obese, while Pima Indians living as subsistence farmers in rural Mexico are lean, show the differential effect of the environment in genetically similar groups.

# Medical Aspects of
# Obesity and Weight Loss

# 84

# Medical Complications of Obesity in Adults

## F. XAVIER PI-SUNYER

Obesity is of public health concern because of its association with medical complications that lead to increased morbidity and mortality (see Chapter 76). Both the National Institutes of Health and the World Health Organization define obesity as a body mass index (BMI) of 30 kg/m$^2$ or greater and overweight as a BMI of 25–30 kg/m$^2$. The most common complications associated with obesity are insulin resistance, diabetes mellitus, hypertension, dyslipidemia, cardiovascular disease, gallstones and cholecystitis, respiratory dysfunction, and increased incidence of certain cancers.

## DIABETES MELLITUS

There is a strong positive correlation between the average weight in a population and the presence of type 2 (non-insulin-dependent) diabetes mellitus. In a male population divided into groups with BMIs of 25.0 to 26.9, 29 to 30, and greater than 35, the risk for diabetes (compared to a population with BMIs less than 21) increases 2.2-, 6.7-, and 42-fold, respectively. The severity of the obesity is a determinant, as is the length of time obesity has been present.

The pathogenesis of the diabetes is related to the insulin resistance caused by the obesity, which tends to increase in severity as BMI rises. Primarily sensitive to the action of insulin are muscle, adipose, and liver tissue. As excess fat accumulates in the body, the ability of insulin to act at the cellular level is impaired. The cellular effect is manifested both at the insulin receptor and postreceptor levels. There is a downregulation of insulin receptors, with a decrease in both the number of receptors at the membrane surface and the affinity of the insulin for the receptors. These changes lower the ability of circulating insulin to bind to the receptors and to initiate the signals that lead to the many intracellular actions of insulin.

More importantly, there are also postreceptor abnormalities in obese individuals, so that the signals for initiating glucose transport, glucose oxidation, and, particularly, glucose storage as glycogen are impaired. The net effect is to decrease glucose entrance into and use by insulin-sensitive cells. This effect is particularly true in muscle. The islet cells of the pancreas respond to the resultant increased blood glucose levels by making and secreting more insulin. This process continues day in and day out, as long as an individual is overweight. Finally, in those individuals who have the appropriate genetic predisposition to the disease, the B cells of the pancreas cannot keep up with the increased requirements and begin to fail, so that frank diabetes supervenes.

## HYPERTENSION

About one-third of all obese persons are hypertensive. Epidemiological studies have demonstrated that for every 10-kilogram rise in body weight over normal, there is an average increase of 3 mm Hg in systolic and 2 mm Hg in diastolic pressure. In the Framingham Heart Study, for every 19% increase in relative weight, systolic blood pressure increased by 6.5 mm Hg. Some studies have shown even greater effects. The longer the duration of obesity, the greater the risk of developing hypertension. Using data from the U.S. National Health Examination II Survey (in which obesity was defined as a weight for height above the 85th percentile of that of men and women in the third decade of life), the prevalence of hypertension in persons 20% or more overweight was twice that of persons of normal weight. The distribution of body fat is an important determinant of blood pressure risk, with central or intra-abdominal body fat constituting a greater risk than peripheral fat.

The causes for the relationship between obesity and hypertension are not clear, although various mechanisms have been invoked. First, sodium retention may occur because of decreased renal filtration surface. Second, insulin enhances the tubular reabsorption of sodium, and insulin levels are high in obese persons because of the prevailing insulin resistance. Third, a number of studies have suggested an increased catecholamine tone in obesity, leading to hypertension. Fourth, some reports have suggested that plasma renin levels may be inappropriately elevated in obese persons. More information is needed on the pathogenesis of hypertension related to excess fat accumulation.

## STROKE

Directly linked to the increased prevalence of hypertension in obese persons is an increased risk of stroke. In the Framingham Heart Study, for instance, there was a steeply rising curve of stroke with increasing weight. For example, in the male group under 50 years of age, the risk of stroke rose from 22 to 30 to 49 per thousand as relative weights rose from 110% to 129% to higher than 130%, respectively.

## DYSLIPIDEMIA

Obesity is associated with three particular abnormalities of circulating lipids: (1) elevation of triglyceride levels, (2) depression of high-density lipoprotein cholesterol (HDL-C) levels, and (3) increased presence of small, dense low-density lipoprotein (LDL) particles. Hypertriglyceridemia seems to be abetted by both increased production by the liver and decreased clearance of triglycerides at the periphery. Triglycerides are transported predominantly as very-low-density lipoproteins (VLDLs). VLDL production in the liver is increased because of hyperinsulinemia, the high levels of free fatty acids (FFAs) arriving at the liver from the abdominal fat depot, and the glucose precursors available to the liver as glycerol. In addition, with obesity, there is often a decreased activity of lipoprotein lipase at the muscle level. This enzyme hydrolyzes triglyceride and allows it to be cleared from the plasma either into muscle for use as fuel or into adipose tissue for storage. As clearance of triglycerides is decreased, higher circulating levels result. The elevated levels of triglycerides are accompanied by a reduction of the size of LDL cholesterol (LDL-C) particles and increase their atherogenicity, leading to greater coronary heart disease risk.

Since HDL-C levels are low in obese persons, while LDL-C levels are usually only mildly elevated or within normal range, the ratio of LDL-C to HDL-C is always elevated. This combination raises the risk of coronary heart disease.

## CARDIOVASCULAR DISEASE

Coronary heart disease is usually described epidemiologically as cardiovascular disease (CVD), which includes angina pectoris, nonfatal myocardial infarction, and sudden death. These conditions occur more frequently in obese persons. There has been much controversy as to how important obesity is in CVD morbidity and mortality. It is well known, as mentioned earlier, that obesity enhances the risk of hypertension, dyslipidemia and diabetes, all of which are strong, independent risk factors for CVD. When these factors are controlled for in statistical multivariate analysis, obesity often does not emerge as an independent risk factor. This finding is more common in the shorter prospective studies, while in studies carried out for longer than 15 years, obesity consistently shows itself to be an independent risk factor. In addition, many epidemiologists believe that, when assessing obesity risk, it is a mistake to control for just those conditions that are made worse by obesity. In the Nurses' Health Study, the risk of CVD increased two-fold at a BMI of 25.0 to 28.9, and 3.6-fold at a BMI of greater than 29, compared with the group with a BMI below 21.

Cardiac hypertrophy begins with left ventricular dilatation, followed by myocardial hypertrophy. Increased intravascular volume causes systolic dysfunction, with a decline in ventricular contractility. Eventually, heart failure can occur.

## GALLBLADDER DISEASE

A number of changes that occur with obesity predispose an individual to gallstone formation. As cholesterol excretion from the liver increases, the bile becomes supersaturated with cholesterol. Also, the motility of the gallbladder decreases, so that the sac is emptied much less efficiently. Whether this condition is due to a decreased sensitivity to the cholecystokinin released with each meal is unclear. The net effect is to increase the formation of predominantly cholesterol-containing stones. These stones enhance the propensity to gallbladder inflammation, so that acute and chronic cholecystitis is much more common in obese persons. The incidence of this condition is higher in women than in men, partly because the prevalence of obesity is higher in women, but there may be other, as yet undiscovered reasons. The need for surgery to remove diseased gallbladders is much more common in obese persons, and more so in women than in men.

## RESPIRATORY DISEASE

The increased weight of the chest in obese persons leads to poor respiratory motion and also decreased compliance of the respiratory system, so that both vital capacity and total lung capacity are often low. As the overweight becomes more severe, ventilation–perfusion abnormalities impair adequate oxygenation of the blood, even though carbon dioxide escape is adequate. With continued and persistent obesity, sleep apnea, either peripheral or central, may occur. Peripheral apnea is manifested by obstruction of the airway, caused by excess fatty tissue and the relaxation of the pharyngeal and glossal muscles. Central apnea is the result of a cessation of the signals that initiate inspiration. The mechanism for this cessation of signals is unclear but apneic episodes may occur many times during the night, causing significant hyperventilation. The severity of all these abnormalities may lead to progressively more severe hypoxemia and hypercapnia, which in turn may lead to pulmonary hypertension, right heart failure, and cor pulmonale.

## CANCER

The relationships of obesity to various forms of cancer are somewhat unclear, and more data are required. However, there is an association between some cancers and overweight. It is not known whether the association may be due to other relationships, such as a high-fat diet, elevated total calories, or other specific dietary components. However, the associations, leaving causality unclear, have been well described.

In women, higher rates have been described for endometrial, gallbladder, cervical, and ovarian cancers. For breast cancer, premenopausal women who are obese are less at risk, while postmenopausal women are at greater risk. It is possible that some of this postmenopausal effect on breast cancer is related to the increasing estrogenicity that occurs with increasing obesity as women age. This increased estrogenicity is the result of estrogen production in adipose tissue from sex hormone precursors that are soluble in fat and converted there to active estrogen. This combined estrogenicity might affect breast cancer incidence. An increased incidence of colorectal and prostate cancers has been found in obese men. The mechanisms of this effect are unknown, although recent evidence suggests that the increased insulin levels resulting from the insulin resistance of obesity may have mitogenic effects.

## ARTHRITIS AND GOUT

Because of the increased stress on the weight-bearing joints caused by increased weight, degenerative disease of these joints is quite common in obese persons, particularly as the duration and severity of the obesity increases.

There is also an increased incidence of gout in persons who are overweight. Such an association has been found repeatedly in cross-sectional studies. This association of gout and overweight is manifested to a much greater degree in men than in women, in whom higher levels of excess fat are needed for the disease to develop.

## EFFECTS OF FAT DISTRIBUTION

Epidemiological data from many countries have established fat distribution as an important determinant of disease risk (see Chapters 68 and 86). As a result, not only the degree of obesity but also the location of deposited fat are important. Results of available studies suggest that intra-abdominal, or visceral, fat is crucial in this regard. The pathophysiology may be related to the increased lipolytic activity of fat cells in this region, which release large amounts of FFA to the liver and the periphery. The combination of hyperlipacidemia and hyperinsulinemia leads to increased VLDL production, with resultant hypertriglyceridemia. The lipacidemia also inhibits glucose transport and oxidation in muscle, increasing the insulin resistance and the propensity for diabetes. The hyperinsulinemia leads to increased sodium absorption and increases the risk of hypertension.

## CONCLUSION

The medical complications of obesity are considerable. It must be realized that diabetes mellitus, hypertension, dyslipidemia, cardiovascular disease, and stroke—aside from cancer, AIDS, and violence—are the leading causes of morbidity and mortality in the developed world. If cancer, a condition in which obesity often plays a part, is added, obesity is a large contributor to the burden of disease affecting industrialized countries. Whether the effect of these diseases is direct and independent or indirect, through enhancing other risk factors, is essentially irrelevant from a public health perspective. If obesity could be prevented, a very significant and positive impact on chronic disease and mortality would occur.

## FURTHER READING

Bjorntorp, P. (1990). "Portal" adipose tissue as a generator of risk factors for cardiovascular disease and diabetes. *Arteriosclerosis*, *10*, 493–496.—A review of the pathophysiology of central visceral adipose tissue in enhancing health risks.

Després, J. P. (1998). The insulin resistance–dyslipidemic syndrome of visceral obesity: Effect on patients' risk. *Obesity Research*, *6* (Suppl. 1), 8S–17S.—A discussion of the effect of increased visceral obesity on health risk.

Eckel, R. H., & Krauss, R. M. (1998). American Heart Association call to action: Obesity as a major risk factor for coronary heart disease. *Circulation*, *97*, 2099–2100.—A report of the association between obesity and coronary heart disease.

Garfinkel, L. (1985). Overweight and cancer. *Annals of Internal Medicine*, *103*, 1034–1036.—A report from the American Cancer Society Study of the relationship between weight and cancer.

Higgins, M., Kannel, W., Garrison, R., Pinsky, J., & Stokes, J., III. (1988). Hazards of obesity—The Framingham experience. *Acta Medica Scandinavica*, *723*(Suppl.), 23–36.—A review of the effects of obesity as seen in one of the largest and most carefully done longitudinal studies of a population group.

Manson, J. E., Colditz, G. A., Stampfer, M.J., Willett, W. C., Rosner, B., Monson, R. R., Speizer, F. E., & Hennekens, C. H. (1990). A prospective study of obesity and risk of coronary heart disease in women. *New England Journal of Medicine, 322,* 882–889.—An interim report of one of the best ongoing longitudinal studies of heart disease in women.

Manson, J. E., Stampfer, M. J., Hennekens, C. H., & Willett, W. G. (1987). Body weight and longevity: A reassessment. *Journal of the American Medical Association, 257,* 353–358.—A discussion of epidemiological–methodological pitfalls in evaluating the impact of obesity on health.

National Heart, Lung, and Blood Institute. (1998). NHLBI clinical guidelines on the identification, evaluation, and treatment of overweight and obesity in adults. The Evidence Report. *Obesity Research, 6*(Suppl. 2), 51S–209S.—An evidence-based report from the clinical trials literature.

Pi-Sunyer, F. X. (1993). Medical hazards of obesity. *Annals of Internal Medicine, 119,* 655–660.—A review of the medical hazards of obesity.

# 85

# Medical Consequences of Obesity in Children and Adolescents

## WILLIAM H. DIETZ

Childhood obesity is associated with a variety of adverse effects on psychosocial function, skeletal growth, and cardiovascular risk factors. Although several periods in childhood appear critical for the development of obesity, it is not yet clear whether these periods are also associated with an increased risk for the complications of obesity in either childhood or adulthood.

## PSYCHOLOGICAL CONSEQUENCES

The psychosocial consequences of obesity are among the most widespread adverse effects of the disease (see Chapters 20, 70, 71, and 72). Children in kindergarten have already learned to associate obesity with a variety of less desirable traits, and rank obese children as those they like the least. College acceptance rates for obese adolescent girls are lower than those for nonoverweight girls of comparable academic background. Adult women who are obese as adolescents or young adults earn less, more frequently remain unmarried, complete fewer years of school, and have higher rates of poverty than their nonobese peers. Few of these effects occur among obese men. These results persist when controlled for the income and educational level of the young women's parents, their IQ, or their self-esteem at baseline. The social effects of obesity in young adult women therefore appear related to an extension of the discrimination that begins in early childhood (see Chapter 20).

## SKELETAL GROWTH AND MATURATION

Obesity has multiple effects on growth and function in children and adolescents. For example, obese children tend to be taller, their bone ages are advanced, their fat-free mass is increased, and menarche in girls occurs earlier than in the nonobese. The origin of these effects is unclear. Increased height, advanced bone age, and earlier menarche may reflect the auxotrophic effects of increased food intake, whereas the increase in fat-free mass may result from both the increased muscle mass to support the increased weight and the nuclear mass of adipocytes. Because of their larger size, overweight children are frequently perceived and treated as older than they are, much to their confusion. Furthermore, the increased stress of weight may cause bowing of the tibia (Blount's disease) or femur and predispose young children to slipped capital femoral epiphysis.

## CARDIOVASCULAR RISK FACTORS

As in adults, obesity affects blood pressure, lipid levels, and glucose tolerance in children and adolescents. Sixty percent of overweight children as young as 5–10 years of age have at least one of these cardiovascular disease risk factors, and more than 20% have two or more. Obesity appears to be the leading cause of hypertension in children. Lipid profiles are similar to those in adults: low density lipoprotein levels are increased, and high density lipoprotein levels are low.

Increased rates of type 2 diabetes have followed the rapid increases in the prevalence of childhood and adolescent obesity. In some settings, type 2 diabetes now accounts for 30–40% of all new cases of diabetes. Although the prevalence of type 2 diabetes in the general population is low (0.5%), among some Native American groups the prevalence is close to 5%. Pediatric cases of type 2 diabetes generally occur among those 10–19 years of age, with a positive family history of type 2 diabetes, and more frequently among obese females or individuals with acanthosis nigricans. At presentation, cases of type 2 diabetes in children and adolescents may resemble type 1 diabetes, suggesting that the actual prevalence of type 2 diabetes may be somewhat higher than it currently appears.

The most important factor related to the likelihood of obesity-associated hypertension, hyperlipidemia, and glucose intolerance in adults appears to be visceral fat. The few studies of adolescents that have controlled for total body fat have demonstrated an independent association of visceral fat, with unfavorable levels of systolic blood pressure and low- and high-density lipoprotein cholesterol.

## PSEUDOTUMOR CEREBRI, SLEEP APNEA, HEPATIC STEATOSIS, AND POLYCYSTIC OVARY DISEASE

Two of the most malignant consequences of childhood onset obesity are pseudotumor cerebri and sleep apnea. Obesity accounts for a significant proportion of pseudotumor cerebri, although the mechanism remains unclear. The diagnosis is established by a history of headaches and the presence of papilledema. The most important sign of sleep apnea is daytime somnolence. Apnea is rarely mentioned spontaneously by parents, despite their apprehension and clear recognition of the difficulty that their child has breathing at night. If the tonsils are enlarged, a tonsillectomy may cure sleep apnea. However, either unremitting sleep apnea or pseudotumor warrant the aggressive use of a restrictive hypocaloric diet in conjunction with vigorous family therapy.

Recent data from several studies indicate that 5–10% of overweight children and adolescents have modestly elevated liver enzymes. Ultrasound studies of these patients demonstrate increased hepatic fat deposition. Liver biopsies in severe cases have demonstrated steatohepatitis. Alcohol use appears to increase the likelihood of these changes. Liver enzymes normalize with weight reduction.

As in adults, polycystic ovary disease (PCOD) in adolescents is associated with obesity. The pathophysiology of PCOD is complicated; hyperinsulinemia is frequently associated with the syndrome, and hyperandrogenemia may contribute to increased fat-free mass and a male distribution of body fat.

## EFFECTS OF CHILDHOOD OBESITY ON PERSISTENCE INTO ADULTHOOD

The likelihood that obesity present during childhood will persist into adulthood rises with the age of the child, independent of the effect of parental obesity. Several studies have indicated that approximately 70% of overweight adolescents become obese adults. Age-of-onset effects of obesity in childhood or adolescence on either the severity or complications of adult obesity remain uncertain.

Obesity in adolescence appears to entrain a variety of morbid consequences. For example, in a cohort of adults originally studied from the time of their enrollment in elementary school through high school, all-cause and cardiovascular mortality rates were higher among men who were obese in high school, but not among women. The risk of diabetes and subsequent atherosclerosis was greater among both men and women who were obese during high school. Except for diabetes, the risk of death or subsequent morbidity was only modestly attenuated when controlled for the effect of adolescent obesity on adult weight. These results suggested that the effect of adolescent obesity on adult morbidity and mortality was not mediated by the effect of adolescent obesity on adult obesity. Either adolescent obesity had a direct impact on adult morbidity and mortality, or a third factor predisposed individuals to both adolescent obesity and adult disease. Body fat distribution may represent the mechanism whereby obesity present in adolescence affects morbidity and mortality. Body fat distribution is more strongly centralized in adolescent males than in adolescent females. Therefore, one possibility is that the regionalization of fatness that occurs in obese adolescent males may increase the risk of later complications of obesity.

## SUMMARY

The prevalence of obesity and its physiological and psychological complications is increasing among children and adolescents. These findings emphasize the need for effective prevention and treatment programs.

## FURTHER READING

Daniels, S. R., Morrison, J. A., Sprecher, D. L., Khoury, P., & Kimball, T. R. (1999). Association of body fat distribution and cardiovascular risk factors in children and adolescents. *Circulation*, 99, 541–545.—Clinical study of effects of regional fat distribution in adolescents on lipids and blood pressure.

Dietz, W. H. (1998). Health consequences of obesity in youth: Childhood predictors of adult disease. *Pediatrics, 101*(Suppl.), 518–525.—Detailed review of health consequences of childhood obesity, with 84 references.

Fagot-Campagna, A., Pettitt, D. J., Englegau, M. M., Burrows, N. R., Geiss, L. S., Valdez, R., Beckles, G. L., Saadine, J., Gregg, E. W., Williamson, D. F., & Narayan, K. M. V. (2000). Type 2 diabetes among North American children and adolescents: An epidemiologic review and a public health perspective. *Journal of Pediatrics, 136*, 664–672.—Review article regarding the rapid increase in the prevalence of type 2 diabetes in children and adolescents.

Freedman, D. S., Dietz, W. H., Srinivasan, S. R., & Berenson, G. S. (1999). The relation of overweight to cardiovascular risk factors among children and adolescents: The Bogalusa Heart Study. *Pediatrics, 103*, 1175–1182.—Best study of the prevalence of cardiovascular disease risk factors among overweight black and white children and adolescents.

Gortmaker, S. L., Must, A., Perrin, J. M., Sobol, A. M., & Dietz, W. H. (1993). Social and economic consequences of overweight in adolescence and young adulthood. *New England Journal of Medicine, 329*, 1008–1012.—A comprehensive demonstration of the adverse effects of obesity on income and marital status.

Must, A., Jacques, P. F., Dallal, G. E., Bajema, C. J., & Dietz, W. H. (1992). Long-term morbidity and mortality of overweight adolescents: A follow-up of the Harvard Growth Study of 1922 to 1935. *New England Journal of Medicine, 327*, 1350–1355.—The most convincing study of the effects of adolescent obesity on morbidity and mortality in adults.

Strauss, R. S., Barlow, S. E., & Dietz, W. H. (2000). Prevalence of abnormal serum aminotransferase values in overweight and obese adolescents. *Journal of Pediatrics, 136*, 727–733.—Nationally representative data regarding the prevalence of hepatic abnormalities associated with obesity.

Whitaker, R. C., Wright, J. A., Pepe, M. S., Seidel, K. D., & Dietz, W. H. (1997). Predicting obesity in young adulthood from childhood and parental obesity. *New England Journal of Medicine, 337*, 869–873.—The most comprehensive study of the natural history of obesity between birth and young adulthood, controlled for the effects of parental obesity.

# 86

# The Metabolic Syndrome

## JEAN-PIERRE DESPRÉS

### RISK AND THE METABOLIC SYNDROME: BEYOND BODY WEIGHT

Obesity increases the likelihood of metabolic complications such as type 2 diabetes, atherogenic dyslipidemias and cardiovascular diseases (see Chapters 76 and 84). On the basis of these associations, the body mass index (BMI) is commonly used to define obesity following a universally accepted definition. Although the BMI has limitations, studies have shown increased incidence of chronic diseases as a function of progressively increasing BMI. Despite this epidemiological evidence, physicians are confronted in their daily practice with the remarkable heterogeneity of their obese patients. Some patients show a severe deterioration in their risk factor profile, whereas others, who are equally obese, do not have the expected complications. Therefore, obesity is a heterogeneous condition, and physicians must go beyond body weight in order to identify and treat high-risk patients.

In this regard, it is important to emphasize the remarkable early clinical observations of Professor Jean Vague from the University of Marseille, who was the first, after World War II, to suggest that the complications of obesity are more closely related to the regional distribution of body fat then to excess fatness per se. In a remarkable short paper published in 1947, Vague suggested that upper body obesity, a condition which he referred to as android obesity, was the dangerous form of obesity found in patients with hypertension, diabetes, or cardiovascular disease, and that the typical female fat distribution, gynoid obesity, was seldom associated with major complications. It took more than 35 years for Vague's work to receive support from prospective observational studies. In those studies, the proportion of abdominal fat was crudely assessed by the ratio of waist-to-hip circumferences, based on the assumption that a higher ratio would reflect greater accumulation of abdominal fat. This ratio has been shown to be a powerful predictor of the incidence of diabetes and cardiovascular disease in prospective studies (see Chapter 68).

# VISCERAL OBESITY: A CENTRAL COMPONENT
# OF THE METABOLIC SYNDROME

Despite its usefulness in epidemiology, the waist-to-hip ratio is a crude estimate of the proportion of abdominal fat (see Chapter 11). Furthermore, this index does not distinguish between abdominal fat located in the abdominal cavity, the so-called intra-abdominal or visceral adipose tissue, and subcutaneous abdominal fat. With the development of imaging techniques such as magnetic resonance imaging (MRI) or computed tomography (CT), it has been possible to measure precisely abdominal fat accumulation and to distinguish subcutaneous abdominal fat from the fat located in the abdominal cavity (Figure 86.1).

We compared individuals matched for the level of total body fat but differing in their amount of visceral adipose tissue, and found that the subgroup of obese patients with high levels of visceral adipose tissue was characterized by a cluster of complications that increase the risk of type 2 diabetes and coronary heart disease. These patients were characterized by hyperinsulinemia, resulting from a state of insulin resistance, and glucose intolerance, as well as an atherogenic dyslipidemic profile including hypertriglyceridemia, elevated apolipoprotein B (apo B) concentration, low high-density lipoprotein cholesterol (HDL-C) levels (contributing to a substantial increase in the ratio of cholesterol/HDL), and increased proportion of small, dense low-density lipoprotein (LDL) particles (Figure 86.1). These alterations in the plasma were noted despite a lack of difference in plasma LDL cholesterol (LDL-C) concentration.

These apparently normal LDL-C concentrations could mislead physicians in their assessment of risk, since they could mask major differences in the concentration and size of LDL particles. By using gradient gel electrophoresis, which allowed us to measure LDL particle size with great accuracy, we found that visceral obesity is associated with an increased concentration and proportion of small, dense LDL particles. As there is one apo B molecule per LDL particle, Sniderman and colleagues suggested more than 20 years ago that measuring apo B could allow us to detect high-risk individuals with an increased concentration of atherogenic lipoproteins, despite apparently "normal" LDL-C levels. When we measured apo B concentration in viscerally obese patients, we found a 25% increase in the concentration of this apolipoprotein, suggesting a substantial increase in the concentration of atherogenic lipoproteins despite fairly normal LDL-C levels.

These results emphasize that a raised LDL-C concentration is not a common feature of the metabolic syndrome and that measuring total cholesterol and LDL-C is not adequate for the proper assessment of coronary heart disease risk in viscerally obese patients. Furthermore, we found that the reduction in HDL-C concentration found in viscerally obese patients with the metabolic syndrome led to a substantial increase in the ratio of cholesterol/HDL-C, this ratio being a traditional and powerful predictor of the risk of coronary heart disease. Therefore, we have suggested that among individuals with abdominal obesity, hypertriglyceridemia, and low HDL-C concentration, the substantial increase of the ratio of total cholesterol/HDL-C could predict substantially increased risk of coronary heart disease. Thus, the atherogenic dyslipidemia of viscerally obese patients with the metabolic syndrome is not characterized by a marked elevation in LDL-C levels but rather by hypertriglyceridemia, elevated apo B, an increased proportion of small, dense LDL particles, reduced HDL-C concentration, and an increased ratio of cholesterol/HDL-C.

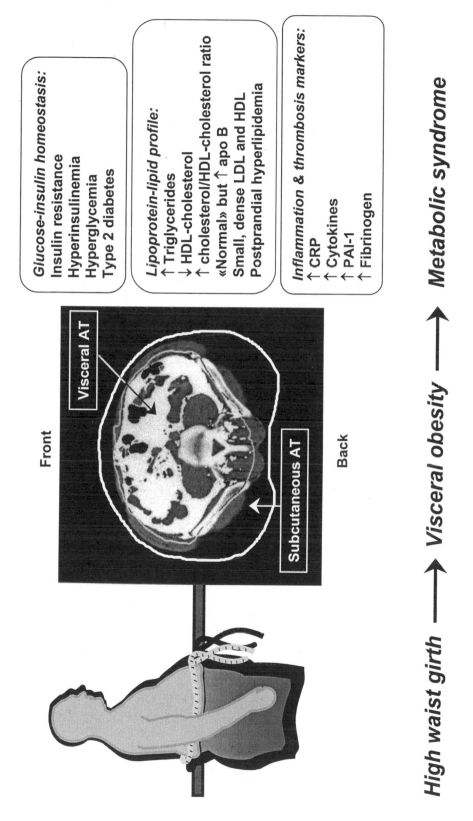

**Glucose-insulin homeostasis:**
Insulin resistance
Hyperinsulinemia
Hyperglycemia
Type 2 diabetes

**Lipoprotein-lipid profile:**
↑ Triglycerides
↓ HDL-cholesterol
↑ cholesterol/HDL-cholesterol ratio
«Normal» but ↑ apo B
Small, dense LDL and HDL
Postprandial hyperlipidemia

**Inflammation & thrombosis markers:**
↑ CRP
↑ Cytokines
↑ PAI-1
↑ Fibrinogen

Front

Visceral AT

Subcutaneous AT

Back

*High waist girth* ⟶ *Visceral obesity* ⟶ *Metabolic syndrome*

**FIGURE 86.1.** Contribution of the waist girth measurement to the assessment of risk associated with visceral obesity. Studies have shown that visceral obesity, which can be crudely estimated from a waist circumference measurement, is associated with a cluster of metabolic abnormalities (metabolic syndrome) that increase the risk of type 2 diabetes and cardiovascular disease.

479

## THE ATHEROGENIC METABOLIC TRIAD:
## BEYOND TRADITIONAL RISK FACTORS

We have also found that the "dysmetabolic" profile found among patients with visceral obesity is associated with a substantially increased risk of coronary heart disease even in the absence of marked elevation in LDL-C levels and traditional risk factors such as type 2 diabetes, hypercholesterolemia, and hypertension. Indeed, we found that a triad of new metabolic markers, including hyperinsulinemia, elevated apo B concentration, and an increased proportion of small, dense LDL particles is associated with a 20-fold increase in the risk of developing a first ischemic heart disease event among asymptomatic middle-age men.

## THE "HYPERTRIGLYCERIDEMIC WAIST":
## A NEW MARKER OF CORONARY HEART DISEASE RISK?

As most clinicians do not have access to these new markers of risk that are features of the metabolic syndrome, we were interested in developing a simple algorithm that would allow clinicians to identify high-risk abdominally obese patients. Based on the significant associations we found between waist circumference and visceral adipose tissue accumulation, fasting insulin, and apo B levels, we believe that measuring waist circumference could provide a good "proxy" variable for the estimation of visceral adipose tissue accumulation as well as fasting insulin and apo B concentrations. Furthermore, it was known that fasting triglyceride concentration is the best predictor of LDL size. Sensitivity and specificity analyses revealed that cutoff values of waist circumference of 90 cm and of fasting triglyceride levels of 2 mmol/liter gave us the best discrimination of carriers–noncarriers of the atherogenic metabolic triad. For instance, middle-age men with waist circumference below 90 cm and fasting triglyceride levels below 2 mmol/liter only had a 10% chance of having the atherogenic metabolic triad. However, men with levels above these had more than 80% chance of simultaneously having hyperinsulinemia, elevated apo B and small, dense LDL particles. There is now a very simple screening tool for the identification of high-risk, abdominally obese, hypertriglyceridemic men with atherogenic features of the metabolic syndrome.

## ADEQUATE SCREENING FOR THE
## HIGH-RISK ABDOMINALLY OBESE PATIENT

Because of its metabolic complications, it has been suggested by the World Health Organization and by the National Institutes of Health that obesity should be considered a disease. On the basis of this recommendation, any healthy women with a BMI $\geq 30$ kg/m$^2$ is "sick," despite an apparently normal risk factor profile. This situation may explain why some disappointing results have been obtained in clinical trials where pharmacotherapy leading to a 10% weight loss only produced modest improvements in the risk factor profile of patients. These trials mainly include healthy, obese women.

We found that a 10% weight loss was associated with a selective mobilization of visceral fat, which could reach 30%, thereby leading to substantial improvements in the metabolic risk factor profile. Therefore, it appears important to focus pharmacotherapy on patients with the highest risk of complications, since they represent the subgroup most likely to benefit from the expected weight loss. Since waist circumference and fasting triglyceride levels allow the identification of a large proportion of high-risk patients, these variables should be included in the medical chart of all patients and considered relevant therapeutic targets (Figure 86.2).

Unfortunately, our lifestyle is rather "toxic" for the metabolic health of our patients, and this is a major barrier to the medical treatment of obesity (see Chapter 78). Most patients are too sedentary and exposed to foods rich in fat and refined sugar, often contributing to a positive energy balance. We recommend an approach in which all relevant aspects will be considered in treatment. First, a healthy diet, including a greater consumption of fruits, vegetables, and fiber, should be recommended, with less products rich in fat and refined sugar. Second, increasing physical activity on a daily basis, without necessarily involving complicated and well-controlled exercise programs, is absolutely necessary

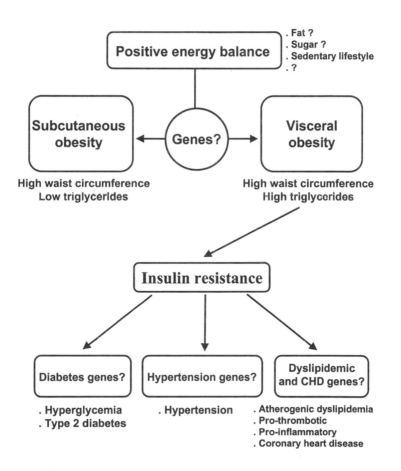

**FIGURE 86.2.** Contribution of visceral obesity and related insulin resistance to the development of various forms of the metabolic syndrome. Depending upon the absence–presence of genetic variants modulating susceptibility to chronic complications, the viscerally obese insulin-resistant patient will develop type 2 diabetes, hypertension, and/or coronary heart disease. This situation may explain why insulin resistance may often, but not always, lead to these chronic complications.

to make the diet more comfortably sustainable by patients (see Chapter 93). The ultimate objective of the modification of energy balance should be to comfortably decrease caloric intake without inducing too much hunger and discomfort. This objective could also be reached by increasing physical activity. More precise evaluation of the risk associated with obesity and better evaluation of therapeutic efficacity beyond body weight could help physicians better identify obese patients with the metabolic syndrome. The patients could ultimately benefit from a pharmacotherapy centered at reducing waist circumference and improving their metabolic risk factor profile rather than normalizing body weight, which is an unrealistic objective.

## ACKNOWLEDGMENTS

This work was supported by the Canadian Institutes for Health Research (Grant Nos. MT-14014 and MGC-15187). Jean-Pierre Després is chair professor of human nutrition and lipidology, which is supported by Parke Davis/Warner–Lambert, Provigo, and by the Foundation of the Québec Heart Institute.

## FURTHER READING

Bray, G. A., Bouchard, C., & James, W. P. T. (1998). *Handbook of obesity.* New York: Marcel Dekker.—A comprehensive, encyclopedia-type document that is an excellent reference handbook.

Després, J. P. (1994). Dyslipidaemia and obesity. *Baillieres Clinical Endocrinology and Metabolism, 8,* 629–660.—A useful review on the dyslipidemic state commonly found in high-risk, abdominally obese patients.

Després, J. P., & Lamarche, B. (1993). Effects of diet and physical activity on adiposity and body fat distribution: Implications for the prevention of cardiovascular disease. *Nutrition Research Reviews, 6,* 137–159.—A review on the effects of diet and physical activity in the management of risk associated with abdominal obesity.

Després, J. P., Moorjani, S., Lupien, P. J., Tremblay, A., Nadeau, A., & Bouchard, C. (1990). Regional distribution of body fat, plasma lipoproteins and cardiovascular disease. *Arteriosclerosis, 10,* 497–511.—Our first comprehensive review of regional body fat distribution and visceral obesity.

Kissebah, A. H., Freedman, D. S., & Peiris, A. N. (1989). Health risk of obesity. *Medical Clinics of North America, 73,* 111–138.—One of the best reviews on the risk of obesity, with a superb discussion of the importance of body fat distribution.

Lamarche, B., Tchernof, A., Mauriège, P., Cantin, B., Dagenais, G. R., Lupien, P. J., & Després, J. P. (1998). Fasting insulin and apolipoprotein B levels and low-density lipoprotein particle size as risk factors for ischemic heart disease. *Journal of the American Medical Association, 279,* 1955–1961.—This paper documents the very high coronary heart disease risk associated with some features of the metabolic syndrome.

Lemieux, I., Pascot, A., Couillard, C., Lamarche, B., Tchernof, A., Alméras, N., Bergeron, J., Gaudet, D., Trembley, G., Prud'homme, D., Nadeau, A., & Després, J. P. (2000). Hypertriglyceridemic waist: A marker of the atherogenic metabolic triad (hyperinsulinemia, hyperapolipoprotein B, small, dense LDL) in men? *Circulation, 102,* 179–184.—This paper emphasizes the importance of "hypertriglyceridemic waist" as a high-risk obesity phenotype.

National Heart, Lung, and Blood Institute, and National Institutes of Health. (1998). Clinical guidelines on the identification, evaluation, and treatment of overweight and obesity in adults:

The evidence report. *Obesity Research*, 6(Suppl. 2), 51S–209S.—An important reference document on obesity, its assessment and management.

Reaven, G. M. (1998). Banting Lecture 1988: Role of insulin resistance in human disease. *Diabetes*, 37, 1595–1607.—A landmark paper on the insulin resistance syndrome: a "must read" article.

Vague, J. (1947). Sexual differentiation, a factor affecting the forms of obesity. *Presse Médicale, 30*, 339–340.—A remarkable paper from a "visionary" who first saw the importance of body fat distribution.

World Health Organziation. (1998). *Obesity: Preventing and managing the global epidemic: Report of a WHO Consultation on Obesity* (WHO/NUT/NCD/97.2). Geneva: Author.—A long awaited and needed document defining obesity.

# 87

# Weight Loss and Risk Factors

## GEORGE L. BLACKBURN

Weight loss is the single most cost-effective treatment for obesity-related comorbid diseases, including the nation's leading cause of morbidity, disability, hospitalization, and mortality—cardiovascular disease. Obesity is closely linked with clusters of the 20-plus identified risk factors that make up various insulin resistance syndromes that are the cornerstones of cardiovascular disease (dyslipidemia, hypertension, abnormalities of coagulation, and endothelial dysfunction) as well as type 2 diabetes (see Chapters 76, 84, and 86).

Reduction of body weight is known to improve the cluster of risk factors associated with a central metabolic syndrome characterized by hyperinsulinemia, dyslipidemia, and obesity; glucose intolerance; and hypertension (see Chapter 86). Hyperinsulinemia is associated primarily with impaired fibrinolysis in subjects with glucose intolerance. A recent study found that excess risk for cardiovascular disease associated with hyperinsulinemia and glucose intolerance may be mediated in part by enhanced potential for acute thrombosis.

Weight loss is known to improve directly or resolve risk factors of cardiovascular disease, that is, serum triglycerides; low-density lipoprotein cholesterol (LDL-C); dense LDL apolipoprotine B particles; (apo B); pattern B; high-density lipoprotein cholesterol (HDL-C); plasminogen activator inhibitor 1 (PAI-1); glucose to insulin ratio; and homeostasis model assessment of insulin resistance (HOMA-ir). Reduction in body weight is also expected to reverse metabolic defects linked to macrovascular complications and microvascular sequelae.

Weight loss as low as 5% of initial body weight can reduce or eliminate disorders associated with obesity. Weight reductions of 10% to 20%, maintained from 2 to 5 years, are known to sustain health benefits. Most obese patients can achieve these goals in 12 to 26 weeks on a balanced hypocaloric diet or on a very-low-calorie diet (VLCD), particularly when combined with regular physical activity and behavior modification. With sustained practice of this new lifestyle, long-term outcomes can be achieved.

Today, successful treatment of obesity has nothing at all to do with reduction to desired weight and maintenance of this weight for 5 years (see Chapter 91). Rather, it has everything to do with a reasonable yet targeted weight loss goal that remains focused on keeping off the amount of body weight necessary to promote health and prevent disease.

Untreated obesity typically ends in morbidity, disability, hospitalization, and mortality from cardiovascular and diabetic complications. Recently, the American Heart Association's Nutrition Committee classified obesity as a major modifiable risk factor for coronary artery disease and redirected their guidelines toward a diet rich in fruits, vegetables, legumes, whole grains, low-fat dairy products, fish, lean meats, and poultry. Five servings of fruits and vegetables and six servings of grains are recommended daily. And, for the first time, two weekly servings of fatty fish, such as tuna or salmon are recommended.

## ADDITIONAL TREATMENT EFFECTS

Modest weight loss (i.e., 5–10% of initial body weight) produces immediate and significant improvements in sense of well-being, self-esteem, energy level, and quality of sleep (see Chapter 90). It improves the metabolic disorder associated with obesity by reducing insulin, blood pressure, fatty acids, and triglycerides. It also reverses insulin resistance, protects against certain cancers, and improves or reverses obesity-related comorbidities, including osteoarthritis, diabetes, and cardiovascular disease.

All successful interventions require exercise components (see Chapter 93). In and of itself, exercise improves the body's ability to convert glucose to energy and has independent, favorable effects on risk factors for cardiovascular disease and diabetes.

Several studies, most notably Dietary Approaches to Stop Hypertension (DASH), underscore the impact and importance of weight loss, dietary patterns, and sodium restriction on health. Other studies have found that a dietary pattern characterized by consumption of foods recommended in current dietary guidelines is associated with decreased risk of mortality in women.

## DIABETES

Weight gain and obesity have been independently associated with hypertension, hyperinsulinemia, and dyslipidemia in individuals at risk for type 2 diabetes. Research has shown that each 5% increase in weight over reported weight at age 20 is linked with a nearly 200% greater risk of developing the cluster of risk factors known as insulin resistance syndrome by middle age.

Obese patients are at increased risk for developing many medical problems, including insulin resistance and type 2 diabetes mellitus. Insulin resistance is commonly observed both in overt diabetes and in individuals prone to, but not yet manifesting, diabetes. In patients with type 2 diabetes mellitus, cardiovascular disease accounts for the majority of morbidity and mortality.

Type 2 diabetes is characterized by abnormalities of insulin action in muscle, adipose tissue, and liver, leading to failure of beta cell function. In the obese patient, these abnormalities of insulin resistance prompt the body to compensate by secreting greater amounts of insulin, which results in hyperinsulinemia. Eventually the patient's body fails to counterbalance the insulin resistance, and hyperglycemia and type 2 diabetes mellitus ensue.

Prior to the end stage of beta cell function, weight loss alone has been shown to reduce hyperglycemia and hyperinsulinemia, and to improve glucose tolerance. Reductions in body weight of 10–20% are known to greatly improve glycemic control in obese, diabetic subjects for 1 to 3 years, even with partial subsequent weight regain (see Chapter 104). Ideally, weight maintenance and exercise will sustain improved insulin sensitivity.

Advances in adjunctive pharmacological treatments, including the new insulin sensitizing medications, offer another way (exceedingly cost-effective) to head off the ravages of cardiovascular disease and diabetes, and improve the quality of life for millions of obese, at-risk individuals.

## HYPERTENSION

The DASH study was the first prospective, randomized trial to compare food-based treatment outcomes to those produced by pharmaceuticals. The study examined the effect on blood pressure of whole dietary patterns rather than individual nutrients. Results showed that the DASH diet quickly and significantly lowered blood pressure. These declines, which rivaled those produced by hypertension medications, started within the first 2 weeks of the study and lasted throughout.

In the absence of sodium restriction, weight loss alone is known to have an independent antihypertensive effect. Studies show that obese and overweight subjects can significantly lower blood pressure by reducing initial body weight by 10%. Weight loss can prevent the onset of hypertension in persons at risk of developing the disease. It also tends to improve left ventricular hypertrophy and other risk factors, including those associated with insulin resistance, diabetes, and cardiovascular disease.

## CARDIOVASCULAR DISEASE

Excess body weight is associated with substantial increases in mortality from all causes, particularly cardiovascular disease (see Chapter 76). More than 5% of the national health expenditure in the United States is directed at medical costs associated with obesity. Modest weight loss is associated with improved results in the risk factors of cardiovascular disease: serum triglycerides; LDL-C; dense LDL particles; apo B; pattern B; HDL-C; PAI-1; glucose to insulin ratio; and HOMO-ir. It is also known to reduce plasma estrogen levels. In obese patients with no indications of hyperlipidemia, momentary coagulation status and antitrypsin III level may be more sensitive risk factors for myocardial infarction than serum lipid levels.

The simultaneous occurrence of insulin resistance and impaired insulin secretion leads to hyperglycemia in type 2 diabetes. The combination of hyperinsulinemia, insulin resistance, and hyperlipidemia best describes the pathophysiology of macrovascular complications, whereas hyperglycemia per se is more closely associated with microvascular sequelae. Indeed, fasting blood glucose values in the upper normal range appear to be important independent predictors of cardiovascular death in nondiabetic, apparently healthy middle-age men.

## GALLSTONE FORMATION

Weight loss in and of itself does not cause gallbladder disease. Dieting and rapid weight loss, however, can increase the risk of gallstone formation in obese individuals—a population with an already increased risk of symptomatic and asymptomatic gallstones.

This greater risk results from supersaturation of biliary cholesterol and gallbladder stasis, both of which can occur during severe caloric restriction. Diets that reduce or eliminate the risk of gallstone formation include 14 g protein and 10 g fat in at least one meal daily (to ensure adequate gallbladder contraction), limit weight loss to 2% of initial body weight per week, and last up to 12 weeks at most. Risk of gallstone disease in obese individuals who reduce their body weight is comparable to that found in the nonobese population.

## SLEEP APNEA

Obstructive sleep apnea (OSA) occurs during deep levels of sleep when soft tissues in the upper airway relax and collapse. This syndrome tends to occur in obese, older patients who have a history of substance abuse. The typical apnea patient is an obese man with systemic hypertension, although about 17% of obese children experience OSA as well.

When the pharyngeal airway collapses during sleep, patients snore. As oxygen saturation drops and snoring becomes more pronounced, they wake up suddenly, usually gasping for breath, then immediately return to sleep. This cycle may recur continuously during the night, leading to fragmented sleep with insufficient rapid eye movement (REM). Like other causes of daytime somnolence, sleep apnea carries an increased risk for accidents and is also associated with heightened risk for resistant hypertension, stroke, cardiac arrythmias, myocardial infarction, and death. Obesity has been shown to be a predisposing factor for the occurrence of bradyarrhythmia in patients with OSA.

Modest weight loss (9% of initial body weight) has been shown to reduce the frequency of airway collapse, improve sleep quality, and reduce daytime somnolence. The degree of improvement, however, often depends on the length of time the condition has been present.

Researchers have yet to identify the mechanism(s) by which weight loss improves OSA. Possible explanations include changes in the anatomy of the airway (increased airway size) or changes in the ventilatory drive (increased activation of upper airway muscles).

## OTHER BENEFITS OF WEIGHT LOSS

Obese patients are at increased risk for complications during and after surgery. A 5–10% reduction in body weight and concomitant diuresis can shorten hospital stays and reduce incidences of postsurgical complications. Modest weight loss improves quality of life in a variety of ways. Depending on existing structural damage, it alleviates low back pain and osteoarthritis, particularly in the knees.

## CURRENT KNOWLEDGE AND FUTURE DIRECTIONS

Obesity research is still in its infancy. Innovations in the ways we address the major modifiable factors in weight control (i.e., satiety using dietary factors and physical activity patterns) are needed. Areas of particular interest include assessment methods; behavioral and psychosocial tools and techniques that restrain energy intake and increase energy expenditure; the design of novel diet and exercise programs, particularly for nonresponders; and the development of strategies that reduce relapse rates and strengthen motivation for compliance.

There is also a great need to address the social and cultural factors that contribute to obesity, and to initiate broad-scale efforts to modify these factors. Community and environmental resources need to be mobilized to reduce food portion sizes, decrease exposure to high-fat foods, and increase opportunities to pursue physical activities during leisure time. Because obesity is difficult to treat, public health efforts need to be directed toward prevention.

## FURTHER READING

Bjornholt, J. V., Erikssen, G., Aaaser, E., Sandvik, L., Nitter-Hauge, S., Jervell, J., Erikssen, J., & Thaulow, E. (1999). Fasting blood glucose: An underestimated risk factors for cardiovascular death: Results from a 22-year follow-up of healthy nondiabetic men. *Diabetes Care, 22*, 45–49.—Among men divided into quartiles of fasting blood glucose level, it was found that those in the highest glucose quartile (fasting blood glucose > 85 mg/dl) had a significantly higher mortality rate from cardiovascular diseases than men in the three lowest quartiles.

Blackburn, G. L. (1999). Benefits of weight loss in the treatment of obesity. *American Journal of Clinical Nutrition, 69*, 347–349.—This paper describes the effect of degree of weight loss on specific disease states and risk factors, and discusses the impact of ethnic background, fat distribution, age, and mode of weight loss on outcome.

Kant, A. K. (2000). Consumption of energy-dense, nutrient-poor foods by adult Americans: Nutritional and health implications: The third National Health and Nutrition Examination Survey, 1988–1994. *American Journal of Clinical Nutrition, 72*, 929–936.—The results suggest that energy-dense, nutrient-poor foods were consumed at the expense of nutrient-dense foods, resulting in (1) increased risk of high energy intake, (2) marginal micronutrient intake, (3) poor compliance with nutrient- and food-group-related dietary guidance, and (4) low serum concentrations of vitamins and carotenoids.

Kant, A. K., Schatzkin, A., Graubard, B. I., & Schairer, C. (2000). A prospective study of diet quality and mortality in women. *Journal of the American Medical Association, 283*, 2109–2115.—These data suggest that a dietary pattern characterized by consumption of foods recommended in current dietary guidelines is associated with decreased risk of mortality in women.

Krauss, R. M., Eckel, R. H., Howard, B., Appel, L. J., Daniels, S. R., Deckelbaum, R. J., Erdman, J.W., Kris-Etherton, P., Goldberg, I. J., Kotchen, T. A., Lichtenstein, A. H., Mitch, W. E., Mullis, R., Robinson, K., Wylie-Rosett, J., St. Jeor, S., Suttie, J., Tribble, D. L., & Bazzarre T. L. (2000). Dietary guidelines: A statement for healthcare professionals from the Nutrition Committee, American Heart Association. *Circulation, 102*, 2284–2299.—The American Heart Association revised its influential dietary guidelines, stressing common sense in choosing one's daily fare and downplaying complicated percentages of fat or nutrients. The focus is toward a diet rich in fruits, vegetables, legumes, whole grains, low-fat dairy products, fish, lean meats, and poultry. Five servings of fruits and vegetables and six servings of grains are recommended daily. And for the first time, two weekly servings of fatty fish, such as tuna or salmon, are recommended.

Meigs, J. B., Mittleman, M. A., Nathan, D. M., Tofler, G. H., Singer, D. E., Murphy-Sheehy, P. M., Lipinska, I., D'Agostino, R. B., & Wilson, P. W. (2000). Hyperinsulinemia, hyperglycemia, and impaired hemostasis: The Framingham Offspring Study. *Joural of the American Medical Association*, 283, 221–228.—Excess risk for cardiovascular disease associated with hyper-insulinemia and glucose intolerance may be mediated in part by enhanced potential for acute thrombosis.

Moore, L. L., Visioni, A. J., Wilson, P. W., D'Agostino, R. B., Finkle, W. D., & Ellison, R. C. (2000). Can sustained weight loss in overweight individuals reduce the risk of diabetes mellitus? *Epidemiology*, 11, 269–273.—Regardless of the amount of weight lost, those who regained the lost weight had no reduction in diabetes risk. A modest amount of sustained weight loss can substantially reduce the risk of diabetes mellitus in overweight individuals.

Polonsky, K. S., Gumbiner, B., Ostrega, D., Griver, K., Tager, H., & Henry, R. R. (1994). Alterations in immunoreactive proinsulin and insulin clearance induced by weight loss in NIDDM. *Diabetes*, 43, 871–877.—In obese subjects and those with subclinical diabetes, weight loss was associated with a reduction in insulin secretion rates, presumably as a result of improvements in insulin sensitivity. In patients with overt diabetes and hyperglycemia, weight loss improved beta cell responsiveness to glucose and was associated with an increase in insulin clearance and a reduction in proinsulin immunoreactivity.

Serdula, M. K., Mokdad, A. H., Williamson, D. F., Galuska, D. A., Mendlein, J. M., & Heath, G. W. (1999). Prevalence of attempting weight loss and strategies for controlling weight. *Journal of the American Medical Association*, 282(14), 1353–1358.—Weight loss and weight maintenance are common concerns for U.S. men and women. Most persons trying to lose weight are not using the recommended combination of reducing calorie intake and engaging in leisure-time physical activity 150 minutes or more per week.

Shick, S. M., Wing, R. R., Klem, M. L., McGuire, M. T., Hill, J. O., & Seagle, H. (1998). Persons successful at long-term weight loss and maintenance continue to consume a low-energy, low-fat diet. *Journal of the American Dietetic Association*, 98, 408–413.—Continued consumption of a low-fat, low-energy diet may be necessary for long-term weight control; persons who have successfully lost weight should be encouraged to maintain such a diet.

Svetkey, L. P., Sacks, F. M., Obarzanek, E., Vollmer, W. M., Appel, L. J., Lin, P. H., Karanja, N. M., Harsha, D. W., Bray, G. A., Aickin, M., Proschan, M. A., Windhauser, M. M., Swain, J. F., McCarron, P. B., Rhodes, D. G., & Laws, R. L. (1999). The DASH Diet, Sodium Intake and Blood Pressure Trial (DASH-sodium): Rationale and design. *Journal of the American Dietetic Association*, 99(Suppl.), S96–S104.—A diet rich in fruits, vegetables, and low-fat dairy foods, and with reduced saturated, total fat and salt can substantially lower blood pressure. This diet offers an additional nutritional approach to preventing and treating hypertension.

Ueki, K., Yamauchi, T., Tamemoto, H., Tobe, K., Yamamoto-Honda, R., Kaburagi, Y., Akanuma, Y., Yazaki, Y., Aizawa, S., Nagai, R., & Kadowaki, T. (2000). Restored insulin-sensitivity in IRS-1-deficient mice treated by adenovirus-mediated gene therapy. *Journal of Clinical Investigation*, 105, 1437–1445.—This data suggests that protein kinase B (PKB) in liver plays a pivotal role in systemic glucose homeostasis and that its activation might be sufficient for reducing insulin resistance even without full activation of phosphatidylinositol 3-kinase (PI3K).

# 88

# Effects of Weight Loss on Morbidity and Mortality

RODOLFO VALDEZ
EDWARD W. GREGG
DAVID F. WILLIAMSON

## BACKGROUND

The concept that, for a given height, there is a range of low-morbidity or low-mortality body weights, is firmly established in epidemiology (see Chapter 76). There is less agreement, however, over the spread of such ranges. Weights within these ranges have been called ideal, desirable, optimal, healthy, or recommended body weights. This general concept has two important implications that constitute the basis of modern weight management guidelines: First, people with body weights outside the recommended range, particularly the overweight, are at risk for chronic disease and even premature death; second, overweight people can lower their health risks by losing weight. Current epidemiological evidence generally supports the first inference but is equivocal about the second. Studies of weight loss are more susceptible than are studies of weight itself to confounder bias, such as underlying illness. Given the high prevalence of overweight and obesity, elucidating the effects of weight loss on health is a priority.

## WHO WANTS TO LOSE WEIGHT AND HOW MUCH?

Table 88.1 demonstrates the widespread desire to lose weight in the U.S. population. About 29% and 43% of adult men and women, respectively, report trying to lose weight. In all body mass index (BMI) categories, women want to lose more weight than men except in the underweight category, where both men and women want to gain weight, but women want to gain much less weight than men (1.2 vs. 5.4 kg). Overall, women want to lose 7.9 kg and men, 4.2 kg.

**TABLE 88.1. Desired Weight Changes in Adult U.S. Men and Women According to Categories of Body Mass Index**

| BMI category[a] | Men | | | | | | Women | | | | |
|---|---|---|---|---|---|---|---|---|---|---|---|
| | Prevalence (%) | % trying to lose weight | Average BMI (kg/m²) | Average desired weight change (kg) | Average desired BMI (kg/m²) | Prevalence (%) | % trying to lose weight | Average BMI (kg/m²) | Average desired weight change (kg) | Average desired BMI (kg/m²) |
| <18.5 | 1.3 | 7.6 | 17.1 | 5.4 | 20.0 | 4.2 | 7.6 | 17.3 | 1.2 | 18.5 |
| 18.5–25.0 | 37.6 | 9.0 | 22.8 | 0.9 | 23.2 | 51.8 | 29.4 | 22.0 | –2.6 | 21.2 |
| 25–30 | 44.2 | 34.9 | 27.1 | –4.1 | 25.8 | 27.0 | 57.5 | 27.2 | –9.3 | 23.7 |
| 30–35 | 12.7 | 57.8 | 31.9 | –12.5 | 28.0 | 11.1 | 66.8 | 32.1 | –18.0 | 25.3 |
| 35–40 | 3.1 | 66.2 | 36.9 | –23.4 | 29.5 | 3.8 | 69.3 | 37.1 | –27.8 | 26.6 |
| ≥ 40 | 1.1 | 70.0 | 44.0 | –40.3 | 31.2 | 2.2 | 72.6 | 44.9 | –44.8 | 27.9 |
| Overall | | 29.1 | 26.4 | –4.2 | 25.2 | | 42.6 | 25.4 | –7.9 | 22.6 |

*Note.* Data from the Behavioral Risk Factor Surveillance System, 1996 and 1998. Sample size is 111,137 men and 152,553 women who self-reported height and weight for those 2 years. Figures are weighted to represent the U.S. population. Each percentage point in prevalence is equivalent to approximately 1 million people.

[a]From top to bottom, respectively, the six BMI categories are classified as underweight, normal, overweight, obesity I, obesity II, and obesity III.

The frequency at which the U.S. population is trying to lose weight is so vast that even minor beneficial effects of weight loss for individuals could translate into important benefits for the population. Conversely, minor harmful effects could become major public health problems. Both beneficial and harmful effects have been reported for weight loss.

## BENEFICIAL AND ADVERSE EFFECTS OF WEIGHT LOSS

Intentional weight loss may exert beneficial effects on health by reducing risk factors associated with obesity (Table 88.2, upper panel). Weight loss reduces risk factors for diabetes and cardiovascular disease, and alleviates conditions such as sleep apnea, chest pain, and low back pain (see Chapter 87). However, intentional loss is not devoid of adverse effects, including gallstone formation and loss of lean body mass (Table 88.2, lower panel). Life-threatening effects of weight loss are rare, and the common, less severe adverse effects may not be enough to deter attempts to lose weight. In cases of obesity and severe obesity (BMIs $\geq$ 30 kg/m$^2$), the benefits of weight loss easily outweigh the risks. In cases of overweight (BMIs = 25.0–29.9 kg/m$^2$), other preexisting conditions, such as comorbidities, are needed for clinicians to recommend treatment for weight loss. Otherwise, weight maintenance should be the strategy of choice.

Both beneficial and harmful effects of weight loss are based largely on short-term studies (weeks or months); hence, it is not clear whether beneficial effects will continue or adverse effects will be reversed over longer periods. However, weight loss studies that follow subjects for long periods do report benefits. For example, the two Trials of Hypertension Prevention (TOHP I, 1993; TOHP II, 1997) and the Trial of Nonpharmacological Interventions in the Elderly (TONE, 1998) have found 21–34% reduction in hypertension and other cardiovascular outcomes associated with rather modest weight losses (2–4%) over periods of 2 to 4 years. In 1999, the Swedish Obese Subjects study (SOS) re-

---

**TABLE 88.2. Reported Beneficial and Adverse Effects of Weight Loss**

Reported beneficial effects of weight loss

- Reduces blood pressure (systolic and diastolic)
- Reduces "bad" (total and LDL) cholesterol and triglycerides
- Increases "good" (HDL) cholesterol
- Reduces the risk of diabetes in high-risk individuals
- Improves glucose metabolism in people with diabetes
- Reduces left ventricular mass and relative wall thickness
- Reduces risk of symptomatic knee osteoarthritis
- Relieves symptoms of dyspnea, and chest and low back pain
- Improves overall physical functioning

Reported adverse effects of weight loss

- Acute cardiac arrest
- Cardiac arrhythmias
- Cardiac electrolyte imbalances
- Gallstones and cholecystitis
- Loss of muscle mass
- Loss of bone density
- Reduced muscle strength

ported the 2-year results of a nonrandomized surgical intervention in very obese subjects (BMI > 40 kg/m²) (see Chapter 102). Surgically treated patients (average weight loss = 28 kg) had significantly lower incidence of hypertension, diabetes, and some lipid abnormalities than matched, conventionally treated patients (average weight loss = 0.5 kg). More recently, the Finnish Diabetes Prevention Study (DPS) reported results of the first randomized, controlled trial testing the effect of lifestyle intervention on the prevention of type 2 diabetes in high-risk (obese and glucose intolerant) individuals (see Chapter 104). The intervention consisted of a personalized and closely supervised 2-year program that included a healthy diet and regular, moderate exercise. By the end of the program, on average, the intervention group lost 3.5 kg and the conventionally treated group lost 0.8 kg. At follow-up, 3–5 years later, the incidence of diabetes was 10% in the intervention group and 22% in the control group, a 58% reduction.

## WEIGHT LOSS AND MORTALITY

Given the physiological benefits of weight loss, it is surprising when research does not show increased longevity. In fact, many studies have found weight loss to be associated with increased mortality, although most did not assess the intentionality of weight loss.

In studies where intentionality of weight loss is discerned, weight loss seems to have either a neutral or a modest positive effect on longevity. In two large prospective studies of women and men in the Cancer Prevention Study I, among women with preexisting chronic conditions, intentional weight loss was associated with a 20% reduction of all-cause mortality and up to a 40% reduction in 13-year mortality related to diabetes and cancer. No association was found with cardiovascular mortality, and no consistent associations were found among women without preexisting conditions. Intentional weight loss in men was found to reduce only the 13-year mortality related to diabetes (by about one-third). There was no association with overall or cardiovascular mortality.

In two recent prospective studies, the Iowa Women's Health Study and the Cardiovascular Health Study, there was no effect of weight loss on all-cause mortality, but in a study of men from Israel, weight loss increased the risk of all-cause mortality.

## METHODOLOGICAL ISSUES IN WEIGHT LOSS STUDIES

Epidemiological studies of weight loss and health must be interpreted with caution due to a series of methodological problems. First, many studies were not designed to test weight loss hypotheses. Second, most studies are not able to distinguish between intentional and unintentional weight loss. Additionally, studies must separate unintentional weight loss due to healthy lifestyles, not necessarily centered around weight management, from unintentional weight losses due to underlying disease. Third, intentional weight loss can be achieved through a variety of approaches and their combinations (e.g., diet, physical activity, drugs, surgery), and each approach may have a different impact on health. Fourth, it is difficult to separate losses of muscle mass from losses of fat mass; the former may have a negative effect on health and the latter a positive one. Fifth, associations of weight loss with ill health can be spurious, because losses are more common among those suffering from obesity-related diseases. Sixth, individuals may be unable to sustain weight loss long enough for some health effects to take place. Seventh, it is possible that not all conditions triggered or aided by excess fat are reversible.

## CURRENT RANDOMIZED, CONTROLLED TRIALS

The U.S. National Institutes of Health is funding two large, multicenter, well-designed, prospective studies of the effects of weight loss on health: the Diabetes Prevention Program (DPP) and the Study of Health Outcomes of Weight Loss (SHOW). The DPP is designed to assess the safety and efficacy of two interventions on the incidence of diabetes in overweight individuals with impaired glucose tolerance. The interventions are an intensive lifestyle program and treatment with metformin, a drug that enhances the glucose-lowering effects of insulin.

The SHOW trial is designed to test the effects of sustained weight loss on the health of obese subjects with type 2 diabetes. The plan is to compare ordinary community care for diabetes with that of intensive lifestyle interventions plus ordinary community care for diabetes.

These two studies, along with the recent DPS from Finland, will help to differentiate the beneficial effects of weight loss from the adverse ones, particularly among high-risk individuals.

## FURTHER READING

Allison, D. B., Zannolli, R., Faith, M. S., Heo, M., Pietrobelli, A., VanItallie, T. B., Pi-Sunyer, F. X., & Heymsfield, S. B. (1999). Weight loss increases and fat loss decreases all-cause mortality rate: Results from two independent cohort studies. *International Journal of Obesity, 23,* 603–611.—Unique study that attempts to differentiate the risks of losing fat versus lean body mass.

Dublin, L. I. (1953). Relation of obesity to longevity. *New England Journal of Medicine, 248,* 971–974.—First paper to examine the epidemiological relationship between weight change and mortality.

Gregg, E. W., & Williamson, D. F. (in press). The relationship of intentional weight loss to disease incidence and mortality. In T. A. Wadden & A. J. Stunkard (Eds.), *Handbook of obesity treatment.* New York: Guilford Press.—Updated review on the issue of weight loss and disease, including a good discussion on methodological issues.

Hamm, P. B., Shekelle, R. B., & Stamler, J. (1989). Large fluctuations in body weight during young adulthood and 25-year risk of coronary death in men. *American Journal of Epidemiology 129,* 312–318.—The first paper on weight cycling and mortality.

Williamson, D. F. (1996). Weight cycling and mortality: How do the epidemiologists explain the role of intentional weight loss? *Journal of the American College of Nutrition, 15,* 6–13.—A critical review of methodological issues regarding weight loss and health.

Williamson, D. F., Pamuk, E., Thun, M., Flanders, D., Byers, T., & Heath, C. (1995). Prospective study of intentional weight loss and mortality in never-smoking overweight U.S. white women aged 40–64 years. *American Journal of Epidemiology, 141,* 1128–1141.—First attempt to relate intentional weight loss to mortality.

# 89

# Metabolic Effects of Exercise in Overweight Individuals

## WIM H. M. SARIS

## EXERCISE, BODY WEIGHT CONTROL, AND ENERGY BALANCE

It is appealing to postulate that exercise may be a key factor in weight control (see Chapter 93). A convincing argument for this regulatory role is the observation that with the exception of sumo wrestlers (who need high body mass for physical combat), the prevalence of obesity is almost zero for athletes. Those who leave sports frequently increase in body weight and fatness. More difficult to prove is the role of inactivity in the etiology of obesity. Furthermore, the public view is that exercise is ineffective for weight control because the amount of exercise required to change weight is too great to be practical, and that the increase in energy raises appetite, thus negating the effect of the additional exercise.

Exercise is linked to power output and heat production, and thus with energy expenditure. According to the laws of thermodynamics, obesity is a result of a positive energy balance in which energy intake has exceeded expenditure over a prolonged period. It is not clear which part of the equation is mostly affected in obesity. There are many factors associated with energy intake, expenditure, and their interaction.

The difference in physical activity between normal and overweight individuals has been examined in a plethora of studies but data are not conclusive. Most studies find no relation between inactivity and obesity, but are severely hampered by methodological problems and unclear definitions of physical activity. A case linking decreased activity with body weight regulation can be made only indirectly with indicators of a sedentary lifestyle, such as cars per household, hours per week watching television, or level of work.

Reduced activity may be balanced partly by the increased energy cost of weight-bearing activities. Moving around with a higher body mass implies a higher energy cost. This was demonstrated in a weight loss study in which each experimental subject wore a vest with weights compensating for his or her weight loss. Subjects' decrease in energy expenditure during weight loss was only half of that of control subjects, who did not compensate for their identical weight loss.

Until recently, methods to quantify physical activity (see Chapters 10, 11, 24, and 25), such as questionnaires, movement counters, or heart rate recorders, were invalid for measuring the small differences in activity that may lead to positive energy balance and ultimately to weight gain. Currently, the doubly labeled water technique is the gold standard for quantifying energy expenditure under free living conditions. Almost no differences in physical activity expressed as a multiple of the resting metabolic rate (RMR) have been found between obese and nonobese subjects, indicating that inactivity is not the prime factor that causes the positive energy balance. However, most studies are cross-sectional and thus use subjects with different genetic and environmental backgrounds.

The interpretation of research is also confused by the fact that "activity" is a complex of minor physical movements, often called "fidgeting," or nonexercise activity thermogenesis (NEAT), normal daily life activities, and more intense movements associated with work and leisure-time activities such as sport. Evidence from secular- and age-trend association studies points to a consistent negative relationship between level of activity and body mass index (BMI). The results from prospective studies are very valid when evaluating the role of inactivity in the etiology of obesity. These studies consistently show higher risks for increased body weight coupled with an inactive lifestyle.

Results of animal studies provide overwhelming evidence of the importance of activity in the regulation of body weight. In addition, the long-term outcome for the treatment of obesity, while generally disappointing, supports the importance of exercise in controlling body weight (see Chapters 93, 106, and 107). Individuals who become regular exercisers (a minimum of three sessions a week), have a fairly good chance of controlling their weight. Those who cease to exercise regain weight.

The main question, then, seems to be settled: Exercise is a key factor in weight control. But questions of considerable importance remain. What is the mechanism by which exercise enhances weight control? Is this just a question of counting the extra calories in the energy balance or does it affect other aspects of metabolism that lead to a better regulation of body weight and body fatness?

## FACTORS LINKING EXERCISE TO WEIGHT CONTROL

### Exercise Expends Energy

Most textbooks on exercise physiology have tables or figures showing the energy costs of recreational activities such as swimming, walking, cycling, and running at different speeds. Since RMR for the average adult is fairly close to 35 ml of oxygen/kg/minute, or 1 kcal/kg/hour, the energy cost of activities is frequently expressed as multiples of RMR. MET is defined as the ratio of the metabolic rate for a specific activity divided by the RMR.

The highest energy expenditure during walking is 9.6 kcal/hour; during running, it is 16.2 kcal/hour; and during breast stroke swimming, it is 19.2 kcal/hour, indicating that in 1 hour of exercise, more energy is expended during running, cycling, and swimming than during walking. However, to expend about 18 kcal/hour for much time, maximal oxygen consumption must be more than 60 ml/kg/minute, possible only for well-trained young subjects. For individuals with a maximum oxygen consumption per unit time ($VO2_{max}$) of 35 ml/kg/minute (the average 40-year-old female is not able to expend more than about 7.2 kcal/kg/hour, corresponding to 70% $VO2_{max}$), fast walking may be as effective as running or cycling. To exercise while covering a certain distance (e.g., from home to office), cycling is most efficient. Walking or running the same distance will cost considerably more energy.

If the net energy expenditure during exercise is calculated by subtracting RMR, the energy cost of exercise varies between 2 and 17 kcal/kg/hour, which means that a person weighing 70 kg can spend somewhere between 130 and 1,200 kcal extra during 1 hour of exercise, depending on the activity and the person's work capacity.

## Exercise Affects Appetite Regulation

Studies on the short-term effects of exercise on appetite and food intake clearly demonstrate accurate compensation due to the sensitizing effects of exercise on physiological responses. However, the physiological responses of lean and obese individuals appear to be different. Lean individuals maintain weight by adjustment of energy intake to increasing expenditure, while obese individuals' intake remains fixed, suggesting an uncoupling of the energy intake from expenditure.

A possible explanation can be found in the postexercise effect of exercise on hunger and satiety. Hunger is typically depressed after intense exercise. Postexercise satiety signals, mainly from the gastrointestinal tract, seem to be potent enough to prevent increased food intake as long as the energy stores in the body are sufficient. In athletes, this phenomenon may become the pathological "exercise-induced anorexia."

Another interesting phenomenon observed in individuals who begin regular exercise is a change toward relatively carbohydrate-rich food choices at the expense of fat. This may also affect hunger and satiety, because equicaloric amounts of carbohydrate have a stronger satiety effect than fat. This finding also implies that exercise does not automatically lead to a postexercise energy deficit if the fat content of the diet is excessive.

## Exercise Affects Macronutrient Balance

The postexercise regulation of body weight can be better understood by taking into account the effects of exercise on carbohydrate and lipid balance, as well as energy balance. Physical training produces several metabolic adaptations that may facilitate weight control. Studies on the relationship between muscle fiber type, carbohydrate–fat oxidation rate, and weight control have made the muscle compartment the focus of attention. About half the energy is expended through skeletal muscle. Sympathetic–adrenergic response and fiber types are influenced by exercise training. Dramatic changes can occur in the skeletal muscle in response to training, which increases the capacity of several metabolic pathways to meet higher performance demands. During exercise, there is a shift to a greater use of fat as fuel to spare glycogen, which is the fuel of preference for the exercising muscle.

Another important adaptation is the increase of insulin sensitivity. Insulin resistance related to obesity diminishes both glucose oxidation and glucose storage in muscle. These lead to a blunting of the facultative thermogenic response to feeding. The postexercise resynthesis of glycogen leads to a decrease in carbohydrate oxidation and a compensatory increase in lipid oxidation.

All these physiological adaptations are focused on one point; the body does not seem to tolerate prolonged carbohydrate imbalance. This difference in sensitivity in maintaining macronutrient balance between carbohydrate and fat suggests that exercise can induce a substantial increase in lipid oxidation, both during and after exercise, at the expense of fat stores. As a consequence, weight maintenance programs using exercise should emphasize diet composition. The beneficial effects will be rather small if the fat–carbohydrate ratio (food quotient) is too high.

Macronutrient balance is also relevant to exercise prescription. Prolonged regular exercise at a moderate intensity level (3 to 6 MET) will maximize the relative lipid content of the fuel mix oxidized, inducing a lipid and energy deficit. Regular low-to-moderate intensity, prolonged-endurance exercise does not invalidate the health benefits caused by exercise.

At this moment no precise conclusions can be drawn regarding the advisable intensity of exercise. Additional factors, in particular long-term adherence, are of major importance. Also, the type of exercise, such as structural versus lifestyle approach, or multiple short bouts versus one long bout, need much more research.

## HOW MUCH EXERCISE IS ENOUGH?

Current public health recommendations are set at a minimum of 150 minutes weekly. However, this may not be enough to prevent long-term weight gain. A meta-analysis based on doubly labeled water studies indicated that among those who spend more than 0.1 MJ/kg body weight/day (around 1,200 kcal) on physical activity, overweight was absent. This represents about 100 minutes of moderate intense activities beyond an estimated 2 hours of daily activities. A first prospective study with a small number of subjects showed a threshold of about 80 minutes daily of moderate activities (walking, cycling) or 35 minutes daily of vigorous activities (jogging, swimming).

These results indicate clearly that the current recommendations may need to be revised. The fact that similar levels of activity emerge from such crude measures of exposure makes this conclusion all the more robust.

## CONCLUSIONS

Although many factors are involved in the delicate balance between energy intake and expenditure, exercise is a key part of weight control. Activity not only facilitates weight reduction through direct energy expenditure but also alters metabolism, so that the release or storage of energy in both muscle and adipose tissue is facilitated. Exercise increases the capacity to oxidize carbohydrate, and especially fat, in muscle by improving free fatty acid metabolism and enhancing tissue insulin sensitivity. In addition, regular exercise induces appetite suppression, with a concomitant preferential intake of carbohydrate, since carbohydrate balance is more tightly regulated than fat balance.

The type (aerobic, strength), intensity (low, moderate, high), and duration (intermittent, short bouts, or long duration) are not yet defined. This is also closely related to other important factors such as compliance (see Chapter 93).

The question on the total amount of exercise for weight control also needs further research. The public health recommendation of 150 minutes weekly may need upward revision. Despite these uncertainties, there is an overwhelming case for the conclusion that physical activity has a strong beneficial effect on metabolism and facilitates energy balance and body weight regulation. Therefore, regular daily physical activity is a prerequisite for healthy body weight control.

## FURTHER READING

Bouchard, C. (2000). *Physical activity and obesity*. Champaign, IL: Human Kinetics.—Recent textbook in which the different aspects of obesity and activity are addressed in detail.

Montoye, H. J., Kemper, H. C. G., Saris, W. H. M., & Washburn, R. A. (1994). *Measuring physical activity and energy expenditure*. Champaign, IL: Human Kinetics.—A handbook of "the state of the art and science" of estimating energy expenditure and physical activity that includes all methods, devices, questionnaires, and Metropolitan Life Insurance Company tables.

Saltin, B., & Gollnick, P. D. (1983). Skeletal muscle adaptability: Significance for metabolism and performance. In L. D. Peach, R. H. Adrian, & S. R. Geiger (Eds.), *Handbook of physiology: Skeletal muscle* (pp. 555–631). Baltimore: Williams & Wilkins.—An overview of the metabolic changes in skeletal muscle during training.

Saris, W. H. M. (1993). The role of exercise in the dietary treatment of obesity. *International Journal of Obesity, 17*, S17–S21.—An overview of the role of exercise during dietary treatment of overweight.

Saris, W. H. M. (1998). Fit, fat and fat free: The metabolic aspects of weight control. *International Journal of Obesity, 22*(Suppl. 2), S15–S21.—Detailed review of the metabolic changes with increasing levels of exercise in the obese.

van Baak, M. A., & Saris, W. H. M. (1998). Exercise and obesity. In P. G. Kopelman & M. J. Stock (Eds.), *Clinical obesity* (pp. 429–468). Oxford, UK: Blackwell Science.—Review of the differences between active and sedentary subjects.

# 90

# Social and Psychological Effects of Weight Loss

## GARY D. FOSTER
## THOMAS A. WADDEN

Many of the effects subjects expect from weight loss are psychosocial in nature, such as improved mood, a better quality of life, or a more positive body image (see Chapter 70). Thus, it is important to review the psychosocial changes that accompany weight loss, so that both practitioners and subjects have realistic expectations. In this chapter, we summarize research findings on the effects of weight loss and weight regain, discuss our clinical impressions of changes in psychosocial functioning that occur with weight loss, and identify areas for further research.

## RESEARCH FINDINGS ON THE EFFECTS OF WEIGHT LOSS AND WEIGHT REGAIN

### Weight Loss

*Mood*

Early studies, conducted before 1970, described adverse emotional reactions during weight loss, including "dieting depression," anxiety, irritability, and nervousness (see Chapter 71). These reports, however, were based on obese psychiatric subjects and lean men. Subsequent studies conducted principally among obese women without psychiatric disturbance revealed that weight loss was associated with improvements in mood or, at a minimum, with no worsening. The most salient difference between early and later studies was the use of behavior therapy in the latter investigations. The positive effect of behavioral treatment has been confirmed in controlled trials; subjects treated with diet combined with behavior therapy showed significantly greater improvement in mood than those treated by diet alone.

## Body Image

Weight loss by a variety of methods is associated with significant improvements in body image (see Chapters 72 and 108). However, there does not appear to be a linear relationship between these two variables: Greater weight loss is not associated with greater improvement in body image. It is troubling that even small amounts of weight regain (2–3 kg) significantly attenuate the improvements in body image that follow weight loss. Interestingly, treatments that do not produce weight loss (e.g., body image therapy, undieting approaches) also result in significant improvements in body image among obese persons. The lack of linear relationship between weight loss and improvements in body image, the partial reversal with minimal weight gain, and the temporary nature of most weight loss efforts suggest that weight loss should not be the principal method to improve body image among the obese.

## Quality of Life

Several studies have documented positive effects of modest weight loss on quality of life (see Chapter 70). In a 12-week study, 30 subjects who lost 6.1 ± 4.0 kg experienced significantly greater improvements than 14 controls who gained 1.3 ± 1.3 kg on three of the eight subscales of the Medical Outcomes Study Short Form-36 Health Survey (SF-36; physical function, physical role, and mental health). Among 487 surgical subjects, who lost approximately 30 kg, and matched controls, who lost 1 kg over 2 years, surgical subjects experienced significantly greater improvements on a scale that assessed the effects of obesity on everyday life, measures of mood, the social introversion scale of the Sickness Impact Profile, and a general health rating index (see Chapters 101 and 102). In a similar sample, sick leave and disability were actually higher in surgical subjects in the first year after treatment, significantly lower in years 2 and 3, and lower, but not significantly so, in year 4. In a study that assessed SF-36 scores before and 18 months after gastric bypass, baseline scores were lower than national norms on all scales except role–emotional. After losing approximately 40 kg, subjects' scores were comparable or better than national norms.

These studies suggest that subjects' weight losses ranging from 6 kg to 30 kg result in significant improvements in quality of life relative to controls. The available literature is compromised by predominantly surgical samples that limit the ability to assess the effects of more typical weight losses of 10% of initial weight.

## Weight Regain

Despite the high prevalence of weight regain, there are few studies of its psychological effects. Subjects in one cross-sectional study reported that weight regain adversely affected their mood, self-esteem, and satisfaction with appearance, although another study found no significant difference in psychological status between persons with or without a marked history of weight cycling. Surprisingly, we found in a prospective study that losing and regaining 21 kg over a 5-year period did not adversely affect mood, binge eating, restraint, or disinhibition. Another study found no changes in weight and eating self-efficacy after weight regain, although the sample was limited to persons seeking a second round of treatment at the same clinic.

## CLINICAL IMPRESSIONS

### Weight Loss

Our clinical impressions are consistent with research findings of positive changes following weight loss but also suggest atypical responses in some subjects. In terms of benefits, obese women who lose weight report almost universally that they are pleased by their improved appearance, their opportunity to buy more fashionable clothes, and their positive feelings about themselves (see Chapters 72 and 108). They are justifiably proud of their weight loss and the hard work required to achieve it, and they enjoy praise from family and friends. Weight loss also brings many women a sense of well-being as their medical conditions improve.

Concomitant with these very positive changes, some subjects, particularly women, experience untoward responses ranging from annoyance to serious distress. One common problem is the increased attention they receive. Such attention and praise are especially difficult for shy patients who are not accustomed to receiving compliments. Some resent being treated so differently based solely on a change in weight.

Attention from the opposite sex, while sought by some, is occasionally disconcerting, particularly to those who have a history of sexual or physical abuse. Weight loss may bring a sense of increased vulnerability, especially when excess weight has served a protective function. It may also change a person's marital, social, and occupational roles. These changes are often positive, although they may not appear to be so. For example, the finding that the divorce rate increased for women who had undergone surgery for obesity was viewed more favorably when studies revealed that these divorces were limited to marriages rated as unsatisfactory before weight loss. These adverse consequences occur in only a minority of subjects, but frequently enough to require that clinicians be alert and intervene promptly.

### Weight Regain

It is difficult to imagine that weight regain is not associated with adverse psychosocial consequences given its public nature and society's negative attributions about the causes of obesity (e.g., lack of willpower, weakness). Our clinical impressions are that as patients regain weight, they experience a variety of emotions, including anger, frustration, shame, and hopelessness. Unfortunately, these emotions prevent subjects from seeking help to stop or reverse their weight gain. Thus, it is important to help subjects identify these potential emotional barriers to seeking additional treatment.

## FUTURE RESEARCH

Current data leave several important questions unanswered: (1) Do most obese subjects experience positive psychosocial changes as a result of weight loss? (2) What is the clinical significance of these changes? (3) What subject or treatment characteristics may modulate specific changes?

We believe these questions may be addressed in several ways. The first is to consider the remarkable heterogeneity of obese persons. Although a variety of factors differentiates obese persons, several factors are especially relevant for the investigation of the psychosocial effects of weight loss. Second is the subject's initial level of psychopathology. It is possible that the greatest harm or benefit may occur in subjects with the highest levels of psychopathology. This may be especially true in subjects with weight-related psychopathology, such as body image disparagement or binge-eating disorder.

Differences in the psychosocial effects of subjects' weight loss may also be related to differences in age of onset and/or the duration of the obesity. The effects of reversing a recent weight gain are likely to differ from those associated with reversing a lifetime history of significant obesity. The circumstances surrounding the onset of obesity may also play a role. Someone who has gained weight during successive pregnancies may feel differently about weight loss than a person who has gained weight after an emotional or physical trauma.

Cognitive factors are another source of significant heterogeneity. Subjects vary greatly in their expectations about changes following weight loss (see Chapter 91). These expectations (e.g., specific goal weight, medical changes, improved social functioning) are likely to affect how subjects view their weight loss. Thus, identical changes in weight may be viewed by different subjects as a "success" or a "failure" depending on their specific cognitive styles. Such characterizations probably modulate changes in self-efficacy and psychological status.

A third general strategy to improve research in this area concerns the use of specific, rather than global, outcome measures. Most researchers use global measures of self-concept or mood. Such measures are less likely to be sensitive to weight loss than those that address psychological or social constructs more closely related to weight, such as body image, perceived health, or size discrimination. Similarly, weight-specific measures of quality of life are likely to be more instructive than overall measures of quality of life.

A significant limitation of the current literature is the inability to assess clinical significance. It is important to know whether statistically significant changes in mean values reflect improvements within a normal range or movement from clinical to subclinical classification. For example, one study reported subjects' significant changes in both anxiety and depression following weight loss, but both were within the normal range 6.3 to 4.6 (depression) and 5.2 to 3.0 (anxiety) within a range of 0 to 21. However, when assessing only those subjects with a clinically significant score > 10), the number of subjects with clinically significant anxiety decreased from 21% to 11%, and those with clinically significant depression decreased from 9% to 4%. Mean values can obscure these important changes in clinical status.

## SUMMARY

Despite the fact that millions of people diet yearly, we know little about whether they achieve the psychosocial outcomes they desire. Moreover, we know even less about whether the failure to lose weight or maintain weight loss may harm, rather than improve, psychological functioning. These questions are central to the responsible and ethical treatment of obese persons and await the concerted efforts of researchers and practitioners.

## FURTHER READING

Foster, G. D., & Wadden, T. A. (1994). The psychology of obesity, weight loss, and weight regain: Research and clinical findings. In G. L. Blackburn & B. S. Kanders (Eds.), *Obesity: Pathophysiology, psychology, and treatment* (pp. 140–166). New York: Chapman & Hall.—A review of the psychosocial consequences of weight loss and weight regain, including clinical descriptions of positive and negative responses to weight loss, as well as suggestions for their clinical management.

Foster, G. D., Wadden, T. A., Kendall, P. C., Stunkard, A. J., & Vogt, R. A. (1996). Psychological effects of weight loss and regain: A prospective evaluation. *Journal of Clinical and Consulting Psychology, 64,* 752–757.—A prospective study examining the psychological effects of losing and regaining 21 kg.

French, S. A., & Jeffery, R. W. (1994). The consequences of dieting to lose weight: Effects on physical and mental health. *Health Psychology, 13,* 195–212.—A review of the physical and psychological consequences of dieting, with particular attention to the methodological issues of defining a "diet."

Jasper, J. (1992). The challenge of weight control: A personal view. In T. A. Wadden & T. B. VanItallie (Eds.), *Treatment of the seriously obese patient* (pp. 411–456). New York: Guilford Press.—An eloquent description of one patient's psychosocial effects of weight loss.

Kushner, R. F., & Foster, G. D. (2000). Obesity and quality of life. *Nutrition, 16,* 947–952.—A comprehensive review of global and obesity-specific measures of quality of life as well as the effects of weight loss on quality of life.

National Task Force on the Prevention and Treatment of Obesity. (2000). Dieting and the development of eating disorders in overweight and obese adults. *Archives of Internal Medicine, 160,* 2581–2589.—A review of the psychological changes following weight loss and the role of dieting in the development of eating disorders.

Smoller, J. W., Wadden, T. A., & Stunkard, A. J. (1987). Dieting and depression: A critical review. *Journal of Psychosomatic Research, 31,* 429–440.—Proposes that factors in addition to behavior therapy, such as the method and frequency of assessment, might have accounted for the differences in results between early and more recent studies.

Wadden, T. A., Sarwer, D. B., Arnold, M. A., Gruen, D., & O'Neil, P. M. (2000). Psychosocial status of severely obese patients before and after bariatric surgery. In H. J. Sugerman & N. J. Soper (Eds.), *Problems in general surgery: Morbid obesity* (pp. 13–22). Philadelphia: Lippincott Williams & Wilkins.—A comprehensive review of psychosocial changes following the surgical treatment of obesity.

# Treatment and Prevention
of Obesity

# 91

# Goals of Obesity Treatment

KELLY D. BROWNELL
ALBERT J. STUNKARD

Establishing the goals of treatment is the first, and in many ways, the most important aspect of the treatment of obesity. These goals consist of improvement of both health and well-being. However, the goals that obese individuals bring to treatment can range from the realistic improvement in health and risk factors to fantasies of marrying the ideal mate and living happily ever after.

Much of the treatment negotiation between the provider and the patient consists of agreeing on the goals of treatment. In some instances, the parties agree from the outset about the desirability of losing weight by modifying food intake and physical activity. The relatively simple task of treatment is then to implement a program that will produce weight loss, reduce risk factors, and improve well-being. At the other extreme are people whose goals are so unrealistic that much of treatment consists of redefining goals to render them potentially achievable. In this redefinition, provider and patient should attempt to achieve (1) shared goals; (2) clear understanding of the responsibility of each part; and (3) reasonable expectations of outcome. In the course of this collaboration, expectations may be lowered, often substantially, in terms of lesser amounts of weight loss. Expectations may also be raised in terms of increased self-esteem, improved body image, and more effective social functioning (see Chapters 70, 72, 90, and 108).

## THE ULTIMATE GOAL

Losing weight is but one means by which individuals can improve health and well-being. Changes in diet and physical activity are beneficial in their own right and can improve an individual's life independent of weight loss (see Chapters 7 and 89). Issues addressed in some programs, such as interpersonal relationships, body image, and self-esteem, can also be important.

Weight change, therefore, is but one means of evaluating progress in obese persons. If a person loses to ideal weight and maintains it, eats a healthy diet, increases activity, and makes changes in psychosocial domains, all is well. However, this is the perfect outcome and perfection is rare. Considering changes in all relevant areas is important in terms of seeing the obese person as more than weight and risk factors.

## INITIAL CONSIDERATIONS

### Whether to Attempt Weight Loss

The goals of obesity treatment differ from those of eating disorders on the issue of dieting. Although various circumstances may make it necessary to defer, modify, or even abandon dieting for some obese individuals, weight loss is the ultimate goal and alleviation of the physical complications of obesity requires it. For the eating disorders, dieting may be the source of the problem and freedom from dieting the goal (see Chapters 14, 15, 16, and 17).

Attempting weight loss is not necessarily an appropriate path for all individuals. Some persons will not lose weight and most will not lose permanently. If chances of success are minimal, pressure to diet will have negative effects. For those who are successful, the rewards can be striking.

In an ideal world, assessments would predict who will succeed. Those with a positive prognosis would receive a treatment matched to their needs; those with moderate prognosis might receive interventions aimed at improving readiness; and those with poor prognosis might be counseled on healthy eating and activity, weight maintenance, and body acceptance.

Unfortunately, we do not live in such a predictable world. The best that we can do is to suggest that practitioners have an honest talk with their patients about the costs of trying to lose weight and patients' levels of readiness (discussed below). Financial costs are one matter, but patients must also be aware of time spent in treatment, the need to be physically active, altered eating habits, and the other concomitants of dieting. If these factors are unfavorable, one option is to defer treatment until they become more favorable. Another is to undertake therapy to resolve barriers to treatment. Such a talk between professional and patient should make possible a decision about whether the patient has a good chance of losing weight and, if so, a specific course of action.

### Readiness

Patients enter treatment with variable levels of readiness (ability and willingness to change lifestyle and attitudes). The concept is useful for discussion between professional and patient, but no valid measures of this construct exist. Brownell developed a Weight Loss Readiness Test (incorporated in The LEARN Program for Weight Management), but psychometric studies have not been done. The test draws from the stages of change model developed by Prochaska, DiClemente, and colleagues, which holds that individuals move through reliable stages when changing behavior, and that treatment must be matched to the individual's current stage. Patients not ready to change require help before they can take action.

## ASSESSMENT GOALS

Assessment of medical variables for the obese patient has been discussed in detail elsewhere (see Chapter 92, the clinical guidelines issued by the National Heart, Lung, and Blood Institute [NHLBI], and the Weighing the Options Report of the Institute of Medicine). A treatment algorithm in the NHLBI clinical guidelines provides decision points for intervention based on body mass index (BMI). Methods for addressing nutrition and physical activity are discussed in Chapters 23 and 24, respectively.

Psychosocial variables can be assessed by defining the areas most likely to be important. These vary from person to person but as a beginning typically include depression, binge eating, and the strength of social support. Methods for measurement are discussed in the book by Allison (cited in Further Reading).

## WEIGHT LOSS GOALS

### The Ideal Weight Flaw

Tables of ideal weights are useful for scientific purposes (see Chapter 76) but in clinical settings lead to goals where perfection (ideal weight) is the chief outcome. Perfection is possible for a rare few, but others are doomed never to reach ideal weight. Height–weight tables have now yielded to BMI tables, but the problem is the same, just with a different metric.

A parallel with exercise might help illustrate this principle. If studies demonstrated that marathon runners had the lowest mortality of those exercising, would we declare marathon running to be the ideal, establish tables of marathon times, show the tables to patients, and foster the notion that anything less is insufficient? This would ignore the epidemiological reality that any increase in activity is beneficial, and the psychological reality that unrealistic goals lead to giving up. Tables of ideal weights (or BMI values) ignore the epidemiological and psychological realities in the obesity field. Small weight losses are beneficial (see Chapters 87 and 88), and unrealistic goals are rampant and lead to giving up, so the concept of ideal weight in clinical practice may be unnecessary and counterproductive.

### Establishing Weight Goals

The concept of reasonable weight loss is often difficult for professionals to accept and may be even more difficult for patients. The problem is well illustrated in a study by Foster and colleagues at the University of Pennsylvania on the goals of treatment identified by obese patients weighing an average of 99 kg before they started treatment. The definition of these goal weights, the percentage of weight loss needed to achieve these losses, and the percentage of patients achieving those goals are listed in Table 91.1.

Weight loss by patients in this trial was actually an above average amount. The mean

**TABLE 91.1. Weight Loss Goals Established by Obese Women Prior to Beginning a Weight Loss Treatment Program, the Percentage of Initial Body Weight and Number of Kilograms Needed To Be Lost to Achieve Each Goal, and the Percentage of Patients Attaining Each Goal after the Program**

| Level of loss and definition | % weight loss needed to achieve | kg loss needed to achieve | % of subjects achieving |
|---|---|---|---|
| *Dream weight* (the ideal) | 38 | 38 | 0 |
| *Happy weight* (less than dream but still satisfying) | 31 | 31 | 9 |
| *Acceptable weight* (not satisfying but reasonable) | 25 | 25 | 24 |
| *Disappointing weight* (better than nothing but clearly disappointing) | 17 | 17 | 20 |

*Note.* Data abstracted from Foster, G. D., Wadden, T. A., Vogt, R. A., & Brewer, G. (1997). What is a reasonable weight loss?: Patients' expectations and evaluations of obesity treatment outcomes. *Journal of Consulting and Clinical Psychology, 65,* 79–85.

weight loss was 16.5% of initial body weight, far above the 10% that is often held out as the goal of treatment. Yet few patients predicted they would be even minimally satisfied with such a loss. Knowing how much weight they are likely to lose might deter many patients from attempting to lose weight, and the weight losses they do achieve might leave them frustrated and prone to relapse.

These findings suggest that setting a goal as to how much a person might ultimately lose may be unnecessary and even contraindicated. Weight losses vary widely among persons and any goal is arbitrary; predicting the weight loss of an individual is still not possible. An alternative is to focus on short-term goals. Among these goals are the modification of the patient's assumptions about body image ("appearance reflects the inner person" and "my appearance is responsible for much of what has happened to me"—see Chapter 108 and the Cash reference in Further Reading). The patient should be reminded frequently about the benefits of modest weight losses and be reinforced when they are achieved.

## BEHAVIORAL AND PSYCHOSOCIAL GOALS

Goals serve the joint purpose of motivating an individual to achieve and providing a standard against which to judge progress. The more frequently a patient establishes and then meets a goal, the more opportunities there are for reinforcement and enhanced self-efficacy. Patients can make progress in many areas aside from weight. Diet, physical activity, and binge eating are several such areas, but others include changes in medical parameters, such as lipids and blood pressure, and in quality-of-life variables (see Chapters 70 and 90). We believe it is important for patients to track their progress in domains affecting their well-being, so that progress can be noted frequently, especially when weight loss is slower than desired. Individuals may sleep better, have more energy, or feel increased confidence around others, to name a few powerful motivators.

## MAINTENANCE GOALS

Since most people do not attain ideal weight when initial treatment ends, the choice must be made to pursue further loss or focus on maintaining what has been accomplished. The latter goal is typically more feasible (see Chapters 106 and 107). One priority must be maintenance of lost weight and prevention of regain, but weight should not overshadow the importance of other changes. Improvements in diet, activity, and other lifestyle areas are victories and should be the focus of maintenance.

## FURTHER READING

Allison, D. B. (Ed.). (1995). *Handbook of assessment methods for eating behaviors and weight related problems: Measures, theory, and research*. Thousand Oaks, CA: Sage.—An impressive, comprehensive book on methods for assessment of all areas pertinent to obesity.

Brownell, K. D. (2000). *The LEARN program for weight management*. Dallas, TX: American Health.—A patient guide, with an emphasis on establishing reasonable weight, nutrition, and activity goals.

Brownell, K. D., & Rodin, J. (1994). The dieting maelstrom: Is it possible and advisable to lose weight? *American Psychologist, 49*, 781–791.—An article that examines potentially positive or negative effects of dieting in the context of treatment for obesity.

Cash, T. F. (1998). *The body image workbook*. New York: Fine Communications.—Excellent description of both body image assumptions that lead people to set unrealistic weight goals and methods of establishing healthier attitudes.

Foster, G. D., Wadden, T. A., Vogt, R. A., & Brewer, G. (1997). What is a reasonable weight loss?: Patients' expectations and evaluations of obesity treatment outcomes. *Journal of Consulting and Clinical Psychology, 65*, 79–85.—Important paper on how individuals seeking treatment for obesity establish highly unrealistic weight loss goals.

Institute of Medicine. (1995). *Weighing the options: Criteria for evaluating weight management programs*. Washington, DC: National Academy Press.—Report from an expert panel dealing with causes of obesity, treatment, and prevention.

McGuire, M. T., Wing, R. R., Klem, M. L., Lang, W., & Hill, J. O. (1999). What predicts weight regain among a group of successful weight losers? *Journal of Consulting and Clinical Psychology, 67*, 177–185.—Data from the National Weight Control Registry showing the extent of effort required to maintain weight loss in a large sample of successful maintainers.

National Heart, Lung, and Blood Institute, National Institutes of Health. (1998). Clinical guidelines on the identification, evaluation, and treatment of overweight and obesity in adults—the Evidence Report. *Obesity Research, 6* (Suppl. 2), 51S–209S.—Authoritative report outlining assessment and treatment guidelines for the management of obesity.

Prochaska, J. O., DiClemente, C. C., & Norcross, J. C. (1992). In search of how people change: Applications to addictive behaviors. *American Psychologist, 47*, 1102–1114.—Important paper summarizing the stages of change model, its application across various areas of behavior change, and data supporting its use.

Stunkard, A. J. (1976). *The pain of obesity*. Palo Alto, CA: Bull.—Classic book on the emotional and social suffering of obese persons that helps practitioners to increase empathy for their obese patients.

# 92

# Clinical Assessment of Obese Patients

ROLAND L. WEINSIER
ROBERT F. KUSHNER

The clinical assessment of patients presenting with obesity is critical for understanding the etiology of the disorder in individual cases and for establishing a reference point for response to therapy. Not all clinical assessments have to be conducted by a physician, although one has to be qualified to rule out neuroendocrine causes of obesity, to assess the presence and extent of comorbidities, to recommend further medical and laboratory evaluation, and to recognize individuals at high risk for complications of obesity and/or its treatment. The clinical assessment consists of a focused medical history, a careful physical examination, and, as appropriate, laboratory studies. In addition, evaluation of readiness, motivation for weight loss, and potential barriers to change need to be appraised.

## MEDICAL HISTORY

The focused medical history should identify the following: (1) potential factors contributing to the individual's obesity (e.g., familial, behavioral, or endocrinological), (2) current medical complications (see Chapter 84), (3) past treatment responses, and (4) factors that should preclude weight reduction intervention. Table 92.1 outlines the factors generally to be considered under each of these categories. Weight cycling (i.e., a history of repeated bouts of weight loss and gain) is common among obesity-prone persons. However, most studies indicate that weight cycling does not cause persistent metabolic abnormalities, such as depressed resting metabolic rate, and should not be a deterrent to subsequent attempts. Although endocrinological abnormalities associated with obesity are listed, it is important to be aware that identifiable endocrine disorders causing obesity are quite uncommon, occurring in less than 1% of cases. When present, the endocrine disorders most likely to cause weight gain (i.e., Cushing's syndrome, hypothyroidism, polycystic ovary syndrome) rarely cause severe degrees of obesity.

When searching for medical complications of the patient's obesity, it is important to

**TABLE 92.1. Factors to be Considered in the Medical History of an Obese Patient**

Factors predisposing to or associated with obesity

- Family history of obesity (number of first-degree relatives)
- Potential endocrinological abnormalities
  - Hypothyroidism (symptoms include cold intolerance, menstrual abnormalities, constipation, weakness)
  - Cushing's syndrome (hypertension, glucose intolerance, menstrual dysfunction, weakness, back pain, compression fractures, bruising)
  - Polycystic ovarian syndrome (reduced/absent menses shortly after menarche, hirsutism)
- Medication-induced weight gain (antidepressants, antipsychotics, antidiabetics, steroid homones, anticonvulsants)
- Lifestyle changes concurrent with onset of weight gain (e.g., job change, marriage/divorce, childbirth, relocation)
- Dietary pattern characterized by dependence on high energy-dense foods
- Sedentary pattern of physical activity

Current medical complications/associates of obesity

- Diabetes, dyslipidemia, hypertension, certain cancers (see Table 92.2)

Past treatment responses

- Pattern of weight cycling (past relapses are not a contraindication to therapy but may provide useful information in planning treatment approach)

History of medical complications of obesity (see Table 92.2)

Factors warranting precaution with or precluding weight reduction

- Most pregnant or lactating women
- Patients with a serious uncontrolled psychiatric illness such as major depression
- Patients with serious illnesses for whom energy restriction might exacerbate illness
- Patients with active substance abuse
- Patients with history of anorexia nervorsa or bulimia nervosa (should be referred for specialized care)

note the following: (1) Not all obese persons have medical complications or are unhealthy; (2) there is still controversy over the extent of the contribution of obesity per se to some medical problems, such as hypertension and hypercholesterolemia; and (3) the known comorbidities of obesity are not evenly distributed among all obese persons. Consequently, one cannot assume that all obese persons are ill, or that their overweight condition is the primary cause of comorbid states when they exist. Nevertheless, when performing the history and physical examination, clinicians should keep in mind the symptoms and diseases listed in Table 92.2 that are directly or indirectly related to obesity.

## PHYSICAL EXAMINATION

### Assessment of Degree of Obesity

The most practical approach for assessing the degree of obesity and medical risk in the clinical setting is measurement of body mass index (BMI) and waist circumference (see Chapter 68). BMI is calculated as weight (in kilograms) divided by height$^2$ (in meters) or,

**TABLE 92.2. Symptoms, Diseases, and Special Problems Associated with Obesity**

Cardiovascular system

Coronary heart disease
Cor pulmonale
Hypertension
Pulmonary embolism
Varicose veins

Gastrointestinal system

Cholelithiasis
Gastroesophageal reflux disease (GERD)
Colon cancer
Hepatic steatosis
Hernias
Nonalcoholic steatohepatitis (NASH)

Integumental system

Cellulitis
Carbuncles
Hygiene problems
Intertrigo
Venous stasis of legs

Musculoskeletal system

Immobility
Low back pain
Osteoarthritis

Genitourinary system

Hypogonadism
Prostate cancer
Urinary stress incontinence

Neurological system

Indiopathic intracranial hypertension
Meralgia paresthetica
Stroke

Psychosocial

Depression
Social/employment discrimination
Work disability

Reproductive/endocrine system

Amenorrhea
Breast cancer
Cushing's syndrome
Diabetes mellitus, type 2
Dyslipidemia
Glucose intolerance
Hypothyroidism
Infertility
Insulin resistance
Uterine cancer
Polycystic ovary syndrome (PCOS)

Respiratory system

Dyspnea and fatigue
Hypoventilation (Pickwickian) syndrome
Obstructive sleep apneas

more conveniently, as weight (pounds)/height$^2$ (inches) × 703. BMI tables are available for quick reference. Classifying obesity by BMI units replaces previous weight–height terminology, such as percent ideal or desirable body weight. The reference values for BMI and waist circumference recommended by the National Heart, Lung, and Blood Institute (NHLBI) and World Health Organization (WHO) are now generally accepted as the standard categorization. A desirable or healthy BMI is 18.5 to 25.0 kg/m$^2$; overweight is 25.0 to 29.9 kg/m$^2$; and obesity is 30 kg/m$^2$ or greater. Risks for several disorders, including type 2 diabetes mellitus, dyslipidemia, hypertension, and cardiovascular disease, are independently associated with excess abdominal fat, which can be clinically defined as a waist circumference greater than 102 cm (> 40 inches) in men and greater than 88 cm (> 35 inches) in women. Measurement of waist circumference is recommended in patients with a BMI between 25.0 and 34.9 kg/m$^2$. The classification of overweight and obesity by BMI, waist circumference, and associated disease risk is shown in Table 92.3.

In some instances, the use of height and weight alone for calculation of BMI as a surrogate measure of body fat may lead to an incorrect estimation of risk. Patients with an unusual body habitus, bodybuilders with increased muscularity, or the elderly with re-

**TABLE 92.3. Classification of Weight Status and Risk of Disease**

| | | Risk of disease[a] | |
|---|---|---|---|
| | | Waist circumference[b] ≤ 35" (88 cm)—women ≤ 40" (102 cm)—men | Waist circumference[b] > 35" (88 cm)—women > 40" (102 cm)—men |
| Weight status | BMI | | |
| Underweight | BMI < 18.5 kg/m$^2$ | | |
| Normal weight | BMI 18.5–24.9 | | |
| Overweight | BMI 25.0–29.9 | + | ++ |
| Obesity (Class I) | BMI 30.0–34.9 | ++ | +++ |
| Obesity (Class II) | BMI 35.0–39.9 | +++ | +++ |
| Extreme obesity | BMI ≥ 40 | ++++ | ++++ |

*Note.* Adapted from National Heart, Lung, and Blood Institute, National Institutes of Health. (1998). Clinical guidelines on the identification, evaluation, and treatment of overweight and obesity in adults: The evidence report. *Obesity Research*, 6(Suppl. 2), 51S–209S.
[a]Risk for type 2 diabetes, hypertension, and cardiovascular disease relative to having a normal weight and waist circumference.
[b]Measure waist circumference just above the iliac crest. An increased waist circumference may indicate increased disease risk even at a normal weight.

duced lean body mass, may be misclassified. Although accurate methods to assess body fat exist, most are impractical and too expensive for routine clinical application. Two methods, skin fold anthropometry and bioelectrical impedance analysis, can be applied in the office setting to estimate the proportions of lean and fat mass. Convenient reference values for percent body fat for men and women are as follows:

| Category | Percent body fat | |
|---|---|---|
| | Men | Women |
| Normal | 10–20 | 20–30 |
| Obese | > 25 | > 35 |

## Medical Examination of the Obese Patient

A comprehensive physical examination should be performed with a high level of suspicion for obesity-related diseases listed in Table 92.2. The following aspects are particularly important when identifying coexistent medical disorders and endocrinological abnormalities. Although identifiable endocrine disorders infrequently account for weight gain and rarely cause obesity, it is nonetheless important to rule out potentially treatable diseases.

• *Blood pressure.* Should be taken using cuff size appropriate for arm circumference (this information is shown on the cuff itself; if in doubt, use larger cuff to avoid spuriously high reading).
• *Skin.* Red to purple depressed striae, hirsutism, acne, and moon facies with plethora suggest Cushing's syndrome; mild hirsutism is also seen in polycystic ovarian syndrome; dry, coarse, cool, and pale skin suggest hypothyroidism; intertrigo, skin mac-

eration, is seen especially in areas of deep skin folds among markedly overweight subjects; cellulitis suggests chronic stasis, especially of lower extremities.

- *Throat and neck*. Crowded oropharynx and large neck circumference (when accompanied by history of loud snoring, gasping, or choking episodes during sleep, excessive daytime sleepiness, and awakening headaches) suggest obstructive sleep apnea.
- *Fat distribution*. Truncal distribution with fat accumulation around the supraclavicular areas and dorsocervical spine (buffalo hump) suggests Cushing's syndrome.
- *Thyroid gland*. Enlargement is suggestive of hypothyroidism.
- *Edema*. Boggy, nonpitting edema of eyes, tongue, hands, and feet suggests myxedema of hypthyroidism; edema localized to lower extremities is common in moderate to severe obesity.
- *Neurological exam*. Slow ankle reflex with delayed relaxation phase suggests hypothyroidism; muscle weakness suggests Cushing's syndrome and hypothyroidism.

## LABORATORY ASSESSMENT

No laboratory test in the obese patient needs to be considered routine and certainly does not replace a good medical history or physical examination. Tests should be dictated by individual findings.

| If suspicion of . . . | Consider . . . |
| --- | --- |
| Cushing's syndrome | 24-hour urine collection for free cortisol (> 150 µg/24 hours; > 3.5 mg/24 hours abnormal) |
| Hypothyroidism | Serum thyroid-stimulating hormone (TSH; normal generally < 5 µU/ml) |
| Diabetes | Fasting serum glucose (normal < 126 mg/dl) |
| Hyperlipidemia | Fasting total cholesterol, triglycerides, high-density lipoprotein cholesterol (HDL-C) |
| Gallstones | Utrasonography |
| Periodic/sleep apnea | Sleep studies (polysomnography) for oxygen desaturation; apnea hypopnea index (AHI), ear, nose, and throat (ENT) exam for upper airway obstruction |
| Polycystic ovarian syndrome | Increase in luteinizing hormone–follicle-stimulating hormone ratio, often > 2.5 |

## READINESS AND MOTIVATION

Assessing a patient's readiness for weight loss and identifying potential barriers for change are important components of the obesity-focused clinical assessment (see Chapter 91). The NHLBI clinical guidelines recommend evaluating the following factors: reasons and motivation for weight loss; previous history of successful and unsuccessful weight loss attempts; family, friends, and work site support; the patient's understanding of overweight and obesity and how it contributes to obesity-associated diseases; attitude toward physical activity, time availability barriers, and financial considerations.

## ASSESSMENT OF RISK STATUS

Information obtained from the medical history, physical examination, and laboratory evaluation is, in the end, synthesized to determine the patient's overall risk status and level of need for clinical intervention. The degree of overweight or obesity using BMI, the presence of abdominal obesity using waist circumference, and the presence of concomitant risk factors or comorbidities are combined with the patient's readiness to determine treatment goals and plans.

## FURTHER READING

Bray G. A. (1993). Fat distribution and body weight. *Obesity Research*, *1*, 203–205.—A discussion of guidelines for healthy body weights and body fat patterns.

Bray, G. A. (1998). Clinical evaluation and introduction to treatment of overweight. In G. A. Bray (Ed.), *Contemporary diagnosis and management of obesity* (pp. 131–166). Newtown, PA: Handbooks in Health Care.—A succinct review of the of the evaluation process and treatment goals for the obese patient.

Han, T. S., van Leer, E. M., Seidell, J. C., & Lean, M. E. J. (1995). Waist circumference action levels in the identification of cardiovascular risk factors: Prevalence study in a random sample. *British Medical Journal*, *311*, 1401–1405.—Large population study supports the association of increased cardiovascular risk factors with increasing abdominal circumferences.

Kushner, R. F., & Weinsier, R. L. (2000). Evaluation of the obese patient: Practical considerations. *Medical Clinics of North America*, *84*, 387–399.—A review of the office-based evaluation of the obese patient.

National Heart, Lung, and Blood Institute, and National Institutes of Health. (1998). Clinical guidelines on the identification, evaluation, and treatment of overweight and obesity in adults: The evidence report. *Obesity Research*, *6*(Suppl. 2), 51S–209S.—Evidence-based guidelines provide 769 references and most current information on patient care aspects of obesity.

National Institutes of Health, National Heart, Lung, and Blood Institute, and the North American Association for the Study of Obesity. (2000). *Practical guide to the identification, evaluation, and treatment of overweight and obesity in adults*. Washington, DC: Department of Health and Human Services, Public Health Service.—Based on the evidence report prepared by the expert panel, the practical guide provides the basic tools needed to assess and manage overweight and obesity appropriately.

Pi-Sunyer, F. X. (1999). Obesity. In M. Shils, J. Olson, M. Shike, & A. C. Ross (Eds.), *Modern nutrition in health and disease* (9th ed., pp. 1395–1418). Philadelphia: Lea & Febiger.—A review of obesity that encompasses classification, assessment of severity, pathogenesis, and therapy.

Weinsier R. L. (1997). Obesity. In D. C. Heimburger & R. L. Weinsier (Eds.), *Handbook of clinical nutrition* (3rd ed., pp. 339–371). St. Louis: Mosby.—An overview of obesity, including guidelines for estimating desirable body weight, etiological factors, disease associations, prevention, and treatment.

Willett, W. C., Dietz, W. H., & Colditz, G. A. (1999). Guidelines for healthy weight. *New England Journal of Medicine*, *341*, 427–434.—A review of the relationship between body weight and morbidity and mortality, and the creation of healthy weight guidelines.

# 93

# Exercise in the Management of Obesity

## STEVEN N. BLAIR
## SCOTT HOLDER

### INCREASING PREVALENCE OF OVERWEIGHT AND OBESITY

At a time when knowledge and interest in diet, nutrition, and exercise are at historically high levels, why does the prevalence of obesity continue to rise? The increase is most likely due to a combination of biological, environmental, and sociocultural factors. Biological factors have not changed over the time of the recent increase in the prevalence of obesity, but these characteristics undoubtedly predispose some individuals to become obese in the presence of an unfavorable environment (see Chapter 78). The primary environmental contributors to the increase in obesity include technological advances that have reduced the need for physical activity at home and work, and greater availability of high caloric density foods that are highly palatable and inexpensive. Possible sociocultural contributors to the rise of obesity are a prevailing mind-set that focuses on quick and simple fixes for problems, a focus on unrealistic ideals of thinness, and overreliance on diet as an approach to weight loss and management.

The primary intervention used for weight reduction continues to be based on a reduction of energy intake (i.e., diet), but increased energy expenditure (i.e., physical activity) is receiving more attention. There also are a variety of pharmacological and surgical options now available for the treatment of obesity. It is imperative that these medical treatments be viewed as adjuncts to increased physical activity and the development of healthy dietary habits if long-term success is to be achieved.

### PHYSICAL ACTIVITY AND WEIGHT MANAGEMENT
#### Prevention, Reduction, and Maintenance of Weight

Physical activity appears to delay or prevent weight gain often associated with aging (see Chapter 81). From 1970 to 1994, we followed 4,599 men and 724 women who received at least three medical examinations at the Cooper Clinic, including assessments of cardiorespiratory fitness by a maximal treadmill test, body weight, and other clinical variables. Change in fitness was calculated as the difference in maximal treadmill time between the first and second visit, and weight change was calculated as the difference in body weight between the first and last examination. The interval between the first and second examination was 1.8 years, and 7.5 years elapsed from the first to the last examination. Individuals who increased their cardiorespiratory fitness over time were much less likely to have significant weight gain during follow-up. For each minute of improvement on the treadmill test from the first to the second examination, women were 10% less likely to have a weight gain of 5 kg, and men were 15% less likely to gain 5 kg. For a weight gain of 10 kg, each minute of improvement in treadmill test time was associated with a 20% lower risk of significant weight gain in both women and men.

Physical activity facilitates the achievement of the negative energy balance necessary for weight reduction to occur, although exercise alone has a relatively minor effect on initial weight loss. A calorie-restricted diet has greater short-term effect on weight loss than does physical activity. Adding regular physical activity to a calorie-restricted diet typically results in a 1- or 2-pound greater weight loss than with diet alone. A general guideline is that 1 pound of body fat yields 3,500 kcal when metabolized. A person weighing 75 kg typically expends approximately 100 kcal to walk 1 mile and would therefore have to walk for 35 miles to expend the energy contained in 1 pound of fat. This example from thermodynamics demonstrates why it is difficult for overweight and obese individuals to lose significant amounts of weight initially through physical activity alone. The low levels of fitness in many overweight people make it unrealistic for them to be highly active, because they do not have sufficient and sustainable calorie-burning capacity. After some initial weight loss and improvement in fitness, overweight persons can exercise at higher levels, burn more calories, and have a larger effect on energy balance.

Even though physical activity contributes only modestly to initial weight loss, activity should be built into weight management programs from the beginning, principally because physical activity is crucial for maintenance (see Chapters 106 and 107). Notable evidence regarding the effect of physical activity on weight loss maintenance comes from data collected by the National Weight Loss Registry from a group of people who lost at least 30 pounds and maintained it for at least 1 year (see Chapter 106). A key finding among these successful maintainers was that they averaged an hour or more of moderate to vigorous physical activity daily. A similar amount of activity required for maintenance in formerly obese individuals has been confirmed by doubly labeled water studies. It is apparent that regular physical activity plays an integral part in the maintenance of weight loss.

Current public health guidelines are that every adult should accumulate 30 or more minutes of moderate intensity activity on most, preferably all, days of the week. However, greater amounts of exercise are probably required to produce substantial weight loss and to maintain large weight losses after they have occurred. Thus, it is reasonable to recommend up to an hour a day of moderate intensity activity.

## Health Benefits of Physical Activity

Regular physical activity provides significant health benefits regardless of body size (see Chapter 89). We followed 21,925 men (30–83 years of age) who completed medical evaluations between 1971 and 1989 (average follow-up of 8 years) to examine the health benefits related to cardiorespiratory fitness and body size. The medical evaluation included anthropometric measurements, a maximal exercise treadmill test, and other clinical assessments. We found that moderate to high levels of cardiovascular fitness provide protection against cardiovascular disease and all-cause mortality in both obese and lean men (Figure 93.1). In fact, fit but obese men had substantially lower death rates than lean but unfit men. Low fitness is more important than fatness as a predictor of mortality.

In addition, regular physical activity is effective in reducing the risk of disorders commonly linked to obesity such as type 2 diabetes, hypertension, gallstones, elevated blood cholesterol, and certain types of cancer.

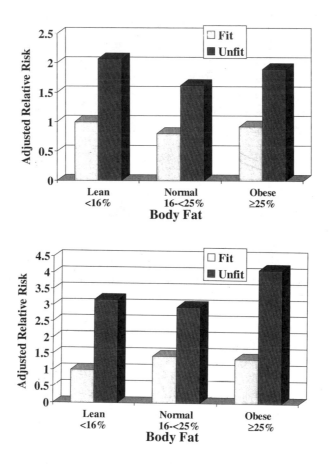

**FIGURE 93.1.** Relative risks (adjusted for single year of age, examination year, smoking habit, alcohol intake, and parental history of heart disease) of all-cause (upper panel) and cardiovascular disease (lower panel) mortality by categories of body fat and cardiorespiratory fitness. The lean, fit men are the reference category for each analysis. Body fatness was assessed by hydrostatic weighing, sum of 7 skin folds, or both. Cardiorespiratory fitness was assessed by a maximal exercise test on a treadmill. Data are based on 21,925 men, ages 30–83 years, who were followed for an average of 8 years after the examination. During follow-up, 428 men died (144 from cardiovascular disease). Data from Lee, C. D., Blair, S. N., & Jackson, A. S. (1999). Cardiorespiratory fitness, body composition, and all-cause and cardiovascular disease mortality in men. *American Journal of Clinical Nutrition, 69,* 373–380.

## Lifestyle versus Traditional Physical Activity

Most weight management programs use prescriptive approaches to alter dietary and exercise behaviors. Physical activity recommendations are often based on the traditional exercise prescription that emphasizes frequency, intensity, time, and type. Individuals are encouraged to engage in 20–40 minutes of moderately vigorous physical activity based on 70% of their maximal heart rate, 3–5 days of the week. This exercise prescription, if followed, is effective in helping individuals prevent weight gain, promote weight loss, enhance maintenance of weight loss, and provide other health benefits. However, poor adherence suggests that the traditional, linear approach to physical activity intervention has not accounted for the environmental and sociocultural contributors to inactivity. Also, many obese individuals are not fit enough initially to engage in 30 minutes of continuous physical activity in a single session.

Reevaluation of previous research and new studies led to altered physical activity guidelines so that people are encouraged to *accumulate* at least 30 minutes of physical activity on most days. This recommendation is consistent with what we call the lifestyle physical activity approach (see Chapter 103), which encourages sedentary people to integrate more physical activity into daily life to offset the reduction in daily energy expenditure caused by increased mechanization. Our controlled studies, and the work of other investigators, show that the lifestyle physical activity approach is as effective as the traditional exercise prescription in improving physical activity, cardiorespiratory fitness, blood pressure, and body composition.

## Brief Overview of the Lifestyle Approach

The lifestyle approach helps individuals use cognitive and behavioral strategies to accumulate 30 minutes of moderate intensity exercise over the course of the day. This approach encourages the accumulation of activity through daily-life routines at home and work, and does not specifically limit activity to scheduled bouts of exercise. An important facet of this approach is to help people alter the traditional mind-set regarding exercise and allow them to adopt a broader definition that focuses on a wider range of options for physical activity. Examples include using the stairs instead of taking the elevator, hand delivering messages at work instead of using email or the phone, parking the car farther away and walking to work or the store, and playing with children or grandchildren.

Conceptually, the lifestyle approach to physical activity is grounded in Prochaska and DiClemente's transtheoretical model, which stipulates that individuals do not change at the same rate and may require different interventions at various times. A variety of cognitive and behavioral strategies are used to tailor the intervention to meet the individual's needs based on level of motivational readiness and other characteristics. Common techniques implemented in our lifestyle intervention include goal setting, self-monitoring, and problem solving regarding barriers to physical activity, along with other traditional cognitive-behavioral skills.

Due to the poor fitness level of obese patients, the lifestyle approach may be a more feasible way to achieve the recommended level of physical activity. The lifestyle intervention is useful for both adults and children, and may be considered an alternative to the traditional gymnasium or structured exercise program.

## SUMMARY AND CONCLUSIONS

In summary, physical activity plays an important role in weight management. It can prevent weight gain often associated with aging, produce moderate increases in weight loss when combined with diet, and contribute to weight maintenance once weight loss has occurred. Regardless of body size or amount of weight loss, increases in physical activity result in significant health benefits. Furthermore, lifestyle activity may allow more initial success for obese individuals than traditional exercise prescriptions.

## FURTHER READING

Andersen, R. E., Wadden, T. A., Bartlett, S. J., Zemel, B., Verde, T. J., & Franckowiak, S. C. (1999). Effect of lifestyle activity vs. structured aerobic exercise in obese women. *Journal of the American Medical Association, 281,* 335–340.—Recent study examining the effectiveness of lifestyle activity in reducing obesity.

DiPietro, L., Kohl, H. W., Barlow, C. E., & Blair, S. N. (1998). Improvements in cardiorespiratory fitness attenuate age-related weight gain in healthy men and women: The Aerobics Center Longitudinal Study. *International Journal of Obesity, 22,* 55–62.—A significant study that demonstrates the role of cardiorespiratory fitness in lessening age-related weight gain.

Dunn, A. L., Marcus, B. H., Kampert, J. B., Garcia, M. E., Kohl, H. W., & Blair, S. N. (1999). Comparison of lifestyle and structured interventions to increase physical activity and cardiorespiratory fitness. *Journal of the American Medical Association, 281,* 327–334.—An excellent examination comparing lifestyle and structured interventions in increasing physical activity.

Lee, C. D., Blair, S. N., & Jackson, A. S. (1999). Cardiorespiratory fitness, body composition, and all-cause and cardiovascular disease mortality in men. *American Journal of Clinical Nutrition, 69,* 373–380.—A significant longitudinal study that demonstrates the health benefits associated with cardiorespiratory fitness regardless of body size.

Leermakers, E. A., Dunn, A. L., & Blair, S. N. (2000). Exercise management of obesity. *Medical Clinics of North America, 84,* 419–440.—Provides a succinct overview of the current role of physical activity, including lifestyle activity, in the role of weight management.

Marcus, B. H., Eaton, C. A., Rossi, J. S., & Harlow, L. L. (1994). Self-efficacy, decision making, and stages of change: An integrated model of physical exercise. *Journal of Applied Social Psychology, 24,* 489–508.—An excellent overview of the cognitive-behavioral skills needed for exercise adoption and maintenance.

Mokdad, A. H., Serdula, M. K., Dietz, W. H., Bowman, B. A., Marks, J. S., & Koplan, J. P. (1999). The spread of the obesity epidemic in the United States, 1991–1998. *Journal of the American Medical Association, 282,* 1519–1522.—Epidemiological examination of obesity prevalence in the United States.

McGuire, M. T., Wing, R. R., Klem, M. L., Seagle, H. M., & Hill, J. O. (1998). Long-term maintenance of weight loss: Do people who lose weight through various weight loss methods use different behaviors to maintain their weight? *International Journal of Obesity and Related Metabolic Disorders, 22,* 572–577.—Provides an in-depth examination of methods of successful maintainers in the National Weight Control Registry.

Pate, R. R., Pratt, M., Blair, S. N., Haskell, W. L., Macera, C. A., Bouchard, C., Buchner, D., Ettinger, W., Heath, G. W., King, A. C., Kriska, A., Leon, A. S., Marcus, B. H., Morris, J., Paffenbarger, R. S., Jr., Patrick, K., Pollock, M. L., Rippe, J. M., Sallis, J., & Wilmore, J. H. (1995). Physical activity and public health: A recommendation from the Centers for Disease Control and the American College of Sports Medicine. *Journal of the American Medical Asso-*

*ciation, 273,* 402–407.—Issues the public health recommendation of "30 minutes or more of moderate-intensity physical activity on most, preferably all, days of the week."

Prochaska, J. O., & DiClemente, C. C. (1983). The stages and processes of self-change in smoking: Towards an integrative model of change. *Journal of Consulting and Clinical Psychology, 51,* 390–395.—The initial article introducing the use of the transtheoretical model of change.

Wing, R. (1999). Physical activity in the treatment of the adulthood overweight and obesity: Current evidence and research issues. *Medicine and Science in Sports and Science, 31,* S547–S552.—An excellent overview of research regarding the role of physical activity in treating obesity.

# 94

# Behavioral Treatment for Obesity

## G. TERENCE WILSON
## KELLY D. BROWNELL

Behavioral weight loss (BWL) treatment has as its primary goals the modification of people's eating habits and level of physical activity. The emphasis is on changing behavior to restrict caloric consumption and increase energy expenditure through physical exercise, thereby producing a negative energy balance and consequent weight loss. BWL treatment has been more intensively researched, and its effects more thoroughly documented, than any other intervention for obesity. Treatment principles and procedures have been clearly specified in "user friendly" treatment manuals for professionals and the public alike. As a result, BWL treatment has been widely disseminated and accepted. Behavioral treatment has for some time now been regarded as a necessary component of any adequate obesity treatment program (see Chapters 91 and 92).

## DESCRIPTION OF TREATMENT

BWL programs are typically administered on a group basis. Current duration of treatment ranges from 4 to 6 months of weekly sessions. A core feature of BWL treatment is self-monitoring, the detailed, daily recording of food intake and the circumstances under which it occurs. This assessment guides selection and implementation of behavioral interventions. Self-monitoring is also part of the behavior change process. Patients use this self-monitoring of performance to evaluate their progress against realistic weight loss goals. Attaining these goals motivates continued adherence to treatment procedures. By learning to identify the personal and environmental influences that regulate their eating, patients can take specific actions to break unhealthy habits. The same behavioral principles are used to encourage increased physical activity (see Chapter 93). Other self-regulatory strategies include stimulus control, which is designed to limit exposure to cues that prompt overeating. For example, patients are instructed to do nothing else while eating (e.g., watch television), so that they remain fully aware of their actions and are not distracted from their consumption goals.

Comprehensive behavioral treatments include several other therapeutic components in addition to self-control strategies for altering eating habits and increasing exercise. There is a focus on improved nutrition. Rigid dieting is discouraged in favor of balanced and flexible food choices designed to reduce consumption of saturated fat and increase complex carbohydrates. Cognitive restructuring is used to identify and modify dysfunctional thoughts and attitudes about weight regulation. Interpersonal relationships are addressed in order to cope with specific triggers for overeating and to increase social support for weight control. Relapse prevention strategies are used to promote maintenance of treatment-induced weight loss (see Chapters 106 and 107). BWL treatment typically emphasizes moderate caloric restriction (1,200–1,500 kcal), but has also been combined with very-low-calorie diets (VLCDs) of 800 calories or fewer (see Chapter 96).

## EVALUATION OF TREATMENT OUTCOME

### Short-Term Effects

The emphasis on systematic and objective evaluation of both short- and long-term effects of intervention is one of the major contributions of the behavioral approach to the treatment of obesity. The results of group BWL programs are consistent and well-established. They induce an average weight loss of 7–10% of initial body weight over the 16- to 24-week treatment phase. Longer treatment duration produces only modest additional weight loss, since the majority of patients appear unable to lose more than 10–15% of their body weight. Combining BWL treatment with a VLCD results in greater initial weight loss but this is rapidly regained. Severe caloric restriction cannot be recommended.

BWL treatment reliably results in improvement in psychological well-being (e.g., reductions in depression, enhanced self-esteem, improvement in body image) and biological variables such as blood pressure and serum lipids.

### Predictors of Weight Loss

Predictors of weight loss have proven elusive. Personality traits, measures of psychopathology, presence of binge eating, dietary restraint, and history of weight cycling have all proven unreliable. The process variables of early weight loss and compliance with self-monitoring are the most useful predictors. Patients who do neither are very poor risks for treatment.

### Long-Term Effects

The problem with BWL treatment, as with other approaches, is that short-term weight loss is not maintained well at long-term follow-up. On average, patients regain approximately one-third of treatment-induced weight lost at 1-year follow-up. Thereafter, for the majority of patients, weight regain continues gradually until weight stabilizes near baseline levels. It should be noted, however, that a minority of patients do succeed in maintaining much of their initial weight loss over a 4-year period (see Chapter 107).

The pace at which weight regain occurs varies across studies, but the pattern is consistent. This is even the case in studies in which specific maintenance strategies have been implemented during the follow-up period. The latter have included relapse prevention training, extended treatment contact, social support, financial incentives, and the provision of portion-controlled foods.

Studies of the psychological changes accompanying weight regain over time have yielded mixed results (see Chapter 90). For example, one prospective study has shown sustained reductions in depression despite weight regain, whereas others have found that depression increases. The long-term effects of BWL treatment on binge eating have not been adequately evaluated.

In contrast to the negative outcomes with adults, BWL treatment for childhood obesity has yielded promising results (see Chapter 103). A family-based program for children (ages 6–12 years), which emphasizes lifestyle change and weight control in both the children and their parents, has shown that 34% of obese children had a decreased percent overweight after 10 years; 30% were no longer obese. Treatment that focused solely on changes in the children's behavior resulted in relapse by the 5-year follow-up. Consistent with other research, obese parents treated in the same program showed the all-too-familiar pattern of initial weight loss followed by relapse. By 5-year follow-up, virtually all had returned to baseline, and at 10-year follow-up, the parents in all groups showed increases in percent overweight.

One explanation of why children but not adults show lasting treatment effects is that it is simply easier to teach healthy eating and activity habits to young children than to adults. A second possibility is that parents can exert external control—including social support and food management—on children and even adolescents living at home. Obese adults who lose weight regain it because the self-control on which they have to rely gradually erodes.

Interpreting long-term weight changes is complex. Return to baseline weight would seem to represent abject failure, and may in fact be so, but must be judged against weights people attain if left untreated or if treated with an alternative approach. If steady weight gain is the norm in such people, as appears to be the case, a return to baseline weight would still represent a benefit.

## Effects on Binge Eating

BWL treatment is also an effective method for binge eating and associated eating disorder psychopathology in obese patients with binge eating disorder (BED, see Chapters 63 and 64). The evidence to date indicates that BWL treatment is as effective as cognitive-behavioral therapy and interpersonal psychotherapy in reducing binge eating, at least in the short-term. The data consistently show that moderate caloric restriction, which characterizes BWL treatment, has a positive effect on binge eating in obese patients. Contrary to criticism of BWL treatment, there is no evidence that moderate caloric restriction exacerbates binge eating in obese patients (see Chapters 17 and 73).

BWL treatment also appears to be comparably effective to cognitive-behavioral therapy in modifying the specific eating disorder psychopathology of dysfunctional concern with body shape and weight. Furthermore, BWL treatment has been shown to produce improvements in general psychological distress and depressed mood in obese patients with BED.

It must be emphasized that available evidence on the effects of BWL treatment on BED consists of short-term studies. Evaluation of the long-term effects of BWL treatment on BED and associated psychopathology is a research priority.

BWL treatment has several potential advantages over specialist psychological therapies such as cognitive-behavioral therapy and interpersonal psychotherapy. It is more disseminable and less costly, and can be used by a wider range of health professionals. Another advantage is that BWL treatment produces significant weight loss in obese BED patients in the short-term. Some studies have shown that obese binge eaters and obese non-binge-eaters respond equally well to BWL treatment in terms of short-term weight loss, whereas other studies have found that comorbid BED might result in a less favorable outcome.

## LIMITS OF BEHAVIORAL TREATMENT

It appears that relapse is attributable to patients' failure to adhere to the self-regulatory strategies they learn in treatment. By definition, for most patients, it appears that weight loss is insufficiently reinforcing to sustain compliance with a pattern of food intake and exercise that promotes a stable weight. Obesity is a chronic condition that may require treatment of indefinite duration. Accordingly, continued contact of one form or another with a treatment program is the best means of maintaining weight loss. But available data show that patients are unwilling to participate in continued, clinic-based sessions over time. Attendance at extended maintenance sessions declines after 6 months in clinical trials. A research priority is developing cost-effective strategies for maintaining patients' motivation to engage in health-promoting, self-regulatory behavior. For example, an intensive, focused, self-help program that provides ongoing social support and direction has shown promise in helping a subset of obese individuals maintain weight loss in long-term follow-ups.

## FUTURE DIRECTIONS

Currently, the problem of maintenance is being pursued using three different strategies. One is to combine BWL treatment with antiobesity medication (see Chapters 99 and 100). Obesity is influenced strongly by genetic factors and, once established, is maintained by several potent biological mechanisms. Pharmacological agents will be directed at these mechanisms or internal environment.

A second approach is to modify the external environment. Genetic influence is only predisposition and not predetermination, but it is expressed in a "toxic" environment that has increasingly exacerbated the risk to the vulnerable person because of the ready availability of convenient, palatable, high-fat foods and a sedentary lifestyle (see Chapter 78). Teaching relevant skills and providing the social support necessary to buffer against these relentless environmental influences will be essential in enhancing long-term maintenance of weight loss.

The third approach is a intensive, individual, cognitive-behavioral treatment that targets psychological processes involved in weight regain. Obese patients often reject modest, albeit healthy, weight loss goals and instead want to change their lives by losing large amounts of weight. Unrealistic weight loss goals lead to failure and disappointment that undermine motivation. Hence, the goal is to promote acceptance of more modest weight goals than patients would ideally wish. It is predicted that patients who are more accepting about themselves in general, and more comfortable with their body image in particular, will be more likely to accept a "reasonable" weight goal (see Chapters 72, 91, and 108).

Behavioral treatment has been used in some form in nearly every approach to weight control. Good, short-term results can be reliably produced, but maintenance is elusive. Behavioral approaches may be sufficient for only some individuals but necessary for all. Whether weight loss is produced by surgical, biological, or behavioral means, fundamental changes in behavioral and cognitive factors are necessary for progress to be sustained. Combining BWL treatment with other, more modern approaches, such as drugs and surgery, is an important area for enquiry.

## FURTHER READING

Agras, W. S., Telch, C. F., Arnow, B., Eldredge, K., Wilfley, D. E., Raeburn, S. D., Henderson, J., & Marnell, M. (1994). Weight loss, cognitive-behavioral, and desipramine treatments in binge eating disorder: An additive design. *Behavior Therapy, 25,* 225–238.—A randomized, controlled trial comparing standard behavioral weight loss and specialty cognitive-behavioral therapy in the treatment of obese patients with BED.

Brownell, K. D. (2000). *The LEARN program for weight management 2000.* Dallas, TX: American Health.—Widely used self-help manual based on cognitive-behavioral principles of change.

Cooper, Z., & Fairburn, C. G. (in press). Cognitive behavioral treatment of obesity. In T. A. Wadden & A. J. Stunkard (Eds.), *Handbook of obesity treatment.* New York: Guilford Press.—An innovative approach to maintenance of weight loss by focusing on psychological processes involved in weight regain.

Epstein, L. H., Valoski, A., Wing, R. R., & McCurley, J. (1994). Ten year outcomes of behavioral family-based treatment of childhood obesity. *Health Psychology, 13,* 373–383.—Summary of successful treatment studies of childhood obesity.

Garner, D. M., & Wooley, S. C. (1991). Confronting the failure of behavioral and dietary treatments for obesity. *Clinical Psychology Review, 11,* 729–780.—Critique of the effectiveness and suitability of dietary and behavioral treatment of obesity.

Jeffery, R. W., Drewnowski, A., Epstein, L. H., Stunkard, A. J., Wilson, G. T., & Wing, R. R. (2000). Long-term maintenance of weight loss: Current status. *Health Psychology, 19,* 5–16.—Comprehensive, up-to-date review of research on the maintenance of weight loss.

Perri, M. G. (1998). The maintenance of treatment effects in the long-term management of obesity. *Clinical Psychology: Science and Practice, 5,* 526–543.—Detailed analysis of the various maintenance strategies that have been used in attempts to prolong weight loss.

Wilson, G. T., & Fairburn, C. G. (1998). Treatment of eating disorders. In P. E. Nathan & J. M. Gorman (Eds.), *A guide to treatments that work* (pp. 501–530). New York: Oxford University Press.—Detailed analysis of the efficacy of pharmacological and psychological therapies, including BWL treatment, for eating disorders.

# 95

# Meal Replacements
# in the Treatment of Obesity

## DAVID HEBER

Since obesity is at epidemic proportions in the United States and elsewhere, efforts to change the food environment, as well as lifestyle and individual appetite and metabolism, will be required to solve this public health problem (see Chapter 78). With fast-food restaurants literally minutes away from most Americans, the urge to eat high-fat and high calorie foods can be easily satisfied. Meal replacements may be one means of helping some people control their weight.

"Meal replacements" are defined as functional foods in the form of drinks or bars meant to replace a meal. They were developed as over-the-counter modifications of the very-low-calorie diets popular in the 1970s, but have more calories and a more complete profile of micronutrients.

Meal replacements have become very popular among consumers; it is estimated that tens of millions of Americans use them each year. In a number of carefully controlled studies described below, meal replacements have proven to be a useful tool in the treatment of obesity by providing patients with reliable and good-tasting alternatives to eating calorically restricted meals. Meal replacements simplify food choices, aid in adherence to dietary regimens, and enable patients to restrict calories more effectively during weight loss and weight maintenance, since the dieter is confident of the number of calories per meal. Often, the estimation of food calories is much less certain. Many patients can sustain this approach without the need for ongoing professional intervention.

Meal replacements are safe and, when used as directed, provide measured amounts of calories, protein, minerals, fiber, and vitamins in the form of either ready-to-drink liquids, powders that are mixed with milk or other liquids, or meal replacement bars. They can be integrated into meal plans that include whole foods and most often provide more nutritional value than the dieter's usual food choices that they replace. After commenting on the nature of obesity and the need to alter the food environment, I briefly review the evidence supporting the use of meal replacements in the treatment of obesity, both alone and with pharmacotherapy.

## THE NATURE OF OBESITY TREATMENT

The scientific understanding of obesity has progressed from the historical view of simple gluttony and lack of willpower to the realization that this complex disorder results from a gene–environment imbalance. Humans have an inherited metabolic efficiency for energy storage resulting from a genetic adaptation to food scarcity but have been exposed over the past few decades to an increasing number of high-fat, high-sugar foods (see Chapters 12 and 83). Modern lifestyles also require less physical activity than man's traditional agricultural and preagricultural lifestyles (see Chapter 93).

While pharmacotherapy and surgery address the patient's ingestive behavior and metabolism, structured functional foods such as meal replacements address the alteration of the food environment as a component of obesity treatment. Since meal replacements are widely available and can be obtained without seeing a physician, they can be used initially with a physician's recommendation but continued without the need for further physician supervision.

## THE EVIDENCE THAT MEAL REPLACEMENTS ARE EFFECTIVE

Meal replacements can be effectively used by following the simple instructions provided in the package insert, and so represent a viable self-care option. In one study of the use of meal replacements in six sites across the United States, our group demonstrated that whereas men could lose 17 pounds over 12 weeks, women lost the same amount of weight over 24 weeks. Of those individuals who remained in the study (about half of all subjects) at 104 weeks, weight loss was maintained.

In a 5-year study conducted at the University of Ulm in Germany, individuals were randomly assigned to receive either a calorically restricted diet consisting of reduced portions of their usual foods or a regimen in which two meals per day were provided as meal replacements. Over 12 weeks, the group using meal replacements lost significantly more weight (16 pounds vs. 3 pounds, $p < 001$) than the group attempting to restrict the intake of favorite foods. Clearly, while both groups were prescribed the same number of calories, adherence was much higher in patients using meal replacements. Of particular interest, this study was continued for 4 years in a subgroup of patients who had significant sustained decreases in blood pressure, insulin, glucose, and triglycerides. In a small subgroup with hypercholesterolemia, cholesterol levels were also reduced.

In a community-based intervention in the city of Pound, Wisconsin, over 170 individuals were followed for 5 years, during which time they were given coupons for meal replacements to substitute for one meal per day. Patients experienced an average weight loss of about 10 pounds, and remarkably, over 90% of participants remained in the program. While there was net weight loss in this city, individuals in surrounding Wisconsin communities gained weight over the same 5-year period. We have recently conducted a demonstration project among 10 primary care physicians in the UCLA Healthcare Network. Physicians found meal replacements to be a useful tool for simplifying their task of initiating a nutrition program for obese patients.

## BEHAVIORAL RATIONALE FOR MEAL REPLACEMENT

Many obese patients find skipping meals easy to accomplish. In fact, many dieters spontaneously forego breakfast in order to postpone their encounters with foods that may trigger bingeing behaviors. The very-low-calorie diet or protein-sparing modified fast was based on the ability of dieters to forego the experience of eating in order to lose weight (see Chapter 96). Participants in these programs often described themselves as "not eating," despite the fact that they were ingesting 500 to 800 calories per day in liquid formula meals.

Meal replacements provide more calories per serving (approximately 220 calories per serving) than very-low-calorie diets (about 110 calories per serving) and are typically incorporated into meal plans using whole foods as well as meal replacements. Many obese patients eat in response to environmental triggers other than hunger cues. By reducing the variety of foods in the diet, meal replacements enable dieters to focus on changing stress- and binge-eating behaviors. Meal replacements can be used to train patients in the skills of stimulus control and relapse prevention by using the meal replacements in situations where bingeing behavior would be likely. For example, patients can be advised to keep meal replacements in their car and to consume these instead of driving into a fast-food restaurant.

## NUTRITIONAL RATIONALE FOR MEAL REPLACEMENT

In order to lose weight, patients must consume fewer calories than they expend. Some patients skip meals altogether. This is not advisable, since subsequent meals often include more calories than those saved by skipping a meal. While fasting may be considered successful if it produces significant weight loss, it can lead to dangerous losses of skeletal and heart muscle. On the other hand, many dieters have misconceptions about the types of foods that reduce calorie intake. Meal replacements often provide fewer calories and less fat than dieters would consume using foods typically eaten during a diet. For example, a delicatessen tuna sandwich made with mayonnaise could supply over 700 calories and 30 grams of fat, while a Chinese chicken salad would provide over 1,000 calories compared to the 220 calories found in a meal replacement. While reducing calories, meal replacements do not sacrifice nutritional value. They typically provide high-quality protein, fiber, vitamins, and minerals, including calcium, which is important for maintaining bone and muscle health.

Meal replacements are typically low in fat but provide necessary protein and carbohydrate. Under hypocaloric conditions, the body still consumes a mixture of fuels, including lipids, which are largely drawn from fat stores when meal replacements with little fat are utilized to create an energy deficit.

## FUTURE DIRECTIONS

The taste and variety of meal replacements have improved over the past decade. One of the complaints of dieters using these products is taste fatigue. The increasing number of flavors, including many different meal bars, and fruit-juice and coffee-flavored drinks, provide the variety that is essential to maintain the interest of the dieter in continued use of meal replacements. As this trend continues, consumers will likely be able to maintain their use of meal replacements better over the long term due to these improvements.

Beyond ready-to-drink liquids and bars is the likely development of many portion-controlled meals that incorporate even more healthy ingredients, including carotenoids and flavonoids found in fruits and vegetables, and even green tea antioxidants. In the very near future, soy-based formulas that provide isoflavones will also be available.

In the future, meal replacements may well be combined with pharmacotherapy (see Chapters 99 and 100). Since the withdrawal of the phentermine–fenfluramine combination as pharmacotherapy for obesity, there has been an increase in the use of meal replacements for obesity treatment. Primary care physicians who have been more reluctant to use pharmacotherapy have expressed increased interest in the meal replacement approaches in our surveys. Because some appetite suppressants and satiety therapies have modest 5–7% weight loss effects, it may be that the combined use of pharmacotherapy and meal replacements will be more effective than either approach alone. In fact, if an additive effect were seen, a 12–14% weight loss would be observed, providing a powerful approach to the amelioration or prevention of common comorbid diseases such as hypertension, diabetes, and hyperlipidemia.

Meal replacements have found a place in both physician-supervised and self-care programs for obesity treatment. They are a healthy alternative for dieters seeking to restrict their calories effectively. As food technologies improve, the taste, texture, and consistency of meal replacements will continue to improve. The term "functional food" has been applied to any food that in some way modifies physiology in addition to providing calorie support. Meal replacements fulfill this definition by both enabling individuals to lose weight effectively and providing healthy nutrition.

## FURTHER READING

Ditschuneit, H. H., Flechtner-Mors, M., Johnson, T. D., & Adler, G. (1999). Metabolic and weight-loss effects of a long-term dietary intervention in obese patients. *American Journal of Clinical Nutrition, 69*, 198–204.—Well-controlled, randomized clinical study that compares meal replacements to usual care, showing impressive weight loss and metabolic effects achieved by meal replacement.

Fletchner-Mors, M., Ditschuneit, H. H., Johnson, T. D., Suchard, M. A., & Adler, G. (2000). Metabolic and weight-loss effects of a long-term dietary intervention in obese patients: A four-year follow-up. *Obesity Research, 8*, 399–402.—Four-year follow-up of patients in the Ditscheneit and colleagues study, again showing beneficial effects of meal replacement.

Goldstein, D. J. (1992). Beneficial health effects of modest weight loss. *International Journal of Obesity, 16*, 397–415.—One of the first discussions of the medical benefits of the modest weight losses produced by most treatments.

Heber, D., Ashley, J. M., Wang, H. J., & Elashoff, R. M. (1994). Clinical evaluation of a minimal intervention meal replacement regimen for weight reduction. *Journal of the American College of Nutrition, 13,* 608–614.—An early, multisite evaluation of meal replacement in clinical settings.

Heber, D., Ingles, S., Ashley, J., Maxwell, M. H., Lyons, R. F., & Elashoff, R. M. (1996). Clinical detection of sarcopenic obesity by bioelectrical impedance analysis. *American Journal of Clinical Nutrition, 64,* 472S–477S.—Study showing the importance of measuring fat-free mass in obese individuals with reduced lean body mass, as opposed to relying on body mass index.

National Heart, Lung, and Blood Institute, and National Institutes of Health. (1998). Clinical guidelines on the identification, evaluation, and treatment of overweight and obesity in adults: The evidence report. *Obesity Research, 6*(Suppl. 2), 51S–209S.—Comprehensive discussion of state-of-the-art methods for clinical intervention with obese patients.

# 96

## Very-Low-Calorie Diets

THOMAS A. WADDEN
ROBERT I. BERKOWITZ

Very-low-calorie diets (VLCDs) reached the height of their popularity in 1988, when Oprah Winfrey revealed to her 12 million viewers that she had lost 67 pounds by consuming a liquid supplement. Use of these diets, however, declined sharply a year later, when Ms. Winfrey announced that she had regained her lost weight and would "never diet again." Now, more than a decade later, interest in liquid supplements is growing again. This chapter provides an overview of VLCDs and recommendations for their use.

### OVERVIEW OF VLCDs

An expert panel convened by the National Heart, Lung, and Blood Institute (NHLBI) recently defined low-calorie diets as those providing 800–1,200 kcal/day and VLCDs as providing < 800 kcal daily. These widely accepted definitions overlook a critical issue, which is the size of the energy deficit induced by a given diet in a given individual. It is inconsistent to require a short, obese woman with a daily energy expenditure of only 1,500 kcal/day to receive extensive medical monitoring while consuming a 700-kcal/day VLCD, and not an obese man with a daily energy expenditure of 3,000 kcal/day on a 1,200-kcal/day low-calorie diet. The energy deficit, weight loss, and potential effects are far greater for the man, although he is not consuming a VLCD. This example illustrates the need to define a VLCD in terms of the energy requirements of the individual. Several investigators have suggested that a VLCD is any diet that provides ≤ 50% of an individual's predicted resting energy requirements.

Regardless of how a VLCD is defined, restricting energy intake further below 800 kcal/day confers only marginal benefit. Three randomized, controlled trials found no significant differences in weight loss between diets providing 800 kcal/day and those with as few as 400 kcal/day. Failure of more restrictive diets to increase weight loss may be attributable to their inducing larger reductions in resting and nonresting energy expenditure, the occurrence of which would thwart weight loss.

## Composition of VLCDs

VLCDs are designed to produce the most rapid weight loss possible while preserving body protein (i.e., muscle mass). This is accomplished with large amounts of dietary protein, usually 70–100 grams/day. Most individuals obtain protein from commercially available powdered-protein diets that are mixed with water and consumed four to five times daily. These diets typically contain egg- or milk-based proteins and provide 50–100 grams/day of carbohydrate, up to 15 grams/day of fat, and 100% of the daily recommended allowance for essential vitamins and minerals. Alternatively, protein may be obtained from a diet of lean meat, fish, and fowl, served in food form (and known as a "protein-sparing modified fast"). This diet must be supplemented with 2–3 grams/day of potassium and a multivitamin. Both dietary approaches require patients to consume 2 liters/day of noncaloric fluid; typically, no other foods are permitted. These two diets produce equivalent weight losses, leaving the choice to personal preference.

## Patient Selection

VLCDs are recommended for individuals with a body mass index (BMI) $\geq 30$ kg/m$^2$; people with lower BMIs can reduce satisfactorily using less aggressive (and expensive) approaches. Medical examination must rule out contraindications that include a recent myocardial infarction; a cardiac conduction disorder; a history of cerebrovascular, renal, or hepatic disease; cancer; type 1 diabetes; or pregnancy. Behavioral contraindications include bulimia nervosa, current major depression (including bipolar disorder), substance abuse disorders, or acute psychiatric illness that would impair dietary adherence.

## Safety

VLCDs are generally safe when administered under appropriate medical supervision that includes a physician visit and blood test approximately every 2 weeks during the period of marked energy restriction. Following these guidelines, no cardiac complications have been reported in patients treated for up to 16 weeks. Patients may experience fatigue, dizziness, muscle cramping, gastrointestinal distress, or cold intolerance during the first few weeks, but these symptoms usually cause only minor discomfort and are easily managed. The most significant complication is increased risk of gallstones, the incidence of which is as high as 26% in some studies. Only a fraction of patients develop symptomatic stones that require treatment. The risk of developing gallstones can be reduced by limiting weight loss to 1.5 kg/week, as well as by prescribing ursodeoxycholic acid.

Anecdotal reports (and one study) suggest that VLCDs may increase the risk of binge eating, particularly when marked energy restriction is terminated and patients resume consumption of conventional foods (see Chapter 73). Paradoxically, binge eating remits dramatically when patients first begin a VLCD. The structured meal plan appears to help control unwanted eating.

## Multidisciplinary Approach

In proprietary programs, such as those offered by Health Management Resources (HMR) and Novartis Nutrition Company (OPTIFAST), VLCDs are usually administered by a multidisciplinary team that may include a physician, a dietitian, a behavioral psychologist, and an exercise specialist. Patients are treated weekly in groups of 10 to 20 persons and are instructed in the modification of eating, activity, and thinking habits. A typical course of treatment lasts 20–30 weeks and includes three principal phases: (1) the VLCD (12–16 weeks); (2) a "refeeding" period in which conventional foods are reintroduced (4–6 weeks); and (3) a weight stabilization phase (4–8 weeks). Costs vary but approach $2,500–3,000. Many programs offer a fourth phase of treatment—long-term weight maintenance. Fewer than 20% of patients participate in such programs despite the clear need to do so.

## RESULTS OF VLCDs

VLCDs induce losses of approximately 20–25% of initial body weight in both men and women during 12–16 weeks of treatment. These reductions are two to three times greater than those produced by a conventional 1,000–1,500 kcal/day balanced deficit diet (BDD) during the same time and are associated with marked improvements in blood pressure, blood glucose, lipids, and other indices of health (including psychological status).

Patients treated by VLCDs regain 35–50% of their lost weight in the year following treatment, even when they receive a comprehensive program of lifestyle modification. Six randomized controlled trials found that long-term weight losses ($\geq$ 1 year) with a VLCD were not significantly greater than those produced by a 1,000–1,500 kcal/day BDD because of the greater weight regain associated with VLCDs. These findings raise questions about the long-term benefits of this approach in view of the intensive (and expensive) medical monitoring required. In addition, cycles of rapid weight loss and regain are demoralizing to dieters, even if they are not associated with clinically significant dysphoria (see Chapter 90). An argument in favor of VLCDs is that they may confer greater improvements in health complications than BDDs during the first 12 to 18 months of treatment and may thus reduce the cumulative disease burden of obesity. There currently are not adequate data to test this hypothesis, although they may be provided by the Study of Health Outcomes of Weight Loss (SHOW) Trial, a 12-year prospective assessment of the effects of intentional weight loss in obese individuals with type 2 diabetes.

## LOW-CALORIE, PORTION-CONTROLLED DIETS

Historically, investigators have focused almost exclusively on the calorie content of VLCDs and overlooked the form and manner in which the diets are consumed. Liquid supplements, in particular, provide obese individuals a choice-free menu of portion-controlled servings that allows them to avoid contact with conventional foods. This approach is likely to facilitate excellent dietary adherence. Moreover, portion-controlled diets provide patients a precise estimate of their calorie intake. By contrast, studies using doubly labeled water have shown that when obese individuals are asked to keep a food record, they typically underestimate their calorie intake by 30–40% (see Chapter 23). Thus, when instructed to eat a 1,200 kcal/day diet, they may actually consume closer to 1,600 kcal/day. Differences in dietary adherence are likely to account for the greater-than-expected weight loss observed in patients who consume a VLCD versus a traditional BDD. From this perspective, it is the provision of portion-controlled servings, not the restriction of energy intake below 800 kcal/day, that is primarily responsible for the efficacy of VLCDs.

Support for this hypothesis is provided by studies that have used a liquid-meal replacement in combination with an evening meal of conventional foods (see Chapter 95). Ditschuneit and colleagues found that patients who were prescribed a 1,200 kcal/day diet of conventional foods lost only 1.2% of initial weight in 3 months, compared with a significantly greater loss of 7.8% in patients who were prescribed a 1,200 kcal/day diet that replaced two meals and one snack per day with a liquid supplement (Slim-Fast). Our research team obtained a 17% loss of initial weight in 4 months with the prescription of a 925 kcal/day diet that included an evening meal of food in combination with four servings/day of a liquid supplement (OPTIFAST). By decreasing the severity of caloric restriction, we were able to reduce medical monitoring from every other week to only twice during the 4 months, thus, substantially reducing the cost of treatment.

## RECOMMENDATIONS

Nearly two decades of research have led our research group to conclude the following concerning the use of VLCDs:

1. The prescription of VLCDs should be discontinued with most patients in favor of low-calorie diets (LCDs) that provide 1,000 kcal/day or more but which retain the use of portion-controlled servings, including liquid supplements and frozen-food entrees (see Chapter 95).

2. All obese individuals who plan to use a portion-controlled LCD to lose 5% or more of initial weight should consult with their physician to ensure that they do not have any contraindications to weight loss. Periodic medical evaluation is recommended to assess potential benefits and side effects of treatment.

3. Whenever possible, a portion-controlled LCD should be combined with a program of lifestyle modification, designed to improve eating and activity habits (see Chapter 94). Increased physical activity is particularly important, given its independent contribution to improved physical health.

4. Prior to treatment, patients should identify a program for facilitating the maintenance of lost weight (see Chapter 107); two approaches merit consideration (in addition to increasing physical activity to 180 minutes or more a week). The first is the long-term (indefinite) use of a liquid supplement to replace one meal and one snack a day. A recent study of this approach reported the maintenance of a 9% reduction in initial weight at 51 months. The second approach is the long-term use of a weight loss medication, as recently reported by Apfelbaum and colleagues (see Chapters 99 and 100).

These recommendations are based on the best information available. While some patients and practitioners may still wish to use a VLCD consisting solely of a liquid supplement, current findings suggest that comparable weight losses and improvements in health may be obtained at a substantially reduced cost by using a portion-controlled LCD that combines a liquid supplement with a daily meal of conventional foods.

## ACKNOWLEDGMENTS

Preparation of this chapter was supported, in part, by Grant Nos. DK56124-01A1 and DK54713 from the National Institutes of Health. We thank Shirley Wang for her editorial assistance.

## FURTHER READING

Apfelbaum, M., Vague, P., Ziegler, O., Hanotin, C., Thomas, F., & Leutenegger, E. (1999). Long-term maintenance of weight loss after a very-low-calorie diet: A randomized blinded trial of the efficacy and tolerability of sibutramine. *American Journal of Medicine, 106*, 179–184.—Patients treated by the combination of a VLCD and sibutramine maintained a loss of approximately 14% of initial weight at 1 year.

Ditschuneit, H. H., Fletchner-Mors, M., Johnson, T. D., & Adler, G. (1999). Metabolic and weight-loss effects of a long-term dietary intervention in obese patients. *American Journal of Clinical Nutrition, 69*, 198–204.—This study describes the superiority of a 1,200 kcal/day meal replacement plan over a traditional 1,200 kcal/day reducing diet.

Fletchner-Mors, M., Ditschuneit, H. H., Johnson, T. D., Suchard, M. A., & Adler, G. (2000). Metabolic and weight-loss effects of a long-term dietary intervention in obese patients: A four-year follow-up. *Obesity Research, 8*, 399–402.—Patients who used a meal replacement product maintained a loss of 9% of initial weight at 51 months.

National Task Force on the Prevention and Treatment of Obesity. (1993). Very-low-calorie diets. *Journal of the American Medical Association, 270*, 967–974.—This article provides a thorough review of the historical development, safety, and efficacy of VLCDs.

Wadden, T. A., Berkowitz, R. I., Sarwer, D. B., Prus-Wisniewski, R., & Steinberg, C. (2001). Benefits of lifestyle modification in the pharmacological treatment of obesity. *Archives of Internal Medicine, 161*, 218–227.—This investigation showed that use of a 1,000 kcal/day meal replacement significantly improved weight loss compared to treatment with a 1,200 kcal/day traditional reducing diet.

Wadden, T. A., Vogt, R. A., Anderson, R. E., Bartlett, S. J., Foster, G. D., Kuehnel, R. H., Wilk, J. E., Weinstock, R. S., Buckenmeyer, P., Berkowitz, R. I., & Steen, S. N. (1997). Exercise in the treatment of obesity: Effects of four interventions on body composition, resting energy expenditure, appetite and mood. *Journal of Consulting and Clinical Psychology, 65*, 269–277.—Consumption of a 925 kcal/day portion-controlled diet induced a loss of 17% of initial weight in obese women. Exercise training did not significantly increase weight loss.

Wing, R. R., Blair, E. H., Marcus, M. D., Epstein, L. H., & Harvey, J. (1994). Year-long weight loss treatment for obese patients with type 2 diabetes: Does including an intermittent very-low-calorie diet improve outcome? *American Journal of Medicine, 97*, 354–369.—Patients who received a VLCD for 3 months on two separate occasions during a 1-year trial lost an average of 16.0 kg on the first VLCD but only 1.4 kg on the second one.

# 97

# Popular Diets

## JOHANNA DWYER
## KATHLEEN MELANSON

## CRITERIA FOR EVALUATING POPULAR DIETS

Consider the criteria discussed below in evaluating whether popular diets are likely to contribute to safe and effective weight control. General categories of weight-reducing diets are shown in Table 97.1. Start by calculating a rough estimate of energy needs, using the approximation shown in Table 97.2.

### Calculated Calorie Deficit Approach

The calorie deficit approach involves active involvement on the part of the dieter in decreasing usual food intake. Energy deficits of 500 calories per day from energy balance levels (calculated as in Table 97.2) will cause a loss of about 1 pound of fat tissue per week. To lose 10 pounds, at least 10 weeks with perfect adherence will be needed. Deficits greater than 500 calories are not recommended for self-initiated efforts.

### Fixed Low-Calorie Reducing Diets

Many diets for weight reduction use fixed calorie levels that limit intake by controlling portion sizes, food composition, menus, choices, and spontaneity in dietary selection. Some people find such eating plans easier to adhere to than the calorie deficit approach. Popular diets of this type include reducing regimens in many diet books and fixed low-calorie diet programs operated by commercial and nonprofit weight loss management groups (see Chapters 95 and 98). They often use prepackaged and portion controlled foods such as low-calorie frozen and canned entrees, and other products available in supermarkets. Common energy levels of such diets range from about 1,200–1,800 kcals, but the problem is that they are often not individualized.

**TABLE 97.1. General Categories of Weight-Reducing Dietary Strategies**

| | |
|---|---|
| Calculated energy deficit | Energy intake = Energy needs − 500 kcal/day |
| Gram counting | Limit total daily grams of fat, protein, carbohydrate, and/or alcohol |
| Fixed energy deficit | |
| Moderate (balanced) calorie diet | Men: ~1,800 kcal/day<br>Women: 1,000–1,200 kcal/day |
| Low-calorie diet (LCD) | 800–1,000 kcal/day |
| Very-low-calorie diet (VLCD) | 600–800 kcal/day |
| Total or partial fasting | Never recommended |

## Gram Counting and Other Strategies

These strategies involve counting and limiting carbohydrate, fat, or protein to a predetermined number of grams. Dietary fat, which provides 9 calories per gram, twice that of protein and carbohydrate, is often targeted for reduction. Many foods high in protein are also high in fat, so when protein gram counting is used, fat intake is also decreased. For those who eat large amounts of sweet foods, counting sugar grams or limiting sugar intakes may produce calorie deficits.

Some diets work by permitting only certain foods. Particularly effective techniques for limiting fat include using leaner cuts of meat (especially among men), increased intake of fat-modified foods, low-fat methods for preparing foods, and combinations of substitution, reduction, and modification of fat-containing foods (popular among women). Abstinence from alcohol is recommended because it is very high in calories (approximately 7 calories per gram absolute alcohol) and not satiating. To determine the caloric contribution of alcohol to intakes, multiply the number of ounces of alcohol consumed by 0.8 and by the proof (the latter is defined as twice the percent alcohol in the product). For individuals used to high-fat omnivorous diets, the adoption of a vegan vegetarian eating plan also often causes weight loss, at least over the short term, owing to the time it takes to become accustomed to low-calorie vegetarian items.

## Moderate Hypocaloric Plans

Moderate hypocaloric plans, often 1,800 calories for men and 1,000–1,200 calories for women, provide the calorie levels used in many of the more responsible commercial weight reduction programs and the sounder weight control books. These regimens are sometimes called "balanced deficit" diets because they are based on relatively balanced deficits in fat, carbohydrate, and protein to achieve the lowered calorie level. Foods may be chosen from ordinary foods and recipes, low-calorie frozen entrees, and other reduced-calorie foods available in supermarkets or through commercial programs.

Structured, moderately low-calorie, nationally franchised weight control programs are operated in a variety of locations, including community settings, work sites, and health care facilities. Although physician consent is required before enrollment, monitoring of changes in metabolic risk factors or other health issues is more difficult than in

**TABLE 97.2. Estimating Energy Needs for Weight Maintenance**

1. Calculate the resting metabolic rate (RMR):
   Male RMR = 900 + 10 (weight in pounds/2.2)
   Female RMR = 700 + 7 (weight in pounds/2.2)

2. Multiply the resulting RMR by an estimate for physical activity level:
   1.2, very sedentary
   1.4, moderately active
   1.8, very active

health care facilities, where medical charts are available and liaison with and referral to health professionals is easier. The advantage of the national commercial programs is that most of them have structured plans, materials, and internet web sites. They emphasize making enduring changes of a healthy nature in lifestyle, nutrition education, and behavioral strategies for real-life situations, and emphasize regular physical activity and exercise. Most of them include weekly meetings, either in groups or with a counselor who may be a registered nurse, licensed practical nurse, registered dietitian, staff member, or a former client who has successfully lost weight and now leads others. The programs vary in their safety, cost, nutritional value of the diets they recommend, effectiveness, and support provided to dieters during and after weight loss. Several programs now provide special meals for those on special diets, such as vegetarian and kosher. Many are now focusing on maintenance efforts; some offer free or lower cost programs to graduates who enroll for maintenance.

Lay-self help programs available at low or no cost include Take Off Pounds Sensibly (TOPS) and Overeaters Anonymous (OA). They have no specific recommended diet plan and recommend that members obtain weight-reduction diets from their health professionals. However, some restrict specific foods such as sugar or white flour. Reasonable, moderately low-calorie diets are also available in some books.

In choosing among the programs, some of the factors to consider are cost, whether the diet provided is nutritionally balanced and adequate, whether it includes choices from all of the food groups (helping to train the patient for weight maintenance), and the provisions for ongoing guidance to maintain weight loss via lifestyle eating behaviors and exercise.

## Low-Calorie Diets

Low-calorie diets (LCDs) provide from 800 to 1,000 calories per day. They require medical supervision, since they have noticeable effects on metabolism and psychological factors. They are best suited for individuals who have significant medical reasons for losing weight rapidly, such as type 2 (non-insulin-dependent) diabetes mellitus, high blood cholesterol and triglycerides, high blood glucose, high blood pressure, and orthopedic problems.

There are two major types of LCDs. First are those based on regular foods that are used in most of the commercial programs. These require vitamin and mineral supplementation (with iron, calcium, vitamin $B_6$, riboflavin, and others) to be adequate, since it is difficult to meet these needs from food sources alone on diets that provide less than 1,200 calories. Many commercial weight control programs now offer liquid meal replacements, prepackaged meals, vitamin supplements, or other products in addition to basic instructions and a LCD. Prepackaged meals or meal replacements reduce the food choices that must be made (see Chapter 95). Some dieters find such preprogramming helpful. However, those who have a significant amount of weight to lose and must remain on the diet for many months may become bored by the limited number of food choices. Because food is provided, the dieter does not practice making daily food choices needed over the long term. Sooner or later, these skills must be learned if relapse is to be avoided. Also, the foods are expensive.

Second are LCDs using specially formulated or fortified food products or meal replacements. Such products now include liquid formulas (usually milk- or soy-based) and dried, canned, or frozen microwavable meals that are available in supermarkets and drugstores, and are becoming increasingly popular. If used according to directions with other low-calorie foods and consumed at levels of 1,100–1,200 calories, they can provide a complete diet, and may provide a helpful and safe low-calorie interlude for those who are able to adhere to the regimen. However, dieters who do not use them as directed (as for only one or two meals per day, and without the recommended supplemental foods) may run the risk of nutrient deficiencies.

## Very-Low-Calorie Diets

Very-low-calorie diets (VLCDs) provide 600–800 calories per day or less (see Chapter 96). Any diet less than 800 calories is below that required for resting metabolism. As energy deficits increase, counterregulatory mechanisms come into play. Resting metabolic rates fall—by as much as 15% in total starvation; lethargy results in decreased physical activity and exercise tolerance, with the end result that the energy deficit is less than anticipated. VLCDs also lead to dramatic shifts in fluid and electrolyte balance, lightheadedness, dizziness, weakness, and feeling faint on standing. Due to the risk of side effects, compromised metabolism, dehydration, ketosis, nutrient deficiencies, and deprivation-induced hyperphagia, VLCDs should not be undertaken without close medical supervision.

VLCDs are not appropriate for self-initiated dieting efforts. They are also inappropriate for most obese children, adolescents under 18 years of age (especially those who are pubertal), pregnant and lactating women, the elderly, persons who are ill, and those with emotional problems.

Clinic- or hospital-based programs are a good option when VLCDs or protein-supplemented modified fasts that require close medical management are used. Access to medical charts, a broad range of health professionals, and professional quality assurance checks are more likely than in commercial settings and are helpful, especially for patients with complex medical problems. Several national programs are available in clinical settings that include VLCDs for initial weight loss followed by LCDs after weight loss has leveled off.

## Total Fasting

Total fasting or starvation (no food intake) is a drastic and inappropriate weight loss strategy for all persons. It causes nutrient deficiency and very large losses in lean body mass, including wasting of the vital organs and muscle, a lowering of resting metabolic rate (15% or more), decreased voluntary physical activity, and intolerance to exercise. Accelerated loss of lean body mass ensues. Once glycogen stores are depleted, carbon skeletons from the glucogenic amino acids are used for glucose synthesis to maintain blood sugar, with resulting increases in protein catabolism. Fasting seems appealing initially because the glycogen depletion and protein catabolism cause saliuresis, kaliuresis, and diuresis, with decreased water balance and weight. Partial or intermittent fasts are also inappropriate because the starvation often results in compensatory binging, or rebound bulimia.

## Composition of the Diet

The composition of the reducing diet affects weight loss, nutrition, and hydration status, especially when energy intake is less than 800 kcals (see Chapters 7 and 8).

Protein is necessary to prevent losses of lean tissue, and the lower the energy intake, the greater the need for protein. High-protein diets (30% calories) that are low in carbohydrate are currently popular. The notion is that carbohydrate consumption above a certain amount will stimulate the release of insulin and promote energy storage and weight gain. However, metabolic fuels are not stored during periods of energy deficits. Most of these diets work because they are ketogenic and hypocaloric (usually about 1,200 kcals).

Carbohydrate levels are important in reducing diets. At least 50–100 grams of carbohydate per day (the amount provided by 4–8 tablespoons of sugar) are needed to spare protein, maintain the blood sugar level, and keep fluid balance at healthy levels. When carbohydrate intake is less than this, insulin levels fall and protein is catabolized to provide the glucogenic amino acids, which can be converted to glucose, the fuel for cells that require glucose. When protein must be catabolized to maintain blood glucose levels, additional water is liberated as the protein is degraded. For each gram of protein or glycogen that is broken down, 3 grams of water are released, leading to large shifts in weight due to changes in fluid balance.

The glycemic index is a term used to describe the rise in blood glucose that results from consumption of a defined amount of carbohydrate relative to the same amount of carbohydrate from a control food (usually 50 g white bread). Consumption of foods with low glycemic indices has been suggested as a tool for treatment and prevention of obesity on the premise that foods whose consumption triggers a rapid, high peak in blood glucose will later produce a rapid drop in blood glucose and blood sugar below levels before eating, with an increase in appetite and food consumption. Although satiety may be transiently affected, longer-term energy intake, and thus weight regulation, may not.

Adequate dietary fiber levels are also important to avoid constipation and to add bulk to the diet.

Electrolytes, including potassium and sodium, must be included, particularly for persons on VLCDs. Diets for weight loss must also incorporate sufficient fluids, vitamins, and minerals to meet the Recommended Dietary Allowance levels. At least 8 glasses of water per day are recommended for patients undergoing weight loss, and more with excessive exercise and/or environmental heat. Vitamin and mineral supplements are recommended for individuals consuming less than 1,200 kcal per day.

## Consumer Issues

The costs of popular diets vary, but costs and effectiveness are not necessarily related. The most expensive plans are not necessarily the most effective or safest. Weight management programs should adhere to ethical business practices in marketing and advertising. Programs should explicitly and fully disclose the physiological and psychological risks associated with weight loss and regain, as well as costs and a realistic estimate of the long-term success of the program after 1 and 5 years.

A good popular diet should include a healthful, nutritious diet plan, physical activity and exercise, and behavior modification in both the weight loss and maintenance phases. When comorbities are present that require simultaneous dietary or medical management, and whenever medications are used, a physician's guidance is also essential.

Long-term maintenance of a healthier weight is essential to reap health benefits but the strategies needed differ from those required for weight loss. Intakes must be lower in energy than those prior to weight reduction, since both resting metabolism and the energy cost of moving the lighter body are less. In general, low-fat, high-fiber, high-carbohydrate, nutritionally adequate patterns and a physically active life that includes exercise and behavior modification in line with lifestyle realities are best for keeping excess weight off (see Chapters 93, 94, and 107).

## AREAS NEEDING RESEARCH

We know enough to assist people in distinguishing between sound and unsound popular diets. However, much remains to be done. We must find ways to help people adopt more realistic targets for their weight reduction efforts. Better regulation of the marketing and advertising of popular diets, including the claims made in popular books, is needed. Means for improving our ability to predict who is likely to benefit the most from different kinds of self-help efforts are needed. Systematic monitoring and reporting mechanisms on both the beneficial and adverse effects of popular self-help dieting programs and long-term effects of weight maintenance are also vital.

## FURTHER READING

Allara, L. (2000). The return of the high-protein, low carbohydrate diet: Weighing the risks. *Nutrition in Clinical Practice, 15*, 26–29.—A recent analysis of current popular diets.

Konnikoff, R., & Dwyer, J. (2000). Popular diets and other treatments of obesity. In T. G. Heffner & D. H. Lockwood (Eds.), *Obesity: Pathology and therapy*. New York: Springer.—Discusses problems of several popular diets.

Melanson, K., & Dwyer, J. (in press). Popular diets for the treatment of overweight and obesity. In T. A. Wadden & A. J. Stunkard (Eds.), *Handbook of obesity treatment*. New York: Guilford Press.—A comprehensive discussion of popular diets.

National Heart, Lung, and Blood Institute, and National Institutes of Health. (1998). Clinical guidelines on the identification, evaluation, and treatment of overweight and obesity in adults: The Evidence Report. *Obesity Research, 6*(Suppl. 2), 51S–209S.—Authoritative guidance on evidence for various weight loss strategies.

Rolls, B. J., & Hammer, V. A. (1995). Fat, carbohydrate, and the regulation of energy intake.

*American Journal of Clinical Nutrition, 62,* 1086S–1096S.—Discussion of the important roles of hunger and satiety in reducing diets.

Willett, W. C., Dietz, W. H., & Colditz, G. A. (1999). Guidelines for healthy weight. *New England Journal of Medicine, 341,* 427–434.—Describes healthy weight targets and their rationale.

Van Itallie, T. B., & Yang, M. U. (1977). Current concepts in nutrition: Diet and weight loss. *New England Journal of Medicine, 297,* 1158–1160.—Classic article on shifts in water balance on various diets.

# 98

# Commercial and Self-Help Weight Loss Programs

## LESLIE G. WOMBLE
## THOMAS A. WADDEN

Obese individuals often turn to commercial or self-help programs to lose weight. These programs serve many more people than do university and hospital clinics. Despite the high demand for commercial and self-help programs, there was little supervision of this industry until the 1990s. This chapter briefly describes commercial nonmedical programs, medically based proprietary interventions, self-help approaches, and web-based programs. It concludes with a discussion of research needs in this area and likely trends in the field.

## ACTIONS OF THE FEDERAL TRADE COMMISSION

In 1990, Congressman Ron Wyden initiated hearings on the misleading and deceptive advertising practices of the commercial weight loss industry. He revealed that few, if any, data support claims that clients can lose all the weight they wanted and keep it off forever. In response to the hearings, the Federal Trade Commission (FTC) stepped up monitoring of these programs. Companies agreed to stop airing questionable ads. They were required to support claims of long-term weight loss with data and to provide a disclaimer that the results reported in testimonials might not be typical.

In 1997, the FTC assembled a panel of academics, industry providers, consumer advocates, and government officials to explore the creation of voluntary guidelines for the disclosure of information concerning weight loss programs. The panel established the Partnership for Healthy Weight Management. Commercial weight loss organizations who join this partnership agree to provide consumers with information to help them identify a program that best fits their needs. This information is summarized in Table 98.1.

## NONMEDICAL WEIGHT LOSS PROGRAMS

Popular nonmedical, commercial programs currently include Weight Watchers, Jenny Craig, and L.A. Weight Loss. These programs vary widely in their approach but generally focus on diet, exercise, and lifestyle modification. Social support is also offered by group (e.g.,Weight Watchers) and individual counseling (e.g., Jenny Craig). In either case, laypeople trained by the company usually provide treatment. Medical care is typically not provided, making these programs most appropriate for individuals who do not have major health problems.

With the exception of Weight Watchers, few data exist to support the effectiveness of nonmedical commercial programs. A recent study showed that Weight Watchers was superior to self-help dieting after 1 year, with weight losses of 5.0 kg and 1.7 kg, respectively. The results, however, may represent a "best case" scenario and cannot necessarily be generalized to the vast number of dieters who enroll in Weight Watchers each year.

**TABLE 98.1. Voluntary Guidelines for Providers of Weight Loss Products or Services**

| Criteria | Description |
|---|---|
| 1. Staff qualifications and central components of the program | • Program content and goals. <br> • Staff's weight management training, experience, certification, and education. |
| 2. Risks associated with overweight and obesity | • Obesity is associated with increased risk of heart disease, diabetes, stroke, etc. <br> • Moderate weight loss (5–10% of initial body weight) can reduce risks. <br> • Weight loss can cause physical changes in the body that are indicative of more serious conditions (i.e., dizziness, interruptions in the menstrual cycle, hair loss). |
| 3. Risks associated with the provider's product or program | • Risks associated with any drugs, devices, dietary supplements, and exercise plans provided in the course of the program or treatment. <br> • Rapid weight loss (> 3 pounds/week or > 0.5% body weight/week) may cause increased risk of developing gallbladder disease. <br> • Very-low-calorie diets (< 800 kcal/day) are designed for rapid weight loss in significantly obese individuals and are medically supervized to minimize risks associated with rapid weight loss. |
| 4. Program costs | • Fixed costs (administrative, entry, or renewal fees, etc.) <br> • Periodic costs (weekly attendance fees, mandatory food purchases, etc.) <br> • Optional costs (optional maintenance program, fees for reentering program) <br> • Any refundable costs |

*Note.* From the Partnership for Healthy Weight Management. (1999). *Voluntary guidelines for providers of weight loss products or services.* Washington, DC: Federal Trade Commission.

In the absence of outcome data showing that more expensive programs are associated with larger weight losses, or better maintenance of weight loss, consumers are advised to beware of commercial programs that require them to purchase food, vitamins, or special services.

## MEDICALLY BASED PROPRIETARY PROGRAMS

Medically based proprietary programs reached the height of their popularity in the late 1980s. They have traditionally combined the use of a very-low-calorie diet (VLCD), providing 400–800 kcal/day, with a multidisciplinary program of lifestyle modification (see Chapter 96). These physician-supervised programs, including OPTIFAST and Health Management Resources (HMR), are recommended for patients with a BMI $\geq$ 30 kg/m$^2$.

The safety and efficacy of both OPTIFAST and HMR have been extensively assessed. Both approaches induce a loss of approximately 20% of initial weight during 4–6 months of treatment. Patients, however, typically regain 35–50% of their lost weight in the year following treatment. This makes it imperative that patients participate in a weight loss maintenance program, as well as consider the cost of these programs, which is typically $2,500–3,000.

## RESIDENTIAL PROGRAMS

Residential weight loss programs, such as the Duke Diet and Fitness Center or the Pritikin Center, are typically administered by a multidisciplinary team that provides nutrition, exercise, and lifestyle modifcation, along with medical management. These interventions are typically very expensive. One week at the Duke Diet and Fitness Center costs $3,095, which does not include housing.

A literature review did not reveal any data to support the short- or long-term superiority of residential programs over outpatient interventions. Consumers need to consider whether residential programs offer unique benefits that justify their substantial costs (which exceed even the most expensive outpatient programs, such as VLCDs).

## SELF-HELP APPROACHES

Self-help programs vary widely in treatment philosophy and techniques. They are organized and conducted by laypersons, all of whom have struggled with their weight or eating. These programs consistently charge no fee or only a nominal one. Self-help is based on the belief that individuals who suffer from the same condition can provide empathy and understanding, as well as specific suggestions for coping with problem eating and activity patterns. Examples of self-help programs include Overeaters Anonymous (OA), Take Off Pounds Sensibly (TOPS), and the Trevose Behavior Modification Program. Few data exist to support the effectiveness of these programs.

Self-help is also available in the form of hundreds of weight loss books and manuals. The most extensively evaluated of these is the *LEARN Program for Weight Management*, which provides a 16-week, step-by-step guide to modifying eating, activity, and thinking habits. Studies have suggested however, that LEARN is more effective when delivered by a health professional than when used on a self-help basis.

## SUPERMARKET SELF-HELP

Supermarket self-help emphasizes reducing calorie intake by using portion-controlled meals. Liquid-meal replacements, such as Slim-Fast, may be purchased at local supermarkets without joining a weight loss program (see Chapter 95). Consumers are free to choose the number of portion-controlled meals they eat per day or week, as well as the number of weeks they choose to diet.

Ditschuneit and colleagues recently showed in a randomized controlled trial that patients who adhered to the Slim-Fast plan lost 11.3% of initial weight during 27 months of treatment. In this study, however, participants met monthly with a nutritionist. They were provided a diet plan, along with sample menus and recipes, and taught to keep food diaries. Consumers who use Slim-Fast products on their own will not receive these interventions, which makes it difficult to generalize the findings of the Ditschuneit study to the average Slim-Fast patron.

## WEB-BASED PROGRAMS

The commercial weight loss industry has entered the web-based economy in the hope of attracting clients who wish to lose weight (see Chapter 110). Web-based programs, including *Nutrisystem.com* and *e-diets.com*, rely on the convenience of the Internet. Unlimited contact and support is provided through on-line chat rooms and 24-hour access to diet and exercise information. Like nonmedical commercial programs, internet interventions vary widely in their approach but generally provide information on diet, exercise, and lifestyle modification. *Nutrisystem.com* requires consumers to purchase prepackaged foods, whereas *e-diets.com* provides customized shopping lists from which consumers choose their own foods. No data exist to support the efficacy of commercial, web-based programs.

## FUTURE RESEARCH

We encourage all commercial programs to collect and publicize the data called for by the Partnership for Healthy Weight Management (see Table 98.1). In addition, we hope that programs will report findings concerning short- and long-term changes in weight and other health outcomes. In collecting such data, providers need to use ecologically valid study designs that test programs or products under the same conditions under which the public will use them. This design stands in contrast to clinical trials that impose more rigorous control and provide more professional contact than do-it-yourself dieters receive. We hope that the provision of such outcome data will become the norm for providers of weight loss products and services, as it already is with companies that manufacture weight loss medications. Only then will consumers be able to make fully informed decisions when selecting a commercial weight loss approach.

## FURTHER READING

Brownell, K. D. (2000). *The LEARN Program for Weight Management 2000.* Dallas, TX: American Health.—A 16-week, step-by-step guide to modifying eating, activity, and thinking habits.

Ditschuneit, H. H., Flechtner-Mors, M., Johnson, T. D., & Adler, G. (1999). Metabolic and weight loss effects of long-term dietary intervention in obese subjects. *American Journal of Clinical Nutrition, 69,* 198–204.—A randomized trial of 100 overweight men and women that compared the Slim-Fast plan to a 1,200–1,500 kcal/day diet of conventional foods.

Latner, J. D., Stunkard, A. J., Wilson, G. T., Jackson, M. L., Zelitch, D. S., & Labouvie, E. (2000). Effective long-term treatment of obesity: A continuing care model. *International Journal of Obesity and Related Metabolic Disorders, 24,* 893–898.—Description and evaluation of the Trevose Behavior Modification Program, a unique, self-help, weight loss program.

Lowe, M. R., Miller-Kovach, K., Frye, N., & Phelan, S. P. (1999). An initial evaluation of a commercial weight loss program: Short-term effects on weight, eating behavior, and mood. *Obesity Research, 7,* 51–59.—A 4-week study comparing Weight Watchers and self-help weight loss programs in 985 women.

Partnership for Healthy Weight Management. (1999). *Voluntary guidelines for providers of weight loss products or services.* Washington, DC: Federal Trade Commission.—A description of the Partnership, including its mission and principles. The Guidelines specify the content of the information that should be provided to prospective patients/clients and the tone of the disclosure.

Presiding Panel. (1997, October 17). *Commercial weight loss products and programs: What consumers stand to gain and lose* (W. C. Gross & M. Daynard, Eds.). Washington, DC: Federal Trade Commission.—Outlines the recent concern of state and federal governments in protecting consumers and improving the information they receive about weight loss products and programs.

Womble L. G., Wang, S. S., & Wadden, T. A. (in press). Commercial and self-help weight loss programs. In T. A. Wadden & A. J. Stunkard (Eds.), *Handbook of obesity treatment.* New York: Guilford Press.—This chapter provides an extensive overview of commercial and self-help weight loss programs, including descriptions of the various types of approaches and reviews of data where available.

# 99

# Current Pharmacological Treatments for Obesity

## LOUIS J. ARONNE

Historically, the pharmacological treatment of obesity has been associated with side effects, abuse, and relapse, leaving most practitioners reluctant to prescribe medications. Newer drugs produced more promising results and were not as habituating, but the short-term treatment paradigm that was utilized ignored health outcomes and resulted in relapse when treatment was discontinued. With the widespread use of phentermine and fenfluramine in the early 1990s, practitioners embraced a chronic treatment model, but overuse, misuse, and poor medical practice were typical. The withdrawal of fenfluramine and dexfenfluramine for safety reasons remains in the minds of many patients and physicians.

Recent guidelines from both the World Health Organization and the National Heart, Lung, and Blood Institute recommend that obesity be considered and managed as a chronic illness (see Chapters 84 and 91). While chronic management with a program of diet, physical activity, and behavior change would be optimal, this is not an effective strategy in all patients, and drugs must be considered.

Body weight is a regulated variable like blood glucose or blood pressure, and attempts at weight loss can be mitigated by counterregulatory systems activated in an attempt to prevent starvation (see Chapter 8). A model of the mechanism includes the brain, the controller; the controlled system, which includes body weight and food intake; and efferent and afferent signaling systems, which are neuronally and hormonally based (see Chapter 1). Current weight loss therapies are active on the efferent side of the feedback loop, and the results of clinical trials must be interpreted in that context. Limited amounts of weight loss can be expected with medication because the afferent system cannot be controlled and its counterregulatory influence limits weight loss. Failure of present medical treatments to produce robust results may reflect an inactive medication or a counterregulating mechanism that impedes weight loss and encourages regain.

Both physicians and patients tend to hold antiobesity pharmaceuticals to unrealistic standards of safety and efficacy. While safety is of utmost importance, medications for many diseases have side effects, but their benefit outweighs the risk. The same standards should apply to antiobesity drugs. Drugs approved for long-term use, sibutramine, a norepinephrine and serotonin reuptake inhibitor that enhances satiety, and orlistat, a lipase inhibitor that reduces fat absorption, have proven effective in large-scale multi-center trials and have side-effect profiles monitored readily by clinicians. In appropriate patients who lose weight on these medications, the associated medical benefit can be significant. The key is to treat patients in whom benefit from weight loss is greatest, those at the greatest medical risk. More than two-thirds of individuals with a body mass index (BMI) greater than 27 have at least one comorbid condition such as diabetes, hypertension, dyslipidemia, coronary artery disease, sleep apnea, and arthritis of the lower extremities (see Chapter 84). Recent studies of up to 2 years duration support the use of medication as an adjunct to lifestyle change and document improvements in comorbidities associated with weight loss and maintenance. In addition, studies document the value of lifestyle interventions in improving outcome when medication is used (see Chapter 94).

## INDICATIONS FOR PHARMACOTHERAPY

Pharmacotherapy is appropriate in individuals who are at medical risk from their obesity and have not responded to conservative management such as diet, exercise, and behavioral change; who have no contraindications to the use of the medication; and who understand the risks, the likelihood of success, and the need for long-term treatment. Guidelines by the National Institutes of Health support the use of medications as an adjunct to lifestyle therapies for patients with a BMI $\geq$ 30 who have no obesity-related comorbidities, and for patients with a BMI $\geq$ 27 if comorbid conditions are present. Patients with a waist circumference greater than 35 inches (women) and 40 inches (men) are also candidates for pharmacotherapy if comorbid conditions are present.

## MEDICAL TREATMENTS CURRENTLY AVAILABLE

### Drugs Approved for Long-Term Use

Sibutramine (Meridia; Knoll Pharmaceuticals, Mt. Olive, NJ), a reuptake inhibitor of serotonin, norepinephrine, and, to a lesser extent, dopamine, was developed initially as an antidepressant. It is typically started at 10 mg/day and the dose is titrated up to 15 mg/day if indicated. A 5-mg capsule is also available. Sibutramine decreases food intake and may increase thermogenesis in some individuals. Studies show that 66% of those who complete 1 year of treatment with 15 mg/day lose more than 5% of total body weight compared to only 29% in a placebo-treated group. Thirty-nine percent of patients lose more than 10% of body weight compared to 6% in a placebo group. A dose-ranging study showed the following mean percent weight loss for those completing a 24-week program: placebo, 1.2%; sibutramine 5 mg, 3.9%; 10 mg, 6.1%; 15 mg, 7.4%. Greater weight losses have been demonstrated in studies with more intensive dietary interventions. Sibutramine has also been shown to inhibit weight regain following a very-low-calorie diet.

The effect of sibutramine on lipids is the same as in placebo-treated patients, with comparable weight loss, although the improvement in triglycerides and high-density lipo-protein (HDL) is somewhat greater than expected based on weight loss alone. Sibutra-mine improves glycemic control in diabetics to the same extent as in placebo-treated patients who achieved comparable weight loss.

The most common adverse events include constipation, dry mouth, headaches, and insomnia. There is a 2% incidence of significant, sustained blood pressure increase in pa-tients taking sibutramine. Meta-analysis of placebo-controlled studies showed average in-creases of 4.1 and 2.4 mm Hg, respectively, in systolic and diastolic pressure. In patients who achieved greater than 5% body weight loss, however, blood pressure was stable or reduced. Patients taking 5 to 15 mg of sibutramine per day have an average increase in pulse rate of 4 beats per minute; patients who lose more than 5% of body weight have a lesser increase. Blood pressure and heart rate changes seen with sibutramine are dose-related and can be managed by decreasing the dose or discontinuing the medication. On-going monitoring of pulse and blood pressure are recommended in patients taking sibutramine. Blood pressure and pulse elevations can be identified clinically. Sibutramine is not recommended in patients with cardiovascular disease or uncontrolled hypertension, is contraindicated in patients taking monoamine oxidase inhibitors, and is relatively con-traindicated in those on other selective serotonin reuptake inhibitors (SSRIs).

A study of patients taking sibutramine showed no relationship between the use of sibutramine and valvular heart disease. Surveillance data do not suggest a relationship be-tween primary pulmonary hypertension (PPH) and the use of sibutramine. A serotonin and norepinephrine reuptake inhibitor (similar to venlafaxine, an antidepressant) rather than a serotonin releaser such as dexfenfluramine and fenfluramine, sibutramine is related to the antidepressant SSRIs, which have not been associated with PPH or valvular heart disease.

Orlistat (Xenical; Hoffman-LaRoche, Nutley, NJ), an inhibitor of gastrointestinal li-pases, acts locally in the gastrointestinal tract. As a result, it has no cardiovascular or cen-tral nervous system side effects. Orlistat blocks about 30% of dietary fat from being ab-sorbed at a therapeutic dose of 120 mg three times daily. A 2-year multicenter trial of orlistat 120 mg three times per day with a hypocaloric diet demonstrated a mean weight loss of 8.8% versus 5.8% in the placebo-treated group. Of patients taking orlistat com-pared to those on placebo, 66% versus 44% lost more than 5% of their initial body weight, and 44% versus 25% lost more than 10% after 1 year. After 2 years, 34% of orlistat-treated patients maintained a 10% weight loss compared to only 17.5% in the placebo group. Orlistat has been shown to prevent weight regain when used for mainte-nance after 6 months of dietary management in patients who had lost at least 8% of body weight. Orlistat-treated subjects regained 33% of their weight loss over 1 year of treat-ment versus 59% regain in the placebo-treated group.

Patients taking orlistat for 1 year showed a small mean reduction in diastolic blood pressure and improvement in lipids attributable to increased weight loss. Orlistat appears to have an independent effect on low-density lipoprotein cholesterol (LDL-C) levels beyond that induced by weight loss. LDL-C levels greater than 130 mg/dl were reduced 8% in the orlistat-treated group at the end of 1 year compared to no change in the placebo-treated group. HDL cholesterol levels were similar in both placebo- and orlistat-treated groups.

Orlistat appears to be helpful in the treatment of diabetes and impaired glucose tol-erance (see Chapter 104). In a trial of orlistat of patients with type 2 diabetes, 49% in the orlistat-treated group compared to 23% in the placebo treated group lost more than 5% of initial body weight after 1 year of treatment. Significant improvements were seen in glycohemoglobin, fasting plasma glucose, total cholesterol, LDL-C, triglycerides, and the

LDL–HDL ratio compared to placebo treatment. Patients with impaired glucose tolerance showed a significant shift into the normal category: 72% of orlistat-treated patients
improved from impaired status to normal, compared to 49% in the placebo-treated
group. Over a mean period of 582 days, only 3.0% of patients progressed from impaired
glucose tolerance to the diabetic category in the orlistat-treated group compared to 7.6%
in the placebo-treated group.

Side effects of orlistat are gastrointestinal in nature and caused by the passage of excess fat through the gut. Many patients have side effects initially, but these diminish over
the first weeks of treatment in most cases. In one trial, only 6% of patients dropped out
because of side effects, and in every trial, more patients dropped out of placebo than
orlistat groups. Patient education about the importance of limiting dietary fat can prevent
side effects; thus, the drug may enhance compliance with a low-fat diet by providing negative feedback to the noncompliant. Multivitamin supplementation is recommended because of a reduction in levels of fat-soluble vitamins. No effects on mineral balance, gallstone, or renal stone formation have been noted.

SSRIs such as fluoxetine and sertraline have not proven effective in long-term studies. Weight regain may occur after 6 months despite ongoing treatment. These drugs,
however, have been shown to be of benefit as an adjunct to the behavioral management
of binge eating disorder (see Chapter 64).

## Drugs Approved for Short-Term Use

Noradrenergic agents such as the Schedule IV drugs phentermine (Ionamin, Fastin,
Adipex) and diethylpropion (Tenuate), and the over-the-counter drug phenylpropanolamine (Dexatrim, Accutrim) are better than placebo in short-term studies. No large-scale,
long-term studies of weight loss or health benefits have been performed. If these drugs are
used for longer than 3 months, the patient must be informed that such use is "off-label"
and has not been studied.

## Over-the-Counter Products

A wide variety of products available to the public, such as chromium picolinate (a trace
mineral), chitosan (a fiber product), L-carnitine, and hydoxycitric acid, show insufficient
efficacy to recommend their use. These products are marketed as "nutritional supplements," with insufficient testing or proof that they work as advertised. Others, such as
the combination of ephedrine (ephedra or mahuang) and caffeine (guarana, kola nut) often seen in "fat-burning products," are effective at inducing weight loss but are not considered safe for unsupervised use at doses typically recommended (75 mg of ephedra base
per day) because of risk for side effects such as tachycardia and hypertension.

## Medications That May Cause Weight Gain and Alternatives

Many commonly prescribed medications are known to cause weight gain as a side effect.
When considering the use of antiobesity medications, attention should be paid to the use
of these medications and the possibility of switching the patient to other medications that
might induce weight loss. For example, sulfonylureas and insulin tend to cause weight
gain. Metformin is often the best first-line drug for the obese diabetic, since it may induce
weight loss, and improve body composition and lipids. The alpha-glucosidase inhibitors

**TABLE 99.1. Potential Targets for New Obesity Treatments**

| Target | Action of drug |
|---|---|
| *Appetite suppressants* | |
| Serotonin (5-$HT_{2C}$ receptor) | Agonist, reuptake inhibitor |
| Norepinephrine ($\alpha_1$ and $\beta_2$) receptors | Agonists, reuptake inhibitors |
| Dopamine (D1) | Agonist, reuptake inhibitor |
| Leptin receptor | Leptin agonist |
| NPY Y1 and Y5 receptors | Antagonists |
| MC3 receptor | Agonist |
| MC4 receptor | Agonist |
| Insulin release | Suppressor |
| MSH | Agonist |
| MCH receptor | Antagonist |
| CRH receptor/binding proteins | Antagonist |
| Urocortin | Antagonist |
| Galanin receptor | Antagonist |
| Histamine (H3) receptor | Antagonist |
| CART receptor | Agonist |
| Amylin | Agonist |
| Apo($A^{IV}$) receptor | Agonist |
| Orexin receptor | Antagonist |
| CCK-A receptor | Agonist |
| GLP-1 receptor | Agonist |
| Bombesin | Agonist |
| *Enhancers of energy expenditure* | |
| Uncoupling proteins | Stimulators |
| Protein kinase A | Stimulator |
| B-3 adrenergic receptor | Agonist |
| *Stimulators of fat mobilization* | |
| Leptin receptor | Leptin agonist |
| B-3 adrenergic receptor | Agonist |
| Growth hormone receptor | Agonist |
| Fatty acid synthease | Inhibitor |
| Protein kinase A | Stimulator |

*Note.* Data from Campfield, L. A., Smith, F. J., Burn P. (1988). *Science, 280,* 1383–1387; Bray, G. A., & Tartaglia, L. A. (2000). *Nature, 404,* 672–677.

acarbose and miglitol may also induce weight loss. Most antidepressants and mood stabilizers cause weight gain, although bupropion often induces weight loss. An anticonvulsant, topiramate can induce weight loss in contrast to the weight gain often seen with other agents, and there are case reports of its use to mitigate the weight gain associated with new antipsychotic agents such as olanzapine. Progesterones, corticosteroids, beta-blockers, and antihistamines, among others, may all cause weight gain.

## FUTURE PHARMACOLOGICAL TREATMENTS

The future of the pharmacological treatment of obesity is particularly promising, with many new drugs in the early stages of development (see Chapter 100). The rapid growth in our understanding of weight-regulating mechanisms will allow us to select more specific targets and permit us to design drug combinations that will be more effective. For example, human trials of recombinant leptin are currently underway. Early clinical trials have shown a mean weight loss of 7.1% in patients on the highest dose, with injection-site reaction being the only major side effect. A recent experiment performed by our laboratory demonstrated that rats with diet-induced obesity experienced synergistic reductions in weight and food intake when sibutramine was coadministered with leptin, suggesting that the plateau phenomenon seen with sibutramine, and probably other efferent treatments, is caused in part by a counterregulatory reduction in the serum concentration of leptin, an afferent signaling hormone. If this finding extends to humans, the combination of an afferent drug (leptin) with an efferent drug (sibutramine, orlistat) might provide encouraging results (see Chapter 6). Other drugs under development include compounds that activate central melanocortin receptors, unbind corticotropin-releasing factor from its binding protein, and beta-agonists that act selectively on skeletal muscle and/or adipose tissue to increase metabolic rate and lipolysis (Table 99.1 on the previous page).

## FURTHER READING

Aronne, L. J. (1999). Drug therapy for obesity: A therapeutic option? *Journal of Clinical Endocrinology Metabolism, 84,* 7–10.—A discussion of the appropriate role for medical therapies.

Bray, G. (1998). *Contemporary diagnosis and management of obesity.* Newtown, PA: Handbooks in Health Care.—An excellent, detailed review of obesity and its treatment.

Bray, G. A., & Greenway, F. L. (1999). Current and potential drugs for treatment of obesity. *Endocrine Reviews, 20,* 805–875.—A comprehensive, authoritative review of medical obesity treatments.

Bray, G. A., & Tartaglia, L. A. (2000). Medicinal strategies in the treatment of obesity. *Nature, 404,* 672–677.—An overview of medical treatment strategies, with an emphasis on those in development.

Campfield, L. A., Smith, F. J., & Burn, P. (1998). Strategies and potential molecular targets for obesity treatment. *Science, 280,* 1383–1387.—A review of potential medical strategies for obesity treatment.

Hvizdos, K. M., & Markham, A. (1999). Orlistat: A review of its use in the management of obesity. *Drugs, 58,* 743–760.—A comprehensive review of the drug.

McNeely, W., & Goa, K. L. (1998). Sibutramine: A review of its contribution to the management of obesity. *Drugs, 56,* 1093–1124.—A comprehensive review of the drug.

National Institutes of Health, National Heart, Lung, and Blood Institute, and the North American Association for the Study of Obesity. *Practical guide to the identification, evaluation, and treatment of overweight and obesity in adults* (2000). Bethesda, MD: Author. (Available online at *www.naaso.org*)—Provides the basic knowledge and tools that physicians need to implement obesity treatment in a clinical setting. The role of medications is discussed.

Schwartz, M. W., Woods, S. C., Porte, D., Seeley, R. J., & Baskin, D. G. (2000). Central nervous system control of food intake. *Nature, 404,* 661–671.—Provides an excellent review of the current understanding of body weight regulation.

World Health Organization. (1998). *Obesity: preventing and managing the global epidemic: Report of a WHO consultation on obesity* (WHO/NUT/NCD/97.2). Geneva: Author.—Discussion of obesity as a chronic illness.

# 100

# Pharmacological Treatments on the Horizon

## STANLEY HESHKA
## STEVEN B. HEYMSFIELD

After two decades during which development of drugs for weight loss appeared to slow, the last few years have brought renewed activity (see Chapter 99). This can be ascribed to several factors that have increased the market potential for new antiobesity treatments. The recognition that the prevalence of obesity is at unprecedented levels and still increasing, approval in the United States of only one new weight-loss drug in the period between 1970 and 1995 (dexfenfluramine), and its subsequent withdrawal because of previously unnoticed adverse effects, all influenced pharmaceutical development priorities. In addition, a spate of discoveries in the field of molecular biology, beginning with the cloning of the *ob* gene in 1994 and the identification of its protein product leptin, have revitalized drug development and the search for promising molecules. And finally, the growing recognition and acceptance that obesity is not a temporary predicament but one that requires long-term treatment has made the commercial potential of successful pharmacological treatment more attractive than ever.

One consequence has been a reevaluation by pharmaceutical companies of drugs currently approved or in development for other indications in which weight loss is a known side effect. The hope is to find a formulation or dosing regimen that will produce clinically significant weight loss. Weight losses are likely to be modest, but the medications vary in mechanisms of action and side-effect profiles, providing physicians and patients with choices.

Also, recent developments in molecular biology, along with the detailed exploration of animal and human genomes, have signaled a paradigm shift in identification of promising molecules. Specific endogenous proteins acting on specific sites can be studied for their effects. The effects are usually not specific or confined to simple disorders but have many seemingly diverse consequences. Still, the new techniques have enabled a more detailed and thorough investigation of mechanisms involved in weight regulation than was previously possible. Consequently, promising new molecules and sites of action have been identified and are being actively investigated.

We first survey variations on pharmacological agents that are in or near clinical trials for weight loss, grouped by their mechanisms of action. A final section mentions some new approaches based on recent molecular discoveries.

## DRUGS TO REDUCE FOOD INTAKE

Currently approved drugs in this category act mainly on serotonergic or adrenergic systems, but some of the most promising new avenues of development are those that explore alternative signaling pathways (see Chapter 1).

Drugs acting on dopamine receptors affect food intake, although the role and interactions of each of the five known receptors are not well understood. Bromocriptine, a D2 agonist that is used in the treatment of prolactinomas, has potential as an antiobesity agent. Ecopipam (SCH 39166), initially studied for its attenuation effects on cocaine-induced euphoria, is a D1/D5 antagonist and may also affect food intake.

Drugs acting on gamma-aminobutyric acid (GABA) offer another pathway for affecting food intake. Topiramate, an FDA-approved antiseizure drug, increases the frequency at which GABA activates its receptors. It has long been used for treatment of certain forms of epilepsy and has shown effects of reduced appetite and sustained weight loss in clinical trials for epilepsy, as well as some promising results in open label trials for treatment of binge eating disorder.

Dating back to the 1980s, numerous reports of psychiatric studies with bupropion, a nontypical antidepressant and smoking cessation drug, have noted weight loss or reduced weight gain. Bupropion enhances noradrenergic and dopaminergic neurotransmitter activity. It has not been shown to increase oxygen consumption and it is conjectured to affect mainly food intake. Since antidepressant medications are often prescribed for long periods of time, extensive data on the safety of bupropion are available. Dose-ranging studies may establish its viability as an antiobesity agent.

## DRUGS TO INCREASE ENERGY EXPENDITURE

One of the most active areas of research has been to discover an agent to increase the rate at which ingested or stored energy is dissipated as heat. In the past, this approach has been frustrated by side effects on sympathetic function, but these may be avoided with a sufficiently selective thermogenic agent.

Beta-3 adrenergic agonists hold considerable promise for selectively and potently stimulating thermogenesis. Several compounds have been investigated in human clinical trials. BRL26830A increased resting energy expenditure (REE) by about 12% and weight loss by 50% over values seen in control subjects. Human studies with Ro-16-8714 and Ro-40-2148 showed increases in REE up to 21%; however, elevations in blood pressure and heart rate were also seen. These agents, among others, were developed on animal $\beta_3$ receptors. At this time, no agent based on the human $\beta_3$ receptor has a clear lead in the development process.

## OTHER PRODUCTS

Cholycystokinin (CCK) is known to cause satiety when injected peripherally in animals and humans (see Chapter 2). Secreted by the gut in response to ingestion of nutrients, it acts both peripherally and centrally. Development of effective CCK analogues is being actively pursued and may lead to a successful treatment.

The development and marketing of nonabsorbable fat substitutes such as olestra for use in food preparation present another avenue for reducing caloric intake. Although presently found in only a few products, the number of available foods using nonabsorbable fats is likely to increase as additional experience regarding safety and side effects is gained. Controlled studies with blinded or naive subjects have shown that daily caloric intake tends to drop initially with the introduction of reduced-calorie foods, but compensation subsequently occurs via increased meal volume. The compensation tends to be incomplete, so there is some remaining reduction from usual consumption. Whether this remains the case when consumers consciously select such foods is not known.

Although there continues to be introduced large numbers of herbal and complimentary medicines claiming to be useful for the treatment of obesity, a recent review by Allison and colleagues found little supportive scientific evidence and few prospects for new products.

## COMBINATIONS OF MEDICATIONS AND NOVEL DOSING REGIMENS

The potential utility of combinations of medications has not been explored extensively. The large, robust effects produced by the combination of fenfluramine (a serotonergic agent) and phentermine (adrenergic), initially documented by Weintraub and colleagues in 1992, led to the widespread and successful use of the fen/phen combination, which ended only when adverse effects on valvular function were discovered. However, there is nothing intrinsically dangerous in the use of combinations of medications provided that the combination has been adequately studied. The management of hypertension frequently involves multiple, concomitant medications.

The safety of combination treatment is made more plausible if the medications have different, unrelated mechanisms of action, making potential drug interactions unlikely. Thus, a drug that affects absorption by its action in the gut may probably be safely combined with a centrally acting appetite suppressant. One combination treatment that has attracted interest is the use of very-low-calorie diets (VLCDs) (600–800 kcal/day) to produce initial weight loss followed by medication to prevent regain. Combinations of medication are likely to be more frequently used as more medications become available.

The possible advantages of interrupted or alternating regimens have not been thoroughly studied. Such practice would reduce total exposure to any one compound over a defined period of time, or permit longer treatment periods for equivalent exposure. It may also delay the development of tolerance and possibly reduce cost of medication. This is likely to become a more important consideration as duration of treatment stretches into years.

## NEW MOLECULAR TARGETS FOR THERAPY

The identification of genes whose malfunction causes phenotypic obesity has sparked a surge of research activity in both academic and commercial circles. The possibility of discovering potent and focused signaling pathways and molecular targets for obesity treatment looms on the horizon. These genes are discussed in detail elsewhere in this volume (see Chapters 3, 4, and 5). We mention two that are in pharmaceutical development at present and among the most promising candidates to lead to therapeutic products.

Leptin, administered subcutaneously or intracerebrally, produces dramatic decreases in adiposity in many animal models (see Chapter 6). Clinical trials of leptin in human subjects have shown a dose-dependent weight loss, but of a magnitude insufficient to be of clinical utility. Of particular interest, however, is the preliminary observation that leptin resulted almost entirely in decreases in the fat compartment while conserving the fat-free compartment. Research is continuing with next-generation molecules. Clinical utility and commercial prospects of leptin analogues will be greatly enhanced if a method of delivery other than subcutaneous injection can be employed. AXOKINE, a ciliary neurotropic factor, has also shown antiobesity activity in animals and humans, and appears to activate some of the same pathways as leptin.

Two melanocortin receptors, MC3-R and MC4-R, are involved in the regulation of body weight in animals. MC4-R, in particular, appears to be in a pathway shared by leptin and agouti gene function, and may be at a crucial nexus in the pathways that regulate human adiposity. Animals lacking the MC3 receptor tend to produce more fat for a given amount of food. These receptors appear to be promising targets for drug therapy, especially if a combination of drugs can be found to work on both receptors in the desired manner.

## CONCLUSIONS

Predicting the future is risky business, as punters and politicians well know. Predicting which pharmacological products currently in clinical or preclinical development will make it to market is no less a gamble. Products in development must clear many hurdles and survive many critical decision points before they reach the new-drug-application stage. Much of the information brought to these decisions is proprietary, subject to confidentiality agreements, business considerations, and often unknown to all but senior officers of the company, much less independent clinical investigators. This makes prognostication especially difficult; yet in view of the range and volume of research activity in this area, we remain optimistic about the future of pharmacological treatments for obesity.

## FURTHER READING

Allison, D. B., Fontaine, K. R., Heshka, S., Mentore, S. B., & Heymsfield, S. B. (2001). Alternative treatments for weight loss: A critical review. *Critical Reviews in Food Science and Nutrition*, *41*, 1–28.—Scholarly review of alternative treatments for obesity.

Bray, G. A., & Greenway, F. L. (1999). Current and potential drugs for treatment of obesity. *Endocrine Reviews*, *20*, 805–875.—A thorough, scholarly review of current and potential pharmacological agents.

Heymsfield, S. B., Greenberg, A. S., Fujioka, K., Dixon, R.M., Kushner, R., Hunt, T., Lubina, J. A., Patane, J., Self, B., Hunt, P., & McCamish, M. (1999). Recombinant leptin for weight loss in obese and lean adults: A randomized, controlled, dose-escalation trial. *Journal of the American Medical Association, 282,* 1568–1575.—The first clinical trial of human recombinant leptin in man.

Kordik, C. P., & Reitz, A. B. (1999). Pharmacological treatment of obesity: Therapeutic strategies. *Journal of Medicinal Chemistry, 42,* 181–201.—A review of strategies for the discovery of antiobesity drugs.

Nature Insight—Obesity. (2000). *Nature, 404,* 631–677.—A collection of reviews on the molecular biology of obesity, including approaches to medicinal treatment.

# 101

# Surgery for Obesity:
# Procedures and Weight Loss

WALTER J. PORIES
JOSEPH E. BESHAY

Obesity becomes a serious disease when it is *morbid*, that is, when the body mass index (BMI) exceeds 40 kg/m$^2$, equivalent to 100 pounds of excess weight. The 5 million Americans who are so afflicted are not only limited by their bulk but also have a high prevalence of diabetes, hypertension, coronary and peripheral vascular disease, congestive heart failure, obstructive sleep apnea, mechanical arthropathy, endocrine disorders, infertility, and cancers of the endometrium, prostate, and breast (see Chapters 76 and 84). In addition, the morbidly obese often suffer disabling psychological and socioeconomic consequences as a result of their excess weight (see Chapters 20 and 71). Although diet, exercise, behavioral therapies, and some recent medications are effective for many obese individuals, the results are disappointing in the morbidly obese.

## SURGERY, THE TREATMENT OF CHOICE

Today, surgery remains the only proven effective therapy for long-term control of morbid obesity (see Chapter 102). Candidates include individuals with a BMI > 40 or those with a BMI > 35 who also present with any of comorbidities of obesity as outlined earlier. Contraindications to surgery include unacceptably high operative risk, unresolved substance abuse, high likelihood of noncompliance with postoperative follow-up, significant uncontrolled emotional disease such as depression or history of suicidal attempts, failure to understand the procedure, or unrealistic expectations from the operation.

## A VARIETY OF SURGICAL PROCEDURES

Surgery for obesity can be broadly divided into those procedures that

- Limit the stomach's capacity for food (restrictive procedures: vertical banded gastroplasty and gastric banding)
- Interfere with digestion (malabsorptive procedures: jejunoileal bypass) or
- A combination of both: Roux-en-Y gastric bypass, biliopancreatic diversion, and duodenal switch.

The gastric bypass is, by far, the most widely performed bariatric operation in the United States today. That operation and the other, less common procedures are outlined below.

### Gastric Restrictive Procedures

#### *Vertical Banded Gastroplasty*

Vertical banded gastroplasty limits intake with a 30 ml. proximal stapled pouch and delays emptying with a small outlet buttressed by a strip of nonexpandable synthetic material (Figure 101.1). As with most obesity surgery procedures, weight loss for vertical banded gastroplasty is greatest in the first year following the procedure. After that, weight stabilizes, with slight tendency toward later weight gain. Although the proponents of the operation reported losses of 40–50% of excess weight 4 years after operation, too many patients were lost in follow-up to provide reliable data. Patients classified as *sweet eaters* were particularly prone to failure because they continued to consume high-calorie liquid or meltable foods such as ice cream or milkshakes, which rapidly traverse the stoma. Although complication rates of 15% were reported, also based on faulty follow-up, most bariatric surgeons have given up on the operation because of the high rate of staple line disruption and occlusion of the gastric outlet due to erosion or tipping of the synthetic band. Other complications include ulcer formation in the gastric pouch, which occurs in less than 10% of patients and is usually easily treated with $H_2$ blockers or proton pump inhibitors. Other serious but rare complications include subphrenic abscess formation, stomal obstruction secondary to stricture formation, and band migration or erosion. Although many patients have been revised to other bariatric operations such as the gastric bypass, others continue to do well. As this procedure is purely restrictive, the potential for malabsorption is less because the stomach and duodenum are not excluded. However, it is still important to supplement these patients with multivitamins, especially B complex vitamins, since deficiencies have been reported in rare patients.

#### *Gastric Banding*

Gastric banding (Figure 101.1) involves the application of a small belt just below the esophagus to create a small, proximal gastric reservoir with a limited outlet. The diameter of that outlet can be adjusted by inflating or deflating a small bladder inside the "belt" through a small subcutaneous reservoir. The concept has several advantages: The operation avoids the vitamin and mineral deficiencies of the malabsorptive procedures; the sur-

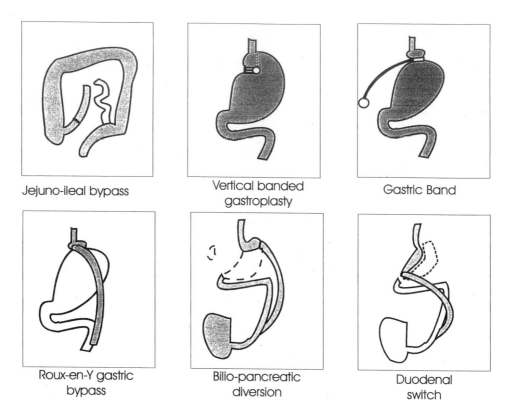

Jejuno-ileal bypass     Vertical banded gastroplasty     Gastric Band

Roux-en-Y gastric bypass     Bilio-pancreatic diversion     Duodenal switch

**FIGURE 101.1.** Varieties of bariatric procedures.

gery can be performed through minimal incisions with a laparoscope; and the size of the outlet can be repeatedly adjusted in the outpatient setting to suit patient needs.

Several models of the restrictive, adjustable bands are now under evaluation. The procedure carries a minimal mortality of $0 - < 1\%$. Reports of weight loss following this procedure are varied but have been reported as high as 55–65% at 3 years. The variation in reported weight loss may be attributed to difference in surgical technique and the type of restrictive device used. Recent studies have demonstrated little difference in complication rate between open and laparoscopic techniques. Early complications following this procedure include 10–15% solid food intolerance, but this can generally be managed by band deflation. The most common operative complication, reported in 13% of the patients in one large study, is the slipping of the band. This process occurs when the expanding proximal pouch pulls additional stomach above the belt, eventually leading to the occlusion of the outlet. Most of these patients require reoperation. Recent reports indicate that placing the band closer to the esophagus and stabilizing its position with additional stitches can avoid the slippage. Other complications include stomach perforation during the operative dissection, intra-abdominal infection, and pulmonary embolism. As with all purely restrictive procedures, patients can beat the surgery by consuming large quantities of soft, high-calorie foods. Overall, the initial results of this new approach are promising.

## Gastric Malabsorptive Procedures: Jejunoileal Bypass

The jejunoileal bypass (Figure 101.1) is included only for historical purposes and to condemn it. The procedure deserves mention because it was the first attempt to control weight through a surgical approach and the first recognition, in 1954, that morbid obesity is a serious enough disease to warrant an operation to control it. The procedure interfered with digestion through the exclusion of the majority of the small bowel from chyme, thus exposing only 14 inches of proximal jejunum and 4 inches of distal ileum to food. The excluded loop was decompressed into the sigmoid colon.

The jejunoileal bypass was the standard surgical treatment for obesity from 1954 to well into the 1970s, and produced significant weight loss in patients. The procedure, however, had to be banned because of its serious nutritional complications, including troublesome diarrhea, metabolic imbalances, liver failure, kidney stones, immune complex reactions, and hypoproteinemia. Some of the complications were due to overgrowth of bacteria in the blind loop of excluded bowel, but others were due to severe malnutrition. Almost all of the patients who underwent these operations have been reconnected or revised to another bariatric procedure. It is not surprising that some of the newer malabsorptive operations listed in the following section, procedures that also exclude more limited lengths of bowel, carry a greater risk of malnutrition than the purely restrictive operations.

## Combined Gastric Restriction and Malabsorption

### Roux-en-Y Gastric Bypass

The Roux-en-Y gastric bypass (Figure 101.1) limits intake with a small 10–30 ml proximal pouch, delays emptying with an 8–10 mm gastroenterostomy, and interferes with digestion by excluding the antrum, duodenum, and proximal jejunum from contact with the flow of food. The procedure also produces a *dumping syndrome* (nausea, flushing, lightheadedness, diarrhea) in over half of the patients upon consumption of a high-sugar liquid meal, particularly in the first year following the procedure. This side effect may actually be a benefit, since it may curtail behavioral problems of sweet binging by aversive conditioning.

The gastric bypass has been shown to produce significant and durable weight loss of up to 14 years duration in a rigorously studied series. Maximum weight loss of 70% of excess body weight is reported approximately 2 years after the operation. After 5 years, patients maintain an average weight loss of 60% of excess body weight. At 10 and 14 years, average weight loss is 55% and 49%, respectively. Early complications include a perioperative mortality of 1.5% in a series that includes many high-risk patients ($< 1\%$ in most current series); wound infections, 3%; anastomotic stenosis, 3%; and subphrenic abscess, 2.5%. The most frequent late complications included vitamin $B_{12}$ deficiency and anemia in as many as 40% of patients, underscoring the need for close follow-up and the supplementation of patients with multivitamins and minerals, especially $B_{12}$, calcium, and iron. Modifications of this procedure to increase the malabsorptive component and improve weight loss by lengthening the limbs of small bowel are being explored. Early data demonstrate improved weight loss in the superobese, but with an increased risk of malnutrition.

The gastric bypass is now widely accepted as the "gold standard" for bariatric sur-

gery because of its low mortality and excellent outcomes, especially in producing full remission of type 2 diabetes mellitus, reversing hypertension, clearing cardiopulmonary
failure, curing pseudotumor cerebri, and restoring a far better quality of life. The recent
demonstration that the operation can be done safely and as effectively with the
laparoscope offers even further encouragement for this successful therapy of a previously
incurable disease.

### Biliopancreatic Diversion

Biliopancreatic diversion, also known as the Scopinaro procedure (Figure 101.1), combines features of the gastric bypass and intestinal bypass with a cholecystectomy and a
gastric resection to produce weight loss greater than that achieved by gastric bypass
alone. In this operation, ingested food, limited in quantity by the reduced gastric reservoir, mixes with digestive enzymes only in the last segment of ileum, establishing
maldigestion and relative malabsorption. Average excess weight loss with this procedure
is reported as high as 70%, maintained for 15 years. Surgical complications, including
gastric perforation, anastomosis site leak, wound dehiscence and infection, occur in approximately 3% of patients. Stomal ulcers occur in up to 15% of patients. Complications
secondary to maldigestion and malabsorption include protein malnutrition, which occurs
in approximately 12% of patients. Anemia due to iron, folate, or $B_{12}$ deficiency occurs in
as many as 35% of patients who are not on *strict* supplementation. With proper
supplementation, this drops to 5%. Of concern are reports of hepatic failure, a serious
complication that occurs infrequently following this operation. Biliopancreatic diversion
is an effective procedure but has potentially serious complications that lead some to reserve it for patients who fail other bariatric procedures. Curiously, patients in Italy appear to fare much better than Americans on a U.S. diet.

### Duodenal Switch

A modification of biliopancreatic diversion, the duodenal switch procedure (Fig. 101.1)
involves vertical resection of the stomach (sleeve gastrectomy), with bypass of the duodenum and proximal ileum. This differs from the biliopancreatic bypass in that the shared
limb of the bypass is approximately twice as long and the pylorus is left intact. Although
long-term follow-up is poor, weight loss with this procedure is reported as high as 70% at
4 years. The most common side effects following this procedure are related to malabsorptive component. Nearly all patients will have more than one bowel movement
daily and complain of frequent bloating and flatulence. Malnutrition is also a concern,
with a 10–20% incidence of anemia. Surgical complications include a 1–2% operative
mortality rate, 1–2% incidence of pancreatitis, and 2–3% incidence of abdominal abscess. Although weight loss is similar to that with biliopancreatic diversion, side effects
related to malnutrition are slightly less with the duodenal switch, largely because the
shared limb of the bypass is longer.

## CONCLUSIONS

Morbid obesity is a serious and increasingly common disease that poses significant health
risks. Surgery is presently the only effective, long-term therapy. Three procedures, vertical

banded gastroplasty, gastric banding, and gastric bypass, have been studied extensively and shown to produce significant and sustained weight loss. Although we commonly gauge the success of a procedure by the amount of weight loss, we must not disregard the benefits that lie beyond this (see Chapter 102). Following gastric bypass, 90% of patients with preoperative type 2 diabetes mellitus or glucose intolerance will return to euglycemia. Hypertension, sleep apnea, osteoarthritis, and percentage of body fat all improve significantly. These effects are seen with many bariatric procedures but are studied most extensively in gastric bypass patients. The biliopancreatic bypass is perhaps for those patients who fail safer bariatric procedures.

## FURTHER READING

Balsiger, B. M., Murr, M. M., Poggio, J. L., & Sarr, M. G. (2000). Bariatric surgery: Surgery for weight control in patients with morbid obesity. *Medical Clinics of North America, 84,* 477–489.—A review article of several bariatric procedures.

Capella, J. F., & Capella, R. F. (1996). The weight reduction operation of choice: Vertical banded gastroplasty or gastric bypass? *American Journal of Surgery, 171,* 74–79.—A comparison of gastric bypass and vertical banded gastroplasty.

Consensus Development Conference Panel. (1991). Gastrointestinal surgery for severe obesity: Consensus Development Conference Statement. *Annals of Internal Medicine, 115,* 956–961.—National Institutes of Health consensus conference recommendations for treatment of severe obesity.

Grace, D. M. (1992). Gastric restriction procedures for treating severe obesity. *American Journal of Clinical Nutrition, 55,* 556S–559S.—A comparison of various restrictive procedures.

O'Leary, J. P. (1992). Gastrointestinal malabsorptive procedures. *American Journal of Clinical Nutrition, 55,* 567S–570S.—A comparison of various malabsorptive procedures.

Pories, W. J. (1997). The surgical approach to morbid obesity. In D. C. Sabiston, Jr. (Ed.), *Textbook of surgery: The biological basis of modern surgical practice* (15th ed., pp. 933–945). Philadelphia: Saunders.—A good discussion of obesity, its complications, and surgical treatments. Also addresses accuracy of the BMI.

Sugerman, H. J., Kellum, J. M., Engle, K. M., Wolfe, L., Starkey, J. V., Birkenhauer, R., Fletcher, P., & Sawyer, M. J. (1992). Gastric bypass for treating severe obesity. *American Journal of Clinical Nutrition, 55,* 560S–566S.—More detailed discussion of gastric bypass and comparison to vertical banded gastroplasty.

# 102

# Surgery for Obesity: Psychosocial and Medical Outcomes

## JARL S:SON TORGERSON
## LARS SJÖSTRÖM

With surgery, unlike other strategies for treating obesity, large and long-standing weight losses can be achieved in a majority of eligible patients (see Chapter 101). There are also substantial improvements in cardiovascular risk factors and health-related quality of life. Perioperative mortality associated with surgical treatment is less than 0.5%. Against this background, obesity surgery as a therapeutic approach is justified in its own right.

A fundamental problem in all obesity treatment is the lack of unequivocal scientific evidence showing beneficial effects of weight loss on mortality. On the contrary, several observational epidemiological studies indicate that weight reduction is related to increased mortality, even in subjects who are obese at baseline. A detailed analysis of this apparent paradox is beyond the scope of this chapter. However, since surgically induced weight loss is maintained long-term, it can serve as a model for the effects of voluntary weight reduction on obesity-related mortality. This is in fact the scientific credo of the on-going intervention, Swedish Obese Subjects (SOS) study, in which the effects of surgery (substantial weight loss) or conventional treatment (weight-stable control group) on mortality in 2,000 matched patient pairs will be followed over 20 years.

## PSYCHOSOCIAL OUTCOME

Health-related quality of life (HRQL) is a broad concept that includes aspects of functional limitations in daily life as well as mental well-being (see Chapter 70). Both disease-specific and generic instruments are used to measure different HRQL dimensions. Compared to normal-weight subjects, obese individuals suffer from a reduced HRQL. In fact, it is as poor as in patients with cancer recurrence. Many obese persons who seek treatment view the poor quality of life as the most disabling aspect of their disease. Consequently, it is important to include measures of HRQL in obesity trials.

## Health-Related Quality of Life in the SOS Study

In the SOS, a battery of different questionnaires has been used to assess a wide range of HRQL aspects. The results are remarkably similar irrespective of HRQL dimension. The patients had very poor HRQL at baseline. In the control group, the ratings remained stable over time. Among the surgically treated patients, there were dramatic improvements in HRQL after 6 and 12 months, followed by a modest decline 2 to 4 years after surgery.

Let us exemplify with the OP-scale, which is an instrument that specifically measures obesity-related psychosocial problems (e.g., being bothered when going to a restaurant, trying on and buying clothes or having intimate relations with a partner). At baseline, between 40% and 80% of patients felt uncomfortable in these very common situations. After 2 and 4 years, the fraction of bothered subjects was substantially reduced to between 10% and 45%.

Depression was assessed by the Hospital Anxiety and Depression (HAD) scale. After surgery, a marked reduction in the prevalence of depression was especially evident among patients losing more than 25% in weight. In this group, the combined prevalence of probable and possible depression was reduced from 23.6% at baseline to 4.2% after 2 years and 7.0% after 4 years. Among subjects who lost less weight (0–25%) the corresponding figures were 26.7%, 11.4%, and 16.0%, respectively.

A general finding in the SOS study is that improvements in different HRQL aspects are related to the degree of weight loss. Patients losing more than 30 kg had stable improvements in HRQL, while deterioration was seen in patients with smaller weight reductions. Subjects losing less than 10 kg tended to return toward baseline levels.

## Socioeconomic Effects of Obesity Surgery

Narbro and colleagues analyzed the number of days lost due to sick leave and disability pension following obesity surgery in the SOS study. The year before inclusion, the surgically treated group lost 104 days and the control group, 107 days. There was a 50% increase in lost days in the surgically treated group the first postoperative year, mainly due to normal convalescence. During the second and third postoperative years, significantly less days were lost in the surgically treated group than in the control group.

In accordance with these results, a number of studies show that employment rates increase after obesity surgery. In a retrospective study Näslund found an 81% employment rate in a group of surgically treated patients compared to 65% among patients still on the waiting list.

## MEDICAL OUTCOME

Profound weight loss is achieved with surgical treatment and as a consequence, most obesity-related cardiovascular risk factors and comorbidities are ameliorated or cured.

## Effects on Mortality

There is no unequivocal evidence that weight loss reduces mortality in the obese (see Chapters 76 and 88). However, there are very promising results concerning the subgroup of patients with type 2 diabetes. Pories and colleagues followed 154 surgically treated obese type 2 diabetics for 9 years and a non-surgically-treated but otherwise comparable group ($n = 78$) for 6 years (see Chapter 101). The incidence of death per patient-year of follow-up was 4.5 times larger among the controls than in the surgically treated group. Mortality data are not yet available from the SOS study.

## Obesity Surgery and Type 2 Diabetes

There are strong pathophysiological and epidemiological links between obesity and diabetes. Consequently, obesity surgery has a dramatic impact on the incidence of type 2 diabetes and on the metabolic control in already-afflicted individuals.

Data from the SOS study showed that the 2-year incidence of diabetes was 6.3% in the weight-stable control group, but only 0.2% in the surgically treated group that lost on average 28 kg. After 8 years, the incidence was 3.6% among surgically treated patients (weight loss 20 kg) and 18.5% among controls that increased on average 0.7 kg in weight. This profound reduction in diabetes incidence is further supported by data from the Pories group on obese patients with impaired glucose tolerance (IGT). They found the rate of conversion from IGT to diabetes to be 4.72 cases per 100 person-years in a weight-stable control group compared to 0.15 cases in a surgically treated group.

Obese patients with established type 2 diabetes or IGT also have great benefit from surgery. Pories and colleagues have reported that 82.9% of patients with diabetes and 98.7% of patients with IGT reverted to euglycemia and maintained normal levels of glucose and glycosylated hemoglobin after 1–14 years' follow-up. A further analysis of patients that did not revert to euglycemia showed that in about 40% of patients this was due to technical failure (e.g., staple line breakdown). The other patients who failed to revert were older and had suffered from diabetes longer than subjects who succeeded. It is noteworthy that among SOS patients with diabetes, the 2-year recovery rate was 73% in the surgically treated group and 19% among weight-stable controls.

## Cardiovascular Effects

There are several reports of the beneficial effect of obesity surgery on blood pressure and hypertension. Typically, hypertension is resolved or improved in two-thirds to three-fourths of surgically treated patients. From the SOS study, we know that the 2-year incidence of hypertension was 9.9% in the control group and 3.2% in the surgically treated group. However, after 8 years, the corresponding figures were 25.8% and 26.4%, respectively. Thus, in spite of a maintained weight loss of 20 kg (16.5%), there was no long-term reduction in the incidence of hypertension. A further analysis revealed that the rapid increase in pulse pressure with aging usually seen in obese subjects was slowed down in the surgically treated group, in spite of the relapse in blood pressure. Since increasing pulse pressure is seen as a consequence of increasing arterial stiffness, it has been associated with an increased intima–media thickness (IMT) and with increased morality. The reduced pulse pressure observed in SOS may indicate an improved cardiovascular state.

Karason and colleagues have examined cardiac function following obesity surgery. Compared to a lean reference group, the obese had higher blood pressure levels, increased left ventricular mass, and relative wall thickness at baseline. Furthermore, both the systolic (left ventricular ejection fraction) and diastolic (E/A ratio) function were decreased. All these variables were improved 1 year after surgery but remained unchanged in the obese controls. Karason also examined IMT of the carotid bulb. The IMT progression rate was almost identical in the surgically treated and lean groups, and about three times slower than in the obese controls. Although this was a small study, the results are very important, since they indicate an effect of voluntary weight loss on the atherosclerotic process.

It is also important that obesity surgery can reduce serum lipid levels. Data from the SOS showed that the 2-year incidence of hypertriglyceridemia was 7.7% in the control group compared to 0.8% in the surgically treated group. A favorable effect of surgery was also observed for high-density lipoprotein cholesterol, while there was no effect on hypercholesterolemia. Elevated levels of plasminogen activator inhibitor 1 (PAI-1) have been related to an increased cardiovascular risk. A study by Sylvan and coworkers showed that 15 years after jejunoileal bypass surgery, subjects' PAI-1 levels were in the normal range and significantly reduced compared to a group of non-treated obese controls.

## Miscellaneous

Obstructive sleep apnea (OSA) is an important predictor of morbidity and psychosocial disturbances in the obese. Several research groups have shown that obesity surgery reduces OSA symptoms such as snoring, apneas, and daytime sleepiness.

The obese often suffer from pain in weight bearing joints. In the SOS study, the prevalence of joint pain at baseline was higher among surgically treated patients than among controls. Nevertheless, a 4-year follow-up showed that the prevalence was significantly reduced in the surgically treated group, while the situation was unchanged in the weight-stable control group. For instance, the prevalence of patients with aching knee joints causing intermittent impairment in working capacity was reduced from 39% to 16% after surgery.

## CLOSING REMARKS

Surgery is currently the only treatment that results in sustained (> 10 years) and substantial (> 15%) weight loss in the obese. The achieved weight loss has profound positive effects on the full spectrum of medical and psychosocial consequences of obesity. As we see it, this clearly indicates that the current therapeutic tradition has to be changed so that more obese patients receive surgery. In the foreseeable future, surgery will probably be the only really efficient treatment option for patients with severe obesity (BMI > 40 kg/m$^2$).

We do not yet know whether intentional weight loss results in a reduction of mortality in the obese. Given the often dramatic improvements in morbidity and cardiovascular risk that follow surgery, it seems reasonable that weight reduction is also beneficial with respect to mortality. We hope that in the years to come, the SOS study will shed further light on this pivotal issue.

## FURTHER READING

Karason, K., Wikstrand, J., Sjöström, L., & Wendelhag, I. (1999). Weight loss and progression of early atherosclerosis in the carotid artery: A four-year controlled study of obese subjects. *International Journal of Obesity*, *23*, 948–956.—The first study to show positive effects of weight loss on atherosclerosis.

Kral, J. (1998). Surgical treatment of obesity. In P. G. Kopelman & M. J. Stock (Eds.), *Clinical obesity* (pp. 545–563). Oxford, UK: Blackwell Science.—A comprehensive review of the outcome of obesity surgery.

MacDonald, K. G., Long, S. D., Swanson, M. S., Brown, B. M., Morris, P., Dohm, G. L., & Pories, W. J. (1997). The gastric bypass operation reduces the progression and mortality of non-insulin-dependent diabetes mellitus. *Journal of Gastrointestinal Surgery*, *1*, 213–220.—An important study showing reduced mortality in diabetic subjects following obesity surgery.

Narbro, K., Ågren, G., Jonsson, F., Larsson, B., Näslund, I., Wedel, H., & Sjöström, L. (1999). Sick leave and disability pension before and after treatment for obesity: A report from the Swedish Obese Subjects (SOS) study. *International Journal of Obesity*, *23*, 619–624.—Data from the SOS study on the economic consequences of obesity surgery.

Näslund, I. (1996). Effects of weight reduction on the somatic, psychosocial and social complications of morbid obesity. In A. Angel, H. Anderson, C. Bouchard, D. Lau, L. Leiter, & R. Mendelson (Eds.), *Progress in obesity research* (Vol. 7, pp. 679–686). London: John Libbey.—A review covering important information on the psychosocial outcome of obesity surgery, with special reference to the SOS study.

Pories, W. J., Swanson, M. S., MacDonald, K. G., Long, S. B., Morris, B. S. N., Brown, B. M., Barakat, H. A., Israel, G., & Dolezal, J. M. (1995). Who would have thought it?: An operation proves to be the most effective therapy for adult-onset diabetes mellitus. *Annals of Surgery*, *222*, 339–352.—Important long-term data on the effects of obesity surgery on the metabolic control in diabetic patients.

Sjöström, C. D., Lissner, L., Wedel, H., & Sjöström, L. (1999). Reduction in incidence of diabetes, hypertension and lipid disturbances after intentional weight loss induced by bariatric surgery: The SOS intervention study. *Obesity Research*, *7*, 477–484.—A 2-year report from the SOS study showing dramatic improvements in cardiovascular risk factors.

Sjöström, C. D., Peltonen, M., Wedel, H., & Sjöström, L. (2000). Differentiated long-term effects of intentional weight loss on diabetes and hypertension. *Hypertension*, *36*, 20–25.—A report from the SOS study showing a relapse in blood pressure in spite of a maintained substantial weight loss.

Sjöström, L. (2000). Surgical intervention as a strategy for treatment of obesity. *Endocrine*, *13*, 213–230.—The latest update of results from the SOS study.

Sullivan, M., Karlsson, J., Sjöström, L., & Taft, C. (in press). Why quality-of-life measures should be used in the treatment of patients with obesity. In P. Björntorp (Ed.), *International textbook of obesity*. Chichester, UK: John Wiley.—A comprehensive review of health-related quality of life in obesity.

# 103

# Management of Obesity in Children

## GARY S. GOLDFIELD
## LEONARD H. EPSTEIN

The prevalence of childhood obesity has doubled in the past 20 years and approximately one-fourth of children ages 6–11 and adolescents ages 12–18 are obese, making childhood obesity one of the most serious pediatric health problems in the Unites States (see Chapters 77 and 85). Several reasons underlie the need to treat pediatric obesity. First, obesity tracks throughout development such that obese children are more likely than lean children to become obese adults. Second, pediatric and adolescent obesity are related to subsequent morbidity and mortality more than 50 years later, even controlling for adult weight. Third, pediatric obesity is associated with adverse medical conditions such as cardiovascular risk factors, asthma, and orthopedic problems, as well as deleterious psychosocial consequences, including teasing, body dissatisfaction, and poor self-esteem.

There are also behavioral, biological, and financial reasons to treat pediatric obesity. It may be easier to mobilize family support for children than for adults. Children also have not had the unhealthy eating and activity patterns as long as adults; thus, their habits may be more amenable to change. Treatment of pediatric obesity can take advantage of growth and increases in lean body mass. Instead of shrinking adipose cells, treatment at an early age prevents the development of excess adipose cells. Finally, the economic costs of obesity and related comorbidities have been estimated to be over $70 billion, or 7% of national health care expenditures (see Chapter 82). Given the limited effectiveness of treatment for obese adults, early intervention that prevents obese children from becoming obese adults may not only improve health and prevent disease, but it may also be especially cost-effective (see Chapter 112).

## COMPONENTS OF TREATMENT

### Diet

The goal of any weight loss therapy is to achieve negative energy balance in which energy expenditure exceeds energy intake. Negative energy balance can be achieved much more rapidly by caloric reduction than by increased energy expenditure; thus, dietary therapy represents a cornerstone of obesity treatment (see Chapter 78). General goals involve reducing and stabilizing caloric intake, reducing fat intake, and improving nutrient density while providing adequate calories for growth and development. Ideally, dietary interventions should adjust caloric intake based on age, degree of overweight, and general activity level, with younger and less obese children having no or smaller calorie restriction, and older or more obese children having more caloric restriction. More severe caloric restrictions (e.g., very-low-calorie diets) have been used with older and very obese children.

We use the traffic-light (or stoplight) diet, which is designed to guide eating patterns to meet age recommendations of the Food Guide Pyramid, thereby increasing the nutrient density of the diet. It groups foods into the colors of a stoplight based on nutrient density and dietary fat: GREEN foods (go) with 0–1 grams of fat per serving are represented by fruits and vegetables; YELLOW foods (caution) contain 2–5 grams of fat per serving and typically represent the staples of the diet that supply basic nutrition; and RED foods (stop) have more than 5 grams of fat per serving or high simple carbohydrate content (e.g., candy). The Stoplight diet maximizes choice of healthy foods based on individual and familial preferences from foods commonly available. There is generally a limit on the number of RED foods consumed each week, and families are asked to eat these RED foods outside of the home, to increase stimulus control over healthy eating. While restriction of unhealthy foods is one goal, there is also an emphasis on healthy foods.

The ideal therapy would facilitate lasting behavior change as caloric intake is reduced. A number of factors about the structure of the dietary program may be important for long-term success. For example, should substitute versions of high-fat–low-nutrient density be encouraged? While these can reduce dietary fat and calories, they may not change food preferences, which would be a desirable goal. How much structure is useful? A highly structured program may provide dietary information and even food, but children and families may not learn to eat better and develop self-regulation skills.

A final issue relates to the long-term effects of food deprivation on dietary change. Food is very reinforcing for obese children, and restriction may paradoxically increase the reinforcing value of food, making long-term adherence difficult. Parents may also use food as a reward for good behavior and to alleviate negative mood states, such as anger, boredom, stress, or depression. This may increase the reinforcing value of food, making it more difficult to maintain healthy eating patterns over time. Thus, it is important to provide training in behavioral hygiene for families.

## Physical Activity

Activity complements dietary interventions to accelerate and improve maintenance of weight loss (see Chapter 93). The combination of diet plus exercise produces greater reductions in weight status than exercise or diet alone.

Exercise programs can be divided into structured exercise programs or lifestyle activity. Structured programs generally focus on increasing the duration and/or intensity of aerobic exercise, with the exercise implemented in one exercise bout. Lifestyle exercise provides more choice of how children obtain their physical activity, with children having options of many physical activities and control over how they are distributed. While the choice may be to engage in highly structured exercise, lifestyle activity allows the child the option to engage in different activities every day at varying intensities, with the activity spread over multiple bouts.

Observational studies of child and adolescent physical activity suggest that children spontaneously engage in brief bouts of high-intensity physical activity, and that they find this more reinforcing than more extended bouts of high-intensity physical activity. Thus, it may be useful to develop programs based on patterns of activity that are normally observed. There are individual differences in preference for lifestyle or structured aerobic programs, and some children may begin with lifestyle exercise and then change to aerobic exercise. Providing a choice of exercise programs may enhance adherence. While the immediate goal of the intervention should be to increase activity, a secondary goal should be to increase the reinforcing value of physical activity, so that children want to keep being active after the formal program ends.

Obese children find sedentary activity more reinforcing than their nonobese peers, and allocation of time to sedentary activities such as watching television can reduce time to be physically active and prompt eating. Developing methods to reduce sedentary behavior is becoming more common.

## Behavior Change

It is essential to discover the best way to acquire and maintain improved eating and activity behaviors (see Chapter 94). One key decision is whether, or how, to involve the parents. Parental participation can range from minimal involvement to implementation of the child intervention, to more intense involvement in which both parents and children attempt to change diet and activity. The extent of parent involvement will depend on the age of the child, but the more the parent is involved, the greater the opportunity for changing the environment and providing support.

Parents' modifications of the shared family environment are called stimulus control, for example, decreasing access to high-fat, energy-dense foods by not bringing them into the house, or limiting access to television viewing by moving the set to a less desirable place in the home, can reduce intake of unhealthy foods and time spent in sedentary behavior. Socializing around physical activity and keeping exercise clothing and equipment easily accessible are examples of how to arrange the environment to promote physical activity. Stimulus control procedures can facilitate healthy changes not only in parents and children but also in other family members.

Parental modeling of healthy eating and activity behaviors are a central part of the child's environment. Parents should model the behaviors and attitudes they want their child to repeat. Parents can model behavioral hygiene by not using food as a reward or to alleviate negative moods, or missing meals to reduce intake.

Self-monitoring is an important self-regulatory skill and a powerful method for enhancing awareness of eating and activity. Both child and parent can record eating and activity throughout treatment, and are instructed to record the behavior immediately, whenever possible, to maximize accuracy. Children and overweight parents should also record their daily weights on a weight graph to provide feedback on weight changes. Self-monitoring not only promotes the awareness necessary for behavior change, but also the feedback from recording can reinforce behavior change and identify areas that need more attention. Self-monitoring is a strong predictor of long-term weight maintenance in parents and children.

Parents can also support their children by using positive reinforcement to facilitate acquisition and maintenance of behavior changes. Praise and contracting are widely used techniques. Parents are taught to be specific regarding behaviors for which they praise their children and to use praise consistently. Children are taught the importance of praise and encouraged to praise their parents for desirable behaviors such as exercising together, and so on.

Contingency contracting involves the delivery of a reinforcer for meeting behavioral change goals. Both parent and child can be reinforced for meeting eating or activity goals. Items to be used as reinforcers can emphasize social interaction and time spent in activities that may improve the parent–child relationship; use of reinforcers such as food, money, or gifts is discouraged. Although it is important for spouses and siblings to provide support for all the behaviors that the children are striving to change, teaching children to reinforce parental behavior changes may enhance the efficacy of a reinforcement system.

Including parents is a critical component of treatment. We use a family-based intervention involving the active participation of at least one parent. In many families, one or both parents are obese and could benefit from weight loss, but even having nonobese parents model appropriate behaviors and restructure the family environment offers substantive benefits. Hence, parents are expected to participate fully and to undergo the same behavior changes required of the obese child. With the exception of very young children, parents and children should be seen separately to maximize the degree of children's responsibility.

Recent research from Golan and associates provides new insights on the importance of including parents. These investigators found that targeting parents as the sole agents of change (children did not participate) produced greater reductions in child percent overweight and dropout at 12-month follow-up compared to the standard intervention of treating children only. Another finding of this study was that the reduction in percent overweight observed in children in the parent-only condition was achieved without the use of a calorie-restricted diet, suggesting that programmed caloric restriction may not be necessary for weight loss when a family-based intervention is employed.

## RESULTS OF CHILD TREATMENT

There is considerable variability in the results of pediatric obesity treatments based on the types and length of the interventions and characteristics of the subjects. The most powerful treatments show 25% decreases in percent overweight over 1 year, with several studies from different laboratories showing successful maintenance at 4-, 5-, and 10-year intervals. These weight changes are associated with decreased percent overweight and important changes in the percentage of children who do not meet percent overweight criteria for obesity. There is considerably less data on parents and other family members who may or may not participate in treatment. In the short term, it appears that participating parents and children are equally successful in weight control, but over the long term, children show better maintenance. Other family members who do not participate in weight control programs also may benefit, but research is limited and the characteristics of children or nonparticipating parents is not known.

## CONCLUSION

Because the prevalence of childhood obesity is increasing (see Chapters 76 and 77), better access to empirically verified treatments is needed to prevent adult obesity and associated comorbid medical conditions. Diet, physical activity, and behavior change represent the core elements of comprehensive pediatric obesity treatment. Interventions should focus on development of healthy eating and activity habits in children that persist beyond the structured intervention to maintain health during development.

## FURTHER READING

Brownell, K. D., Kelman, S. H., & Stunkard, A. J. (1983). Treatment of obese children with and without their mothers: Changes in weight and blood pressure. *Pediatrics, 71*, 515–523.—A well-controlled study that demonstrates the importance of including both parents and children in treatment, and that separating parents and children in treatment enhances outcome.

Colditz, G. A. (1999). Economic costs of obesity and inactivity. *Medicine and Science in Sports and Exercise, 31*(Suppl.), S663–S667.—A detailed examination of the economic burden of obesity and inactivity, with estimated total costs derived from the cost of treatment of comorbidity, indirect costs caused by lost productivity, and foregone earnings caused by premature mortality.

Dietz, W. H., & Gortmaker, S. L. (1985). Do we fatten our children at the television set?: Obesity and television viewing in children and adolescents. *Pediatrics, 75*, 807–812.—The best documentation that television viewing is prospectively and cross-sectionally related to obesity.

Epstein, L. H., Myers, M. D., Raynor, H. A., & Saelens, B. E. (1998). Treatment of pediatric obesity. *Pediatrics, 101*, 554–570.—A comprehensive review of the treatment of pediatric obesity.

Epstein, L. H., Valoski, A. M., Vara, L. S., McCurley, J., Wisniewski, L., Kalarchian, M. A., Klein, K. R., & Shrager, L. R. (1995). Effects of decreasing sedentary behavior and increasing activity on weight change in obese children. *Health Psychology, 14*, 109–115.—A well-controlled study that establishes the importance of decreasing sedentary behavior in obesity treatment.

Epstein, L. H., Valoski, A. M., Wing, R. R., & McCurley, J. (1994). Ten year outcomes of behavioral family-based treatment for childhood obesity. *Health Psychology, 13*, 373–383.—The first paper to present data from well-controlled studies demonstrating the long-term efficacy of behavioral, family-based treatment.

Epstein, L. H., Wing, R. R., Koeske, R., & Valoski, A. (1985). A comparison of lifestyle exercise, aerobic exercise and calisthenics on weight loss in obese children. *Behavior Therapy, 16*, 345–356.—A well-controlled demonstration of the importance of increasing activity levels in the treatment of childhood obesity.

Golan, M., Weizman, A., Apter, A., & Fainaru, M. (1998). Parents as exclusive agents of change in the treatment of childhood obesity. *American Journal of Clinical Nutrition, 67*, 1130–1135.—A well-controlled study in which treating parents alone was a more effective intervention than treating children directly; treatment effects were established without caloric reduction.

Rolland-Cachera, M. F., Deheeger, M., & Guilloud-Bataille, M. (1987). Tracking the development of obesity from one month of age to adulthood. *Annals of Human Biology, 14*, 219–229.—A thorough analysis of the developmental pattern of obesity from infancy to adulthood.

Stark, O., Atkins, E., Wolff, O.H., & Douglas, J. W. B. (1981). Longitudinal study of obesity in the National Survey of Health and Development. *British Medical Journal, 283*, 13–17.—The best demonstration that obese children are at risk of becoming obese adults.

Whitaker, R. C., Wright, J. A., Pepe, M. S., Seidel, K. D., & Dietz, W. H. (1997). Predicting obesity in young adulthood from childhood and parental obesity. *New England Journal of Medicine, 337*, 869–873.—Provides data for the mutual influence of child weight and parental obesity on the risk of a child becoming obese in adulthood.

# 104

# Treatment of Obesity in Patients with Type 2 Diabetes

## RENA R. WING

Diabetes is a major health problem in the United States that affects approximately 16 million Americans and costs $50 billion per year. Most individuals with diabetes have type 2 diabetes (previously called "non-insulin-dependent diabetes"); approximately 60–90% of these individuals are overweight (see Chapter 84).

Weight loss is recommended for obese patients with type 2 diabetes because weight loss reduces hyperglycemia and improves abnormalities in hepatic glucose production, insulin sensitivity, and insulin secretion (see Chapter 87). Although there appears to be a dose–response relation between weight loss and improvements in glycemic control, even modest weight losses of 15–30 pounds produce long-term improvements in glycemic control.

Weight loss and maintenance are difficult to achieve in overweight patients with diabetes. In fact, recent data from a variety of weight loss interventions suggest that weight loss and maintenance may be an even greater problem for diabetic than for nondiabetic individuals. Efforts are therefore needed to develop more effective interventions for these patients.

## BEHAVIORAL WEIGHT CONTROL FOR PATIENTS WITH TYPE 2 DIABETES

For the most part, weight loss strategies for obese patients with diabetes parallel those used with nondiabetics and involve a combination of diet, exercise, and behavior modification (see Chapters 93 and 94). This section highlights some of the differences in the treatment of diabetic versus nondiabetic individuals.

## Need for Medical Monitoring

Caloric restriction produces dramatic, immediate improvements in glycemic control; 3–7 days of dieting can decrease fasting glucose from 220 to 170 mg/dl. Since most patients with diabetes are treated with oral medication or insulin, these sudden changes in glycemic control require careful adjustments in medication to prevent hypoglycemic reactions. Before starting patients on low-calorie diets, it may be helpful to stop or reduce these medications. Blood glucose levels should be monitored frequently to permit further adjustments in medications. Since many patients with diabetes are also being treated for hypertension and/or hyperlipidemia, medications for these conditions must also be adjusted during weight loss.

Some investigators have observed poorer weight losses in insulin-treated than in other patients with diabetes; our data do not support this. We find no differences in weight loss among subjects treated with diet only, oral medication, or insulin, perhaps because of the frequent adjustments in the medication regimen.

## Dietary Regimen

The major dietary goal for obese patients with type 2 diabetes is to decrease caloric intake. The magnitude of the caloric deficit appears to be related to the degree of improvement in glycemic control, independent of weight loss. In our treatment programs, we have used both balanced diets of 1,000–1,500 kcal/day and very-low-calorie diets (VLCDs; 400 kcal of lean meat, fish, or fowl, or liquid formula diets) in combination with behavior modification. We found that the use of VLCDs increased the magnitude of initial weight loss, the percentage of patients achieving significant weight loss, and the initial improvements in glycemic control. Like other investigators who have studied VLCDs with nondiabetic subjects, unfortunately, we found no significant differences in weight loss at 1-year follow-up for subjects treated with VLCDs versus balanced, low-caloric diets (see Chapter 96). However, subjects treated with the VLCD had better long-term improvements in glycemic control than subjects treated with a balanced, low-calorie diet. Since this finding was not replicated in a second study, further research is needed to determine whether VLCDs have a long-term impact on glycemic control. Recently, we have also shown that prescribing VLCDs for 1 day each week, or for 5 days every 5 weeks, may improve weight loss and glycemic control.

There are also questions regarding the macronutrient composition of the diet for individuals with diabetes. Given their increased risk of cardiovascular disease, a low-fat diet is advised; however, some studies have shown that low-fat, high-carbohydrate diets actually worsen triglyceride levels and glycemic control in individuals with diabetes. These studies have utilized weight maintenance regimens. In a study conducted with a calorie-restricted weight loss diet, we found that emphasizing low dietary fat intake (< 20% of calories from fat) increased weight loss in patients with type 2 diabetes, with no adverse effects on glycemic control or lipid levels.

## Exercise

The other key component of a weight loss regimen for individuals with diabetes is exercise (see Chapter 93). As with nondiabetic subjects, diabetics have better long-term weight losses when treated with the combination of diet plus exercise rather than diet alone (see Chapters 93, 106, and 107). Exercise, independent of weight loss, also reduces insulin resistance and in some studies improves glycemic control; these benefits are observed primarily in individuals with milder or newly diagnosed diabetes. In a randomized controlled trial, we found that obese patients with diabetes randomly assigned to a diet plus exercise regimen lost significantly more weight than those in the diet-only condition at 10-week, 20-week, and 1-year follow-up. Moreover, self-reported level of activity at 1 year was related to improvements in glycosylated hemoglobin, independent of weight loss. However, other randomized trials have failed to show greater improvements in glycemic control in patients assigned to a diet plus exercise compared to a diet-only regimen.

Since many overweight diabetics are older and suffer from other health problems, increasing exercise may be difficult and adherence may be poor. Gradual changes in activity level and low-intensity exercise such as walking clearly make the most sense for these older, sicker individuals (see Chapter 93 for discussion of exercise adherence).

## Self-Glucose Monitoring and Behavioral Self-Regulation

Self-glucose monitoring enables diabetic patients to monitor their glucose levels accurately and adjust insulin as needed to achieve normal glycemic control. It has been suggested that the feedback from glucose monitoring regarding the effect of diet and exercise on blood sugar control should produce greater success at self-regulation. Unfortunately, controlled trials of glucose monitoring have not supported this hypothesis. There is no evidence that type 2 diabetic patients who are taught to monitor their blood sugar adhere better to their diet and exercise regimen, lose more weight, or achieve better glycemic control than subjects given comparable attention and education but not taught glucose monitoring. Clearly, the information obtained from glucose monitoring is useful to the physician in adjusting diabetes medication, but this technique does not appear to lead automatically to increased self-regulatory behavior on the part of the diabetic patient.

## Frequent Contact

Recently, researchers have stressed that obesity is a chronic disease that may require lifelong treatment (see Chapters 84, 91, and 92). This chronic disease model is particularly appropriate for obese individuals with diabetes. Our most recent weight loss programs for patients with diabetes involved weekly contact for a full year. The program produced our most successful outcomes to date. However, when treatment was stopped at the end of the year, subjects regained weight. Thus, some type of ongoing intervention model must be developed (see Chapter 107).

## COMBINING BEHAVIORAL TREATMENT AND WEIGHT LOSS MEDICATIONS

Currently, there are two medications that have FDA approval for weight loss (see Chapter 99). Both appear helpful when used in combination with a lifestyle modification program in the treatment of obese patients with type 2 diabetes. Orlistat is a lipase inhibitor that selectively inhibits the absorption of dietary fat. In a yearlong study in patients with diabetes, individuals treated with orlistat and a reduced-calorie diet lost 6.2 kg versus 4.3 kg in patients given a placebo. The orlistat-treated group also achieved somewhat better long-term improvements in glycemic control and even more positive changes in lipid levels. The other weight loss medication available at present is sibutramine, which is a norepinepherine and serotonin reuptake inhibitor. Diabetic patients treated with sibutramine and a 700 kcal/day deficit diet lost 7.3% of their body weight at 12 months versus 2.4% in patients given a placebo. Improvements in glycemic control did not differ between the two groups, a surprising finding given the large difference in weight loss. Further studies are needed using these and other weight loss medications in combination with more structured behavioral weight loss programs.

## WEIGHT CONTROL IN THE PREVENTION OF TYPE 2 DIABETES

The prior sections have emphasized the importance of weight loss in the treatment of patients with diabetes. However, it should be noted that weight loss and exercise may also be important in preventing this disease. Numerous prospective studies have shown that obesity is related to the risk of developing type 2 diabetes (see Chapters 76 and 86). Upper-body fat distribution and low activity levels are also important independent modifiable risk factors for diabetes.

Given this, it is reasonable to hypothesize that weight loss and/or increased physical activity might prevent or delay the occurrence of diabetes in individuals at risk for this disease. In a recent study, individuals with impaired glucose tolerance were treated in a weight loss and exercise program. Participants in the intervention group lost approximately 2.3–3.7% of their initial body weight, whereas weight increased by approximately 0.5–1.7% in untreated subjects. These modest weight losses had marked effects on the incidence of diabetes. Only 11% of individuals in the intervention program developed diabetes over the 6-year follow-up compared to 22% in a nonrandomized control group. Moreover, improvements in glucose tolerance were significantly correlated with weight loss and increased physical fitness. This and several other recent studies strongly support the suggestion that weight loss and increased physical activity may reduce the risk of developing diabetes. A controlled clinical trial (diabetes prevention program) testing whether such lifestyle intervention can prevent or delay diabetes in high-risk individuals is currently under way.

## FURTHER READING

Diabetes Prevention Program Research Group. (1999). Design and methods for a clinical trial in the prevention of type 2 diabetes. *Diabetes Care, 22*, 623–634.—Describes the methods being used in an ongoing, multicenter trial to determine whether it is possible to delay or prevent the development of diabetes in high-risk individuals.

Hamman, R. F. (1992). Genetic and environmental determinants of non-insulin-dependent diabetes mellitus (NIDDM). *Diabetes/Metabolism Reviews, 8*, 287–338.—Reviews the research on the genetic and environmental determinants of non-insulin-dependent diabetes mellitus.

Kelley, D., & Goodpaster, B. (1999). Effects of physical activities on insulin action and glucose tolerance in obesity. *Medicine and Science in Sports and Exercise, 31*, S619–S623.—Reviews studies on the effects of exercise on glucose and insulin metabolism.

Kelley, D. E., Wing, R., Buonocore, C., Sturis, J., Polonsky, K., & Fitzsimmons, M. (1993). Relative effects of calorie restriction and weight loss in non-insulin-dependent diabetes mellitus. *Journal of Clinical Endocrinology and Metabolism, 77*, 1287–1293.—Assesses the relative effects of weight loss versus caloric restriction on glycemic control, insulin secretion and sensitivity, and hepatic glucose output in type 2 diabetics.

Kriska, A. M., & Bennett, P. H. (1992). An epidemiological perspective of the relationship between physical activity and NIDDM: From activity assessment to intervention. *Diabetes/Metabolism Reviews, 8*, 355–372.—Reviews literature on exercise and non-insulin-dependent diabetes mellitus.

Tuomilehto, J., Knowler, W. C., & Zimmet, P. (1992). Primary prevention of non-insulin-dependent diabetes mellitus. *Diabetes/Metabolism Reviews, 8*, 339–353.—Discusses determinants of diabetes and the results of intervention studies to reduce the risk of diabetes.

Vinik, A. I., Wing, R. R., & Lauterio, T. J. (1997). Nutritional management of the person with diabetes. In D. Porte & R. S. Sherwin (Eds.), *Ellenberg and Rifkin's diabetes mellitus* (5th ed., pp. 609–652). Old Tappan, NJ: Appleton & Lange.—Discusses issues related to the dietary component of treatment interventions for patients with diabetes.

Wing, R. R. (1993). Behavioral treatment of obesity: Its application to type 2 diabetes. *Diabetes Care, 16*, 193–199.—Reviews progress made in the behavioral treatment of type II diabetes.

Wing, R. R. (1997). Behavioral approaches to the treatment of obesity. In G. Bray, C. Bouchard, & W. P. T. James (Eds.), *Handbook of obesity* (pp. 855–873). New York: Marcel Dekker.—Review of behavioral weight loss literature and strategies to promote adherence to diet and exercise intervention.

Wing, R. R. (2001). Weight loss in the management of type 2 diabetes. In H. H. R. Gerstein (Ed.), *Evidence based diabetes care* (pp. 252–276). Ontario: Decker.—Reviews the empirical literature in order to develop and support evidence-based messages on the effects of weight loss on glycemic control in diabetic patients.

# 105

# Weight Loss Programs for Minority Populations

## JOHN P. FOREYT

The prevalence of obesity among minority populations in the United States generally exceeds that of the majority white population (see Chapters 75 and 79). Among females, for example, approximately 22% of whites, 37% of African Americans, and 34% of Mexican Americans are obese (body mass index > 30). Among males, 20% of whites, 21% of African Americans, and 23% of Mexican Americans are obese. All these figures appear to be increasing as new data become available. We are losing, not winning, the obesity war.

Obesity is a major risk factor affecting mortality and morbidity, including hypertension, type 2 diabetes, coronary heart disease, stroke, gallbladder disease, osteoarthritis, sleep apnea and respiratory problems, and some cancers, including endometrial, breast, prostate, and colon cancer (see Chapters 76, 79, and 84). Although some data suggest that these relationships may be less strong in minority populations than in the white population at this time, these differences may be only temporary, while these populations are undergoing current epidemiological transitions. Other methodological issues, such as selective nonresponsiveness to surveys or cohort effects, also may be responsible for the observed differences.

## DETERMINANTS OF OBESITY

Poverty and lower levels of education are associated with higher levels of obesity, and these factors affect proportionately more individuals in minority populations than in the white population. Different minority populations appear to share a preference for high-fat diets and low patterns of physical activity, and in general seem to be less concerned about weight than the white population. Minorities typically have less access to health care, including counseling about potentially effective weight management strategies. The primary factor associated with higher levels of obesity in minorities appears to be lower socioeconomic status (see Chapter 79).

## COGNITIVE-BEHAVIORAL TREATMENT OF OBESITY

Cognitive-behavioral interventions for the treatment of obesity have been the state of the art for over 30 years (see Chapter 94) and focus on lifestyle change, including a healthy diet and exercise program aimed at achieving a realistic weight goal and maintenance of weight loss. The primary components of current interventions include (1) self-monitoring eating and exercise patterns, and the cognitive patterns associated with those behaviors; (2) modifying the antecedent barriers associated with inappropriate eating and exercise patterns; and (3) restructuring the consequences of the inappropriate behaviors. Building social support is also an important component of the intervention.

Cognitive-behavioral interventions are usually conducted in groups of about 10 individuals and the weekly meetings last about an hour. The groups are typically led by a health care professional, such as a registered dietitian. The intervention usually lasts about 4 to 6 months. The average obese individual loses about 22 pounds and maintains two-thirds of the loss at measurement 1 year later. However, without continued contact, the average individual gains back most of the initial weight lost over the following year or two (see Chapters 94 and 107). Trends in the cognitive-behavioral treatment of obesity include better screening of individuals who would be most likely to benefit, matching of individuals to specific treatments, increasing the length of intervention, building stronger social support systems, and combining cognitive-behavioral interventions with other approaches such as very-low-calorie diets (VLCDs), pharmacotherapy, and gastric bypass surgery.

## TREATMENT OF OBESITY IN MINORITY POPULATIONS

Few controlled, long-term studies have been reported on the treatment of obesity in minority populations (see Chapter 79). Minorities participate far less in formal treatment programs than do whites. In two large clinical trials, African American women lost less weight than did white women when enrolled in the same obesity treatment program. In the control group, African American women gained more weight than did their white counterparts. In another study, Mexican American women achieved about half the weight loss typically seen in white women over an equal time period.

Among the growing number of published pilot studies and descriptions of clinic-, hospital-, community center-, and church-based intervention programs for minorities, the majority are not randomized, controlled investigations, are of short duration or lacking in details, and do not readily lend themselves to interpretation or evaluation. For example, the Bariatrics Clinic at Howard University, Washington, DC, reported the results of their 7-week culturally sensitive, behavioral intervention program with 14 low-income, obese African American women and 2 men. Patients had an average weight loss of 14 pounds after 7 weeks. Another example is the PATHWAYS program, a church-based weight loss intervention for urban African American women at risk for type 2 diabetes.

The program, administered by trained lay volunteers, resulted in average weight losses of 10.0 pounds ($n$ = 15) at 14 weeks compared to a gain of 1.9 pounds in the control group ($n$ = 18). A helpful, annotated bibliography of many of these pilot programs specifically designed to achieve weight reduction in minorities is published in the National Institutes of Health/National Heart, Lung, and Blood Institute clinical guidelines (see Further Reading).

Long-term, controlled studies of weight reduction programs for minorities are scant. In a 1-year, double-blind, placebo-controlled, multicenter trial examining the safety and efficacy of sibutramine, an antiobesity drug, 36% of the 224 obese patients with hypertension were African American. Changes in body weight were similar among African American and white participants. Other efficacy and safety profiles for sibutramine among African Americans and whites were also similar. In Mexico, a 6-month, double-blind, placebo-controlled, single-center study of 69 obese patients resulted in a weight loss in sibutramine-treated patients of 10.27 kg and 1.26 kg in the placebo group. A randomized investigation using a very-low-calorie diet (VLCD) compared weight losses of black and white patients with type 2 diabetes. At 1-year follow-up, blacks had smaller weight losses than whites regardless of treatment assignment (7.1 kg in blacks vs. 13.9 kg in whites). A 6-month, randomized controlled trial for older (55–79 years) African American patients with type 2 diabetes ($n$ = 64) resulted in improved glycemic and blood pressure control and better weight losses in the treatment group compared to the usual-care controls.

## CONVENTIONAL VERSUS CULTURALLY RELEVANT INTERVENTIONS

Cognitive-behavioral interventions for the treatment of obesity are typically conducted in groups of unrelated individuals. Such an approach may be less relevant with many minority populations, which place high value on extended families, such as grandmother/mother/daughter/granddaughter. Interventions that exploit intergenerational ties may be more effective than conventional approaches.

The primary dietary intervention in conventional programs includes an emphasis on the U.S. Department of Agriculture (USDA) food pyramid and the basic food groups. With minority populations, programs might have more success if they focused on the special dietary problems of the participants, including concerns related to lactose intolerance; low intake of fresh fruits, vegetables, and fiber; the use of "soul" food; and frequent snacking. Some minority groups have their own folk systems of food classification that could be incorporated into, rather than excluded from, dietary programs. Individuals who have poor nutritional status, such as insufficient calcium and iron, will require special intervention. The church, the extended family, and other social factors may play a more prominent role in relation to the development and maintenance of dietary habits than is currently emphasized in conventional programs.

Barriers to change need to be recognized and addressed. Poverty, higher acceptable weight standards associated with health risks, and lack of knowledge of the relationship between obesity and some cancers may play a more prominent role in treatment.

Current counseling methods with members of minority groups that typically rely on didactic approaches may be less effective than more indirect strategies, such as emphases on storytelling, more role playing, linking of folk beliefs to current scientific facts, sharing experiences, and more active learner participation.

## PUBLIC HEALTH APPROACHES

The higher prevalence of obesity in minorities compared to the white population would be lessened by reducing the socioeconomic differences. However, the prevalence of obesity among whites continues to climb. Public health approaches to treating obesity appear to be the most logical choices for achieving significant reductions in this serious risk to health (see Chapters 111 and 112). Several approaches that might be helpful in reducing obesity in the population, including that of minorities.

Education is one necessary key to weight management. Required health education in the schools that includes information about the management of obesity, equal access to treatment, increased availability of healthy foods (especially fruits and vegetables), and more opportunities for physical activity would help individuals to manage their weight better.

Limiting access to unhealthy foods may also help control obesity at the societal level (see Chapters 111 and 112). Excise taxes on foods high in fat may not be such a farfetched idea, especially if healthier foods, including fruits and vegetables, were subsidized and available at lower costs. Limiting advertisements on television for high-fat foods or placing warning labels on them, similar to strategies used in this country for the sale of cigarettes, might be effective.

Evaluating food labeling and how it might more effectively be modified to influence minorities, especially those loyal to certain brand names, should be a priority. School breakfast and lunch subsidy programs disproportionately affect minorities. Modifying these programs has the potential to affect the development of lifelong dietary habits, especially in the very young.

## SUMMARY AND CONCLUSIONS

The prevalence of obesity in minority populations is generally higher than in the white population. The lack of strong social pressure to lose weight, despite an awareness of the health risks of obesity, and little physical activity contribute to the problem. Published data suggest that relatively few minorities participate in formal intervention programs compared to whites. Among those who do join obesity treatment programs, attrition is higher and weight losses are lower than among white participants given the same interventions. Relatively few intervention programs have been designed specifically to treat obese minorities. The design of such programs requires a behavioral analysis of the factors and barriers that affect weight within a culturally relevant context. Both clinical and public health approaches are urgently needed to combat this growing threat to the health of minority populations in this country.

## ACKNOWLEDGMENT

Preparation of this chapter was supported by Grant No. DK-57177 from the National Institutes of Health (NIH), National Institute of Diabetes and Digestive and Kidney Diseases (NIDDK).

## FURTHER READING

Agurs-Collins, T. D., Kumanyika, S. K., Ten Have, T. R., & Adams-Campbell, L. L. (1997). A randomized controlled trial of weight reduction and exercise for diabetes management in older African American subjects. *Diabetes Care, 20,* 1503–1511.—An example of a culturally sensitive intervention program for older African Americans with type 2 diabetes.

Cuellar, G. E., Ruiz, A. M., Monsalve, M. C., & Berber, A. (2000). Six-month treatment of obesity with sibutramine 15 mg; A double-blind, placebo-controlled monocenter clinical trial in a Hispanic population. *Obesity Research, 8,* 71–82.—A double-blind, placebo-controlled, parallel, prospective clinical study of the safety and efficacy of sibutramine in 69 obese Mexican patients in Mexico City.

Kaul, L., & Nidiry, J. J. (1999). Management of obesity in low-income African Americans. *Journal of the National Medical Association, 91,* 139–143.—An example of a hospital-based, culturally sensitive intervention program for low-income African Americans.

Kumanyika, S. K. (1994). Obesity in minority populations: An epidemiologic assessment. *Obesity Research, 2,* 166–182.—An excellent review of the issues relating to the prevalence, health implications, prevention, and treatment of obesity in minorities in the United States.

Kumanyika, S. K., Obarzanek, E., Stevens, V. J., Hebert, P. R., & Whelton, P. K. (1991). Weight-loss experience of black and white participants in NHLBI-sponsored clinical trials. *American Journal of Clinical Nutrition, 53,* 1631S–1638S.—An examination of race-specific weight loss results from two randomized, multicenter trials: the Hypertension Prevention Trial (HPT) and the Trials of Hypertension Prevention (TOHP).

McMahon, F. G., Fujioka, K., Singh, B. N., Mendel, C. M., Rowe, E., Rolston, K., Johnson, F., & Mooradian, A. D. (2000). Efficacy and safety of sibutramine in obese white and African American patients with hypertension: A 1-year, double-blind, placebo-controlled, multicenter trial. *Archives of Internal Medicine, 24,* 2185–2191.—An assessment of the efficacy and safety of treatment with sibutramine for achieving and maintaining weight loss in African American and white patients with controlled hypertension.

McNabb, W., Quinn, M., Kerver, J., Cook, S., & Karrison, T. (1997). The PATHWAYS church-based weight loss program for urban African American women at risk for diabetes. *Diabetes Care, 20,* 1518–1523.—An example of a culturally sensitive, church-based, weight loss intervention for low income, urban African Americans at risk for type 2 diabetes.

National Institutes of Health/National Heart, Lung, and Blood Institute. (1998). *Clinical guidelines on the identification, evaluation, and treatment of overweight and obesity in adults* (NIH Publication No. 98-4083). Washington, DC: U.S. Government Printing Office.—The appendix of this excellent, evidence-based publication includes an annotated bibliography of studies specifically designed to achieve weight reduction in minority populations.

Solomons, N. W., & Kumanyika, S. K. (2000). Implications of racial distinctions for body composition and its diagnostic assessment. *American Journal of Clinical Nutrition. 71,* 1387–1389.—Thoughtful discussion of the implications of a study reporting racial differences in body composition of blacks and whites.

Wing, R. R., & Anglin, K. (1996). Effectiveness of a behavioral weight control program for blacks and whites with NIDDM. *Diabetes Care, 19,* 409–413.—A behavioral intervention program based on the use of a very-low-calorie diet for patients with type 2 diabetes.

# 106

# Characteristics of Successful Weight Maintainers

RENA R. WING
MARYLOU KLEM

Long-term maintenance of weight loss is clearly difficult to accomplish. However, some individuals are successful in losing weight and maintaining the loss over the long term. This chapter reviews the research on the prevalence of weight loss maintenance and the characteristics of individuals who have achieved it.

## PREVALENCE OF WEIGHT LOSS MAINTENANCE

Few studies have assessed the prevalence of weight loss maintenance. Currently, there is no accepted criterion for successful maintenance (how much weight must be lost and how long it must be maintained).

In 1959, Stunkard and McLaren-Hume concluded that < 5% of obese individuals are able to lose weight and maintain it. This pessimistic conclusion, derived from a sample of 100 patients, was based on only one weight loss attempt. Other investigators, reporting results in clinical treatment programs, have found that 13–22% of individuals maintain a weight loss of ≥ 5 kg at 5 years.

Estimates of maintenance have also been made from community samples. Recently, researchers used a random-digit dial telephone survey to determine the point prevalence of weight loss maintenance in a nationally representative sample of 500 adults in the United States. Maintainers were defined as those who, at the time of the survey, had maintained for at least 1 year a weight loss of ≥ 10% of their maximum adult weight. Fourteen percent of the sample as a whole and 21% of those with a history of obesity were currently 10% below their highest weight, had reduced intentionally, and had maintained a 10% weight loss for at least 1 year. These data contrast the belief that no one ever succeeds at weight loss maintenance.

## THE NATIONAL WEIGHT CONTROL REGISTRY

In order to learn more about successful weight loss maintenance, James Hill and Rena Wing established the National Weight Control Registry (NWCR). In order to be eligible for the registry, an individual must have lost at least 30 pounds and kept it off at least 1 year. Currently, there are over 3,000 individuals in the registry, and these participants far exceed these minimum criteria. On average, NWCR members have lost 66 pounds and kept it off 6 years. Other findings of particular interest about these members are as follows:

• Of NWCR members, 55% report losing weight with some type of assistance (a commercial program, a nutritionist, a physician), but the other 45% report losing weight entirely on their own.

• Among members, 46% became overweight before age 11 and 25% became overweight between ages 12 and 18; hence, the presence of childhood-onset obesity did not preclude success. Similarly, 46% of the sample had one biological parent who was overweight, and 27% had two overweight parents. Despite a possible genetic predisposition to obesity, they were able to lose weight and maintain it.

• Over 90% of the members had tried previously to lose weight; thus, these successful weight losers were previously "unsuccessful losers." This finding suggests that it may be more appropriate to identify differences between successful and unsuccessful weight loss *attempts* rather than between successful and unsuccessful weight losers.

## BEHAVIOR CHANGES ASSOCIATED WITH SUCCESSFUL WEIGHT LOSS MAINTENANCE

### Physical Activity

Physical activity has been the factor most consistently related to weight maintenance, as seen in different types of studies (see Chapters 89, 93, and 107). Studies comparing successful maintainers to regainers have consistently shown differences in physical activity. In one study, 90% of successful maintainers reported exercising at least three times per week for 30 minutes or more, compared to only 34% of weight regainers. Among individuals who initially used exercise to lose weight, another study found that 100% of weight maintainers, and only 53% of weight regainers, were still exercising at 50% or more of their original activity level.

Only one study quantified the amount of activity of successful maintainers. Researchers with the NWCR found that participants reported expending 2,826 kcal per week through physical activity, an amount equivalent to walking 4 miles per day. When registry members were classified according to their initial method of weight loss (organized program, liquid-formula diet, or on their own), there were no differences between the groups in total energy expenditure. Individuals who had lost weight on their own were most likely to report high levels of vigorous activity such as running or weight-lifting. Nonetheless, the similarity of activity levels among individuals who initially used such different methods to lose weight is noteworthy.

Randomized clinical trials also provide evidence for the role of physical activity in weight loss maintenance. In many (but not all) of these studies, subjects randomly assigned to diet plus exercise treatment conditions have shown better maintenance of weight loss than subjects assigned to diet-only or exercise-only conditions. A recent clinical trial has demonstrated, however, that adding exercise recommendations to treatment protocols is not a panacea. Seventy-seven obese women were randomly assigned to receive a 48-week behavioral weight loss program that included (1) aerobic exercise, (2) strength training, (3) aerobic exercise plus strength training, or (4) no exercise training. Contrary to expectations, follow-up one year after treatment indicated no differences in the groups' success at weight maintenance: All had regained 35–55% of their initial weight loss, and post hoc analyses indicated that subjects in the exercise conditions were no more likely than subjects in the diet-only group to be currently exercising on a regular basis. However, when self-described regular exercisers were compared to subjects not exercising on a regular basis (collapsing across treatment groups), regular exercisers had significantly greater mean weight loss at follow-up (12.1 kg vs. 6.1 kg) and had regained less weight between end of treatment and follow-up (5.5 kg vs. 8.4 kg). Thus, while the impact of regular exercise on successful weight maintenance has been demonstrated, the issue remains of how best to help patients comply with exercise recommendations.

## Dietary Factors

The earliest studies of successful maintainers surveyed participants about the types or kinds of food they were eating and found some indication of altered eating habits. Compared to regainers, weight maintainers were more likely to report restricted intake of candy and chocolate, and diets low in sugar, fat, and red meat. Recent studies have further quantified the dietary habits of successful maintainers. Individuals in the NWCR were asked to complete the Block Food Frequency Questionnaire. Registry participants reported consuming a low-calorie (1,380 kcal/day), low-fat (24% of calories from fat) diet. Registry members had similar, if not higher, intake of selected nutrients (vitamins A, C, E and calcium) when compared to a national sample of U.S. adults and to the Recommended Daily Allowances (RDAs) issued by the U.S. Department of Agriculture. Thus, as a group, they were eating a healthy diet high in fruits, vegetables, and low-fat calcium products.

While maintainers appear in general to be eating low-fat diets, this pattern may differ according to the method used to lose weight. Individuals in the registry who lost weight through bariatric surgery reported higher levels of daily fat intake (34.8%) and lower levels of protein and carbohydrate intake than did those who had lost a comparable amount of weight (mean = 120 pounds) through other means. While biases in self-reports of energy intake may explain this difference, it is also possible that gastric surgery creates physiological changes that affect dietary selection (see Chapters 101 and 102). If such differences truly exist, their impact on the health consequences of weight loss maintenance (e.g., serum cholesterol levels) or probability of continued weight maintenance should be explored.

## Behavioral Strategies

The mainstay of behavioral weight loss programs is self-monitoring, and there is evidence that successful maintainers continue to monitor their weight and eating behaviors on some level (see Chapter 94). Maintainers report that they must continue to be conscious of the quantity and type of food consumed, as well as the level of activity necessary to stay at reduced weight. They are more likely than relapsers or controls who have never been overweight to weigh themselves at least once a week and to regulate dietary fat intake by modifying meat preparation, avoiding fried foods, and substituting low-fat for high-fat foods. Specifically, within the NWCR, at least one-third of participants reported using strategies such as limiting intake of certain types of food or portion sizes and counting calories or fat grams, and 72% reported weighing themselves at least once a week. Taken together, these findings certainly imply that maintainers remain vigilant regarding their weight and food intake.

## PSYCHOLOGICAL CONSEQUENCES OF SUCCESSFUL WEIGHT LOSS MAINTENANCE

People maintain substantial weight losses (e.g., average weight loss of NWCR members is 66 pounds) through a combination of low energy intake and high activity levels, and thus might be considered "chronic dieters." It has been suggested that chronic dieting can lead to emotional problems and disordered eating (see Chapters 15, 16, and 17). While research on this issue is limited, available data suggest that psychosocial problems are not an inevitable outcome of successful maintenance of weight loss (see Chapter 90). Anecdotal evidence from early studies of weight maintainers suggested that subjects felt "more confident," "self-assured," and "more capable of handling their problems." Psychological functioning and disordered eating have been assessed in NWCR members and compared to levels of functioning in psychiatric- and community-based samples. Levels of distress and depressive symptoms in the maintainers were similar to the levels observed in community samples and much lower than those found in psychiatric samples. Rates of binge eating, self-induced vomiting, and disinhibition were also much lower than rates found in samples of patients with eating disorders. Of NWCR members, 85% also reported that weight loss and maintenance had improved their quality of life, level of energy, physical mobility, general mood, self-confidence, and physical health, while only 20% reported more time spent thinking about weight and 14% more time spent thinking about food. A possible explanation of these findings could be that psychologically healthy individuals are more likely either to be successful at weight loss or to volunteer for studies. At the very least, these findings suggest that psychological dysfunction is not an inevitable consequence of successful maintenance and in all likelihood, maintenance improves well-being.

## FACTORS ASSOCIATED WITH WEIGHT REGAIN

Since many individuals who lose weight subsequently regain, investigators have suggested that metabolic changes associated with weight loss may predispose individuals to regain (see Chapters 8 and 12). For example, it has been suggested that there may be a greater than expected decrease in metabolic rate that would make these individuals vulnerable to weight regain. Although some studies have found resting metabolic rate to be reduced in formerly obese individuals, most studies have found that it is appropriate to the reduced, lean mass. For example, investigators found no evidence of decreased resting metabolic rate in the reduced obese subjects in the NWCR compared to weight-matched controls with no history of weight loss.

Several studies have found that successful weight losers have higher respiratory quotients than weight-matched controls. These data indicate that there may be decreased fat oxidation in reduced obese individuals (which would predispose them to regain weight), or this could result from the low-fat diet often consumed by successful weight losers.

Other studies have focused on behavior changes as factors associated with weight regain. When NWCR participants were followed for 1 year, 35% gained 5 pounds or more. Risk factors for weight gain included more recent weight loss (< 2 years vs. > 2 years), larger initial weight losses (> 30% of maximum weight vs. < 30%), and higher depression, dietary disinhibition, and binge-eating levels at entry into the registry. Moreover, those who gained over the 1-year interval reported greater decreases in physical activity, greater increases in percentage of calories from dietary fat, and greater decreases in dietary restraint. Thus, weight regain appears to be due in large part to failure to maintain behavior changes.

# CONCLUSION

Recent studies have indicated that there are indeed individuals who are successful at long term weight loss and maintenance. These individuals appear to be characterized by continued consumption of a low-calorie, low-fat diet, high levels of physical activity, and overall vigilance regarding their weight.

## FURTHER READING

Kayman, S., Bruvold, W., & Stern, J. S. (1990). Maintenance and relapse after weight loss in women: Behavioral aspects. *American Journal of Clinical Nutrition, 52*, 800–807.—Compares behavioral and psychological characteristics of successful weight loss maintainers, regainers, and controls.

Klem, M. L., Wing, R. R., McGuire, M. T., Seagle, H. M., & Hill, J. O. (1997). A descriptive study of individuals successful at long-term maintenance of substantial weight loss. *American Journal of Clinical Nutrition, 66*, 239–246.—Describes characteristics of individuals in the NWCR.

McGuire, M. T., Wing, R. R., & Hill, J. O. (1999). The prevalence of weight loss maintenance among American adults. *International Journal of Obesity, 23*, 1314–1319.—Random-digit dialing survey of the prevalence of successful maintenance of weight loss.

McGuire, M. T., Wing, R. R., Klem, M. L., Lang, W., & Hill, J. O. (1999). What predicts weight regain among a group of successful weight losers? *Journal of Consulting and Clinical Psychology, 67*, 177–185.—Examines variables associated with weight regain in the NWCR.

Wadden, T. A., Vogt, R. A., Andersen, R. E., Bartlett, S. J., Foster, G. D., Kuehnel, R. H., Wilk, J., Weinstock, R., Buckenmeyer, P., Berkowitz, R. I., & Steen, S. N. (1997). Exercise in the treatment of obesity: Effects of four interventions on body composition, resting energy expenditure, appetite, and mood. *Journal of Consulting and Clinical Psychology, 65*, 269–277.—Randomized, controlled trial of the effects of aerobic and resistance training on long-term maintenance of weight loss.

Wing, R. (1999). Physical activity in the treatment of the adulthood overweight and obesity: Current evidence and research issues. *Medicine and Science in Sports and Exercise, 31*, S547–S552.—Recent review of the relationship between physical activity and weight loss.

# 107

# Improving Maintenance in Behavioral Treatment

## MICHAEL G. PERRI

Poor maintenance of treatment-induced weight loss represents a critical problem in the management of obesity (see Chapter 94). Individuals who complete behavioral weight loss programs lose on average about 9% of their body weight but regain about half of the lost weight within 1 year and nearly all of it within 5 years. Nonetheless, a significant proportion of participants in behavioral programs (approximately 20%) succeed in sustaining 50% or more of their lost weight over 4 years. Moreover, an increasing number of studies provide data about the effectiveness of specific methods to enhance maintenance (see Chapter 106). Knowledge of the research on maintenance strategies can provide the clinician with useful information for long-term treatment planning in the care of obese clients.

## UNDERSTANDING THE MAINTENANCE PROBLEM

The "maintenance problem" in obesity treatment stems from a complex interaction of physiological, environmental, and psychological variables. Physiological factors such as reduced metabolic rate, resulting from sustained dieting, prime the obese person to regain lost weight. Continuous exposure to an environment rich in tasty, high-calorie foods, combined with a dieting-induced, heightened sensitivity to palatable foods, further predisposes the individual to setbacks in dietary control (see Chapter 78). Most obese persons cannot sustain the substantial degree of psychological control needed to cope effectively with this unfriendly combination of environment and biology (see Chapter 83). Furthermore, following weight loss treatment, there are fewer reinforcers to help patients maintain adherence to changes in diet and activity. The most reward-

**TABLE 107.1. Effects of Maintenance Strategies Implemented or Continued after Initial Behavioral Treatment**

| Maintenance strategy | Beneficial effect observed 6 to 12 months after initial treatment | Beneficial effect observed 13 or more months after initial treatment |
| --- | --- | --- |
| Extended treatment | | |
| Continued weekly or biweekly group treatment sessions up to 1 year | Yes | Yes |
| Therapist contact by mail + phone | Yes | Unknown |
| Telephone prompts by nontherapists | No | Unknown |
| Skills training | | |
| Relapse prevention training during initial treatment | No | Unlikely |
| Relapse prevention training combined with posttreatment therapist contacts | Yes | Unknown |
| Social support training | | |
| Peer support training | No | Unlikely |
| Social support training for clients recruited with friends or relatives | Yes | Unknown |
| Food provision | | |
| Provision of no-cost, portion-controlled meals | Yes | No |
| Optional purchase of portion-controlled meals | No | Unlikely |
| Financial incentives | | |
| Financial incentives for weight loss | No | No |
| Financial incentives for exercise | No | No |
| Exercise | | |
| Supervised group exercise | No | No |
| Use of personal trainers | No | No |
| Home-based exercise | Yes | Unknown |
| Short-bout exercise + home exercise equipment | Yes | Unknown |
| Multicomponent posttreatment programs | | |
| Therapist contact + increased exercise | Yes | Yes |
| Therapist contact + social support | Yes | Yes |
| Therapist contact + increased exercise + social support | Yes | Yes |

ing element of treatment, weight loss, typically ends with the cessation of intervention. As a result, many individuals perceive a high "cost" associated with continued dietary control, while experiencing diminished "benefits" in terms of little or no additional weight loss. Thus, discouragement is common. Small, posttreatment weight gains often lead to patients' attributions of personal ineffectiveness that can result in hopelessness and giving up.

## MAINTENANCE STRATEGIES

The use of strategies designed to maintain the changes accomplished in initial treatment may improve long-term outcome. The maintenance methods that have been evaluated include extended treatment, skills training, social support, food provision, financial incentives, exercise, and multicomponent programs. Table 107.1 provides a summary of the effects of these strategies on the maintenance of lost weight as tested in controlled studies with 6- to 24-month follow-up.

### Extended Treatment

In general, the longer obese clients remain in contact with treatment providers, the longer they adhere to necessary behaviors. "State-of-the-art" behavioral programs typically include 6 months of weekly group sessions followed by extended treatment regimens, with 6 to 12 months of additional therapist contact. Extended treatment programs enable obese individuals to maintain 80-100% of the weight they lose during the initial intervention. Without continuing contact, clients typically maintain only 50-60% of their initial losses.

Extended treatment provides clients with the opportunity for professional assistance in negotiating obstacles to maintenance. Extending the length of treatment offers a relatively straightforward approach to improving outcome. Alternatives to continuing, in-person treatment sessions include therapist contacts by telephone and mail, as well as the use of telephone reminders to prompt clients to engage in key behavioral strategies such as self-monitoring. In general, additional counseling via telephone and mail appears to have a beneficial impact on adherence and the maintenance of lost weight. However, the use of simple telephone prompts by nonclinicians has not been effective.

### Skills Training

Training in specific cognitive-behavioral strategies may minimize setbacks following treatment. Clients can be taught to recognize situations that pose "high risk" for a lapse; problem solving can then be employed to generate ways of coping with high-risk situations; clients can be taught cognitive restructuring techniques to overcome the sense of failure that accompanies lapses in self-control. Teaching relapse prevention techniques during initial therapy does *not* have a beneficial effect on long-term progress. However, combining relapse prevention training and professional contacts during follow-up seems to improve maintenance. To prevent a relapse, clients may need the assistance of a health care professional at the time they are experiencing an initial slip or lapse.

### Social Support

Self-help groups such as TOPS (Take Off Pounds Sensibly) and OA (Overeaters Anonymous) are available to assist overweight people with ongoing social support, but little is known about the effectiveness of these groups as aids to maintaining lost weight (see Chapter 98). Several studies have examined the use of partners, peers, family members, and friends in the management of obesity. Some research has indicated that *cooperative* partners can have a beneficial impact on outcome. Other studies have suggested that groups of obese individuals can be taught how to run their own peer support groups and that such groups may have a positive impact on the maintenance of lost weight. In addition, recruiting obese clients to participate in treatment together with small groups of friends or family members and then training them to make use of social support has shown promising results in the short-term maintenance of lost weight.

## Food Provision

Some obesity researchers have suggested that better long-term results might be obtained by directly altering the environment of obese individuals rather than relying on clients themselves to make required dietary changes. Similar to the approach of commercial programs such as NutriSystem, some studies have examined the effectiveness of providing clients with portion-controlled meals. The provision of no-cost, portion-controlled meals has been shown to improve weight loss during both initial treatment and a 12-month maintenance period. The mechanism primarily responsible is better adherence to decreased energy intake. Unfortunately, the benefits of this approach are limited. When food provision ends, clients regain weight, and when offered the opportunity to purchase portion-controlled meals, few do so.

## Financial Incentives

The consequences of eating and exercise behaviors represent important environmental influences on weight control. Thus, some researchers have examined the impact of providing monetary incentives for weight loss. Results generally indicate no benefit from the provision of financial incentives, even when very strong monetary contingencies are applied (e.g., $25 per week for maintenance of a 14-kg weight loss).

## Exercise

Regular exercise produces many benefits for overweight individuals, including increased energy expenditure and improvements in mood and self-concept (see Chapters 89 and 93). However, most controlled trials have failed to show that the combination of diet plus exercise produces greater maintenance of lost weight than diet alone. The modest effects of exercise (particularly supervised group exercise) on long-term weight may be due to poor or inconsistent exercise adherence. Consequently, attention has turned to improving exercise adherence in obesity treatment. Several approaches have been evaluated, including home-based exercise (rather than supervised group exercise), the use of short rather than long bouts of exercise (e.g., four 10-minute bouts vs. one 40-minute bout), the provision of home exercise equipment, the use of personal trainers, and posttreatment programs focused exclusively on exercise adherence. Improvements in adherence and weight loss have been observed with home-based exercise programs and with short-bout exercise regimens combined with home exercise equipment (i.e., motorized treadmills). Although the use of personal trainers increases attendance at supervised exercise sessions, improved weight loss has not been demonstrated. Similarly, posttreatment programs with an exclusive focus on exercise adherence are not sufficient to improve long-term weight outcome. Successful maintenance programs require attention to energy intake as well as energy expenditure.

## Multicomponent Posttreatment Programs

The ideal maintenance program would involve matching treatment methods to the specific needs of particular clients. However, an empirical database describing those procedures best suited to particular clients is not yet available. Consequently, multicomponent programs have been developed with the expectation that some aspect of a multifaceted approach will benefit each individual. Empirically tested, multicomponent posttreatment programs have included ongoing professional contacts, training in problem-solving or relapse prevention skills, social support, and high-frequency exercise. Several studies have demonstrated that weight loss treatments supplemented with multicomponent maintenance programs produce better long-term results than treatments without maintenance programs. However, while multicomponent programs are appealing to clients and therapists, adding facets such as social support, skills training, or increased exercise opportunities may not produce benefits beyond the positive effects produced by extended therapy.

## CONCLUSION

The long-term management of obesity presents a daunting challenge to health care professionals. For most obese individuals, the successful management of obesity will require the implementation of maintenance strategies over long periods of time. Thus, professionals must be prepared to aid the obese client in identifying effective methods to sustain the behavioral changes needed for long-term success. Equipped with a variety of strategies to enhance the persistence of changes in diet and exercise, clinicians will be better able to assist their clients in the long-term management of obesity.

## FURTHER READING

Cooper, Z., & Fairburn, C. G. (in press). Cognitive behavioral treatment of obesity. In T. A. Wadden & A. J. Stunkard (Eds.), *Handbook of obesity treatment*. New York: Guilford Press. A cognitive-behavioral analysis of weight regain in obesity treatment.

Jakicic, J. M., Winters, C., Lang, W., & Wing, R. R. (1999). Effects of intermittent exercise and use of home exercise equipment on adherence, weight loss, and fitness in overweight women: A randomized trial. *Journal of the American Medical Association, 282*, 1554-1560. Outcome study showing the benefits of short bouts of exercise and the use of home exercise equipment.

Jeffery, R. W., Drewnowski, A., Epstein, L. H., Stunkard, A. J., Wilson, G. T., Wing, R. R., & Hill, D. R. (2000). Long-term maintenance of weight loss: Current status. *Health Psychology, 19*(Suppl.), 5-16. A comprehensive review of the long-term effects of obesity treatments.

Jeffery, R. W., Wing, R. R., Thorson, C., Burton, L. R., Raether, C., Harvey, J., & Mullen, M. (1993). Strengthening behavioral interventions for weight loss: A randomized trial of food provision and monetary incentives. *Journal of Consulting and Clinical Psychology, 61*, 1038-1045. Outcome study documenting the impact of food provision and monetary incentives on weight loss.

Kramer, F. M., Jeffery, R. W., Forster, J. L., & Snell, M. K. (1989). Long-term follow-up of behavioral treatment for obesity: Patterns of weight gain among men and women. *International Journal of Obesity, 13*, 124-136. Long-term study documenting the patterns of weight change following behavioral treatment.

Perri, M. G., & Corsica, J. A. (in press). Improving the maintenance of weight lost in behavioral treatment of obesity.  In T. A. Wadden & A. J. Stunkard (Eds.), *Handbook of obesity treat-ment*. New York: Guilford Press. A comprehensive review of research on maintenance strate-gies.

Perri, M. G., McAllister, D. A., Gange, J. J., Jordan, R. C., McAdoo, W. G., & Nezu, A. M. (1988). Effects of four maintenance programs on the long-term management of obesity. *Journal of Consulting and Clinical Psychology, 56*, 529-534. Outcome study documenting the benefits of posttreatment maintenance programs.

Perri, M. G., Martin, A. D., Leermakers, E. A., Sears, S. F., & Notelovitz, M. (1997). Effects of group- versus home-based exercise in the treatment of obesity. *Journal of Consulting and Clin-ical Psychology, 65*, 278-285. Outcome study demonstrating the benefits of home-based exer-cise.

# 108

## The Management of Body Image Problems

### THOMAS F. CASH

### THE NATURE OF BODY IMAGE AND BODY IMAGE PROBLEMS

Body image is a clinically important, multifaceted psychological concept that refers to persons' perceptions, attitudes, and experiences about the body, especially its appearance (see Chapter 72). It has clear effects on psychosocial functioning and quality of life; individuals who are dissatisfied with their appearance are susceptible to impaired self-esteem, social self-consciousness and anxiety, depression, eating disturbances, and sexual difficulties. Body image disturbances may be viewed on a continuum from relatively benign discontent to experiences of intense preoccupation and distress. The latter may reflect severe clinical conditions, such as somatic delusional disorder, body dysmorphic disorder, anorexia nervosa, bulimia nervosa, and gender identity disorder (see Chapter 21).

In the United States, body image dissatisfaction has increased, certainly among women and perhaps among men. Concurrently, the population has become heavier. Women's body image concerns, especially displeasure with weight and shape, are so prevalent they have been termed "normative discontent." Immersed in cultural messages that "looks are everything," people aspire to physical ideals that are extreme and seldom attainable (see Chapter 19).

Psychological investment in one's physical appearance comes at a price. The internalization of lofty standards can undermine self-worth as one's body fails to meet ideals. Body image development is also influenced by familial and peer modeling of values about appearance, and by the interpersonal reactions to one's body. For example, appearance-related teasing and criticism can exert lasting deleterious effects on body image. From such experiences, people acquire guiding assumptions or schemas about the psychosocial importance of their looks. Such assumptions are pivotal in the meaning that individuals attach to experiences in everyday life. To manage body image discomfort, people employ a variety of cognitive and behavioral strategies, including avoidant and compensatory actions, as well as efforts to alter the body to conform to personal ideals.

As Rosen has discussed earlier in this volume (Chapter 72), overweight and obese individuals clearly experience a more negative body image than do thin persons. Their degree of body image disparagement is related to experiences of weight stigmatization during childhood, adolescence, and adulthood. Weight loss does lead to body image improvements. Still, research suggests that among formerly overweight or obese persons, all is not lost. Often they retain "phantom fat"—a vulnerable view of their body that remembers the adverse experiences that come with the condition.

## BODY IMAGE TREATMENT: COGNITIVE-BEHAVIORAL COMPONENTS

Because negative body image is a widespread problem that may impair quality of life, professionals have developed various psychotherapeutic treatments. Among these, cognitive-behavioral treatment (CBT) has emerged as an effective, empirically sound intervention. Cash's CBT program for a negative body image has gone through four generations of development. The first was a treatment manual from a study in 1985 by Butters and Cash. The second version was Cash's published audiotape program available to mental health practitioners: *Body-Image Therapy: A Program for Self-Directed Change*. The third version of the program was his 1995 self-help book for the public: *What Do You See When You Look in the Mirror?: Helping Yourself to a Positive Body Image*. The most recent refinement of the program, based on empirical data and client feedback, is *The Body Image Workbook: An 8-Step Program for Learning to Like Your Looks*. It is presented in a user-friendly format and contains over 40 "Self-Discovery Helpsheets" and "Helpsheets for Change." The elements of this version of the program are summarized as follows:

• The workbook's introduction explains the nature of body image problems and offers an overview of the program, including its empirical foundations. Severe problems (e.g., body dysmorphic disorder, eating disorders, and clinical depression) that require professional assistance are discussed.

• *Step 1* involves baseline assessments with a series of scientific measures of key facets of body image—for example, the Multidimensional Body Self-Relations Questionnaire, the Situational Inventory of Body Image Dysphoria, and the Body Images Ideal Questionnaire. Using interpretations provided for the calculated assessment profile, participants then set specific goals for change.

• *Step 2*, a psychoeducational aspect of the program, delineates the nature of body image and the causes of body image problems. Participants learn how developmental and historical events, including the acquisition of body image attitudes based on cultural and social experiences, serve as diatheses for later difficulties. They then learn how these vulnerabilities are activated and unfold in day-to-day thoughts, feelings, and behaviors that often become self-perpetuating. The self-discovery process also includes mirror-exposure activities and an autobiographical summary of participants' own body image development. Completing a "Body Image Diary," participants learn to monitor their current body image experiences by attending to and recording the precipitants of distress and the associated effects on their thought processes, emotions, and subsequent behaviors. This diary is used systematically throughout the program.

• *Step 3* teaches "Body and Mind Relaxation," which integrates muscle relaxation, diaphragmatic breathing, mental imagery, and positive self-talk to promote skills for managing emotions caused by dysphoric body image. These skills are then applied in desensitization exercises to foster body image comfort in relation to physical and contextual stimuli that provoke body image distress.

• *Step 4* identifies dysfunctional "appearance assumptions"—beliefs or schemas that impact daily body image experiences. Derived from Cash and Labarge's Appearance Schemas Inventory, examples of these problematic assumptions are as follows: "If I could look just as I wish, my life would be much happier." "Physically attractive people have it all." "If people knew how I really look, they would like me less." "I should do whatever I can to always look my best." "The only way I could ever like my looks would be to change them." Participants learn to become cognizant of the ongoing operation of these assumptions, and to question and refute them.

• *Step 5* enables participants to identify particular cognitive distortions in body-related thought processes and offers strategies for modifying them. Such distortions include comparing one's appearance to more attractive persons, thinking of one's looks in dichotomous extremes (e.g., ugly or good-looking; fat or thin), assuming that other people share a negative view of one's looks, and arbitrarily blaming one's appearance for life's difficulties and disappointments. Participants extend their diary keeping to incorporate cognitive restructuring exercises, in order to correct their cognitive distortions and to witness the emotional and behavioral consequences.

• *Step 6* helps participants to develop specific behavioral strategies for altering avoidant behaviors related to poor body image—avoiding activities (e.g., exercising, going without makeup, or having sex), situations (e.g., the beach or gym), or people (e.g., attractive individuals) that might engender self-consciousness and body image distress. Participants also target and modify "appearance-preoccupied rituals" such as repeated mirror checking or excessive grooming regimens. These self-tailored strategies typically involve graduated exposure and interventions for response prevention.

• *Step 7* applies the metaphor of interpersonal relationship satisfaction (i.e., a good marriage or friendship) to facilitate a proactive, positive relationship with one's body. Participants engage in prescribed exercises for "body image affirmation" and "body image enhancement"—for example, reinforcing activities that pertain to physical fitness and health, sensate enjoyment, and grooming for pleasure rather than for the concealment or reparation of perceived flaws. Thus, whereas Step 6 largely targets negatively reinforced behaviors (i.e., situational avoidance and compulsive habits), Step 7 emphasizes the acquisition of body-related activities through positive reinforcement by creating experiences of mastery and pleasure.

• *Step 8* concludes the program by having participants retake body image assessments and receive feedback about the changes they have achieved. Participants then set goals for further needed changes. From a perspective of relapse prevention, they learn to identify and prepare for situations (e.g., difficult interpersonal situations) that place them at future risk for body image dysphoria.

## THE EFFECTIVENESS OF BODY IMAGE COGNITIVE-BEHAVIORAL THERAPY

Numerous studies attest to the effectiveness of body image CBT carried out as individual therapy, group therapy, and self-administered treatment (see Chapter 72). Outcomes include increased body satisfaction; less investment in appearance; reduced experiences of body image distress; fewer avoidant and compulsive behaviors; and generalization of positive effects to self-esteem, social functioning, sexual experiences, depressive symptoms, and eating pathology. Follow-up evaluations beyond several months are lacking, so whether these favorable changes are lasting remains unknown.

Although most body image CBT studies have been conducted with college women who experience extreme dissatisfaction, outcomes are comparable regardless of participants' weight. Rosen's clinical trials have confirmed the efficacy of body image CBT with two additional, important populations: individuals with body dysmorphic disorder and obese persons. His latter study enrolled participants who had been repeatedly unsuccessful with weight loss and wished to feel better about themselves without dieting. Evidence of their improved body image without subsequent weight gain refutes assumptions that overweight or obese individuals must lose weight to improve their body image, and that better body image acceptance will lead to weight gain.

In our thinness-preoccupied and fat-phobic society, adiposity is a stigmatizing condition across the lifespan. Given the fact that dieting interventions are only moderately efficacious vis-à-vis the long-term maintenance of weight loss and that subsequent weight regain produces a substantial deterioration of body image, there are good reasons to consider body image CBT as an adjunctive or alternative treatment for obese persons. Such treatment might facilitate more appropriately moderate goal setting for weight loss and help stabilize binge eating and maladaptive dysphoria related to being obese.

## CONCLUSIONS

The quality of our embodied lives can be heightened or diminished by the views we hold of our own physical appearance. Many people, often women, invest their self-worth in the size and appearance of their body and attempt to conform to exacting cultural standards of beauty. Body image dissatisfaction can compromise self-esteem, emotional health, social and sexual well-being, and adaptive eating behaviors. People who are overweight or obese can have an especially damaged body image. The continued pursuit of scientific knowledge concerning how body image problems develop and can be prevented and overcome is imperative.

## FURTHER READING

Butters, J. W., & Cash, T. F. (1987). Cognitive-behavioral treatment of women's body image dissatisfaction. *Journal of Consulting and Clinical Psychology, 55*, 889–897.—Early protocol for managing body image disturbance.

Cash, T. F. (1996). The treatment of body image disturbances. In J. K. Thompson (Ed.), *Body image, eating disorders, and obesity: An integrative guide for assessment and treatment* (pp. 83–107). Washington, DC: American Psychological Association.—A detailed overview of the cognitive-behavioral treatment of body image.

Cash, T. F. (1997). *The body image workbook: An 8-step program for learning to like your looks.* Oakland, CA: New Harbinger.—The author's structured program for body image change, for both self-help and therapists' use.

Cash, T. F. (2000). Body image assessments (*www.body-images.com*).—The author's web site provides access to his validated measures of body image.

Cash, T. F., & Pruzinsky, T. (Eds.). (1990). *Body images: Development, deviance, and change.* New York: Guilford Press.—Delineates theory and research on body image and its development, assessment, and treatment.

Cash, T. F., & Roy, R. E. (1999). Pounds of flesh: Weight, gender, and body images. In J. Sobal & D. Maurer (Eds.), *Interpreting weight: The social management of fatness and thinness* (pp. 209–228). Hawthorne, NY: Aldine de Gruyter.—Reviews the literature on body image and obesity, with implications for intervention.

Friedman, M. A., & Brownell, K. D. (1995). Psychological correlates of obesity: Moving to the next research generation. *Psychological Bulletin, 117,* 3–20.—Critically reviews the literature on individual psychosocial differences associated with obesity.

Milkewicz, N., & Cash, T. F. (2000, November). *Dismantling the heterogeneity of obesity: Determinants of women's body images and psychosocial functioning.* Poster presentation at the convention of the Association for Advancement of Behavior therapy, New Orleans, LA.—Investigation of determinants of body image and psychosocial adjustment among obese, formerly obese, and stable, average-weight women (available from the author).

Rosen, J. C., Orosan, P., & Reiter, J. (1995). Cognitive behavior therapy for negative body image in obese women. *Behavior Therapy, 26,* 25–42.—Describes an investigation of the efficacy of body image therapy for obese persons.

Rosen, J. C., Reiter, J., & Orosan, P. (1995). Cognitive-behavioral body image therapy for body dysmorphic disorder. *Journal of Consulting and Clinical Psychology, 63,* 263–269.—Describes an investigation of the efficacy of body image therapy for persons with body dysmorphic disorder.

Thompson, J. K., Heinberg, L. J., Altabe, M., & Tantleff-Dunn, S. (Eds.). (1999). *Exacting beauty: Theory, assessment, and treatment of body image disturbance.* Washington, DC: American Psychological Association.—An extensive, scholarly volume on body image.

# 109

# Nondieting Approaches

## GARY D. FOSTER

During the last decade, dieting has come under attack by a growing movement that contends that "diets don't work" and that their physical and psychological ill effects far outweigh any fleeting benefits (see Chapters 15, 16, and 17). This movement—often referred to as "nondieting," "antidieting," or "undieting"—has gained support from professionals and nonprofessionals alike. This paradigm shift has left both practitioners and their obese patients in a quandry about how to manage weight and health. Should practitioners advise their overweight patients "to diet or not to diet"? Although the lack of data precludes a conclusive answer to this question, this chapter reviews the assumptions of the nondieting movement, the goals and methods of nondieting programs, and the research evaluating their efficacy.

## ASSUMPTIONS

The growing discontent with dieting and a search for alternative approaches is based on three basic premises: (1) Dieting confers a host of harmful physical and psychological effects; (2) dieting does not result in sustained weight loss; and (3) basic assumptions about the causes and consequences of overweight are incorrect.

### Dieting Is Harmful

First, the nondieting movement contends that dieting has significant medical and psychological consequences, including binge eating, reductions in metabolic rate, depression, irritability, low blood pressure, dizziness, food and weight preoccupation, social isolation, and diminished body image and self-esteem. Dieting is seen as a behavioral endorsement of the cultural norms that overvalue thinness and scorn obesity (see Chapters 19 and 20). Weight cycling—repeated cycles of dieting, weight loss, and regain—is believed to magnify the ill effects of dieting and may even lead to the very conditions (e.g., heart disease) that dieting seeks to improve.

## Dieting Is Ineffective

A second principle of the nondieting movement is that diets fail to produce their most desired outcome—long-term weight loss. It is argued that, in the long term, dieters usually end up weighing more, not less, after a diet. The negative consequences of dieting, described earlier, are even more disturbing given that dieters will not experience any sustained weight loss. Thus, dieting is viewed as a treatment that is both harmful and ineffective.

## Basic Assumptions Are Incorrect

A third tenet of the nondieting movement is that fundamental assumptions about the causes and consequences of overweight are incorrect. The genetic determinants of body weight are emphasized. The lack of efficacy of behavioral treatments is viewed as support for the biological, rather than the behavioral, basis of obesity. The nondieting movement also challenges the assumption that being overweight is unhealthy. It raises the possibility that the relationship between overweight and medical conditions can be explained by a third factor, such as repeated dieting, inactivity, or smoking to suppress appetite.

## PROGRAM GOALS AND METHODS

### Goals

These three beliefs have given rise to a number of "nondieting" approaches. These programs differ in their specific methods, but all generally seek to (1) increase awareness about dieting's ill effects; (2) encourage the use of internal cues such as hunger and fullness to guide eating behavior; (3) enhance knowledge about the biological basis of body weight; (4) improve self-esteem and body image through self-acceptance rather than weight loss; and (5) increase physical activity.

### Methods

Most programs begin by having participants examine their weight and dieting histories to underscore the untoward consequences and ineffectiveness of dieting. Information on the strong genetic influences on body weight is used to underscore the fact that weight cannot be easily changed and to debunk the notion that everyone can or should be the same size and weight.

Participants are encouraged to modify their eating behaviors by (1) abandoning dieting behaviors (e.g., going long periods of time without eating, avoiding forbidden foods, and getting weighed frequently); (2) rating hunger and fullness before, during, and after eating; and (3) choosing foods based on a model of healthy eating, such as the Food Guide Pyramid, rather than on calories and weight loss. Some programs make specific energy and macronutrient recommendations, while others suggest that participants eat whatever internal signals dictate. Similarly, some programs suggest keeping food records, while others view record keeping as dieting behavior. Suggestions for physical activity include having participants move their bodies in ways that they enjoy. This often involves changing long-standing beliefs about the type of activities in which overweight persons should not engage (e.g., dancing, jumping rope).

A principal technique for improving self-esteem and body image is to have participants engage in behaviors *now* rather than "putting life on hold," until they lose weight (e.g., taking a cruise, going to a high school reunion, or wearing certain types or colors of clothing). Participants are also encouraged to identify and counter their own antifat attitudes.

## EMPIRICAL SUPPORT

Most of the early studies on nondieting programs were descriptive in nature and showed significant improvements in participants' mood and self-esteem. Some studies reported weight losses of approximately 2 kg over 8 weeks, while others found weight gains of approximately 6 kg in 10 weeks. These studies were helpful in collecting initial data about novel approaches but provided no comparisons to traditional dieting approaches. More recent, controlled evaluations have shown greater improvements in mood and some measures of eating-related psychopathology when compared to dieting and wait-list controls. In addition, both the nondieting and weight loss groups lost small amounts of weight (< 3 kg). Participants in studies that used some elements of nondieting coupled with moderate restriction (1,800 kcal/day) showed better weight loss at 1 year than those assigned to a more traditional and restrictive weight loss approach (1,200 kcal/day). It is interesting to note that in at least one study, nondieting participants continued to lose weight during follow-up, while those receiving the standard dieting treatment gained weight. The available studies are limited by small sample sizes, short interventions, and incomplete follow-up.

## A CRITICAL VIEW

### Strengths

A major strength of the nondieting movement is its continued emphasis on the long-term ineffectiveness of dieting. Although regular physical activity and continued participant–practitioner contact following treatment significantly improve the maintenance of weight loss in the year following treatment, weight regain is the most frequent long-term outcome of dieting. Clearly, new approaches that are not based on the current paradigm of dieting are needed. The nondieting movement has provided one such alternative.

Perhaps the greatest strength of the nondieting movement is the affirmation of a person's worth, no matter what he or she weighs. This message is so counterculture that it can seem ridiculous to suggest that overweight persons should like themselves or that overweight does not result from a lack of character or willpower. Such stereotypes are not only inaccurate but they are also cruel. Like other forms of discrimination and prejudice, they should not be tolerated.

## Weaknesses

The most significant weakness of the nondieting approaches is the lack of scientific support. It is troubling that the number of nondieting books increases daily despite the dearth of controlled studies to demonstrate their effectiveness. Overweight persons deserve better. They are entitled to know the short- and long-term results of alternative treatments, so they can make informed decisions about their health and weight.

The nondieting movement also suffers from a lack of empirical support for some of its basic tenets. For example, the putative ill effects of dieting are inconsistent with a large body of literature demonstrating that dieting and weight loss are typically quite positive among obese persons receiving standard cognitive-behavioral treatment (see Chapter 90). In addition, the belief that weight is not a risk factor for disease or premature death is contrary to multiple studies that have controlled for mediating factors. Some data do suggest that being "healthy" may be more influenced by the degree of fitness than the degree of overweight. However, these findings are far from conclusive. Thus, it seems misleading, perhaps even irresponsible, to state unequivocally that excess weight has no adverse effects on health.

## Challenges

Given these strengths and weakness, the nondieting movement, as well as the entire scientific community with an interest in the health of overweight persons, is faced with a series of challenges. One is to evaluate nondieting approaches in controlled clinical trials. Such trials will need to define clearly what is meant by "dieting" and "nondieting," since nondieting approaches and standard behavioral interventions for weight loss have more in common than might be thought (e.g., eating a variety of foods in moderation, using stimulus control, increasing physical activity). Optimal interventions are likely to last at least 6–12 months and include follow-up evaluations $\geq 2$ years. If health at any weight is the desired paradigm shift, it will be essential to provide comprehensive measures of medical and psychosocial outcomes.

In addition to the larger issue of relative efficacy, it would be useful to identify which persons might benefit most from nondieting approaches (e.g., overweight persons who have never dieted, overweight persons who have dieted unsuccessfully, those at risk for eating disorders). A final challenge is to decrease the distance between dieting approaches, typically used by professionals in the obesity field, and nondieting approaches, typically used by those in the eating disorders field. This division has sometimes resulted in misunderstandings that can lead to hostility and hyperbole (see Chapter 17). Overweight persons would be better served by active collaboration between the two fields.

## SUMMARY

The development of nondieting approaches represents an exciting development in the care of overweight persons. These approaches should be carefully evaluated before being widely disseminated. Such information will help overweight persons make informed decisions about managing their health and weight. Whether the ultimate decision is to diet or not to diet, health care professionals should help overweight persons believe that weight is just one factor that describes them—it does not define them.

## FURTHER READING

Blair, S. N. (1991). *Living with exercise: Improving your health through moderate physical activity.* Dallas, TX: American Health.—An excellent guide for making small and sustainable changes in physical activity.

Foster, G. D., & Johnson, C. (1998). Facilitating health and self-esteem among obese patients. *Primary Psychiatry, 5,* 89–95.—A review of how obese patients are treated in the medical setting and ways to make office settings more receptive to obese patients.

Foster, G. D., & McGuckin, B. G. (in press). Nondieting approaches: Principles, practices and evidence. In T. A. Wadden & A. J. Stunkard (Eds.), *Handbook of obesity treatment.* New York: Guilford Press.—A comprehensive review of the assumptions, methods, and research of nondieting approaches.

Garner, D. M., & Wooley, S. C. (1991). Confronting the failure of behavioral and dietary treatments for obesity. *Clinical Psychology Review, 11,* 729–780.—A landmark paper that reviews the discontent with dieting approaches.

Johnson, C. (1995). *Self-esteem comes in all sizes: How to be happy and healthy at your natural weight.* New York: Doubleday.—A superb self-help book for creating weight-independent self-esteem.

Lyons, P., & Burgard, D. (1990). *Great shape: The first fitness guide for large women.* Palo Alto, CA: Bull.—An exceptional book to help large women move their bodies in way that is enjoyable.

The following papers, all from the same 1999 issue of *Journal of Social Issues* (Vol. 55) represent the current thinking of nondieting approaches from variety of perspectives. This is the single, best resource of information on the nondieting movement from leaders in the field.

Berg, F. M. (1999). Health risks associated with weight loss and obesity treatment programs. *Journal of Social Issues, 55,* 277–297.

Cogan, J. C., & Ernsberger, P. (1999). Dieting, weight and health: Reconceptualizing research and policy. *Journal of Social Issues, 55,* 187–205.

Ernsberger, P., & Koletsky, R. J. (1999). Biomedical rationale for a wellness approach to obesity: An alternative to a focus on weight loss. *Journal of Social Issues, 55,* 221–260.

McFarlane, T., Polivy, J., & McCabe, R. E. (1999). Help, not harm: Psychological foundation for a nondieting approach toward health. *Journal of Social Issues, 55,* 261–276.

Miller, W. C. (1999). Fitness and fatness in relation to health: Implications for a paradigm shift. *Journal of Social Issues, 55,* 207–219.

# 110

# Obesity and the Internet

## KEVIN R. FONTAINE
## DAVID B. ALLISON

The internet is having a substantial impact on daily life. Every day, thousands of new persons come "on-line" and are given near-instantaneous access to a wealth of information (and misinformation) that few dreamed possible even a decade ago. The exponential growth of the internet in conjunction with the increasing trend toward taking more personal responsibility for one's own health and health care has meant that the "web" has become an important source of health information. In this chapter, we briefly and selectively outline the obesity-related resources available on the internet. We will also highlight recent efforts to incorporate web technologies to promote weight control and obesity prevention, identify key issues, and offer some speculative recommendations for the use of this powerful technology.

## OBESITY-RELATED RESOURCES ON THE INTERNET

A search of key words such as "obesity," "nutrition," and "weight loss" on any search engine (e.g., Yahoo, WebCrawler) will unleash thousands of resources. Generally speaking, the resources can be divided into four categories: (1) academic resources, (2) obesity-related organizations, (3) chat groups and social support resources, and (4) commercial services and products. Table 110.1 presents a small selection of some prominent obesity-related web sites.

## THE INTERNET AS A THERAPEUTIC TOOL

In addition to its value as an information repository, the internet holds great promise as a technology to promote weight loss, long-term weight control, and obesity prevention. An example of the application of web technologies to the problem of obesity is the Shape Up

**TABLE 110.1. Selection of Obesity-Related Resources Available on the Internet**

| Web site | Description |
| --- | --- |
| American Dietetic Association (*www.eatright.org*) | Provides information on nutrition and weight control |
| American Obesity Association (*www.obesity.org*) | Provides education for general public and health professionals, and advocates for rights of obese persons |
| International Obesity TaskForce (*www.iotf.org*) | Provides education and advocates that obesity be viewed as a worldwide epidemic |
| National Association to Advance Fat Acceptance (*www.naafa.org*) | Advocates on behalf of obese persons to improve quality of life and reduce discrimination |
| National Heart, Lung, and Blood Institute (*www.nhlbi.nih.gov*) | Provides resources for health professionals and the general public |
| New York Obesity Research Center (*http://cpmcnet.columbia.edu/dept/obesectr/NYORC/*) | Provides information about the National Institutes of Health–funded New York Obesity Research Center and a useful set of links |
| North American Association for the Study of Obesity (*www.naaso.org*) | Interdisciplinary society that develops, extends, and disseminates knowledge in the field of obesity |
| Obesity Medications and Research News (*www.obesity-news.com*) | Provides general information on obesity and drug treatment |
| Shape up America! (*www.shapeup.org*) | Provides general information and an interactive weight control and physical activity program |

America! Program. Founded by former U.S. Surgeon General, C. Everett Koop, this initiative involves a coalition of industry and health experts, with the goals of promoting understanding of the importance of maintaining a healthy weight and increased physical activity, providing scientifically based information on how to achieve a healthy weight, and advancing healthy weight and physical activity as major public health priorities.

Moreover, federally funded efforts have been initiated to develop and pilot-test interactive web-based programs to (1) help prevent weight regain in person's that have weight-reduced; (2) promote changes in the dietary and physical activity practices of African American girls, a group at high risk of becoming obese; and (3) prevent pregnancy-induced obesity among minority women. It is hypothesized that by incorporating web-delivered components such as education on healthy eating and physical activity, self-monitoring, and on-line individual consultations, we will be able to enhance adherence and retention, and thereby increase the efficacy of weight management protocols. The findings from both Shape Up America! and these research projects will inform the field and generate further ideas on how to apply web technologies to the problem of obesity. To date, however, data pertaining to the efficacy of internet-based approaches to the problem of obesity are lacking.

## KEY ISSUES

Although the internet is a valuable resource for obesity-related information and holds great promise as a technology to promote weight control, it is not without drawbacks. First, as with any media, there is a danger that some of the information presented on the net is inaccurate or even potentially harmful (e.g., an ill-advised diet). There is perhaps a tendency among many users of the internet to assume that information presented electronically is somehow less prone to inaccuracy than information presented conventionally. However, if anything, the ease and efficiency with which information can be posted in cyberspace means that misinformation is likely. This may be especially so with regard to diet- and obesity-related chat rooms, where the validity of shared information and experiences cannot be verified. Second, and ironically, spending hours searching the internet to obtain information on how to control one's weight may in fact promote obesity (see Chapters 85, 93, and 103); that is, the time spent acquiring information could have been used to address one's weight more directly (e.g., exercise, cook healthy meals, etc.). People can become trapped in the belief that by searching the internet for obesity-related information, they are doing something tangible to address their weight, when they are not. Indeed, the impact of increased use of the internet on our already sedentary lifestyles may have a deleterious effect on weight and health. Third, the use of the web to deliver weight control interventions should not deter us from continuing to develop new and better ways to promote weight control; that is, obesity researchers and clinicians need to be careful to avoid the trap of simply using the web as a way to "repackage" current weight loss techniques and strategies that are of demonstrably limited efficacy. This would be reminiscent of efforts in the past to promote weight control by using more primitive repackaging techniques (e.g., bibliotherapy, audiocassettes). In short, the web should augment, not be a substitute for, the creation of innovative techniques to promote successful weight management.

Although the potential drawbacks of using the internet in the service of weight control and prevention should be kept in mind, the web also holds great promise in facilitating our ability to provide treatment-related information to obese individuals. The potential advantages of using the web include (1) the ability to reach literally thousands of persons at very low cost, (2) 24-hour access to the services provided, (3) the ability to facilitate the delivery of algorithms that match individuals to particular programs and treatment strategies, (4) frequent monitoring and the ability to send participants individualized feedback, and (5) the ability for persons to participate in treatment relatively anonymously. As noted earlier, several recently funded research efforts are evaluating whether these potential advantages can be exploited to produce better outcomes than standard treatment delivery methods.

## RECOMMENDATIONS

The internet has the potential to contribute greatly both to individual and societal efforts to stem the growing tide of obesity. However, as we have speculated, it may also actually

**TABLE 110.2. Potential Research Questions Related to Obesity and the Internet**

- Is the internet a reliable/useful source for conducting surveys on obesity-related topics? If so, under what circumstances?
- Does internet use promote physical inactivity and obesity?
- How can the quality of obesity-related information available on the internet be improved?
- What new weight management techniques can be developed that exploit the interactive capabilities of the internet?

have the potential to contribute to the problem. As such, we offer the following recommendations:

1. Users should evaluate all information critically and prefer information that has a firm scientific basis.
2. Information contained on web sites from well-respected organizations (e.g., American Dietetic Association, American Heart Association) should be preferred to that from less credible sources.
3. Obtaining obesity-related information and support from the web should not be at the expense of actually making the behavioral and psychosocial changes required for weight control.
4. Researchers and clinicians should not view the internet as simply another means to deliver treatment, but as a potential avenue with which to develop creative new ways to promote sustained behavior change and weight control. In Table 110.2 we suggest some research questions that need to be addressed by future work.

The potential of the internet to promote health, weight control, and well-being is limitless. However, if we are to make the most of this powerful technology, we need to evaluate carefully its strengths and weaknesses, and realize that it is simply a tool, not a substitute for "the torture of thought and effort."

## FURTHER READING

Ferguson, T. (1998). *Health online*. Reading, MA: Addison-Wesley. Provides a useful introduction to accessing health-related information via the internet.

Greeno, C. G., Wing, R. R., & Shiffman, S. (2000). Binge antecedents in obese women with and without binge eating disorder. *Journal of Consulting and Clinical Psychology, 68*, 95-102. Reports on the use of handheld computers to measure mood and appetite in a samples of binge-eating and non-binge-eating women.

Leaffer, T., & Gonda, B. (2000). The internet: An underutilized tool in patient education. *Computers in Nursing, 18*, 47-52. Describes the impact of a pilot study designed to increase internet use among senior citizens.

Maxwell, B. (1998). *How to find health information on the internet*. Washington, DC: Congressional Quarterly. A very user-friendly introduction to using the internet and accessing health-related information.

Winzelberg, A. J., Eppstein, D., Eldridge, K. L., Wilfley, D., Dasmahapatra, R., Dev, P., & Taylor, C. B. (2000). Effectiveness of an internet-based program for reducing risk factors for eating disorders. *Journal of Consulting and Clinical Psychology, 68*, 346-350. Reports on the use of computer-assisted health education program that addresses body dissatisfaction and weight–shape concerns among 60 college-age women.

# 111

# Public Health Approaches to the Management of Obesity

## ROBERT W. JEFFERY

The purpose of this chapter is to discuss the treatment of obesity from a public health perspective. Its primary thesis is that there are important differences between the medical and public health views of the problem and that these differences have implications for treatment.

Public health interventions for obesity should not simply be thought of as medical interventions disseminated on a larger scale. A public health perspective leads to consideration of environmental strategies that are quite different from those used in clinical management of obesity (see Chapter 112). Here, the success of the current generation of community programs for obesity control is described and alternative public health approaches are proposed.

## PUBLIC HEALTH VERSUS MEDICAL MODELS

Differences between medical and public health models begin with the definition of "obesity" itself. From a medical perspective, obesity is an individual-level variable. Patients are obese because their body fatness is high compared with population norms or biological ideals. From a public health perspective, however, "obesity" is defined in terms of average fatness in the population as a whole or the percentage of the population that exceeds a certain fatness level (prevalence). Obesity is a public health problem when its prevalence in a population is higher than that in other groups.

Public health and medical models also differ in the emphasis given to causal variables. The medical model searches for causes in variables that differ between individuals, including individual differences in genetics and in acquired characteristics (biological, psychological, and behavioral) that make some individuals susceptible to obesity.

The public health model recognizes individual differences as a source of variability, but to determine why some populations are more obese than others, the focus is on factors outside the individual, in particular, population exposure to environmental conditions that promote obesity (see Chapter 78).

It is not totally clear what specific types of exposure contribute to population obesity. Plausible suspects are a high energy-density food supply that is high in palatability and low in cost, and the widespread availability of labor-saving technologies that have eliminated the need for physical activity as part of everyday life. The main driving force behind the prevalence of obesity in the population is exposure to environmental conditions that promote high energy intake and a sedentary lifestyle (see Chapters 78 and 83). The extent to which specific individuals are affected by this exposure, however, is dictated to a large degree by individual differences in susceptibility (see Chapters 3, 4, and 5).

## MODELS FOR INTERVENTION

Interventions derived from the medical model aim to alter individual susceptibilities, treating the environment as a constant. In some, the aim is to modify biological susceptibility through pharmacological or surgical methods. In others, still within the same framework, the focus is to strengthen people's ability to cope with an adverse environment by providing education and skills training to develop psychological and behavioral adaptations.

Public health interventions for obesity can also be approached from an individual perspective. Indeed, virtually all public health efforts to date have been in this domain. These efforts have focused on disseminating education and behavioral skills training programs to wide audiences at a low unit cost. Among these strategies are school-based education programs for youth, mass media education, work site interventions, home correspondence approaches, and community programs involving multiple components.

The results of these public health interventions for obesity have not yet been impressive. The general population is acutely aware of the problem of obesity, and a high proportion of people report taking direct action to control their weight. Individual programs have also been successful in inducing large numbers of people to participate, and those who do usually achieve some weight loss. Nevertheless, at the population level, these programs have so far had only a negligible effect on the prevalence of obesity.

## TARGETING THE ENVIRONMENT

An unexplored aspect of the public health model of obesity targets the environment rather than the individual as the focus of change. The focus is to reduce the exposure of the entire population to factors that promote obesity.

A wide range of strategies have been employed in public health to address population exposure to disease-promoting agents. By way of illustration, and to stimulate further inquiry, six strategies that may have applicability to population obesity are discussed briefly here. For purposes of illustration, constant exposure to inexpensive but highly palatable food is singled out as an obesity-causing agent, although similar arguments would be applicable to other environmental exposures as well.

## Modifying Environmental Abuse Potential

The first of these public health strategies is to reduce the abuse potential of the environment (see Chapter 112). People are exposed to many potentially harmful substances in the environment, so efforts are made to reduce the potential for harm by imposing environmental safety standards. Successful examples of this strategy include mandating safety glass in automobiles and regulating the lead content of paint. Two possible strategies for obesity are suggested. One strategy would be to regulate the energy density of food products, so that their consumption in normal quantities would be less likely to contribute to obesity. A second would be to regulate the size of the packages in which high-calorie foods are sold, in an effort to reduce the likelihood that purchasers will consume too much of such a product.

## Controlling Advertising

A second public health strategy is to control advertising practices (see Chapter 112). The principle is to limit the ability of special interest groups to encourage the use of products by population groups for whom these products would constitute a significant hazard, or to require that factual information be provided to help consumers make wiser decisions about their use of these products. The limitation of cigarette advertising is a current example of such a strategy, as is the recent addition of health warning labels on alcoholic beverages. For obesity, three possible uses of this strategy are suggested. One is to improve nutrition labeling or product packaging, so that people are better able to assess whether food products have abuse potential; some progress is being made in this area. A second is to directly restrict the promotion of high-fat food items (e.g., the advertising of high-fat foods on children's television programs). A third is to tax food advertizing and to use these revenues to support nutrition messages designed by groups that do not have commercial interests in what people eat.

## Controlling Sales Conditions

A third public health strategy is to control the conditions under which products are sold. The purpose is to limit exposure to hazardous substances either in vulnerable subgroups or in the population as a whole. Children are a particularly vulnerable group for a variety of products; thus, there are minimum age laws for the use of tobacco, alcohol, and automobiles. We also recognize that unlimited access to alcohol poses a threat to the general population; in most jurisdictions, there are restrictions on the number of outlets and the hours of sale. Similar restrictions might be directed at products that contribute to obesity. For example, high-fat, low-nutrient foods could be removed from school vending machines and publicly supported school lunch programs (recent trends are clearly in the opposite direction), and the number of outlets for distribution of foods with high abuse potential might be reduced through licensing policies.

## Controlling Prices

The fourth public health strategy is to control exposure by controlling price. Excise taxes on alcohol and tobacco, for example, are in place partly because they reduce consumption. An analogous strategy might be adopted with respect to food energy. An excise tax on calories would increase the cost of higher-calorie foods and act as a disincentive to consumption of these foods. For producers, it would encourage the development of a wider array of products with lower energy content.

## Improving Environmental Controls

A fifth public health strategy is imposing environmental controls to minimize adverse consequences. These strategies recognize both the risks of certain products and the likelihood of their use, and would be an attempt to modify the environment so as to reduce the degree of harm. Successful examples of environmental control strategies are roadway and home engineering standards, which reduce the likelihood that individual carelessness will result in dire consequences. For obesity, environmental control strategies might focus on exercise. Exercise is protective against obesity. Policies that increase the availability and affordability of exercise participation might have a positive influence on population obesity.

## Improving Public Health Education

The final strategy is public health education. It is clear that educational strategies exhorting individuals to change their behavior will have limited utility as either a clinical or a public health approach. However, education can also have other functions: It can destigmatize the problem of obesity and accurately portray the costs and probability of success of alternative treatment options. In addition, it can help develop a greater awareness of the broad environmental conditions that contribute to the problem and the potential that exists for changing the environment.

One problem in discussing environmental interventions for obesity is that data to support these ideas are scarce. However, the results of a recent study bear on one of these issues. The study examined two environmental interventions in increasing purchases of low-fat snacks from vending machines in 12 work sites and 12 high schools. Vending machines in each site were randomized to one of 12 treatment conditions for a 1-month period each over the course of 2 years. Low-fat snack items were sold at the same price as high-fat items or at a 10%, 25%, or 50% price reduction. Low-fat products were given no promotion or were encouraged by (1) clear labeling or (2) labeling and attractive advertising signs. Results showed increases in the proportion of low-fat-item sales of 9%, 39%, and 93%, with increasing price reductions for low-fat items. Sales increases of about 10% were seen with promotional labeling. Importantly, vending machine profits were not reduced by any of the interventions. Although this study was limited in scope, it makes the important point that substantial changes in food purchases can be achieved in defined populations by changing the food environment. Moreover, it suggests that such changes may be economically feasible.

## CONCLUSIONS

Medical and public health models of obesity differ in the way they define the problem of obesity, in the variables that are emphasized in their etiological models, and in treatment approach. The medical model focuses on individual-difference variables, whereas the public health model also incorporates the manipulation of a broad range of environmental influences. To date, public health interventions have focused largely on mass dissemination of individual-oriented change strategies. These strategies have not been markedly effective. An area that deserves further study is whether environmental strategies, some of which have been quite successful in other health domains, might not also be successfully applied to the management of obesity as a population problem.

## FURTHER READING

Flegal, K. M., Kuczmarski, R. J., & Johnson, C. L. (1998). Overweight and obesity in the United States: Prevalence and trends, 1960–1994. *International Journal of Obesity*, 22, 39–47.—National surveys documenting temporal trends in obesity prevalence.

French, S. A., Jeffery, R. W., Story, M., Breitlow, K. K., Baxter, J. S., Hannan, P., & Snyder, M. P. (2001). Pricing and promotion effects on low fat vending snack purchases: The CHIPS study. *American Journal of Public Health*, 91, 112–117.—A randomized trial examining the effects of price reduction and educational signage on the purchase of low-fat snacks from vending machines in work sites and high schools. This study is one of the first to examine the effects of environment on eating behavior.

Jeffery, R. W., Forster, J. L., French, S. A., Kelder, S. H., Lando, H. A., McGovern, P. G., Jacobs, D. R., & Baxter, J. E. (1993). The Healthy Worker Project: A work-site intervention for weight control and smoking cessation. *American Journal of Public Health*, 83, 395–401.—Results of a 2-year work site intervention program for obesity and smoking that used a combination of education and payroll-based incentives. It is unique among work site studies in its use of a randomized design and assessment of results based on the entire workforce rather than just program participants.

Jeffery, R. W., & French, S. A. (1999). Preventing weight gain in adults: The Pound of Prevention study. *American Journal of Public Health*, 89, 747–751.—The first large trial examining the effects of a low-intensity educational intervention in reducing the rate of weight gain with age.

Jeffery, R. W., Gray, C. W., French, S. A., Hellerstedt, W. L., Murray, D., Luepker, R. V., & Blackburn, H. (1995). Evaluation of weight reduction in a community intervention for cardiovascular disease risk: Changes in body mass index in the Minnesota Heart Health Program. *International Journal of Obesity*, 19, 30–39. An evaluation of the results of both the Minnesota Heart Health Program and the Stanford Five-Cities Project (see Taylor et al., below). These two studies represent the state of the art in community trials conducted during the 1980s.

Luepker, R. V., Perry, C. L., McKinlay, S. M., Nader, P. R., Parcel, G. S., Stone, E. J., Webber, L. S., Elder, J. P., Feldman, H. A., Johnson, C. C., Kelder, S. H., & Wu, M. for the CATCH Collaborative Group. (1996). Outcomes of a field trial to improve children's dietary patterns and physical activity: The Child and Adolescent Trial for Cardiovascular Health (CATCH). *Journal of the American Medical Association*, 275, 768–776.—Results of a large, school-based intervention for reducing dietary fat intake, increasing physical activity, and losing weight.

Schmitz, M. K. H., & Jeffery, R. W. (2000). Public health interventions for the prevention and treatment of obesity. *Medical Clinics of North America*, 84, 491–512.—Review of public health interventions for prevention and treatment of obesity.

Taylor, C. B., Fortmann, S. P., Flora, J., Kayman, S., Barrett, D. C., Jatulis, D., & Farquhar, J. W. (1991). Effect of long-term community health education on body mass index. *American Jour-*

*nal of Epidemiology, 134,* 235–249.—Findings on obesity from the Stanford Five-Cities Project, a 10-year research project designed to reduce cardiovascular risk factors in entire communities.

Wadden, T. A., & Stunkard, A. J. (1985). Social and psychological consequences of obesity. *Annals of Internal Medicine, 103,* 1062–1067.—A review of the social–psychological correlates of obesity, prepared for an National Institutes of Health–sponsored consensus conference on the topic.

# 112

# Public Policy and the Prevention of Obesity

## KELLY D. BROWNELL

## THE NEED FOR BOLD ACTION

We are losing the war on obesity. Its prevalence is rising in country after country, with no signs of reversal (see Chapters 74, 75, 76, and 77). The primary cause, environmental factors leading to poor diet and physical inactivity, are growing worse (see Chapter 78). In all likelihood, its prevalence will continue to increase. This dire situation argues for taking bold action and making fundamental breaks from existing approaches.

Prevention of obesity is of massive public health importance. Obesity, once established, carries with it significant medical and psychosocial morbidity, and is most difficult to treat. Treatment is expensive and can be questioned on grounds of poor efficacy, not to mention effectiveness. As noted in Chapter 78, the number of cases of obesity reversed by treatment is minuscule compared to the number of new cases entering the obese population. It is clear that treatment will not influence prevalence at the national level.

## BREAKING FROM THE MEDICAL MODEL

Whether the focus is on treatment or prevention of obesity, it is logical to base an approach on causes. It is now common to explain obesity with a combination of biological, environmental, and individual variables. This stance issues forth from a medical model, in which causes are sought for individual cases (see Chapter 111), and does not readily lead to clear notions for either treatment or prevention. This may explain in part why modern treatment for obesity is based relatively little on theory or on studies of causal factors.

Breaking from the medical model to consider a public health model focuses attention on why the population is overweight and what can be done at the population level to reverse increasing prevalence. Cost-effectiveness is a key consideration, and prevention becomes a priority. Unfortunately, there has been little discussion of the prevention of obesity, much less research on environmental contributors to the problem and the impact of preventive interventions.

The absence of research on cause makes it difficult to specify what is to be prevented. In the broadest sense, eating and activity must change, but much more specificity is needed if interventions are to be designed in more than a haphazard fashion. The government needs to fund more research on causal factors that might lead to means for prevention (see Chapter 78).

## SPECIFIC POLICY RECOMMENDATIONS

The main call in this chapter is for recognition that (1) powerful environmental forces are causing the obesity epidemic; (2) current approaches have little hope of affecting prevalence; (3) there is need for bold action; and (4) intervention with public policy offers the most immediate and perhaps most powerful means to have an impact.

Specific policy recommendations can only be made in a tentative fashion because of the absence of supporting research. Based on a public health model, Jeffery (see Chapter 111), has proposed such recommendations. More follows here. Whether these recommendations are optimal remains to be seen, but the ideas may provide a basis for testing environmental change. Here, six policy proposals are outlined.

### Enhance Opportunities for Physical Activity

Because declining physical activity is a key contributor to increasing obesity, every opportunity to make physical activity more available, desirable, and rewarding must be taken. In concert with educational, family, and community interventions that are being tested, public funding to increase activity opportunities is prudent. Building additional recreation centers and bike paths, and enhancing physical activity in schools would be logical places to begin. Coalitions between scientists, public health advocates, legislators, and grassroots organizations around issues of common interest would facilitate this movement. Efforts to convert rails to trails are an example of such an issue.

### Regulate Food Advertising Aimed at Children

The average child in the United States sees 10,000 food advertisements per year, 95% of which are for fast foods, sugared cereals, soft drinks, or candy. The most intrepid parents have difficulty competing. Efforts were made several decades ago by grassroots groups and the Federal Trade Commission to limit the number of food advertisements during cartoon television hours (Saturday morning), but fierce opposition, particularly from the cereal companies, blocked this movement. Even today, to limit advertising is a difficult policy to sell.

An alternative may be to mandate equal time for pronutrition messages with some specified number of advertisements for poor foods. A precedent exists for smoking. In the 1960s and 1970s, some public health advocates lobbied for a ban on all forms of cigarette advertising. Instead, the Fairness Doctrine was implemented and mandated equal time for antismoking messages to offset inducements to smoke from television advertisements. The antismoking messages had the desired effect, to the point that tobacco companies no longer found television advertising to be cost-effective. In what was a brilliant maneuver, the tobacco companies agreed voluntarily to end all television advertising in exchange for freedom to market in other ways.

It is possible that an equal-time approach would affect food choices. I propose legislation that would mandate equal television time for pronutrition messages and provide funds to develop effective advertising campaigns. Additional research would be necessary to determine whether forms of advertising other than television should be addressed.

## Prohibit Fast Foods and Soft Drinks from Schools

It is alarming that (1) many schools have fast-food franchises in school cafeterias; (2) schools without such franchises are selling much the same food; (3) school systems enter into contracts with soft drink companies that provide financial incentives for increasing sales; and (4) television designed specifically for schools (e.g., Channel One) has a heavy concentration of advertising for products such as fast foods (see Chapter 78).

Many possible means might exist for changing these influences. One dramatic means would be to prohibit soft drinks and fast foods from schools. Such a move would likely create great resistance on the part of students and even their parents, especially if it were justified on the grounds of improving health. An alternative rationale would be to note than poor nutrition interferes with learning. Foods low in nutrition and high in fat and sugar supplant foods that might enhance energy, alertness, mental acuity, and other factors consistent with learning and performance.

## Restructure School Lunch Programs

Consistent with the previous point would be to restructure school lunch programs in a way that increases consumption of healthy foods. Food service in schools, sometimes run internally and other times subcontracted to large companies such as Sodexho Marriott is considered a support service (such as custodial or grounds) rather than central to the educational mission of the institution. If food service becomes education, the entire context changes.

Food service as education would involve more than a mandate that the menu meet nutritional criteria. It would involve education about nutrition, input from people trained in education of this type, involvement of students and parents, and integration of this education with other aspects of education (e.g., health education and physical education). For education to be engaging and therefore effective, the foods themselves must be appealing, and there must be criteria for ensuring that students acquire basic knowledge.

## Subsidize the Sale of Healthy Foods

Currently, it is more convenient and less expensive to eat in an unhealthy than in a healthy fashion. Combined with the fact that many foods low in nutrition score high in taste because of fat, sugar, and salt, this maximizes the likelihood of poor nutrition and creates barriers to healthy eating. This must be reversed if there is any hope of dealing with obesity.

If healthy foods were reduced greatly in price, say, if all fruits and vegetables were reduced by 50% or more, a number of positive changes might occur. People sensitive to price might increase consumption of such foods. Food manufacturers could bring technology to bear on preparing, packaging, and delivering attractive versions of healthy foods, perhaps maintaining a profit margin similar to what now exists for unhealthy foods. Fast-food restaurants could develop fast and convenient items that, if priced attractively, could compete with items currently available.

An additional way to spur the sale of healthy foods is to support their promotion. Advertising fast foods, soft drinks, and so on, dwarfs advertising for healthy foods (see Chapter 78). Creative advertising campaigns should be developed and funded to support the consumption of classes of products (e.g., fruits and vegetables).

## Tax Foods with Poor Nutritional Value

The least attractive proposal is to tax foods low in nutrient density. From experience, this highly controversial practice is viewed by some as punitive. However, the feasibility of the concept might depend on how it is justified.

Taxes might very well be a means for reducing consumption of unhealthy foods, but the price increment necessary to provoke changes might be unacceptable. If a tax were imposed for the sake of raising revenues to be used in the service of a perceived benefit, say, funding nutrition education programs, supporting subsidies of healthy foods, or building exercise facilities, it might be seen as having virtuous rather than punitive aims.

In a review of taxes imposed on soft drinks and snack foods, Jacobson and Brownell noted that more than a dozen states in the United States have such taxes—in all cases small ones. Enacted to raise revenue, not to change consumption, these taxes have been acceptable to both the public and food producers. Collectively, they raise approximately $1 billion per year. Jacobson and Brownell note that in no case are the funds earmarked for programs related to nutrition or physical activity. Such earmarking could provide enormous benefit. Taxes used in the service of a good cause could become good causes themselves, and might therefore be acceptable.

## SUMMARY

With obesity spiraling out of control, innovative action is necessary and must extend beyond more work on biology, pharmacology, and traditional treatments, perhaps focusing much more on prevention. Prevention, however, must be defined more broadly than application of traditional treatment methods to larger groups of people. Considering public policy as a means for reducing the number of people affected by obesity may be the bold action necessary to have an impact on rising prevalence.

## FURTHER READING

Brownell, K. D. (1994, December 15). Get slim with higher taxes [Editorial]. *The New York Times*, p. A-29.—One of the early calls to consider public policy as a means for reversing the rising prevalence of obesity, based on the assumption that the environment is the cause, and that medical and personal responsibility models are ineffective.

French, S. A., Jeffery, R. W., Story, M., Hannan, P., & Snyder, M. P. (1997). A pricing strategy to promote low-fat snack choices through vending machines. *American Journal of Public Health*, 87, 849–851.—Important study showing that reducing prices of healthy foods in vending machines increases their sales.

French, S. A., Story, M., & Jeffery, R. W. (2001). Environmental influences on eating and physical activity. *Annual Review of Public Health*, 22, 63–89.—Excellent review that deals with environmental contributors to obesity and focuses on both diet and physical activity.

Horgen, K. B., & Brownell, K. D. (1998). Policy change as a means for reducing the prevalence and impact of alcoholism, smoking, and obesity. In W. R. Miller & N. Heather (Eds.), *Treating addictive behaviors* (2nd ed., pp. 105–118). New York: Plenum Press.—Overview of the effects of legislation and regulation targeted at diet, smoking, and alcohol consumption.

Horgen, K. B., Choate, M., & Brownell, K. D. (2001). Food advertising: Targeting children in a toxic environment. In D. G. Singer & J. L. Singer (Eds.), *Handbook of children and the media* (pp. 447–462). Thousand Oaks, CA: Sage.—Comprehensive review of the extent of food advertising aimed at children and its impact on individuals and the culture at large.

Jacobson, M. F., & Brownell, K. D. (2000). Small taxes on soft drinks and snack foods to promote health. *American Journal of Public Health*, 90, 854–857.—Review of taxes imposed on snack foods and soft drinks, with the recommendation that the funds be earmarked for nutrition programs.

Nestle, M. (2000). Soft drink "pouring rights": Marketing empty calories. *Public Health Reports*, 115, 308–319.—Paper showing trends in soft drink consumption, with a critical view of marketing aimed at children and practices in the schools.

Nestle, M., & Jacobson, M. F. (2000). Halting the obesity epidemic: A public health policy approach. *Public Health Reports*, 115, 12–24.—One of the few papers recommending that the obesity epidemic be addressed with specific changes in public policy.

Wadden, T. A., Brownell, K. D., & Foster, G. D. (in press). Obesity: Confronting a global epidemic. *Journal of Consulting and Clinical Psychology*.—Paper discussing etiology, treatment, and prevention of obesity, and covering approaches based in both medical and public health models.

# Index